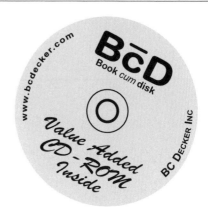

TRAVELERS' MALARIA

PATRICIA SCHLAGENHAUF-LAWLOR, Ph.D.

Research Scientist,
Division of Epidemiology and Communicable Diseases,
WHO Collaborating Center on Travel Health,
Institute for Social and Preventive Medicine,
University of Zürich,
Zürich, Switzerland

2001
BC Decker Inc.
Hamilton • London

BC Decker Inc
20 Hughson Steet South
P. O. Box 620, L.C.D. 1
Hamilton, Ontario L8N 3K7
Tel: 905-522-7017; 1-800-568-7281
Fax: 905-522-7839; 1-888-377-4987
E-mail: info@bcdecker.com
Website: www.bcdecker.com

01 02 03 / FP / 9 8 7 6 5 4 3 2 1
ISBN 1-55009-157-3
Printed in Canada

Sales and Distribution

United States
BC Decker Inc
P.O. Box 785
Lewiston, NY 14092-0785
Tel: 905-522-7017 / 1-800-568-7281
Fax: 905-522-7839 / 1-888-377-4987
E-mail: info@bcdecker.com
Website: www.bcdecker.com

Canada
BC Decker Inc
20 Hughson Street South
P.O. Box 620, L.C.D. 1
Hamilton, Ontario L8N 3K7
Tel: 905-522-7017 / 1-800-568-7281
Fax: 905-522-7839 / 1-888-377-4987
E-mail: info@bcdecker.com
Website: www.bcdecker.com

Foreign Rights
John Scott & Company
International Publishers' Agency
P.O. Box 878
Kimberton, PA 19442
Tel: 610-827-1640
Fax: 610-827-1671
e-mail: jsco@voicenet.com

U.K., Europe, Scandinavia,
Middle East
Harcourt Publishers Limited
Customer Service Department
Foots Cray High Street
Sidcup, Kent
DA14 5HP, UK
Tel: 44 (0) 208 308 5760
Fax: 44 (0) 181 308 5702
E-mail: cservice@harcourt_brace.com

Australia, New Zealand
Harcourt Australia Pty. Limited
Customer Service Department
STM Division
Locked Bag 16
St. Peters, New South Wales, 2044
Australia
Tel: (02) 9517-8999
Fax: (02) 9517-2249
E-mail: stmp@harcourt.com.au
Website: www.harcourt.com.au

Japan
Igaku-Shoin Ltd.
Foreign Publications Department
3-24-17 Hongo
Bunkyo-ku,Tokyo,
Japan 113-8719
Tel: 3 3817 5680
Fax: 3 3815 6776
E-mail: fd@igaku.shoin.co.jp

Singapore, Malaysia, Thailand,
Philippines, Indonesia, Vietnam,
Pacific Rim, Korea
Harcourt Asia Pte Limited
#09/01, Forum
583 Orchard Road
Singapore 238884
Tel: 65-737-3593
Fax: 65-753-2145

Notice: The authors and publisher have made every effort to ensure that the patient care recommended herein, including choice of drugs and drug dosages, is in accord with the accepted standard and practice at the time of publication. However, since research and regulation constantly change clinical standards, the reader is urged to check recent publications and the product information sheet included in the package of each drug, which includes recommended doses, warnings, and contraindications. This is particularly important with new or infrequently used drugs.

This book is dedicated with love to my family

Marcel
Sarah and Seán

CONTRIBUTORS

J. KEVIN BAIRD, Ph.D.
Director, Parasite Diseases Program,
United States Naval Medical Research Unit #2,
American Embassy Jakarta,
Jakarta, Indonesia

CARRIE BEALLOR, M.D., C.C.F.P., D.T.M. & H.
University Health Network Centre for
Travel & Tropical Medicine,
Toronto, Canada

YNGVE BERGQVIST, Ph.D.
Associate Professor, Analytical Chemistry,
Dalarna University College,
Borlänge, Sweden

GERD-DIETER BURCHARD, M.D.
Institute of Tropical Medicine and Medical
Faculty Charité, Humboldt-University,
Spandauer Damm,
Berlin, Germany

JEANINE BYGOTT, M.B.B.S., B.Med.Sci.,
F.R.A.C.G.P., D.T.M. & H.
Senior Registrar, Tropical Medical Bureau,
Dublin, Ireland

ASHLEY M. CROFT, M.D.
Consultant, Public Health Medicine,
Surgeon General's Department, Whitehall,
London, United Kingdom

VALERIE D'ACREMONT, M.D., D.T.M.H.
Travel Clinic Clinician
Lausanne, Switzerland

JOHN A. FREAN, M.B. B.Ch., M.Med.,
D.T.M. & H., M.Sc.
Senior Lecturer and Senior Pathologist,
Department of Clinical Microbiology
and Infectious Diseases,
School of Pathology;
University of the Witwatersrand,
Johannesburg, South Africa

GRAHAM FRY, M.B., F.R.C.S.I., D.T.M. & H.
Lecturer, Tropical Medicine,
University of Dublin Trinity College;
Medical Director, Tropical Medical Bureau;
Dublin, Ireland

MAIA FUNK-BAUMANN, M.D.
Division of Epidemiology and Prevention of
Communicable Diseases
World Health Organization Collaborating
Centre for Travelers' Health
Institute for Social and Preventive Medicine
Travel Medicine
University of Zurich
Zurich, Switzerland

ROBERT A. GASSER Jr., M.D.
Assistant Professor, Department of Medicine,
Uniformed Services University of the
Health Sciences,
Bethesda, Maryland;
Program Director,
Infectious Diseases Fellowship,
Walter Reed Army Medical Center,
Washington, DC, and
National Naval Medical Center,
Bethesda, Maryland

KATIE G. GEARY, M.D.
Specialist Registrar in Public Health Medicine,
Surgeon General's Department, Whitehall,
London, United Kingdom

BLAISE GENTON, M.D., Ph.D., M.Sc.,
D.T.M.H.
Privat Dozent
Head of Travel Clinic
Consultant in Tropical Diseases
Basel, Switzerland

A. RUSSELL GERBER, M.D.
Chief, Epidemiology and Surveillance Unit
Office of Medical Services, Peace Corps
Washington, D.C., U.S.A.

MARTIN P. GROBUSCH, M.D., M.Sc.,
D.T.M. & H.
Department of Infectious Diseases, Charité,
Humboldt University,
Berlin, Germany

CHRISTOPH F.R. HATZ, M.D.
Associate Professor, Swiss Tropical Institute,
Basel, Switzerland

MARGARETHA ISAÄCSON, M.B. B.Ch.,
M.D., D.Sc. (Med), D.P.H., D.T.M. & H,
F.A.C.T.M.(Hon)
Emeritus Professor of Tropical Diseases,
Department of Clinical
Microbiology and Infectious Diseases,
School of Pathology,
University of the Witwatersrand,
Johannesburg, South Africa

TOMAS JELINEK, M.D.
Consultant, Department of Infectious Diseases
and Tropical Medicine,
University of Munich,
Munich, Germany

KEVIN C. KAIN, M.D., F.R.C.P.C
Associate Professor, University of Toronto,
Department of Medicine,
Toronto General Hospital,
Toronto, Canada

KENT E. KESTER, M.D., F.A.C.P.
Chief, Clinical Vaccine Development Program
Department of Immunology
Walter Reed Army Institute of Research
Assistant Professor, Department of Medicine
Uniformed Services University of
Health Sciences
Bethsada, U.S.A.

JAY KEYSTONE, M.D., M.Sc. (CTM), F.R.C.P.C.
Professor of Medicine, University of Toronto;
Staff Physician,
Centre for Travel and Tropical Medicine,
Toronto General Hospital,
Toronto, Canada

PHYLLIS KOZARSKY, M.D.
Associate Professor of Medicine, Infectious
Diseases, Department of Medicine,
Emory University School of Medicine,
Atlanta, Georgia, U.S.A.

HANS O. LOBEL, M.D.
Center for Disease Control,
Atlanta, U.S.A.

LOUIS LOUTAN, M.D., M.P.H.
Travel and Migration Medicine Unit
Department of Community Medicine
University Hospital of Geneva
Geneva, Switzerland

ANNE E. McCARTHY, M.D., F.R.C.P.C.,
D.T.M. & H.
Assistant Professor, University of Ottawa;
Consultant Tropical Medicine and Infectious
Diseases Canadian Forces Health Services;
Director, Tropical Medicine and International
Health Clinic,
Ottawa Hospital, General Campus,
Ottawa, Canada

KIMBERLY MORAN, M.D.
Walter Reed Army Medical Center
Washington (DC), U.S.A.

PATRIC MUENTENER, M.D.
(formerly) Division of Communicable
Diseases,
Institute for Social and Preventive Medicine
University of Zurich
Zurich, Switzerland

HANS. D. NOTHDURFT, M.D.
Department of Infectious Diseases and
Tropical Medicine,
University of Munich,
Munich, Germany

AAFJE E.C. RIETVELD, M.D., M.Sc., M.P.H.,
MEDICAL OFFICER
Roll Back Malaria, World Health Organization
Geneva, Switzerland

PATRICIA SCHLAGENHAUF, B.Sc.(Pharm),
M.P.S.I., Ph.D.
Research Scientist, Division of Epidemiology
and Communicable Diseases,
WHO Collaborating Center on Travel Health,
Institute for Social and Preventive Medicine,
University of Zürich,
Zürich, Switzerland

ELI SCHWARTZ, M.D., D.T.M. & H.
Sackler School of Medicine,
Tel-Aviv University, Tel-Aviv, Israel;
The Center for Geographic Medicine,
Sheba Medical Center,
Tel-Hashomer, Israel

G. DENNIS SHANKS, M.D., M.P.H.
Uniformed Services, University Health
Sciences, Armed Forces Research
Institute of the Medical Sciences,
Bangkok, Thailand

ROBERT STEFFEN, M.D.
Professor of Travel Medicine
Division of Epidemiology and Prevention of
University of Zurich
Communicable Diseases, Institute of Social
and Preventative Medicine
Zurich, Switzerland

DIETER STÜRCHLER, M.D., M.P.H.
Professor, Basel University,
Department of Social and Preventive Medicine,
Basel, Switzerland

MATIUS P. STÜRCHLER, M.D.
Institute for Social and Preventive Medicine,
University of Zürich;
Division of Epidemiology and Prevention of
Communicable Diseases,
WHO Collaborating Center for
Travellers' Health;
Zürich, Switzerland

DOMINIQUE TESSIER, M.D., C.C.F.P., F.C.F.P.
Hôpital Saint-Luc, Centre hospitalier
Université de Montréal;
Medical Director,
Medisys Travel Health Clinic,
Montréal, Canada

DAVID C. WARHURST, B.Sc., Ph.D., D.Sc.,
F.R.C.Path
Professor of Protozoan Chemotherapy
London School of Hygiene and Tropical
Medicine
Co-Director PHLS Malaria Reference
Laboratory
London, England

Contents

FOREWORD

Malaria imposes a staggering burden on society. It is currently endemic in 105 countries and territories, and causes an estimated 300 million episodes of clinical disease each year, resulting in more than a million deaths. Over 90% of deaths occur in Africa, and young children face the highest risk of dying from malaria. Travelers, to and from endemic areas, are increasingly threatened by the disease, and imported malaria is frequently reported in malaria–free countries.

Malaria is a complex disease and its local characteristics are determined by a variety of geographical, environmental, vector, host, and parasite factors. Therefore, this book focuses on travelers in the broadest sense of the word: Tourists, migrants, occupational travelers, and relief groups all have their own particular needs and face different risks with regard to malaria.

The editor, Dr. Patricia Schlagenhauf, has made a major contribution to both travel medicine and malaria control by bringing together a thorough, up-to-date, in-depth overview of the many facets of malaria as they affect travelers. This comprehensive volume is a landmark publication. It includes a global forum of international expert opinions on new approaches to travelers' malaria which, although not exclusively, the recommendations of the World Health Organization (WHO), provide an agenda for international discussion on strategies, means and methods for monitoring, preventing, diagnosing, and controlling the disease.

In 1998 the WHO formed Roll Back Malaria (RBM) — a global partnership with UNDP, UNICEF, and the World Bank. RBM aims to halve the global burden of malaria by the year 2010, through a comprehensive approach involving all sections of society. By reducing malaria in endemic countries, RBM will also reduce the risk to travelers and migrants. We at RBM look forward to working with your towards this goal.

David Alnwick, M.Sc., D.L.S.H.T.M.
Project Manager, Roll Back Malaria
World Health Organization

PREFACE

Travelers' malaria is not a recent phenomenon. Travel and malaria have been inextricably linked since prehistoric times when our hominid ancestors shuffled across continents propagating the plasmodium in alliance with the Anopheles. Today's traveler has many faces: Migrants, tourists (an estimated 5 billion), occupational travelers, and refugee populations constitute an increasingly large and mobile segment of the world population. Travelers' malaria is multidimensional and has become an increasingly intricate subject. This book is a detailed, state–of–the–art insight into a fascinating topic, providing a comprehensive yet, practical reference for health professionals, scientists, and others involved in travel medicine. Experts from various academic, government, and international agencies including the CDC, the Walter Reed Army Institute of Research and opinion leaders world wide, have contributed their expertise to this publication. Particularly welcome are the evidence–based sections defining risk areas for travelers as there is otherwise a dearth of accurate, epidemiological malaria–risk data. The chapters on strategies and personal-protection measures highlight the importance of awareness and practical advice and the key role of anti–mosquito measures stressing the use of the impregnated bednet. The sections pertaining to drugs used for malaria chemoprophylaxis contain the considered opinions of selected experts and offer new approaches to chemoprophylaxis that are worthy of discussion. Several laudable sections in the book examine the growing problem of malaria in migrants and the impact of migrant groups with regard to imported malaria in industrialized countries; perhaps this book will be the impetus to focus on a neglected target group. Other at–risk groups that are discussed in detail include pregnant women, infants, immunocompromised persons, and long- and short-term travelers. The current rapid and exciting progress in malaria research is discussed in detailed chapters — new drugs and combination therapies, evolving techniques for the determination of antimalarial drugs, and rapid malaria tests that will have a major impact on anti–malaria strategies. Malaria in travelers may present differently than the disease in semi–immune residents of endemic areas, and important chapters address the clinical features, diagnosis and treatment of malaria in non–immunes. The status quo of vaccine development is detailed and the mosquito as a traveler is the theme of the chapter dealing with Odyssean malaria. The section on imported malaria reminds us that mosquitoes, plasmodia and indeed, the modern traveler, are not restrained by borders, distance or time–zones. Malaria is mobile and global.

Patricia Schlagenhauf
Zürich
April 20, 2001

ACKNOWLEDGMENTS

One of the most pleasurable aspects of producing a volume of this kind is the interaction and cooperation with colleagues worldwide who share a *passion for the plasmodium* and who are interested in various aspects of travelers' malaria. I would like to express my thanks to all the contributors for their time and effort spent preparing such high-quality chapters and for sharing their particular views on this topic. Gratitude is particularly due to my ISPM colleagues in Zürich, namely Drs. Maia Funk-Baumann, Matius Stürchler, Lorenz Amsler and our chief Prof. Robert Steffen, not just for their praiseworthy chapters but also for their support and helpful discussions in preparing this book. I would like to express my special thanks to Hans Peter Jauss, who changes ideas into illustrations, figures, and tables and who has brought style and innovation to graphic design through years of presentations. Thanks are due to Ruth Lehmann who tracked down some obscure references for Chapter 1 and to Maja Rentsch for Fedex coordination.

Books remain ideas until a publisher brings them to life. Brian Decker brought life to this opus and I am indebted to him for his faith, commitment, and ongoing support. A big "Thank you" to the entire BC Decker Inc team headed by a most competent production editor, Christina Philips.

On a personal note, I am grateful to my family in Ireland, Vera, Mary, and Arthur for their long-distance encouragement, and most of all, I would like to express my gratitude to my immediate family — my husband Marcel and our children Sarah and Seán for their love and support.

ENVOI

The history of malaria contains a great lesson for humanity – that we should be more scientific in our habits of thought, and more practical in our habits of government.

Ronald Ross.
*The Prevention of Malaria.*1911.

Chapter 1

TRAVELERS' MALARIA: SOME HISTORIC PERSPECTIVES

Patricia Schlagenhauf

ABSTRACT

Travelers' malaria. Malaria and travelers. The two subjects have been inextricably linked since the dawn of time. Malaria owes its worldwide distribution to human travelers, be they early hominids, colonists, conquistadores, slaves, explorers, migrants, or tourists. Travelers as military men or colonists were responsible for key discoveries about the malaria life cycle: Charles Louis Alphonse Laveran first sighted the malaria parasite in the blood of a soldier with febrile symptoms during his posting to Algeria in November 1880, and the Briton Ronald Ross demonstrated the complete avian mosquito cycle, far from home, in Calcutta in July 1897. Travelers as Jesuits, colonists, or soldiers are linked with the discovery, refinement, and development of several antimalarial drugs, including quinine and some synthetic antimalarials. The organized war against mosquitoes, the vectors of malaria, was initiated by travelers: explorers, missionaries, and agents of empire spurred by colonist greed or (less often) philanthropic motives. Travelers today are either tourists—an estimated 5 billion per year—or unwilling refugee populations, and although the mode of travel has changed, our plasmodial baggage is essentially that of our hominid ancestors.

Key words: colonists; conquistadores; hominids; quinine; synthetic antimalarials; travelers.

OF MALARIA, BIRDS, MONKEYS, AND EARLY HOMINIDS ON THE MOVE

The epic story of *Plasmodium* spans and antecedes the history of man. Human travel was a key factor in the global dissemination of malaria (Figure 1–1). If we start at the beginning, when our stooped hominid ancestors were more identifiably malarious than human, some very hard-to-answer questions arise: Just how old is malaria? Where did it originate, and how was it propagated? What was the role of human travel in malaria dispersal?

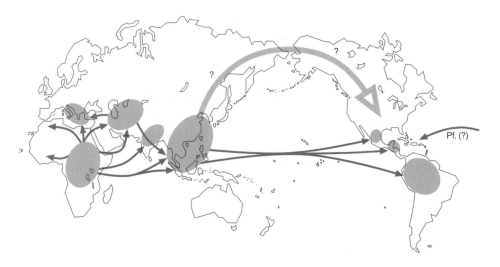

Figure 1–1. Probable routes of spread of malaria in prehistoric and early historic times. (Adapted from Bruce-Chwatt LJ. Paleogenesis and paleo-epidemiology of primate malaria. Bull World Health Organ 1965;2:363–387.)

Bruce-Chwatt, in his 1965 paper "Paleogenesis and Paleo-epidemiology of Primate Malaria," points to the evolution of the *Plasmodium*-like parasite in his statement, "the *Haemosporidia*, which comprise the malaria parasites, have probably evolved from *Coccidia* of the intestinal epithelium of the vertebrate host by adaptation first to tissues of the internal organs and then to life in the circulating cells of the blood."[1] In the adaptation process, the hematosporidia acquired a second invertebrate insect host, and fossil representatives of two-winged insects that date back 150 million years have been found. The oldest line of the malaria parasites lived in reptiles and birds, and the more recent line represents the evolutionary stem of malaria parasites in mammals, including primates and humans. So far, so good; but we then broach the bristly debate on the antiquity of human malaria, and nothing is so simple anymore. Take *Plasmodium falciparum*, the agent of malignant human malaria. There are two schools of thought. One group believes that *P. falciparum* is a relatively new human parasite acquired by a recent host switch from domestic birds perhaps as recently as the onset of agriculture some 5,000 to 10,000 years ago.[2,3] This group also maintains that the virulence of *P. falciparum* may be a consequence of its only recently having become a human parasite. The argument that *P. falciparum* is a recent phenomenon resulting from a lateral transfer between avian and human hosts is also supported by the assertion of Waters and colleagues (based on their analysis of small subunit [SSU] ribosomal ribonucleic acid [rRNA] sequences) that *P. falciparum* is phylogenetically closer to *Plasmodium* species parasitic to birds than to species that parasitize humans or other primates.[4,5]

On the other side of the fence are Escalente and Ayala.[6] They also did an analysis of the SSU rRNA genes of 11 *Plasmodium* species, but they included *Plasmodi-*

um reichenowi, a chimpanzee parasite that was not included by Waters and colleagues in their previous analyses. Escalente and Ayala concluded from this SSU rRNA analysis that the oldest relative of *Plasmodium falciparum* is the chimpanzee parasite *Plasmodium reichenowi* and that the clade formed by these two species is only remotely related to other *Plasmodium* species, including those parasitic to birds and also including other human parasites such as *Plasmodium vivax* and *Plasmodium malariae*. The plot thickens in a later paper, by Escalente and colleagues, describing analyses of conserved regions of the gene coding for the circumsporozoite protein (CSP) in 12 species of *Plasmodium*.[7] The CSP results corroborate the conclusions obtained with the rRNA genes, namely, that *Plasmodium falciparum* and *Plasmodium reichenowi* are phylogenetically very close and that their clade is only remotely related to other *Plasmodium* species. The estimated time point of the divergence of *Plasmodium reichenowi* and *Plasmodium falciparum* is 8 to 9 million years ago, which is consistent with the 6.8 million years commonly assumed for the divergence of the chimpanzee and human lineages. Moreover, Escalente and colleagues maintain that *Plasmodium malariae*, *Plasmodium vivax*, and *Plasmodium vivax*–like species are genetically indistinguishable from three species parasitic to monkeys, and they conclude that it is plausible that *Plasmodium malariae*, *Plasmodium vivax*, and *Plasmodium vivax*–like species are the younger malaria organisms that have only recently become human parasites acquired by lateral host transfer from monkey plasmodia parasites.[7]

WHERE DID MALARIA ORIGINATE?

The cradle of malaria is thought to be Africa, specifically the Ethiopian region,[8] and the host-parasite relationship was probably established there at the dawn of humanity. It is certain that the *Anopheles* species existed there well before the first hominids, and the same is also true in the temperate climates, where the penetration of humans was preceded by that of the insect vector.[1] Malaria is thought to have spread through the African continent by way of the Nile Valley, into the Mediterranean, and thence overland to Asia and north throughout Europe, where epidemics are considered to have had a major impact on civilization. Overall though, Europe suffered much less from malaria than did other parts of the Old World, mainly because it was spared the burden of *Plasmodium falciparum* infections, due to the refractoriness of the main European vector (*Anopheles atroparvus*) against tropical *Plasmodium falciparum*.[1]

Some suggest that Africa may not have been the original site of evolution of primate malaria and point to the forests of Southeast or south-central Asia as the original site[9] where the hominid ancestor invaded the Asian forest environment and acquired the parasites from nonhuman arboreal primates. Some papers strongly suggest that specifically *Plasmodium malariae* and *Plasmodium vivax* came from the original area of Southeast Asia. Following through on this theory, early man (the original traveler) introduced his newly acquired parasites not only into his own group but also into the apes and monkeys of Africa.

Controversy abounds, and wherever malaria originated, the mobile human host traveled and dispersed, taking his malarial baggage along, preceded by the mosquito vectors of the disease. Later, in the era of the ancient civilizations, contacts with tropical Africa were astonishingly wide, and this must have been an important factor in the spread of malaria. Herodotus describes travel across the Sahara to Timbuktu and Lake Chad. Greeks, Persians, and Romans explored East Africa and made excursions to what are now India, Sri Lanka, China, and Indonesia. The Malayan colonization of Madagascar is a striking example of the antiquity of human movements some 4,000 miles away from the nearest starting point.[1] The impressive extent of human travel in these early times was described by Johnson in 1937[10] and was by no means limited to small groups of sailors but rather encompassed huge movements of people across continents. Having gained a foothold, the curse spread, and Europe was not spared. The disease was termed mal'aria, ague, paludisme, Wechselfieber, Dardag Kolle, triasuchka, and likhoradka among other things, depending on the country in which one was afflicted. Popes died, kings sweated, tsars shivered, regional populations were decimated, and armies were laid waste by the tiny *Plasmodium* allied with *Anopheles*. While the Old World shivered, the New World was poised to receive *Plasmodium falciparum*.

TRAVELERS TO AMERICA: COLUMBUS, CONQUISTADORES, SLAVES, AND PLASMODIA

Equally hotly debated is the antiquity of malaria in the New World. Poser and Bruyn[11] discuss this controversy at length in their recent history of malaria, and Desowitz[12] provides an entertaining account of the scenario in his popular book. The issues are the following: Who brought which malaria to the Americas? Did the early traveler bring the plasmodia with him as hidden baggage during the grueling great migration from Asia across the Bering Strait, and did the hardy plasmodia survive the hardships of the postglacial millennia to become established in the indigenous Amerindians (see Figure 1–1)? (This is considered unlikely by many researchers.) Did the Incas, Mayas, and Aztecs suffer malaria before the Spanish conquest? Could prehistoric voyages of Bronze Age Mediterranean groups have brought the disease, or was it brought by Arab traders, Vikings from the malarious areas of northern Europe, or seafaring travelers from Polynesia, Melanesia, and Southeast Asia? (This is considered likely by some experts.) Whoever brought it, there is some conjecture that travelers brought *Plasmodium vivax* and *Plasmodium malariae* to areas in central South America before the "discovery" of the New World by the Spanish. Desowitz[12] describes the elegant sequencing of parasite ribonucleic acid (RNA), which shows that the monkey malaria *Plasmodium simium* of South America is actually the Southeast Asian *Plasmodium vivax* acquired by cross-infection with humans as the original source of the infection. Similarly, *Plasmodium malariae* underwent a name change to *Plasmodium brasilianum* when it infected South American monkeys, and it is conjectured that this *Plasmodium malariae* came to America with isolated groups of seafaring Africans. Others argue that there was no malaria before Columbus and that it appears that Columbus, the Spanish conquistadores, and colonists who brought the slave trade concomitantly introduced *Plasmodium falciparum* to the New World, starting on the island of Hispaniola and thence spreading to the mainland. This Columbus–African slave trade–*P. falciparum* hypothesis has received the most support. By 1510, African slaves were in great demand by Spanish colonists and were shipped in ever increasing numbers to the New World.[11] This late introduction of *P. falciparum* to the New World appears to be the most logical hypothesis when the genetic evidence is considered.[13,14] The genetic polymorphisms (considered to be associated with malaria in other parts of the world) were absent in the aboriginal American populations. The factors that protect against *P. falciparum* require a long time to achieve a frequency high enough in a population to protect against malaria. Estimates for the time required range from 5,000 years[15] to between 50,000 and 100,000 years.[16] Thus, on the basis of a dearth of protective genetic polymorphisms in the New World, it would appear that *P. falciparum* malaria is a relatively recent arrival, brought by European travelers and the slave trade in the 15th century.

TRAVELERS AND THE *PLASMODIUM* LIFE CYCLE

The elucidation of the *Plasmodium* life cycle and the mode of transmission of malaria are historic tales fraught with the controversy of the primacy of discovery (i.e., who was first to see what). Key discoveries are attributed to travelers or to expatriates (often army doctors) working in malarial areas. That malaria is caused by a parasite rather than poisonous gases or miasmas emanating from bogs and swamps was suggested by several individuals, both inhabitants of malarial areas and travelers. John Crawford, a ship's surgeon from Ireland who had appointments in the East India Company and in Guyana, claimed as early as 1807 that malaria was caused "by eggs insinuated without our knowledge, into our bodies" by biting "animalcules and insects (like mosquitoes and fleas)."[17] This wild notion was dismissed contemptuously by proponents of the "bad air"–miasma philosophy. Shortly afterward, however, there was increasing support for the "contagium vivum" concept (i.e., that malaria was caused by microorganisms); in about 1816, a certain Giovanni Rasori was reported to have had the very enlightened opinion that "intermittent fevers are produced by parasites, which renew the paroxysm by the act of their reproduction, which recurs more or less rapidly according to the variety of the species."[11] The identification of the exact organism is attributed to the French army physician Alphonse Laveran, who termed his mobile flagellated organisms "Oscillaria malariae"(Figure 1–2).[18] The protozoa he saw in the blood of malaria patients in 1880 in Constantine, Algeria, are now recognized as the gametocyctes of *Plasmodium falciparum*; from this discovery came Patrick Manson's battle cry, "Follow the flagellum!" Ronald Ross (Figure 1–3), a Briton posted to Calcutta, rose to the occasion and definitively demonstrated the mosquito-malaria connection in an avian model on July 4, 1897. He documented the oocysts (his wonderful "pigmented cells") protruding from the stomach walls of a dapple-wing mosquito.[19]Another great player, who was not necessarily a traveler, must be included in the annals of discovery: Giovanni Batista Grassi, who, in his native Italy in November 1898, recognized the anopheline transmission of human malaria.[20]

TRAVELERS AND ANTIMALARIAL DRUGS

Travelers have played a pivotal role in the discovery and propagation of malaria treatment. Prior to the 17th century, treatment of malaria was based mainly on purging and bleeding. Other cures for the ague ranged from the sublime to the

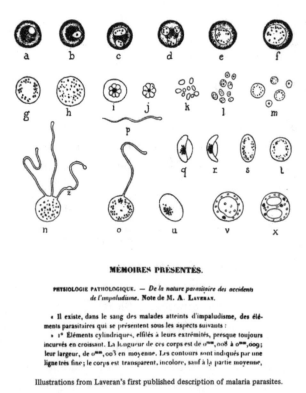

Illustrations from Laveran's first published description of malaria parasites.

Figure 1–2. Illustrations from Laveran's first published description of malaria parasites. (Reproduced with permission from The Wellcome Library.)

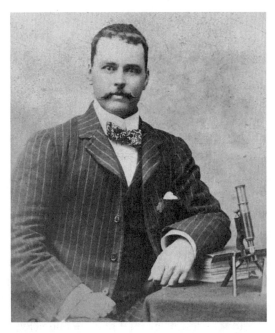

Figure 1–3. Ronald Ross and his portable microscope, Darjeeling, May, 1898. (Reproduced with permission from The Wellcome Library.)

bizarre. They included garlic in sour wine, the wearing of the largest tooth of a fish as an amulet (both for quartan fever), and cool drinks containing cucumber and camphor. Several intriguing references to the value of spiders in the prevention and treatment of malaria date back earlier than Paracelsus; spiders were eaten whole in a pat of butter, or their webs were rolled into pellets.[21] Then came the traveling Jesuits and cinchona bark, and a revolution in malaria treatment began.

Cinchona Bark and Quinine

"In the district of the city of Loja, diocese of Quito, grows a certain kind of large tree, which has a bark like cinnamon, a little more coarse and very bitter: which, ground to powder is given to those who have a fever, and with only this remedy, it leaves them" (Figure 1–4).

Bernabe Cobo (1582–1657), *Historia del Nuevo Mundo*[22]

The history of malaria is fraught with controversy, and the story of cinchona bark and quinine is also debated. Some believe that the Indians of what is now Peru were acquainted with the properties of the fever bark prior to the Spanish conquest,[23] but many historians agree that there is little evidence to suggest that the Peruvian Indians linked the cinchona bark with malarial fevers (if malaria was indeed present prior to the arrival of Columbus). The romantic and often cited story of the cure of the Countess of Chinchon (wife of the viceroy of Peru) of the ague by the use of cinchona bark is considered to be completely fanciful,[24] but all agree that the

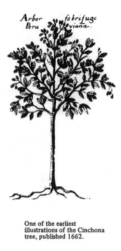

One of the earliest
illustrations of the Cinchona
tree, published 1662.

Figure 1–4. The Cinchona tree. (Reproduced with permission from The Wellcome Library.)

early fame of the bark in Europe was initiated by Jesuit missionary travelers return-ing from the New World. The Jesuit cardinal Juan de Lugo (Figure 1–5) is credited with propagating the use of the bark, especially for the priests in their missionary work. In this context, it was even claimed that Emperor Kang Hsi of China was cured of malaria by Jesuits using cinchona bark.[11] The bark was introduced in England in 1650 and ensured the fame of one Richard Talbor, an apprentice apothecary (Figure 1–6) who cured royal malaria with a secret remedy containing the Peruvian bark.[25] In the 1730s, James Lind, a British naval surgeon, advocated the use of cinchona bark (with great success) to prevent malaria on British ships voyaging to "unhealthy climates." Although not infallible, his potion (infused in spirits) significantly reduced the amount of malaria in the British navy.[26,27] Despite

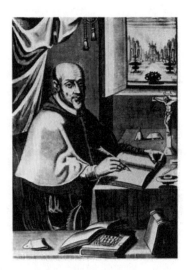

Figure 1–5. Cardinal Juan de Lugo (1583–1660). (Reproduced with permission from The Wellcome Library.)

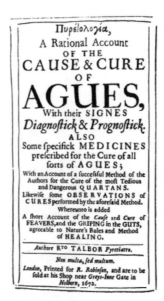

Figure 1–6. Title page of Robert Talbor's *Pyretologia.* Published 1672. (Reproduced with permission from The Wellcome Library.)

the magic of the Peruvian potion, malaria dogged the early explorers; their plight has been traced by Gelfend.[28] Africa was appropriately termed the "white man's grave," and mortality from malaria was particularly high in riverine areas. Mungo Park's exploration of the Niger River in 1805 reduced his group from 45 to 5 (a 91% mortality rate). Gelfend provides a masterly history of African river exploration (Tuckey, Congo River, 1816; Clapperton, Niger River, 1827; Lander, Niger, 1830; MacGregor Laird, Niger, 1832 to 1834; Trotter, Niger, 1841). The mortality for the six major expeditions was 49% and was largely due to malaria and yellow fever.

Travelers with military goals fared no better. British and French armies in the 19th century had more losses from fever than from bullets.[29] During World War I, a flare-up of malaria on the Macedonian front caused a military disaster of historic magnitude, aptly summarized by General Sarrail's frantic telegram to Paris, "Mon armée est immobilisée dans les hôpitaux."[30] There was some effort to use quinine prophylaxis, especially in military campaigns (Figure 1–7), when the bitter taste of the cinchona bark was disguised with wine or spirits. Quinine was often recommended as a tonic (Indian tonic water) by Victorian physicians.[24] (If it were only sufficiently effective, gin and tonic would be a most desirable chemoprophylaxis today!) Thus, cinchona bark and cinchona alkaloids have been a mainstay for hundreds of years.

Synthetic Antimalarials

In many ways, quinine was the instrument of colonialism that permitted European dominance in military campaigns. However, the era of synthetic antimalarials was nigh. The demand for synthetic antimalarial drugs was a response to travel either in

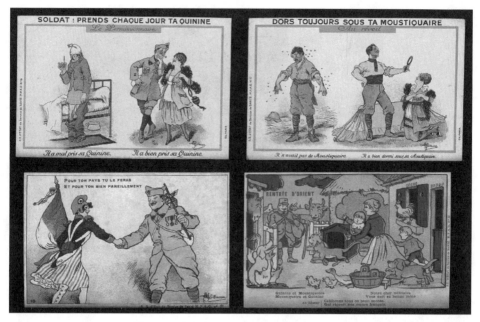

Figure 1–7. Postcards issued by the French Ministry of Health in the First World War. (See Color Plates). (Reproduced with permission from The Wellcome Library.)

the service of the colonizing powers or in times of conflict. War was the spur required to develop many of these new agents; after the Japanese took Java, the cinchona plantations were lost, and quinine supplies became precarious. The main countries involved in the development of synthetic antimalarial compounds were the countries preparing for or engaged in war: Germany, Great Britain, and the United States.[31] Pamaquine, mepacrine, chloroquine, proguanil, pyrimethamine, primaquine, and quinocide were the first synthetic antimalarials developed; then the sulfones and sulfonamides were enlisted. Later came the newer generation, with mefloquine, halofantrine, trioxane derivatives, 8-aminoquinolines, naphthoquinones, and peroxides derived from a traditional Chinese plant, *Artemisia annua*.[32] The latest hope is tafenoquine (from the Walter Reed Army Institute of Research), which promises to provide long-term protection after an initial loading dose (see Chapter 8.7). The race for a vaccine (with or without adjuvation) continues, but so far, the complexity of the wily *Plasmodium* has thwarted efforts on this front; there is still no effective vaccine to protect against any of the malarias in humans.

TRAVELERS AND PREVENTION MEASURES

Long before the details of the *Plasmodium*-human-avian triage were elucidated, travelers used innovative measures for malaria prevention. The use of pyrethrum (*Chrysanthemum cinerariaefolium*) for insecticidal purposes dates back to the ancient Persians and is described in the *Arabian Nights*.[11] Greek and Roman travelers used gauze, muslin, and fishing nets. The early prophylactic use of quinine has been described above. Travelers, as colonists, also approached malaria prevention by going to war on the malaria vector; the drainage of swamps and the control of breeding sites were major factors in malaria risk reduction for expatriates. Sometimes, this approach was successful: Sir Malcolm Watson, inspired by the commercial need to maintain Malayan rubber plantations, filled swamps and greatly reduced malaria in Malaysia.[33] Later, the World Health Organization (WHO) campaigns with insecticides seemed poised for success. Lavicidal oil, Paris green, pyrethrum spray, and dichlorodiphenyltrichloroethane (DDT) heralded possible malaria eradication, but the *Anopheles* species became resistant, the surefire weapons backfired, and the brash fanfare of "eradication" was replaced by "control" whispered against the wind. Bednets have been shown to afford great protection against malaria. In the words of the mercurial malariologist Ronald Ross,[34] "I myself have been infected with malaria only once in spite of nineteen years' service in India and thirteen subsequent malaria expeditions to warm climates; I attribute this good fortune to my scrupulous use of the bed net." Today's travelers are still advised to use a combination of personal protective measures against mosquito bites, and impregnated bednets constitute a cornerstone in malaria prevention strategies.

We began at the dawn of humankind, when our hominid ancestors shuffled slowly across continents, propagating the plasmodia. Now, an estimated 5 billion tourists per year fly to and from malaria-endemic areas in a matter of hours. Unwilling migrants and refugees are forced to travel by need or war. Malaria is mobile as evidenced by the high levels of "imported malaria," by the several recent outbreaks of autochthonous malaria in U.S. areas classified as "malaria free,"[35] and by the transmission of malaria in Europe resulting from the introduction of infected mosquito aircraft stowaways or from the contamination of local European mosquitoes after they feed on infected persons returning from malaria-endemic areas. Despite all our advances in locomotion, our present, rusty antimalaria arsenal consists of ancient antimosquito measures, imperfect prophylactic agents, and therapies based on a traditional Chinese plant, *Artemisia annua*. To date, there is no vaccine. One thing is certain: malaria and travelers will remain inseparable albeit unwilling companions for some time to come.

REFERENCES

1. Bruce-Chwatt LJ. Paleogenesis and paleo-epidemiology of primate malaria. Bull World Health Organ 1965;2:363–387.
2. Hoeprich PD. Host-parasite relationships and the pathogenesis of infectious disease. In: Hoeprich PD, Jordan MC, editors. Infectious diseases. Philadelphia: J.B. Lippincott, 1989.
3. Livingstone FB. Anthropological implications of the sickle cell gene distribution in West Africa. Am Anthropol ;60:533–562.

4. Waters AP, Higgins DG, McCutchan TF. *Plasmodium falciparum* appears to have arisen as a result of lateral transfer between avian and human hosts. Proc Natl Acad Sci U S A 1991;88:3140–3144.

5. Waters AP, Higgins DG, McCutchan TF. Evolutionary relatedness of some primate models of *Plasmodium*. Mol Biol Evol 1993;10:914–923.

6. Escalente AA, Ayala FJ. Phylogeny of the malarial genus *Plasmodium* derived from the rRNA gene sequences. Proc Natl Acad Sci U S A 1994;91:11373–11377.

7. Escalente AA, Barrio E, Ayala FJ. Evolutionary origin of human and primate malaria: evidence from the circumsporozoite protein gene. Mol Biol Evol 1995;12:616–626.

8. Bruce-Chwatt LJ, de Zuleta J. The rise and fall of malaria in Europe. Oxford: Oxford University Press, 1980.

9. Coatney G, Collins RE, Warren M, et al. The primate malarias. Bethesda (MD): U.S. Dept. of Health and Welfare, 1971.

10. Johnson HH. The opening up of Africa. London: Butterworth, 1937.

11. Poser CM, Bruyn GW. An illustrated history of malaria. New York and London: The Parthenon Publishing Group, 1999.

12. Desowitz R. Tropical diseases from 50,000 BC to 2500 AD. London: Flamingo, 1998.

13. Dunn FL. On the antiquity of malaria in the western hemisphere. Hum Biol 1965;37:385–393.

14. Dunn FL. Patterns of parasitism in primates: phylogenic and ecological interpretations with particular reference to hominoidea. Folia Primatol (Basel) 1966;4:329–345.

15. Flint J, Harding RM, Boyce AJ, Clegg JB. The population genetics of the haemoglobinopathies. Baillieres Clin Haematol 1993;6:215–262.

16. Warrell DA. Foreword. In: Poser CM, Bruyn GW. An illustrated history of malaria. New York and London: The Parthenon Publishing Group, 1999.

17. Crawford J. The cause, seat and cure of diseases. Baltimore: Edward J. Coale, 1811.

18. Laveran A. The pathology of malaria. Lancet 1881;2:840–841.

19. Ross R. On some peculiar pigmented cells found in two mosquitos fed on malarial blood. BMJ 1897;2:1786–1788.

20. Grassi B. Mosquitos and malaria. BMJ 1899;2:748–749.

21. Moore W. On cobwebs as a remedy for malarious fevers. Ind Med Gaz 1886;1:326.

22. Haggis AW. Fundamental errors in the early history of cinchona. Bull Hist Med 1941;10:417–459, 568–592.

23. Gray J. An account of the Peruvian or Jesuit's bark. Philos Trans R Soc 1737;40:81–86.

24. Greenwood D. The quinine connection. J Antimicrob Chemother 1992;30:417–427.

25. Talbor R. The English remedy or Talbor's wonderful secret for cureing of agues and feavers. London: Joseph Hindmarsh, 1682.

26. Lind J. An essay on the most effectual means of preserving the health of seamen in the Royal Navy. London: Wilson,1762.

27. Lind J. Two papers on fevers and infections. London: Wilson, 1763.

28. Gelfend M. Rivers of death in Africa. London: Oxford University Press, 1964.

29. Melvill CH. The prevention of malaria in war. In: Ross R, editor. The prevention of malaria. 2nd ed. London: Murray, 1911.

30. Sergent ED, Sergent ET. L'Armée d'Orient delivrée du paludisme. Paris: Masson, 1932.

31. Greenwood D. Conflicts of interest: the genesis of synthetic antimalarial agents in peace and war. J Antimicrob Chemother 1995;36:857–872.

32. Schlagenhauf P. In pursuit of the persistent *Plasmodium*. J Travel Med 1998;5:113–115.

33. Harrison G. Mosquitoes, malaria and man: a history of the hostilities since 1880. New York: E.P. Dutton, 1978.

34. Ross R. Memoirs with a full account of the great malaria problem and its solution. London: Murray, 1923.

35. Zucker JR. Changing patterns of autochthonous malaria transmission in the United States: a review of recent outbreaks. Emerg Infect Dis 1996;2:37–43.

Chapter 2

Global Epidemiology of Malaria

Dieter Stürchler

ABSTRACT

Malaria results from encounters between *Anopheles* mosquitoes, *Plasmodium* parasites, and humans, in habitats that range from seashores to highlands and from oases to cities. Transmission varies locally; it is stable and intense in tropical forest areas but unstable, seasonal, or interrupted in arid and highland areas. Malaria is endemic in 101 countries: in 61, *Plasmodium falciparum* and *Plasmodium vivax* co-occur; in 28 others, mainly in tropical Africa, *Plasmodium falciparum* occurs but *Plasmodium vivax* is absent; and in 12 countries in North Africa, Latin America, and Western Asia, the reverse is true. The current range of *Plasmodium falciparum* is between latitudes 31° north and 31° south; that of *Plasmodium vivax* is between latitudes 37° north and 31° south. Malarious areas, though delineated on maps, have open borders that infective *Anopheles* and humans can cross. *Plasmodium* infections and malaria disease are different entities. Infections are seen in semi-immune people in areas of stable transmission. Their characteristics include low-density parasitemia, a low manifestation index, and an immune response that controls parasite biomass. Of 2.28 billion persons at risk worldwide, some 185 million are infected, for a crude point prevalence of 8%. *Plasmodium falciparum* accounts for about four-fifths of infections; the remaining fifth is due to *Plasmodium vivax*, *Plasmodium ovale*, and *Plasmodium malariae*. Africa carries 83% of *Plasmodium falciparum* infections while Australasia carries 74% of *Plasmodium vivax* infections. In travelers, migrants, infants, and other nonimmune persons, exposure is inadequate for inducing a controlling immune response. In these nonimmune individuals, virtually all infections become clinically manifest. The number of cases is difficult to estimate, one obstacle being the lack of a universal case definition. Based on incidences in control groups included in intervention trials, the annual global number of malaria cases in the year 2000 was 657 million, with falciparum malaria accounting for 71% (465 million). Depending on access to care, time to treatment, and drug resistance, the case-fatality ratio of falciparum malaria is 0.1% to 10%. Using 0.3% as a center case-fatality ratio (CFR), the global number of malaria deaths is 1.4 million per year. The malaria situation has deteriorated in the past decade, and malaria is on the world health agenda as a leading target for control. Impregnated bednets and prompt treatment of falciparum malaria are control tools that should be made universally available.

Key words: *Anopheles*; drug resistance; insecticide resistance; malaria cases; *Plasmodium falciparum*; *Plasmodium* infection; *Plasmodium malariae*; *Plasmodium ovale*; *Plasmodium vivax*; travelers.

INTRODUCTION

"Each year millions of people die from malaria, and many more are incapacitated: there are perhaps 100 times as many cases as there are deaths. Since each case produces a certain physical disability, the economic losses due to malaria are very great..."

World Health Organization Expert Committee, 1959[1]

Following the Eighth World Health Assembly in 1955, the World Health Organization (WHO) embarked on a malaria eradication program, which by the late 1960s brought malaria cases to a historic low. Countries that eliminated malaria at that time (with year of certification) included most Caribbean islands (1965 to 1973), the United States (1970), Mauritius (1973), Bulgaria (1965), Hungary (1964), Italy (1970), the Netherlands (1970), Poland (1967), Portugal (1973), Romania (1967), Yugoslavia (1973), Israel (1967), and Taiwan (1965). Malaria has resurged, however,[2] and is today being put back onto the agendas of international and nongovernmental organizations, ministries of health, and research institutions.

The epidemiology of malaria has been reviewed.[3–7] Here, the focus is on international health, with sections on mosquitoes, habitats, parasites, human hosts, and malaria's impact on public health.

VECTORS AND TRANSMISSION OF MALARIA

Biology and Behavior of *Anopheles* Mosquitoes

That only female mosquitoes suck blood and that only *Anopheles* females transmit human malaria was established in 1898, by R. Ross in India and by B. Grassi, A. Bignami, and G. Bastianelli in Italy.[8] Of about 3,000 mosquito species, about 400 are *Anopheles* species.[9,10] Travelers can distinguish *Anopheles* females from other mosquitoes by observing the biting position, which in *Anopheles* is at an angle to the surface (while the body is kept straight), or by inspecting palps, which are clearly longer than feathery antennas. The taxonomy of *Anopheles* can be confusing; important features are hairs, colors, and wing patterns. Identically appearing adults can represent sensu stricto (ss) species or sibling species called complexes or sensu lato (sl) species.

After a blood meal, *Anopheles* females begin to produce eggs. After deposition of eggs at breeding sites, four larval stages and a nymph stage follow. Development, which needs water, takes 7 to 20 days. Under optimal conditions, populations can explode. Breeding sites are seasonal or perennial and include ponds (Figure 2–1), canals (Figure 2–2), fields, lagoons, cisterns, wells, drains, and cans. An unusual breeding site in Latin America is the water in tree bromeliads.[11]

With increasing distance from breeding sites, the number of *Anopheles* and the risk of receiving infective bites are decreasing. In Dakar, Senegal, for example, the density of *Anopheles arabiensis* females in the rainy season decreased from about 400 per 100 rooms up to 160 m from a breeding site to about 20 per 100 rooms 800 to 900 m away from the site.[12] Irrigation projects and deforestation have a profound impact on breeding sites. Unlike *Culex*, *Anopheles* does not breed in polluted water.

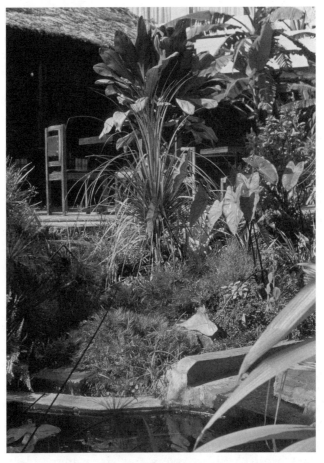

Figure 2–1. A pond where malaria transmission can occur, in a hotel garden in the city of Nairobi. The pond is an ideal mosquito breeding site although fish in the pond may help to keep down the number of larvae. (Courtesy of D. Stürchler.) (See Color Plates)

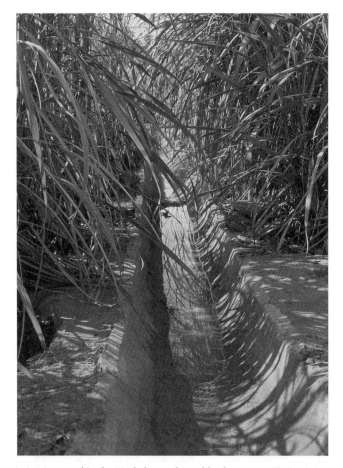

Figure 2–2. An irrigation canal in the Zimbabwean lowveld, where transmission is intense. To keep the canal from becoming a breeding site, it must frequently be flushed and permitted to dry out. (Courtesy of D. Stürchler.) (See Color Plates)

Tropical *Anopheles* have life spans of 3 to 30 days. Temperate *Anopheles* live longer or hibernate. The 15°C summer isotherm marks their survival limit.[13] Some *Anopheles* extend north as far as Scandinavia, Russia (*Anopheles messeae* of *Anopheles maculipennis* complex), and Canada (*Anopheles freeborni, Anopheles quadrimaculatus*) while the southern range ends in northern Argentina (*Anopheles darlingi*), South Africa (*Anopheles gambiae* sl), and northern Australia (*Anopheles farauti* sl) (Table 2–1).[14–18]

Anopheles have flight ranges of several hundred meters, on occasion perhaps more. In a capture-recapture experiment, a range of 7 km was observed.[19] Adults can be carried long-distance by winds,[20] trucks, boats,[21,22] trains,[23] airplanes,[24] baggage,[25–27] or cargo.[28] The eggs and larvae of *Aedes albopictus* have been shipped to other continents by means of old tires.[29]

Anopheles are active from sunset to sunrise. Nocturnal biting can have one to three peaks.[15] Females seek meals indoors (endophagic) or outdoors (exophagic),

Table 2–1. **Some Malaria Vectors: Habitat and Insecticide Resistance**

Region and Vector	Range, Habitat, and Insecticide Resistance
Tropical Africa	
A. funestus	Widespread S of Sahara; prefers clean, shaded freshwater bodies (e.g., swamps, ditches, wet fields); R to pyrethroids.
A. arabiensis*	S of Sahara in savanna and arid areas in dry season; breeds in sunlit pools, irrigated fields, roofs; R to pyrethroids.
A. gambiae ss*	Most efficient vector, S of Sahara to South Africa in humid season; breeds in sunlit pools, wet fields; R to DDT and pyrethroids.
A. melas*	Common on W African coast; breeds in lagoons and mangrove swamps.
A. merus*	E African coast; breeds in brackish or saltwater lagoons.
North and Latin America	
A. albimanus	Texas and Florida to Ecuador; breeds in fresh or brackish water (e.g., ditches, pools, lagoons); R to DDT.
A. darlingi	Mexico to Argentina, mainly in warm and humid forests; breeds in water with floating vegetation (e.g., water hyacinth [*Eichornia* sp]); R to DDT.
Australasia	
A. culicifacies sl	Arabian peninsula to China and SE Asia in rural areas; breeds in river pools, rice fields, gem mine pits; R to DDT and pyrethroids.
A. dirus/balabacensis	SE Asia in forest areas, around camps; breeds in shady pools.
A. minimus	India to Southeast Asia and Taiwan; prefers flowing waters (e.g., foothill streams, irrigation ditches).
A. punctulatus/ farauti†	From Moluccas to SW Pacific and Queensland; breeds in fresh, brackish, and man-made and polluted water collections.
A. stephensi	Egypt to Far East, mainly urban; breeds in man-made habitats (e.g., wells, cisterns); R to pyrethroids.
Europe	
A. maculipennis sl‡	Mediterranean basin to England, Scandinavia, and Russia; breeds in fresh or brackish water; *A. sacharovi* R to DDT in Greece.

A. = *Anopheles*; DDT = dichlorodiphenyltrichloroethane; E = east; R = resistant; S = south; SE = South East; sl = sensu lato; ss = sensu stricto; SW = southwestern; W = west.
* These species are included in the *Anopheles gambiae* complex.
† A taxonomically difficult group; includes *Anopheles punctulatus* sl, *Anopheles faraunti* sl, and *Anopheles koliensis*.
‡ Includes the competent vectors *Anopheles sacharovi* and *Anopheles labranchiae*, the poor vectors *Anopheles atroparvus* and *Anopheles messeae*, and the nonvector *Anopheles maculipennis* ss.
Data from World Health Organization,[14] Zimmerman RH,[15] Tadei WP et al.,[16] Nájera JA,[17] and Coetzee M et al.[18]

on humans (anthropophilic) or mammals (zoophilic), and rest indoors (endophilic) or outdoors (exophilic) for 24 to 48 hours to digest the blood meal. Exophilic species are more difficult to control with residual insecticides than endophilic species.

Malaria Transmission

The word "transmission" means the mode by which *Plasmodium* gets from one host to another. Vector-borne transmission is cyclic as it requires the malaria parasite to go through a sexual phase. Endemic, airport, and introduced malaria are transmitted in this way. Malaria can also be transmitted through parasitized red blood cells; this mode is called acyclic because it goes directly from host to host.

Transmission without Anopheles

In febrile patients without a history of stay in a malarious area or airport perimeter,[24,30] malaria remains a possibility to be considered. Acyclically transmitted malaria includes post-transfusion malaria,[31,32] post-transplantation malaria,[30-37] needlestick malaria,[38-40] dialysis and heparin locks malaria,[41,42] malaria in intravenous drug users,[43-45] experimental (induced) malaria,[46-51] and congenital malaria.[52-56]

In industrial countries that exclude recent travelers to malarious areas from blood donation, the risk of transfusional malaria is small, probably < 1 per million units transfused.[32] In developing countries, the risk of transfusional malaria is much higher,[57] and adventurous travelers should be aware of this risk.

Infective and Competent Anopheles

Some 40 to 60 Anopheles species are receptive to human malaria parasites. Most receptive females are noninfectious. In fact, the proportion of infectious Anopheles females (the sporozoite index) is 2% to 5% in tropical Africa and 0.5% to 2% in other malarious areas. This index varies by species and season (Table 2–2).[58]

Some two dozen Anopheles species are considered competent malaria vectors. These species are highly anthropophilic and have life spans that are clearly longer than the entomological pre-patent period (Table 2–3).[4,6] Vectorial capacity can be measured by the number of Anopheles mosquitoes that become infective after feeding on a human carrier.

Resistant Anopheles

In 1939 in Switzerland, Paul Müller discovered the insecticidal properties of dichlorodiphenyltrichloroethane (DDT). Today, indoor house spraying is still an effective means to reduce transmission by endophilic Anopheles species.[59] Unfortunately, Anopheles has acquired resistance to insecticides. The number of resistant Anopheles species has increased from 0 in 1947 to 1950 to 67 in 1981 to

Table 2–2. Proportion of *Anopheles* Females Positive for *Plasmodium* Antigen*

Anopheles sp	No. Examined	% Infected with Plasmodium	
		Plasmodium falciparum	Plasmodium malariae
A. gambiae	1,441	0.8–2.1	0–0.3
A. arabiensis	8,200	0.5–0.8	0.1
A. funestus	3,617	1.4–3.5	0–0.1

A. = Anopheles.

* In enzyme-linked immunosorbent assay (ELISA), captured on resting sites or by human baits, in an area of tree savanna in southern Senegal, 1992–1995.

Data from Fontenille D, Lochouarn L, Diagne N, et al. High annual and seasonal variations in malaria transmission by anophelines and vector species composition in Dielmo, a holoendemic area in Senegal. Am J Trop Med Hyg 1997;56:247–253.

Table 2–3. **Days Needed by** *Plasmodium* **to Complete Development in** *Anopheles,* **by Ambient Temperature**

Plasmodium sp	Days Needed for Development					
	26°C	*24°C*	*22°C*	*20°C*	*18°C*	*16°C*
P. vivax	9	11	14	19	30	slow
P. falciparum	11	14	19	28	slow	arrested
P. malariae	14	18	24	36	slow	arrested

P. = Plasmodium.
Data from Molyneax L,[4] and Mouchet J et al.[6]

1985.[60] Of concern is resistance to pyrethroids such as permethrin and deltamethrin, which have a low toxicity and a low bioaccumulation profile. Resistance to permethrin is reported for *Anopheles gambiae* sl in West Africa,[61] *Anopheles funestus* in South Africa,[62] and *Anopheles culicifacies* in Sri Lanka[63] (see Table 2–1).

Impregnated bednets are a valuable and effective alternative.[64] Knowledge is limited on the efficacy of nets impregnated with insecticides to which vectors are resistant. It seems that such nets retain activity.[65] Personal behavior can reduce exposure as well, as the following experiment demonstrated.[66] In 1942 in the southwestern Pacific, General G.C. Kenney assigned two squadrons to wear either long trousers and long-sleeved shirts or shorts and T-shirts. After 1 month, there were 2 malaria cases in the squadron wearing long clothes and 62 cases in the squadron wearing short clothes.

Seasons and Epidemics

Transmission is stable when at the same level throughout the year. This pattern is seen in warm and humid climates. Unstable transmission is characterized by pronounced seasonal variations or by interruptions for 3 to 9 months.[7,67] Typical settings are high plateaus and dry savannas. Under conditions of unstable transmission, malaria epidemics can occur, possibly confounded by mobile populations (such as refugees who carry new parasite strains or transmigrants who are immunologically naive to local strains), new breeding sites made by humans, and natural disasters such as floods (Table 2–4).[68–79]

Malaria Habitats

A habitat is a place whose soil, slope, light, and humidity support a set of plants and animals. Malaria habitats have been grouped by "strata," a few examples of which follow.

Rain Forests. Along roads in the Amazon rain forest, there is a constant coming and going of loggers, miners, farmers, and narcotics traffickers, with risks of epidemics and the emergence of antimalarial resistance. Nocturnal work and sleep-

Table 2–4. **Recent Malaria Epidemics, by Location and Setting**

Location and Setting	Year	Cases	Remarks	Reference
Tropical Africa				
Ethiopia, highlands	1958	> 3,000,000	Pf, CFR 5–10%	68
Somalia, Balcad town	1987–88	1,100	Pf, emerging resistance	69
Ethiopia, civil war	1990	> 500,000		70
Kenya, highlands	1994	> 30,000	Pf, attack rate ~50%	71
Kenya, floods	1998	23,400	Pf, attack rate ~40%	72
Latin America				
Cuba, Haitian refugees	1992	235	Pf, attack rate ~2%	73
Haiti, hurricane	1963	75,000		74
Australasia				
India, Thar Desert	1994	?	1,000 deaths	75, 76
Sri Lanka, irrigation scheme	1994–95	> 130	Pf and Pv	77
Sri Lanka, after control	1968	~1,000,000	Pv	78
Thailand, Karen refugees	1984	9,600	Pf, attack rate ~100%, CFR 0.3%	79

Pf = *Plasmodium falciparum*; Pv = *Plasmodium vivax*; CFR = case-fatality ratio; ~ = approximately.

ing outdoors enhances exposure. *Plasmodium* infections have a point prevalence of 1% to 5% and a 12-month period prevalence of 50% to 95%, with about equal shares of *Plasmodium falciparum* and *Plasmodium vivax*. Frequent use of antimalarials keeps down mortality and the CFR.[80–82]

Highlands. In Africa near the equator, *Plasmodium falciparum* and *Anopheles* reach altitudes of 2,500 m;[83] elsewhere in Africa, 2,200 m is hardly exceeded.[71,84,85] The Tigray region of northern Ethiopia is at an altitude of 1,800 to 2,200 m. The main transmission season is September to November (after the summer rains), the main malaria vector is *Anopheles arabiensis*, and the main parasite is *Plasmodium falciparum*. The incidence of clinical malaria is significantly higher in children living at an altitude of 1,800 to 1,900 m than in children living at 2,000 to 2,200 m; it is also higher in children living close to small dams than in those living 8 km or more from dams.[86] In Zimbabwe, areas at < 600 m in the northwest and southeast of the country have perennial transmission, with a disease incidence of 4 in 1,000 per year. *Plasmodium falciparum* accounts for 90% of cases. The high plateau (> 1,200 m), which runs from northeast to southwest and hosts the cities of Harare and Bulawaio, has little or no transmission. People from the high plateau experience heavy exposure and the risk of severe malaria when visiting the lowveld (see Figure 2–2). In suitable years, the main vector, *Anopheles gambiae* sl, ascends to the highveld or hibernates along the way, causing epidemics.[87] In Yunnan province of China, *Plasmodium vivax* reached 2,500 m,[88] and in the Bolivian altiplano, *Plasmodium malariae* was recorded at up to 2,500 m.[89] In the highlands of Irian Jaya, *Plasmodium falciparum*, *Plasmodium vivax*, and *Plasmodium ovale* all reach elevations of 1,500 m.[90,91]

Oases. Surprisingly, local transmission of *Plasmodium falciparum*, *Plasmodium vivax*, and *Plasmodium malariae* can take place in oases. Examples are oases in African[92–94] and Arabian[95] deserts. Despite their isolation, oases close to highways such as the trans-Sahara highway are receptive for imported malaria.

Islands. Due to sustained control measures, many islands are kept malaria free despite the presence of competent vectors—again, a vulnerable situation. On La Réunion, malaria was officially declared eradicated in 1979. While cases continue to be imported, mostly from Madagascar and the Comoros, introduced malaria has not occurred.[96] Similarly, all Caribbean islands except Haiti and the Dominican Republic are free of local malaria. Occasional outbreaks and cryptic infections do occur, however. On Grenada, 58 *Plasmodium malariae* infections were reported in 1978.[97] In 1991, Trinidad and Tobago recorded a *Plasmodium vivax* outbreak that involved 9 persons, and in 1994 to 1995, *Plasmodium malariae* caused 22 cases.[98,99] Travelers have contracted malaria on the islands of Lombok and Bali, Indonesia.[100] On Lombok, the parasitemia point prevalence was 6% in 2,258 residents screened, and *Plasmodium falciparum*, *Plasmodium vivax*, and *Plasmodium malariae* were found.[101] Guam, in the malaria-free Marianas, had small malaria outbreaks in 1966 and 1969 as well.[102]

Coastlines. Contrary to the common belief that winds prevent transmission, coastlines are not free of malaria. On the Pacific coast of Colombia, transmission occurs throughout the year. The point prevalence of infections is about 10%, and both *Plasmodium vivax* and *Plasmodium falciparum* have shares of about 45%, with mixed and *Plasmodium malariae* infections accounting for the remainder.[103] On African coasts, effective vectors are available (see Table 2–1), and transmission can be intense and stable. In coastal areas of West Africa, the point prevalence of *Plasmodium falciparum* parasitemia in preschool children is 30% to 50%. Children have two to three febrile illnesses per year, every third febrile illness is due to malaria, and the mortality is 8 per 1,000 per year.[104]

Nature Parks. The Krüger National Park and other game parks in Mpumalanga province of South Africa are popular tourist destinations. *Plasmodium falciparum* is endemic in the area, and chloroquine-resistant *Plasmodium falciparum* occurs. The South African health authorities advise continuous chemoprophylaxis from October to May, when risks are highest. Tourists visit from Western Europe, North America, Australia, and New Zealand. The diversity of their countries of origin parallels the diversity of their prophylactic regimens.[105]

Tourist Resorts. Many pamphlets suggest that popular tourist destinations in potentially malarious areas will be malaria free. Surprisingly few studies are available to substantiate this. Vivax malaria has occasionally been reported from Acapulco on the Pacific coast of Mexico[106] and from Cancun on the northeast tip of the Yucatán peninsula.[107] Falciparum malaria imported from the seemingly malaria-free Caribbean island of Guadeloupe has also been reported.[108] In Thailand, many areas frequented by tourists are indeed malaria free, but risks exist in areas bordering Myanmar, in Tak province, and Cambodia, in Trat province, where ruby trading is important and the popular island of Koh Chang is located. In both provinces, the incidence of clinical malaria is 50 to 80 per 1,000 per year.[109–111]

Disaster Areas. Floods increase the risks of vector-borne diseases. An example is the massive 1998 falciparum malaria epidemic in northeastern Kenya (see Table 2–4), which began approximately 3 months after heavy rainfalls that followed a 2-year period of drought. Using a disaster-adapted case definition of fever plus the presence of *P. falciparum* on a thin blood smear, an attack rate of approximately 390 per 1,000 was found, and mortality was estimated about 1 per 1,000 per day.[72]

Development Areas. In the Thar desert of western Rajasthan in India, heavy rainfalls or irrigation schemes may both explain the occurrence of epidemic malaria.[75,76,112,113] The construction of dams in Sri Lanka has been associated with the appearance of new breeding sites and epidemic malaria.[114]

Cities. While many cities in Latin America are free of transmission, urban malaria exists in tropical Africa, including city centers (see Figure 2–1). Brazzaville is a city located at the southern fringe of the African rain forest. Inhabitants receive about 20 infective bites per person per year. The prevalence of *Plasmodium* infections varies by borough and is 10% to 80% in schoolchildren. *Plasmodium falciparum* is dominant, but *Plasmodium malariae* and *Plasmodium ovale* also occur. Severe falciparum malaria is age dependent and has an incidence of 0.1 to 1 per 1000 per year.[115] Urban malaria exists in India as well.[116,117] ("Calcutta is now intensely malarious. Malarial infections are detected in every month.")[117] Every third fever case is attributed to malaria, and *Plasmodium falciparum* accounts for every third case.

MALARIA EXPOSURE

Exposure describes the risk of receiving viable *Plasmodium* parasites. It is characterized by time and intensity. Time can be short, intermittent, or continuous. Exposure time and risk of malaria in travelers are correlated.[118] However, exposure of a few hours such as at stopovers at an airport can be sufficient for infection. Intensity of exposure is influenced by housing (such as proximity to breeding sites and mosquito screens) and behavior (nocturnal activities such as fishing or visits to bars, clothing such as T-shirts or shorts, and the use of bednets).

Exposure in Travelers

Are malaria risks in travelers the same as malaria risks in local populations?[119] If groups with the same living conditions and protective measures can be compared, the answer is yes. Statistics of imported malaria suggest that areas of intense transmission are often high-risk areas for tourists as well. In 1999, when a new malaria focus was recognized around Punta Cana on the southeast coast of Haiti, rising numbers of malaria cases in locals were quickly followed by malaria in visitors.[120] Similarly, in the wake of the 1997 El Niño event and heavy floods, an upsurge of falciparum malaria in northeast Kenya was reflected by malaria in tourists.[72,121]

In short-term visitors to single destinations, arrival and departure dates by and large define the exposure period. In frequent visitors and in visitors to multiple destinations, however, the period of exposure is much less well defined. Antisporozoite antibodies are evidence of past exposure[122] (see Chapter 4). Antibodies to *P. falciparum* sporozoites are detected in 1% to 5% of travelers.[123,124]

A history of past or planned exposure is important for malaria diagnosis and prevention. A minimum set of questions includes where, when (season), how (type of travel and accomodation), and how long? In travelers likely to change itinerary at the last minute, risk evaluation should be adjusted accordingly. (See also Chapter 4.)

Exposure in Local Populations

Most local populations experience unprotected and continuous exposure. This repeated antigenic stimulation can trigger polyclonal and autoimmune responses. A surrogate measure of exposure is the time spent in a malarious area. A quantitative measure is the entomological inoculation rate (EIR), which indicates the number of infectious bites an unprotected person receives in a night at a given place. If measured in a representative period, it can be extrapolated to a year and expressed as number of bites per person per year. In areas of intense transmission, the EIR can reach 900 per person per year or 2 to 3 per person per day.[125] Such figures imply that most of these infections do not become manifest. In low-transmission areas, EIRs of 1 to 30 per person per year are common. Like the sporozoite index, the EIR varies with season and *Anopheles* and *Plasmodium* species (Table 2–5).[58]

Table 2–5. **Entomological Inoculation Rates in Tree Savanna in Southern Senegal, 1992 to 1995**

| | | Infectious Bites/Person/Year | | | | | |
| | | P. falciparum | | | P. malariae | | |
Anopheles *sp*	No. *of* Anopheles Examined	Yr 1	Yr 2	Yr 3	Yr 1	Yr 2	Yr 3
A. gambiae	1,441	33	10	8	3	0	2
A. arabiensis	8,200	18	48	81	3	8	11
A. funestus	3,617	173	20	46	5	0	3

A. = *Anopheles*; P. = *Plasmodium*.
Data from Fontenille D, Lochouarn L, Diagne N, et al. High annual and seasonal variations in malaria transmission by anophelines and vector species composition in Dielmo, a holoendemic area in Senegal. Am J Trop Med Hyg 1997;56:247–253.

Given local variabilities, the number of exposed people is difficult to quantify. A surrogate measure is the census of people living in a malarious area, where known unexposed segments are subtracted. Because malarious areas were amazingly stable in the last three decades,[126,127] the method is supposed to provide reasonable estimates.[128–131] Of about 6 billion people in 2000, I estimate that 38% (46% of those ≤ 14 years of age and 35% of those > 14 years of age) or 2.28 billion were exposed (Table 2–6). A decade ago, the proportion was 40%.[132] Of these, two-thirds (1.52 billion) live in Australasia, 29% (656 million) live in Africa, and 5% (108 million) live in Latin America.

Table 2–6. Year 2000 Estimates of Exposures and Infections, Overall and by *Plasmodium* Species*

Location	Census (×10⁶)		All Exposed (×10⁶)		All Infected (×10⁶)		Pf (×10⁶)	Pv (×10⁶)	Po (×10³)	Pm (×10³)
	≤ 14 yr	> 14 yr	≤ 14 yr	< 14 yr	≤ 14 yr	> 14 yr				
Africa										
North†	56	89	4	7	0.03	0.005	0.005	0.03	0	1
Tropical‡	303	369	287	349	118	14	120	4	2,000	6,000
Southern§	7	9	4	5	0.6	0.08	0.7	0.01	0	19
Subtotal	366	467	295	361	119	14***	121	4	2,000	6,000
Latin America										
Caribbean‖	12	27	3	4	0.06	0.009	0.07	0	0	0
Central#	52	87	17	25	2	0.3	0.02	2	0	0
South**	114	228	19	38	2	0.5	0.8	2	0	10
Subtotal	178	342	39	69	4	1	1	4	0	10
Australasia										
West††	138	209	55	71	5	0.5	2	3	0	80
Central‡‡	463	889	427	813	30	5	17	20	20	180
Southeast§§	116	205	48	82	5	0.8	4	1	40	100
East‖‖	409	1,114	4	11	0.05	0.01	0.001	0.05	0	1
Pacific##	8	22	2	3	1	0.1	0.8	0.2	1	9
Subtotal	1,134	2,439	536	980	41	6	24	23	60	370
Rest of world	208	821	0	0	0	0	0	0	0	0
World	1,886	4,069	870	1,410	164	21	146	31	2,000	6,000

Pf = *Plasmodium falciparum;* Pv = *Plasmodium vivax;* Po = *Plasmodium ovale;* Pm = *Plasmodium malariae.*
* For age groups ≤ 14 and > 14 years of age. All numbers in table are rounded. For method, see Stürchler D.[236]
† Algeria, Egypt, Libya, Morocco, Tunisia, Western Sahara.
‡ 49 countries.
§ Botswana, Namibia, South Africa, Zimbabwe.
‖ 24 countries.
Belize, Costa Rica, El Salvador, Guatemala, Honduras, Mexico, Nicaragua, Panama.
** 14 countries.
†† 25 countries.
‡‡ Bangladesh, Bhutan, India, Maldives, Nepal, Pakistan, Sri Lanka.
§§ 10 countries.
‖‖ 8 countries.
23 countries.
*** = Pf.

PLASMODIUM PARASITES

Malarious Areas

Although the French physician C.L.A. Laveran[135] discovered malaria parasites in 1880 in Constantine, Algeria, reports on the geography of malaria before 1945 should be interpreted in the context of that time, when diagnoses were rarely confirmed parasitologically. For instance, in 1945 to 1949, 4,241 malaria cases were reported in the United States. Of 498 cases appraised, only 55 (11%) were confirmed, of which only 19 were classified as indigenous, and it was concluded that "the malaria morbidity statistics during this period were grossly misleading."[136] A well-intended signboard in a malarious area (Figure 2–3) should not be taken literally; infected *Anopheles* and humans *do* cross borders.

Despite these limitations, risk mapping (Figures 2–4 and 2–5)[127,137] is an extremely useful tool for prevention and control. By comparing past[86,126,133,134] and present situations, vulnerable areas can be identified. Malaria is currently endemic in 101 countries. In 61 countries, *P. falciparum* and *Plasmodium vivax* co-occur. In Haiti, the Dominican Republic, and 26 countries in tropical Africa, *Plasmodium falciparum* is present but *Plasmodium vivax* is absent. In 12 countries, *P. vivax* occurs but *Plasmodium falciparum* does not; these countries are Algeria, Argentina, Armenia, Azerbaijan, El Salvador, Iraq, Mauritius, Morocco, Paraguay, South Korea, Syria, and Turkey. *Plasmodium ovale* and *Plasmodium malariae* do not have territories of exclusivity; they co-occur with *Plasmodium falciparum*, *Plasmodium vivax*, or both.

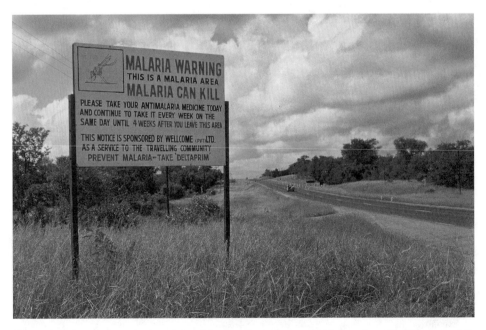

Figure 2–3. A malaria notice board for visitors to the malarious Zimbabwe lowveld. (Courtesy of D. Stürchler.)

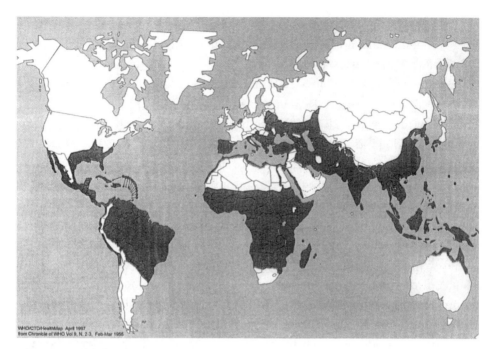

Figure 2–4. Global malarious areas in 1946, according to the World Health Organization (WHO). (Reproduced with permission from Chronicle World Health Organ 1955;9.)

Malaria situation, 1999

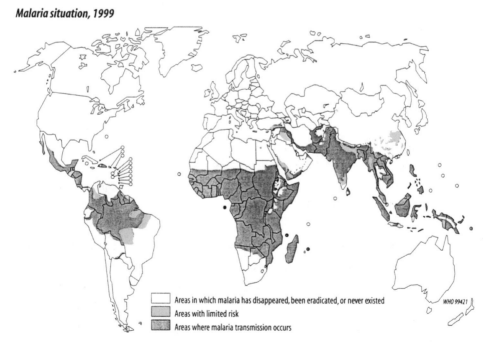

Figure 2–5. Global malarious areas in 1999, according to the World Health Organization (WHO). (Reproduced with permission from World Health Organization. Communicable Diseases 2000. WHO/CDS/2000.1.)

Thus, *Plasmodium falciparum*, the tropical parasite, occurs in 89 countries. Its range is bound to the north by latitudes 18.5° in Mexico (Tabasco), 30.5° in Egypt (Nile delta), 28° in India (Assam),[138] and 25° in China (Yunnan) and to the south by latitudes 28° in Brazil (Santa Catarina), 31° in South Africa (Mpumalanga, formerly KwaZulu-Natal), and 19.5° in Vanuatu (Tanna Island).[139,140] In the past, its range went further north but not much further south. In North America, *P. falciparum* reached Florida and the Mississippi River delta (latitude 30°north), possibly the Southwest, and New York City (45° north), this latter location being corroborated by recent evidence of local transmission.[141] In Europe, *P. falciparum* was present in southern Portugal (38.5° north), Corsica (43° north), Sicily, the Greek mainland, and the Danube delta in Romania (45° north). In Asia, it reached the Henan and Anhui provinces of central China (latitude 35° north).[142]

Plasmodium vivax is present in 73 countries. It is a parasite of both tropical and temperate climates. In West Africans who lack the Duffy blood group, it is absent. Its prevalence increases toward the Horn of Africa, where some ethnicities express the blood group. Its current range is bound by latitudes 26° north in Mexico (Sinaloa), 35° in Morocco (Mediterranean coast), 37° in Turkey (Anatolia), and 33° in southern China and by latitudes 28° south in Argentina (Corrientes), 31° in South Africa, and 19.5° in Vanuatu. In the past, *P. vivax* probably reached latitudes 45° north in the Great Lakes region,[143] 47.5° in the French Bretagne,[144,145] 52° in British York and Kent,[146] 53° on the Zuider Zee (Netherlands),[147] 61.5° in the Russian oblast of Arkhangelsk,[89] 44° in the Yili valley of Xinjiang,[148] and 52° in the Amur valley of Manchuria. In the south, it extended to 33° in Argentina (Mendoza), 32° in South Africa (East Cape), and 15° to 16° in Australia (Northern Territory and Queensland).[149]

Plasmodium ovale is present in 34 countries. Its core area is tropical Africa.[150,151] A separate focus, now well supported by new diagnostic techniques, is in Southeast Asia.[152–154] Its northern limit runs from latitude 16° north in Senegal[155] to 12° at the Horn of Africa, 19° in India (Orissa),[156] and to the Philippines. Its southern limits are South Africa (26°), Madagascar, Irian Jaya (5°), and Papua New Guinea (10°). Interestingly, *P. ovale* seems absent from most Indonesian islands, including Java, Kalimantan, Sulawesi, and Sumatra.[157]

Plasmodium malariae is present in 58 countries. It occupies a broad tropical and subtropical area of low endemicity, with pockets of high endemicity. Its current range is bound to the north by latitudes 27° in India (West Bengal) and 44° in China (Xinjiang) and to the south by latitudes 28° in Argentina (Corrientes). In the past, *P. malariae* may have occurred in the Mediterranean basin and the southern United States.

(See also Chapter 3, "Geographic Distribution of Malaria at Traveler Destinations.")

Biology

Plasmodia are protozoan parasites. There are 110 to 120 *Plasmodium* species. Of these, four (*Plasmodium falciparum, Plasmodium vivax, Plasmodium ovale,* and *Plasmodium malariae*) occur in humans, about 20 occur in monkeys,[89] about 20 in rodents and bats, about 30 in birds, and about 40 in reptiles. *Plasmodium falciparum* is phylogenetically related to bird plasmodia.

Sexual reproduction begins when infected humans develop male and female gametocytes. *Anopheles* females take up these gametocytes, and the sexual cycle is completed in *Anopheles* when viable sporozoites invade the salivary gland. This development (entomological pre-patent period) takes 9 to 36 days (see Table 2–3).[4,6] It is slowed or arrested by ambient temperatures < 20°C (*P. falciparum* and *Plasmodium malariae*) or < 16°C (*Plasmodium vivax*). *Plasmodium* is not transmitted transovarially.

During a blood meal, infectious *Anopheles* females inject sporozoites into humans. *Plasmodium malariae* and *Plasmodium falciparum* are nonrelapsing while *Plasmodium vivax* and *Plasmodium ovale* are relapsing. *Plasmodium malariae,* if untreated, can persist for decades.[158,159]

Resistance

Resistance is the ability of plasmodia to survive inhibitory or parasiticidal drug concentrations (see Chapter 9). It is directed against one antimalarial (monoresistance) or more than one structurally unrelated (multiresistance) or related (cross-resistance) antimalarial. Poor compliance or underdosing do not constitute resistance.[160]

Chloroquine-resistant *Plasmodium falciparum* appeared in the 1950s in South America and Southeast Asia. Its spread in Africa was closely monitored.[161] In 2000, it was recorded or rampant in 76 (85%) of 89 countries where *P. falciparum* is endemic. Only countries north of the Panama Canal and the Arabian peninsula are exempt. In tropical Africa, the emergence of chloroquine resistance has been associated with a significant increase of malaria mortality.[162] Antifol-resistant *P. falciparum* is widespread in the Amazon basin, Southeast Asia, and the southwestern Pacific; in tropical Africa, where antifols are an affordable alternative to chloroquine, its current low prevalence is monitored with apprehension.[163,164] Mefloquine-resistant *P. falciparum* is currently relevant only in border areas of Thailand, Myanmar, and Cambodia.[166] In other *P. falciparum*–endemic areas, mefloquine resistance is sporadic but prone to change.[165,167,168]

In 1989, chloroquine-resistant *Plasmodium vivax* was reported in Papua New Guinea.[169] It now occurs in Irian Jaya,[170] parts of Southeast Asia,[171] and Latin America.[172] Since the 1950s, strains of *P. vivax* that tolerate standard doses of primaquine have been known from Southeast Asia and the southwestern Pacific. Primaquine-resistant *P. vivax* is now reported in nonimmune people in Guatemala[173] and Somalia.[174]

To prevent resistance, drug combinations were developed in the 1980s;[175–178] these drugs were criticized for their discordant and long elimination half-lives.[179,180] However, pressing needs have renewed interest in combination products,[181,182] creating similar controversy about their use.[183] New insights into the occurrence of resistance may come from the multiplicity of clones and from the intensity of transmission[184] (Table 2–7).

MALARIA INFECTIONS

Parasitemia, demonstrated by microscopy of thick and thin blood films, is firm evidence of infection. New diagnostic tools include microscopy of buffy coat, test strips that capture proteins or enzymes of one or more *Plasmodium* species,[185] and nucleic acid amplification tests (see Chapters 12 and 13). The latter are able to detect subpatent parasitemias.[186–188]

Infections in Semi-immune Persons

Semi-immune persons can carry parasitemia subclinically. Depending on the intensity and duration of exposure, a carrier state is reached in 0.5 to 10 years[7,189] (see Table 2–7). High antibody titers to asexual blood stages are suggestive of this condition. Children in transition to semi-immunity often present with enlarged spleens. Interruption of exposure by season, control measure, or migration seems to go along with a loss of semi-immunity.[190] Semi-immune persons living outside of malarious areas should take preventive measures when visiting malarious homes.[191]

Asexual parasitemias in semi-immune persons are often of low density or submicroscopic. When intercurrent illnesses or pregnancy tips the balance in favor of

Table 2–7. **Levels of Malaria Exposure, Immune Response, and Malaria Morbidity**

	Mostly Semi-immunes	*Some Semi-immunes*	*Mostly Nonimmunes*
Exposure	Perennial and intense, in tropical forest areas	For > 3 mo/yr, in areas with 1–2 rainy seasons	For 0–3 mo/yr, in highlands and dry areas
Infecting bites/ person/yr	365–900	12–365	0–12
Yr to semi- immunity	< 5	5–10	Mostly not reached
Children point prevalence	50–75%	10–49%	0.1–9%
Fevers due to malaria	30%	10% (dry season) to 80% (wet season)	< 10% (dry season) to > 80% (epidemic)
No. of clones/ parasitemia	3	2	1
Risk of drug resistance	Low	Moderate	High

parasite biomass, a critical parasite density (pyrogenic threshold) builds up, and clinical malaria ensues. In *Plasmodium falciparum*, the critical density is commonly set at 500 to 20,000 asexual parasites per microliter.[192] The mean duration of *P. falciparum* infections in a population of approximately 4,100 Papuans was 146 days in infants and small children and 53 to 57 days in adolescents and adults.[193] Single clones may have higher turnover rates.

Neonates born to semi-immune mothers by being protected from maternal antibodies frequently carry subclinical *Plasmodium* infections. In contrast, congenital malaria disease occasionally occurs in nonimmune neonates.[55]

The only way *Anopheles* females become infected is by picking up gametocytes in a blood meal. In stable transmission areas, the principal sources of gametocytes are preschool children. Migrants carrying gametocytes have caused outbreaks of falciparum and vivax malaria in the United States[194] (including California,[195,196] Florida,[197] Georgia,[198] Michigan,[199] New Jersey,[200] New York,[141,201] and Texas[202]), in Europe (including France[203,204] and Italy[205]), and in central Asia.[206] This form of malaria, transmitted by local *Anopheles* mosquitoes to residents of nonmalarious areas, is referred to as introduced malaria.

Reservoirs of Infection

Reservoirs are secure places where plasmodia can thrive and multiply. Humans and *Anopheles* are the accepted malaria reservoirs. Their shares of parasite biomass are unknown. Monkeys are not considered a reservoir of human malaria.[207] In South America, the monkey plasmodia *Plasmodium brasilianum* and *Plasmodium simium* are morphologically identical to *Plasmodium malariae* and *Plasmodium vivax*, respectively. In Brazil, *Plasmodium brasilianum* is prevalent in monkeys, and zoonotic infections are suspected in Indian populations.[208–210] A monkey reservoir would be at variance with the thought that *Plasmodium malariae* came to Latin America with pre-Columbian Australasians, that *Plasmodium vivax* arrived with Christopher Columbus, and that *Plasmodium falciparum* came with post-Columbian African slaves.[211]

Susceptible and Refractory Humans

Not all exposed humans become infected. Nutritional factors (such as iron, protein, and vitamin A) and the genetic makeup of the host modulate susceptibility to infection and disease. ("It would take a book to tell of the blood and malaria; suffice it to say where malaria has been a long companion of a people, there is funny blood.")[211] Innate resistance works by inhibiting *Plasmodium* attachment, invasion, development, release, or other mechanism. Altered hemoglobins, enzymes, and blood groups are involved. West Africans who lack the Duffy blood group are refractory to *Plasmodium vivax*.[212,213] Melanesians who lack the red blood cell band-3 membrane protein (ovalocytosis) seem to be protected from

Plasmodium invasion.[214–217] Sickle cell hemoglobin heterozygotes have lower *Plasmodium falciparum* parasite densities, are less prone to severe malaria and malaria anemia, and have lower post-therapeutic relapse rates than homozygotes.[218–220] Deficiency of the red blood cell enzyme glucose-6-phosphate dehydrogenase (G6PD) offers partial protection against *P. falciparum* infection and disease.[221–223] Conversely, people with sickle cell anemia (HbSS) are particularly susceptible to falciparum malaria, and people with α-thalassemia are prone to vivax malaria.[224] Histocompatibility (human leukocyte antigen [HLA]) genes seem to control immune response to *Plasmodium* antigens.[225,226]

Clearly, ethnic background is important not only for malaria prevention in susceptible individuals but also for evaluation of drug metabolism and drug safety (pharmacogenetics).

Mixed and Intercurrent Infections

Mixed infection means the presence of more than one *Plasmodium* species in a host; up to nine different clones can coexist.[227] With the use of nucleic acid amplification tests that identify up to three times more mixed infections than conventional methods,[228] the proportion of mixed infections is likely to increase. Models suggest that *Plasmodium malariae* can reduce coexisting peak *Plasmodium falciparum* parasitemia by as much as 50%.[229] In contrast, mixed infections in 2,162 individuals in a field study in Papua New Guinea were found to have a chance distribution.[228] Perhaps the most practical aspect of mixed infections is that when in doubt, one should rule in coexisting low-level *P. falciparum* infection ("in dubio pro falciparo").

Intercurrent infections are infections newly acquired by a parasitemic host. Chance associations can occur with other common conditions such as pneumonia,[230,231] measles,[232] bacterial meningitis,[233] diarrheal disease, or human immunodeficiency virus (HIV) infection. In a febrile semi-immune person presenting with *Plasmodium* parasitemia, intercurrent infections must therefore be ruled out. Parasite density can help to separate malarial disease from a *Plasmodium* infection associated with an intercurrent infection. Intercurrent infections with the same agent are called superinfections. Immunity against superinfection is called premunition.

Prevalence and Incidence of Infection

The percentage of persons with parasitemia at a given time (slide positivity rate) is a point prevalence. If malaria suspects are examined, this measure is not representative of the population. Also, single blood smears are inadequate to detect parasitemias that oscillate around detection level.[234] The cumulative percentage of people who are infected at least once in a period is a period prevalence (annual parasite index).[235]

The prevalence of asexual parasitemias or splenomegalies in children 2 to 9 years of age is used to class levels of endemicity as hypoendemic (< 10%), mesoendemic (11% to 50%), hyperendemic (persistently 51% to 75%), or holoendemic (persistently 75%).

From 1970 to 2000, publications were reviewed to update infection point prevalence estimates by age group and *Plasmodium* species.[236] Because representative data for those > 14 years of age were not available for many countries, values in this group were arbitrarily set at one-tenth of the median values in persons ≤ 14 years of age. By this method, approximately 185 million people were estimated to be infected in the year 2000, for a global prevalence of 8% (see Table 2–6). *Plasmodium falciparum* accounted for 79% (146 million) of infections, *Plasmodium vivax* for 17% (31 million), *Plasmodium malariae* for 3% (6 million), and *Plasmodium ovale* for 1% (2 million). Africa carried 83% of *Plasmodium falciparum* infections, and Australasia carried 74% of *Plasmodium vivax* infections. The median infection prevalence in children in tropical Africa was 30%, with broad variability by age and area. Variability is exemplified by 1,848 Kenyan children in whom the infection (> 95% *Plasmodium falciparum*) prevalence ranged from 42% in infants to 83% in preschool children.[192] In Latin America and Australasia, prevalences in children were 1% to 10%. A typical example is Nicaragua, with a *Plasmodium vivax* infection prevalence of 8%.[237]

Incidence is the rate by which *new* species, strains, or clones are acquired during the observation period (e.g., a year or person-times). Incidence data are available in control groups in intervention trials. New infections are difficult to distinguish from relapses; this is now possible with nucleic acid amplification tests.

In tropical Africa, *Plasmodium falciparum* infections have incidences of 800 to 3,000/1,000/yr or 1 to 3/person/yr (Table 2–8).[237–246]In Latin America, rates of reported infections per 1,000 per year were highest in Guyana (450), Surinam (350), and French Guyana (300).[247] Near Iquitos in the Amazon part of Peru, *Plasmodium vivax* and *Plasmodium falciparum* infections reached incidences of 826 and 166/1,000/yr, respectively, in a population of virtually 100% bednet users.[243] In the southwestern Pacific, rates of reported infections per 1,000 per year peaked in the Solomon Islands (370), Vanuatu (200), and Cambodia (80).

MALARIA DISEASE

In nonimmune people who are not taking antimalarials, virtually all *Plasmodium* infections (including low-density parasitemias)[49] become apparent, for a manifestation index of 100%. Nonimmune people are virtually never long-term carriers of gametocytes and are therefore not involved in cyclic transmission, including that of resistant plasmodia (see Chapter 6).

Table 2–8. Incidence of *Plasmodium* Infections in Control Groups in Intervention Trials

Location	Population	Species	No. Examined	Weeks of Follow-Up (pwks)	Incidence/ Person/ Year*	Reference
Africa						
Gabon	Children	Pf	140	12	0.8	238
Kenya	Children	Pf	221	~6 (1,096)	9.6	239, 240
	Adults	Pf	54	10	2.7	
Zambia	Adults	Pf	111	10	1.9	241
Latin America						
Brazil	Children, adults	Pf	85	78 (14,799)	0.4	242
		Pv	127		0.7	
Nicaragua	Children, adults	Pv	5,125	~16	0.2	237
Peru	Children, adults	Pv	1,400	52	0.8	243
		Pf	1,400	52	0.2	
Australasia						
Indonesia	Men	Pf	41	28 (837)	0.8	244
		Pv	41	28 (806)	1.0	
Thailand	Children, adults	Pf 38%, Pv 62%	249	78	1.5	245, 246
		Pv	101	~ 25	0.4	
		Pf	101	~ 25	0.2	

Pf = *Plasmodium falciparum*; Pv = *Plasmodium vivax*; pwks = person-weeks; ~ = about.
* Pwks × 52 provided corresponding rates/yr.

Incubation, Persistence, and Progression

In short-term and frequent travelers, the shortest possible incubation period is of particular interest (Table 2–9, which includes data from experimental infections).[4,49,50,248] In *Plasmodium falciparum*, it is 5.5 days. In persons returned home and forgetting past exposure, long incubation periods and *Plasmodium* persistence are of equal interest. In *Plasmodium falciparum*, incubation periods of 6 to 18 months are unusual but are on record,[89,249–251] and in endemic areas, this species can persist well beyond the transmission season.[252] Benign malarias can take 12 months to first manifestation.[206,253–256] In a person with a history of past febrile illness, a relapse can mimic a primary attack, particularly in *Plasmodium vivax* strains that exhibit different relapse patterns.[116]

Some 90% of malaria attacks in travelers occur at home.[251,257] By 3 months after returning home, more than 90% of falciparum cases and a majority of vivax cases have become manifest[258] (Table 2–10).[251]

For the first one to two parasitemia cycles, uncomplicated falciparum malaria and benign malarias are indistinguishable clinically and have fever as the lead symptom. Soon, however, evolution splits the two into malignant and benign forms, making "malaria" a disease syndrome. In malignant or falciparum malaria, sequestration and blocking of the microcirculation of vital organs create an emergency. "The prin-

Table 2–9. **Plasmodium Pre-patent Periods, Incubation Periods, and Longevities**

	Pre-patent Period* (d)		Incubation Period (d)				
	Short	Long	Short[†]	Usual	Long	Relapse	Longevity (mo)
P. falciparum	6	25	7	12	365	No	18
P. vivax	8	27	10	14	365	Yes	60
P. ovale	12	20	14	14	365	Yes	52
P. malariae	14	59	21	28	210	No	630

d = days; *P.* = *Plasmodium.*
* Time to first microscopic detection of asexual blood forms (patency) or positive subinoculation trial.
[†] Assuming a subpatent erythrocytic cycle of 2 days (*P. falciparum*) or 3 days (*P. vivax*).
Data from Molyneaux L,[4] Stürchler D et al.,[49,50] and Beaudoin RL.[248]

ciple is that patients everywhere who are suspected of having malaria must receive full treatment without delay."[259] In contrast, untreated vivax and other benign malarias go on to produce synchronized parasitemia and classic fever patterns.

Disease Incidence

Imported malaria (see Chapter 18) and endemic malaria in Latin America seem reasonably well reported. In tropical Africa, however, more than 90% of cases are not reported. Problems with surveillance include lack of access to health facilities and lack of accepted case definitions of adequate specificity and sensitivity.[260–272] I propose that the following simple set of widely available core parameters be included in any malaria case definition:

> **Setting.** Consider exposure intensity and duration: Which season? Which local risk level? How long does the patient live in the area? Are there nocturnal activities? Is there use of bednets?
>
> **Age and presumed immune status.** Infants less than 6 months of age, primigravid females,[52,53,273,274] and visitors should be considered high-risk groups.
>
> **History.** Take a history of fever and medications: Number of days febrile? Number of days since fever? How many lifetime malaria episodes? Current antimalarial medications? Antipyretics? Vomiting?
>
> **Physical status.** Examine the patient for vital signs, body core temperature, and comorbidities such as pneumonia, measles, bacterial meningitis, and typhoid fever.
>
> **Follow-up of treatment response.** Depending on the class of antimalarial and the sensitivity of the local strain, it takes 1 to 3 days for core temperature to fall and remain at $< 37.5°C$.[275–280a] An overnight stay or a follow-up visit is therefore needed to evaluate treatment success or failure.

If supported by resources and cost effectiveness analysis, laboratory confirmation should always be sought, but tests should not deter caregivers from prompt treatment of suspected falciparum malaria.

Table 2–10. **Proportion of Imported Malaria Cases Diagnosed between Arrival and Onset of Symptoms, United States, 1995**

| | % of Cases Diagnosed | | | |
Interval	Plasmodium falciparum (n = 367)	Plasmodium vivax (n = 432)	Plasmodium ovale (n = 21)	Plasmodium malariae (n = 3 1)
Before arrival	12	5	5	3
0–4 weeks	80	35	19	45
1–3 months	6	20	9	16
3.1–6 months	1.2	15	33	13
6.1–12 months	0.5	20	24	16
> 1 year	0.3	5	10	7

Data from Centers for Disease Control—United States. MMWR Morb Mortal Wkly Rep 1999;48 Suppl 1:1–24.

Tropical Africa, with powerful vectors and a malicious parasite, is expected to bear a high disease toll. For this region, the incidence of clinical malaria in children was estimated to be 1 per person per year.[280a] This estimate corresponds to results in control groups in recent intervention trials (Table 2–11)[192,237,239,281–287] but is at variance with a continued malaria vaccine trial in West Africa, where the disease in controls had an incidence of < 0.1 per person per year.[281,282] Surprisingly, an earlier careful review reported an attack rate of 1 to 2 per person per year in African adults.[288] High disease rates are also reported outside of tropical Africa. In western Thailand, in a low-transmission area with a high manifestation index, the disease incidence was about 1 per person per year,[289] and in the

Table 2–11. **Incidence of Malaria Disease in Longitudinal Studies in Endemic Areas**

Location	Population	Species	No. Followed	Weeks Followed	Incidence/ Person/Yr	Reference
Africa						
Gambia	Children	Pf	136 and 203	104	up to 0.01	281, 282
Kenya	Children	Pf	1,848	34	1	192
Kenya	Children	Pf	78	6	6	239
Sierra Leone	Children	Pf	~400	48	1.3	283
Tanzania	Children	Pf	123	52	0.3–2.5	284
	Children	Pf	312	52	0.8	285
Latin America						
Guatemala	General	Pv	341	52	0.2	286
Nicaragua	General	Pv	12,831	16	0.2	237
Australasia						
Thailand	Migrants	Pf, Pv	135	38	0.6	287

Pf = *Plasmodium falciparum;* Pv = *Plasmodium vivax;* ~ = approximately.

Amazon part of Peru, falciparum and vivax malaria together reached a combined attack rate of 1 per person per year.[243]

Disease incidences applied to exposed populations provide malaria case estimates (Table 2–12). With annual incidences per person aged ≤ 14 years of 1.0 in Africa, 0.2 in Latin America, and 0.5 in Australasia, and with one-tenth of these rates in adults, the predicted number of cases in the year 2000 was 657 million. The scenario includes the idea that at least one of all the infections occurring in a year produces disease. It suggests that the situation has deteriorated since 1992, when the estimate was 282 million cases.[236]

Nonimmune people can experience high disease incidence rates as well. When the French cruiser *Marseillaise* docked in Dakar in 1917, 440 of 598 crew members came down with falciparum malaria, for an attack rate of 74%.[290] In 1942, Australian and U.S. troops in the southwestern Pacific experienced attack rates of up to 1,500 per 1,000 per year and CFRs of up to 30%, with quinine in short supply.[66] Despite chemoprophylaxis, the incidence of falciparum malaria in a French humanitarian corps working in central Africa was 31 per 1,000 per month.[291] In unprotected short-term travelers to tropical Africa, Asia, and Latin America, the attack rate per 1,000 persons per month is estimated to be 15 to 24, 0.3 to 4, and ≤ 0.5, respectively[292,293] (see Chapter 18).

Further Impact

Anemia and other malaria-related morbidities; out-of-pocket expeditures for transportation, care, and drugs; the number of days lost from home, school, or work; and the years of life spent with disability after the survival of cerebral malaria are further measures of the impact of malaria that are not discussed here in any detail. Malaria illness lasts 1 to 6 days in children and 5 to 9 days in adults.[288,294]

Table 2–12. **Year 2000 Malaria Case Estimates***

Location	Exposed (Million) ≤ 14 yr	> 14 yr	Disease Incidence/ Person/Yr ≤ 14 yr Low	Core	> 14 yr Low	Core	Malaria Cases (Million) Low[†]	Core[†]	Falciparum Cases (Million) Low[‡]	Core[‡]	Malaria Deaths (Million) Low[§]	Core[§]
Africa	295	361	0.2	1.0	0.02	0.1	66	331	60	298	0.06	0.9
Latin America	39	69	0.1	0.2	0.05	0.02	7	9	Few	1	Few	Few
Australasia	536	980	0.25	0.5	0.125	0.05	257	317	135	166	0.1	0.5
World	870	1,410	—	—	—	—	330	657	195	465	0.2	1.4

* For persons ≤ 14 and > 14 years of age, of those exposed, malaria cases, falciparum cases, and malaria deaths, using low and moderate disease incidence rates.
† By applying incidence estimates of the previous column to exposed persons.
‡ By applying the proportions of *Plasmodium falciparum* in Table 2–6 to malaria cases.
§ By applying case-fatality ratios (CFRs) of 0.1% (low) or 0.3% (core) to falciparum cases.

Between 3% and 21% of survivors of severe falciparum malaria may suffer from permanent neurologic or sensory deficits.[280a] Disability-adjusted-life-years (DALYs) are a measure of disease burden that combines years of life lost due to premature death and years of life lived while disabled.[295] In 1990, DALYs totaled approximately 1,379 million worldwide. Malaria ranked eighth among infection syndromes and caused 31.7 million (2.6%) DALYs, to which children aged 0 to 4 years contributed 73% (23.2 million).

Malaria Deaths

Virtually all malaria deaths are due to *Plasmodium falciparum*. Risk factors include (1) delay between the onset of illness and the start of treatment and (2) treatments that are inadequate because of product choice, dosing, or route. Depending on access to care and patient mix, falciparum malaria has a CFR of 0.01% to 25%.[251,296–300] In northern Thailand, in a population of 4,728 people with good access to diagnosis and care, there were 5,776 clinical cases of falciparum malaria in 2 years; 303 (5%) were severe, and of these patients, 11 died, resulting in a CFR of 0.2% (all cases) or 3.6% (severe cases) and a mortality rate of 1.2 per 1,000 per year.[289] In 15 southern provinces of Vietnam, 383,102 malaria cases (the majority caused by *Plasmodium falciparum*) were reported in 1989. Of these, 5,019 (1%) were severe and 1,069 patients died, resulting in a CFR of 0.3% (all cases) or 21% (severe cases).[301] Despite high-technology medicine, CFRs in travelers seem amazingly close to CFRs in malarious areas with a range of 0.4% to 10%.[302–304]

CFRs applied to falciparum malaria cases can provide estimates of the number of malaria deaths. With CFRs of 0.3%, the annual number of malaria deaths is 1.4 million (see Table 2–12). Deaths directly *and* indirectly attributable to malaria are estimated by a comparison of pre- and postcontrol situations. This method provides overall mortality estimates of 10 per 1,000 per year, with local variations by a factor of 10.[300] After a careful review of 129 publications, malaria mortality in Africa was estimated to be 5 per 1,000 per year.[288] In a meta-analysis, falciparum malaria mortality in tropical Africa in 1995 was estimated to be 9, 2, 1, and 0.1 per 1,000 in the respective age groups of 0 to 4, 5 to 9, 10 to 14, and > 14 years.[305]

Appropriate treatment regimens and the shortening of treatment delays are strategies likely to reduce CFRs and malaria mortality. Shortening treatment delays is difficult in remote tropical areas. Ways to overcome delays include the home use of suppositories, which avoid overdosing and vomiting,[306] and training mothers how to self-treat their children.[307]

FORECASTING MALARIA EPIDEMIOLOGY

Rainfall, surface water, ambient temperature, vegetation, and other environmental variables that influence malaria transmission are amenable to satellite observation and to analysis by a geographic information system (GIS).[308] For accurate surveillance and forecasting, satellite data with high spatial (~1 km) and temporal (> 2 orbits in 24 hours) resolution are required. A geographic information system is now used to combine epidemiologic and entomological data, with the aim of mapping malaria risks in Latin America,[309] Africa,[67,119,310] and Australasia.[311,312] It is also used for forecasts. It was predicted that of 5 million Kenyan children less than 5 years of age and at risk, 400 per day would develop clinical malaria warranting hospital care, and that about 70 would die.[67]

CONCLUSION

The evidence presented points to a clear deterioration in the past decade of major indicators of the world malaria situation, including the number of deaths, cases, and infections; the level of resistance to antimalarials; and the level of resistance to insecticides. Malaria must be rolled back onto the world health agenda as a leading target for control. Promising control tools with universal application are impregnated bednets and prompt (possibly presumptive) treatment of falciparum malaria (if not at home, then at least at the nearest health center).

REFERENCES

1. World Health Organization. Expert committee on hygiene and sanitation in aviation. WHO Tech Rep Ser 1959;174:1–62.
2. World Health Organization. World malaria situation, 1988. World Health Stat Q 1990;43:68–79.
3. Spencer HC. Epidemiology of malaria. Clin Trop Med Commun Dis 1986;1:1–28.
4. Molyneaux L. The epidemiology of human malaria as an explanation of its distribution, including some implications for its control. In: Wernsdorfer WH, McGregor I, editors. Malaria: principles and practice of malariology. Edinburgh: Churchill Livingstone, 1988. p. 913–998.
5. Molyneaux L, Muir DA, Spencer HC, et al. The epidemiology of malaria and its measurement. In: Wernsdorfer WH, McGregor I, editors. Malaria: principles and practice of malariology. Edinburgh: Churchill Livingstone, 1988. p. 999–1089.
6. Mouchet J, Carnevale P. Les vecteurs et la transmission. In: Danis M, Mouchet J, editors. Paludisme. Paris: Ellipses, 1991. p. 35–59.
7. Marsh K. Malaria—a neglected disease? Parasitology 1992;104:S53–S69.
8. Dobson MJ. The malaria centenary. Parassitologia 1999;41:21–32.
9. World Health Organization, White GB. Malaria vectors. Training and information materials on vector biology and control. Geneva: World Health Organization, 1991.
10. World Health Organization, Rozendaal JA. Vector control. Geneva: World Health Organization, 1997.
11. Gadelha P. From "forest malaria" to "bromeliad malaria": a case-study of scientific controversy and malaria control. Parassitologia 1994;36:175–195.

12. Trape JF, Lefebvre-Zante E, Legros F, et al. Vector-density gradients and the epidemiology of urban malaria in Dakar, Senegal. Am J Trop Med Hyg 1992;47:181–189.

13. Reiter P. Malaria and global warming in perspective? Emerg Infect Dis 2000;6:438–439.

14. World Health Organization. Geographical distribution of arthropod-borne diseases and their principal vectors. Geneva: World Health Organization, 1989; WHO/VBC/89.967. p. 1–134.

15. Zimmerman RH. Ecology of malaria vectors in the Americas and future direction. Mem Inst Oswaldo Cruz 1992;87 Suppl 3:371–383.

16. Tadei WP, Thatcher BD, Santos JMM, et al. Ecologic observations on anopheline vectors of malaria in the Brazilian Amazon. Am J Trop Med Hyg 1998;59:325–335.

17. Najera JA. Malaria control. Geneva: World Health Organization, 1999; WHO/CDS/RBM/99.10. p. 1–126.

18. Coetzee M, Craig M, Le Sueur D. Distribution of African malaria mosquitoes belonging to the *Anopheles gambiae* complex. Parasitol Today 2000;16:74–77.

19. Charlwood JD, Alecrim WD. Capture-recapture studies with the South American malaria vector *Anopheles darlingi*, root. Ann Trop Med Parasitol 1989;83:569–576.

20. Mothiron C, Alemanni M, Manigand G, et al. Paludisme après un séjour à la Guadeloupe. Presse Med 1990;19:1504.

21. Ellis ME. Vivax malaria acquired in Trinidad, a malaria free area. BMJ 1986;292:1048–1049.

22. Merritt A, Ewald D, van den Hurk AF, et al. Malaria acquired in the Torres Strait. Commun Dis Intelligence 1998;22:1–2.

23. Fox E, Bouloumie J, Olson JG, et al. *Plasmodium falciparum* voyage en train d'Ethiopie à Djibouti. Med Trop 1991;51:185–189

24. Guillet P, Germain MC, Giacomini T, et al. Origin and prevention of airport malaria in France. Trop Med Int Health 1998;3:700–705.

25. Rizzo F, Morandi N, Riccio G, et al. Unusual transmission of falciparum malaria in Italy. Lancet 1989;1:555–556.

26. Mantel CF, Klose C, Scheurer S, et al. *Plasmodium falciparum* malaria acquired in Berlin, Germany. Lancet 1995;346:320–321.

27. Robert Koch Institut. Fallbericht: In Deutschland erworbene Malaria tropica. Epidemiol Bull 1998;11:73–74.

28. Peleman R, Benoit D, Goossens L, et al. Indigenous malaria in a suburb of Ghent, Belgium. J Travel Med 2000;7:48–49.

29. Guillet P, Nathan M. *Aedes albopictus*, une menace pour la France? Med Trop 1999;59:49–51.

30. Lusina D, Legros F, Estève V, et al. Paludisme d'aéroport: quatre nouveaux cas dans la banlieue de Paris durant l'été 1999. Eurosurveillance 2000;5:76–80.

31. Wells L, Ala FA. Malaria and blood transfusion. Lancet 1985 June 8;1317–1319.

32. Centers for Disease Control. Transfusion-transmitted malaria—Missouri and Pennsylvania, 1996–1998. MMWR Morb Mortal Wkly Rep 1999;48:253–256.

33. Holzer B, Glück Z, Zambelli D, et al. Transmission of malaria by renal transplantation. Transplantation 1985;39:315–316.

34. Lefrère F, Besson C, Datry A, et al. Transmission of *Plasmodium falciparum* by allogenic bone marrow transplantation. Bone Marrow Transplant 1996;18:473–474.

35. Turkmen A, Sever MS, Ecder T, et al. Posttransplant malaria. Transplantation 1996;62:1521–1523.

36. Fischer L, Sterneck M, Claus M, et al. Transmission of malaria tertiana by multi-organ donation. Clin Transplant 1999;13:491–495.
37. Nüesch R, Cynke E, Jost MC, et al. Thrombocytopenia after kidney transplantation. Am J Kidney Dis 2000;35:537–538.
38. Bourée P, Fouquet E. Paludisme par inoculation accidentelle. Bull Soc Pathol Exot 1978;71:297–301.
39. Haworth FLM, Cook GC. Needlestick malaria. Lancet 1995;346:1361.
40. Public Health Laboratory Service. Needlestick malaria with tragic consequences. Commun Dis Rep CDR Wkly 1997;7:247.
41. Bayahia R, Balafrej L, Cadi Soussi M. A propos de quatre cas de paludisme à *Plasmodium falciparum* chez des patients hémodialysés. Sem Hôp Paris 1992;68:380–381.
42. Abulrahi HA, Bohlega EA, Fontaine RE, et al. *Plasmodium falciparum* malaria transmitted in hospital through heparin locks. Lancet 1997;349:23–25.
43. Baker JE, Crawford GPM. Malaria: a new facet of heroin addiction in Australia. Med J Aust 1978;2:427–428.
44. Senaldi G, Castelli F, Chelazzi G, et al. *Plasmodium vivax* malaria in a drug addict in Italy. Trans R Soc Trop Med Hyg 1985;79:738–739.
45. Gonzalez Garcia JJ, Arnalich F, Peña JM, et al. An outbreak of *Plasmodium vivax* malaria among heroin users in Spain. Trans R Soc Trop Med Hyg 1986;80:549–552.
46. Rieckmann KH, Beaudoin RL, Cassells JS, et al. Use of attenuated sporozoites in the immunization of human volunteers against falciparum malaria. Bull World Health Organ 1979;57 Suppl:S261–S265.
47. Yang BL, Wan WJ, Wang WR, et al. Experimental studies on the biological characteristics of *Plasmodium vivax* in South Yunnan. J Parasitol Parasitic Dis 1986;4:101–104.
48. Austin SC. The history of malariotherapy for neurosyphilis. Modern parallels. JAMA 1992;268:516–519.
49. Stürchler D, Just M, Berger R, et al. Evaluation of $(5.1\text{-NANP})_{19}$, a recombinant *Plasmodium falciparum* vaccine candidate, in adults. Trop Geogr Med 1992;44:9–14.
50. Stürchler D, Berger R, Rudin C, et al. Safety, immunogenicity, and pilot efficacy of *Plasmodium falciparum* sporozoite and asexual blood-stage combination vaccine in Swiss adults. Am J Trop Med Hyg 1995;53:423–431.
51. Collins WE, Jeffery GM. A retrospective examination of sporozoite- and trophozoite-induced infections with *Plasmodium falciparum*: development of parasitologic and clinical immunity during primary infection. Am J Trop Med Hyg 1999;61 Suppl:S4–S19.
52. Brabin BJ. The risks and severity of malaria in pregnant women. Geneva: World Health Organization, 1991; World Health Organization Applied Field Research in Malaria Reports No. 1. p. 1–34.
53. Steketee RW, Wirima JJ. Malaria prevention in pregnancy: the effects of treatment and chemoprophylaxis on placental malaria infection, low birth weight, and fetal, infant and child survival. Am J Trop Med Hyg 1996;55 Suppl:S1–S100.
54. Fischer PR. Congenital malaria: an African survey. Clin Pediatr 1997;36:411–413.
55. Balaka B, Agbere AD, Bonkoungou P, et al. Paludisme congénital-maladie à *Plasmodium falciparum* chez le nouveau-né à risque infectieux. Arch Pediatr 2000;7:243–248.
56. Zenz W, Trop M, Kollaritsch H, et al. Konnatale Malaria durch *Plasmodium falciparum* und *Plasmodium malariae*. Wien Klin Wochenschr 2000;112:459–461.

57. Kabiru EW, Kaviti JN. Risk of transfusion malaria in Nairobi. East Afr Med J 1987;64:825–827.

58. Fontenille D, Lochouarn L, Diagne N, et al. High annual and seasonal variations in malaria transmission by anophelines and vector species composition in Dielmo, a holoendemic area in Senegal. Am J Trop Med Hyg 1997;56:247–253.

59. Roberts DR, Manguin S, Mouchet J. DDT house spraying and re-emerging malaria. Lancet 2000;356:330–332.

60. Shidrawi GR. A WHO global programme for monitoring vector resistance to pesticides. Bull World Health Organ 1990;68:403–408.

61. Chandre F, Darrier F, Manga L, et al. Status of pyrethroid resistance in *Anopheles* gambiae sensu lato. Bull World Health Organ 1999;77:230–234.

62. Hargreaves K, Koekemoer LL, Brooke BD, et al. *Anopheles funestus* resistant to pyrethroid insecticides in South Africa. Med Vet Entomol 2000:14:181–189.

63. Karunaratne SH. Insecticide cross-resistance spectra and underlying resistance mechanisms of Sri Lankan anopheline vectors of malaria. Southeast Asian J Trop Med Public Health 1999;30:460–469.

64. Choi HW, Breman JG, Teutsch SM, et al. The effectiveness of insecticide-impregnated bed nets in reducing cases of malaria infection: a meta-analysis of published results. Am J Trop Med Hyg 1995;52:377–382.

65. Darriet F, N'guessan R, Koffi AA, et al. Impact de la résistance aux pyréthrinoïdes sur l'efficacité des moustiquaires imprégnées dans la prevention du paludisme: resultants des essays en cases expérimentales avec la deltaméthrine SC. Bull Soc Pathol Exot 2000;93:131–134.

66. Joy RJT. Malaria in American troops in the south and southwest Pacific in World War II. Medical Hist 1999;43:192–207.

67. Snow RW, Gouws E, Omumbo J, et al. Models to predict the intensity of *Plasmodium falciparum* transmission: application to the burden of disease in Kenya. Trans R Soc Trop Med Hyg 1998;92:601–606.

68. Fontaine RE, Najjar AE, Prince JS. The 1958 malaria epidemic in Ethiopia. Am J Trop Med Hyg 1961;10:795–803.

69. Warsame M, Wernsdorfer WH, Huldt G, et al. An epidemic of *Plasmodium falciparum* malaria in Balcad, Somalia, and its causation. Trans R Soc Trop Med Hyg 1995;89:142–145.

70. Abose T, Yeebiyo Y, Olana D, et al. Re-orientation and definition of the role of malaria vector control in Ethiopia. Geneva: World Health Organization, 1998; WHO/Mal/98.1085. p. 1–38.

71. Malakooti MA, Biomndo K, Shanks GD. Reemergence of epidemic malaria in the highlands of western Kenya. Emerg Infect Dis 1998;4:671–676.

72. Brown V, Issak MA, Rossi M, et al. Epidemic of malaria in north-eastern Kenya. Lancet 1998;352:1356–1357.

73. Bawden MP, Slaten DD, Malone JD. Falciparum malaria in a displaced Haitian population. Trans R Soc Trop Med Hyg 1995;89:600–603.

74. Najera JA, Kouznetzsov RL, Delacollette C. Malaria epidemics. Detection and control, forecasting and prevention. Geneva: World Health Organization 1998, WHO/MAL/98.1084. p. 1–81.

75. Bouma MJ, van der Kaay HJ. Epidemic malaria in India and the El Niño southern oscillation. Lancet 1994;344:1638–1639.

76. Bouma MJ, van der Kaay HJ. Epidemic malaria in India's Thar desert. Lancet 1995;346:1232–1233.

77. Amerasinghe PH, Amerasinghe FP, Konradsen F, et al. Malaria vectors in a traditional dry zone village in Sri Lanka. Am J Trop Med Hyg 1999;60:421–429.

78. World Health Organization. Activités antipaludiques: les 40 dernières années. World Health Stat Q 1988;41:64–71.

79. Decludt B, Pecoul B, Biberson P, et al. Malaria surveillance among the displaced Karen population in Thailand, April 1984 to February 1989, Mae Sot, Thailand. Southeast Asian J Trop Med Public Health 1991;22:504–508.

80. Cruz Marques A. Migrations and the dissemination of malaria in Brazil. Mem Inst Oswaldo Cruz 1986;81 Suppl II:17–30.

81. Camargo LMA, Ferreira MU, Krieger H, et al. Unstable hypoendemic malaria in Rondonia (western Amazon region, Brazil): epidemic outbreaks and work-associated incidence in an agro-industrial rural settlement. Am J Trop Med Hyg 1994;51:16–25.

82. Guarda JA, Asayag CR, Witzig R. Malaria reemergence in the Peruvian Amazon region. Emerg Infect Dis 1999;5:209–215.

83. Garnham PCC. Malaria epidemics at exceptionally high altitudes in Kenya. BMJ 1945;11:45–47.

84. Lindsay SW, Martens WJM. Malaria in the African highlands: past, present and future. Bull World Health Organ 1998;76:33–45.

85. Mouchet J, Manguin S, Sircoulon J, et al. Evolution of malaria in Africa for the past 40 years: impact of climatic and human factors. J Am Mosq Control Assoc 1998;14:121–130.

86. Ghebreyesus TA, Haile M, Witten KH, et al. Incidence of malaria among children living near dams in northern Ethiopia: community incidence survey. BMJ 1999;319:663–666.

87. Taylor P, Mutambu SL. A review of the malaria situation in Zimbabwe with special reference to the period 1972–1981. Trans R Soc Trop Med Hyg 1986;80:12–19.

88. Chen GG. An epidemiological investigation of malaria in Weixi county, Yunnan province. Chin J Epidemiol 1985;6:208–210.

89. World Health Organization. Parasitologie du paludisme. WHO Tech Rep Ser 1969;433:1–76.

90. Anthony RL, Bangs MJ, Hamzah N, et al. Heightened transmission of stable malaria in an isolated population in the highlands of Irian Jaya, Indonesia. Am J Trop Med Hyg 1992;47:346–356.

91. Bangs MJ, Purnomo, Anthony RL. *Plasmodium ovale* in the highlands of Irian Jaya, Indonesia. Ann Trop Med Parasitol 1992;86:307–308.

92. Benzerroug EH, Janssens PG, Ambroise-Thomas P. Etude séroépidémiologique du paludisme au Sahara algérien. Bull World Health Organ 1991;69:713–723.

93. Develoux M, Chegou A, Prual A, et al. Malaria in the oasis of Bilma, Republic of Niger. Trans R Soc Trop Med Hyg 1994;88:644.

94. Kenawy MA, Beier JC, El Said S. First record of malaria and associated *Anopheles* in El Gara oasis, Egypt. J Am Mosq Control Assoc 1986;2:101–103.

95. Sebai ZA. Malaria in Saudi Arabia. Trop Doct 1988;18:183–188.

96. Denys JC, Isautier H. Le maintien de l'éradication du paludisme dans l'île de la Réunion (1979–1991). Bull Epidemiol Hebdom 1992;20:89–90.

97. Tikasingh E, Edwards C, Hamilton PJS, et al. A malaria outbreak due to *Plasmodium malariae* on the island of Grenada. Am J Trop Med Hyg 1980;29:715–719.

98. Chadee DD, Beier JC, Doon R. Re-emergence of *Plasmodium malariae* in Trinidad, West Indies. Ann Trop Med Parasitol 1999;93:467–475.

99. Chadee DD, Kitron U. Spatial and temporal patterns of imported malaria cases and local transmission in Trinidad. Am J Trop Med Hyg 1999;61:513–517.

100. Munckhof WJ, Grayson ML, Turnidge JD. Malaria acquired in Bali. Med J Australia 1995;162:223.

101. Fryauff DJ, Baird JK, Candradikusuma D, et al. Survey of in vivo sensitivity to chloroquine by *Plasmodium falciparum* and *P. vivax* in Lombok, Indonesia. Am J Trop Med Hyg 1997;56:241–244.

102. Nowell WR. Vector introduction and malaria infection on Guam. J Am Mosquito Control Assoc 1987;3:259–265.

103. Gonzalez JM, Olano V, Vergara J, et al. Unstable, low-level transmission of malaria on the Colombian Pacific coast. Ann Trop Med Parasitol 1997;91:349–358.

104. Velema JP, Alihonou EM, Chippaux JP, et al. Malaria morbidity and mortality in children under three years of age on the coast of Benin, West Africa. Trans R Soc Trop Med Hyg 1991;85:430–435.

105. Waner S, Durrhiem D, Braack LEO, et al. Malaria protection measures used by in-flight travelers to South African game parks. J Travel Med 1999;6:254–257.

106. World Health Organization. *Plasmodium vivax* infection among tourists to Puerto Vallarta, and Acapulco, Mexico—New Mexico, Texas. MMWR Morb Mortal Wkly Rep 1985;34:461–462.

107. Bradley D. Malaria in Mexico and the Dominican Republic. Eurosurveill Wkly 2000;6:1–2.

108. Poinsignon Y, Arfi C, Sarfati C, et al. Accès palustre au retour d'un voyage aux antilles françaises. Discussion du mode de transmission. Med Trop 1999;59:55–57.

109. Thimasarn K, Jatapadma S, Vijaykadga S, et al. Epidemiology of malaria in Thailand. J Travel Med 1995;2:59–65.

110. Hill DR, Behrens RH, Bradley DJ. The risk of malaria in travelers to Thailand. Trans R Soc Trop Med Hyg 1996;90:680–681.

111. Kidson C, Singhasivanon P, Supavej S. Mekong malaria. Southeast Asian J Trop Med Public Health 1999;30 Suppl 4:1–101.

112. Tyagi BK, Chaudhary RC, Yadav SP. Epidemic malaria in Thar desert, India. Lancet 1995;346:634–635.

113. Akhtar R, McMichael AJ. Rainfall and malaria outbreaks in western Rajasthan. Lancet 1996;348:1457–1458.

114. Wijesundera M de S. Malaria outbreaks in new foci in Sri Lanka. Parasitol Today 1988;4:147–150.

115. Trape JF. Malaria and urbanization in central Africa: the example of Brazzaville. Trans R Soc Trop Med Hyg 1987;81 Suppl 2:1–42.

116. Adak T, Sharma VP, Orlov VS. Studies on the *Plasmodium vivax* relapse pattern in Delhi, India. Am J Trop Med Hyg 1998;59:175–179.

117. Mandal B, Mitra NK, Mukhopadhyay AK, et al. Emerging *Plasmodium falciparum* in an endemic area in Calcutta. J Indian Med Assoc 1998;96:328–329.

118. Stürchler D, Naef U, Fernex M, et al. Malaria and mosquitoes: how often for how long? Trans R Soc Trop Med Hyg 1990;84:780.

119. Lengeler C, Genton B. Cartographie du paludisme: les nouveaux outils et leur utilisation. Med Hyg 2000;58:1094–1097.

120. Robert Koch Institut. Zum aktuellen Malariarisiko in der Dominikanischen Republik (Update). Epidemiol Bull 2000;19:155.

121. Public Health Laboratory Service. Rise in falciparum malaria imported from East Africa. Commun Dis Rep CDR Wkly 1998;8:177–178.

122. Miller KD, Campbell GH, Nutman TB, et al. Early acquisition of antibody to *Plasmodium falciparum* sporozoites in nonimmune temporary residents of Africa. J Infect Dis 1988;158:868–871.

123. Cobelens FGJ, Verhave JP, Leentvaar-Kuijpers A, et al. Testing for anti-circumsporozoite and anti-blood-stage antibodies for epidemiologic assessment of *Plasmodium falciparum* infection in travelers. Am J Trop Med Hyg 1998;58:75–80.

124. Nothdurft HD, Jelinek T, Blüml A, et al. Seroconversion to circumsporozoite antigen of *Plasmodium falciparum* demonstrates a high risk of malaria transmission in travelers to East Africa. Clin Infect Dis 1999;28:641–642.

125. Hay SI, Rogers DJ, Toomer JF, et al. Annual *Plasmodium falciparum* entomological inoculation rates (EIR) across Africa: literature survey, internet access and review. Trans R Soc Trop Med Hyg 2000;94:113–127.

126. World Health Organization. Status of malaria eradication during the first semester of the year 1970. Wkly Epidemiol Rec 1971;46:97–109.

127. World Health Organization. Communicable diseases 2000. Geneva: World Health Organization, 2000; WHO/CDS/2000.1.

128. World Health Organization. World malaria situation 1986–1987. Wkly Epidemiol Rec 1989;64:241–254.

129. Pan American Health Organization. Status of malaria programs in the Americas. Bull Pan Am Health Organ 1988;22:92–103.

130. Kondrashin AV, Rashid KM, editors. Epidemiological considerations for planning malaria control in the WHO South-East Asia region. New Delhi: World Health Organization Regional Office for South-East Asia, 1987. p. 1–411.

131. Kondrashin AV. Malaria in the WHO Southeast Asia region. Indian J Malariol 1992;29:129–160.

132. Institute of Medicine. Malaria. Obstacles and opportunities. Washington (DC): National Academy Press, 1991.

133. Russel PF. World-wide malaria distribution, prevalence and control. Am J Trop Med Hyg 1956;5:937–965.

134. Wernsdorfer WH. The importance of malaria in the world. In: Kreier JP, editor. Malaria. Vol. 1. Epidemiology, chemotherapy, morphology, and metabolism. New York: Academic Press, 1980.

135. Laveran CLA. Note sur un nouveau parasite trouvé dans le sang de plusieurs malades atteints de fièvre palustre [reprinted in Rev Infect Dis 1982;4:908–911]. Bull Acad Méd 1880;19:1235–1236.

136. Andrews JM, Quinby FE, Langmuir ADL. Malaria eradication in the United States. Am J Public Health 1950;40:1405–1411.

137. World Health Organization Chronicle. WHO 1955;9. (Courtesy of WHO)

138. Dutta P, Bhattacharyya DR, Dutta LP. Epidemiological observations on malaria in some parts of Tengkhat PHC, Dibrugarh district, Assam. Indian J Malariol 1991;28:121–128.

139. Bourée P, Bonnisseau G, Ratard RC. Etude épidémiologique du paludisme à Tanna (Vanuatu). Bull Soc Pathol Exot 1984;77:459–465.

140. Miles J. Infectious diseases: colonising the Pacific? Dunedin, New Zealand: University of Otago Press, 1997.

141. Layton M, Parise E, Campbell CC, et al. Mosquito-transmitted malaria in New York City, 1993. Lancet 1995;346:729–731.

142. Huang ZS. Analysis on epidemic characteristics of falciparum malaria in south Henan. Chin J Parasitol Parasitic Dis 1987;5:18–20.

143. Fisk GH. Malaria in Canada. Can Med Assoc J 1931;(Dec):679–683.

144. Doby JM. Le paludisme autochtone en Bretagne. Bull Soc Pathol Exot 1992;85: 76–88.

145. Nozais JP. Le paludisme dans le monde méditerrannéen. Bull Soc Pathol Exot 1988;81:854–860.

146. Dobson MJ. Malaria in England: a geographical and historical perspective. Parassitologia 1994;36:35–60.

147. Verhave JP. The advent of malaria research in the Netherlands. Hist Phil Life Sci 1988;10:121–128.

148. Zhou ZJ. The malaria situation in the People's Republic of China. Bull World Health Organ 1981;59:931–936.

149. Spencer M. The history of malaria control in the Southwest Pacific region, with particular reference to Papua New Guinea and the Solomon islands. Papua New Guinea Med J 1992;35:33–66.

150. Lysenko AJA, Beljaev AE. An analysis of the geographical distribution of *Plasmodium ovale*. Bull World Health Organ 1969;40:383–394.

151. Ukpe IS. *Plasmodium ovale* in South Africa. Trans R Soc Trop Med Hyg 1998;92:574.

152. Kawamoto F, Miyake H, Kaneko O, et al. Sequence variation in the 18S rRNA gene, a target for PCR-based malaria diagnosis, in *Plasmodium ovale* from southern Vietnam. J Clin Microbiol 1996;34:2287–2289.

153. Paxton LA, Slutsker L, Schultz LJ, et al. Imported malaria in montagnard refugees settling in North Carolina: implications for prevention and control. Am J Trop Med Hyg 1996;54:54–57.

154. Zhou M, Liu Q, Wongsrichanalai C, et al. High prevalence of *Plasmodium malariae* and *Plasmodium ovale* in malaria patients along the Thai-Myanmar border, as revealed by acridine orange staining and PCR-based diagnoses. Trop Med Int Health 1998;3:304–312.

155. Faye FBK, Konaté L, Rogier C, et al. *Plasmodium ovale* in a highly malaria endemic area of Senegal. Trans R Soc Trop Med Hyg 1998;92:522–525.

156. Jambulingam P, Mohapatra SS, Das LK, et al. Detection of *Plasmodium ovale* in Koraput district, Orissa state. Indian J Med Res 1989;89:115–116.

157. Baird JK, Purnomo, Masbar S. *Plasmodium ovale* in Indonesia. Southeast Asian J Trop Med Public Health 1990;21:541–544.

158. Yu HL, Xu ZJ. A study of 33 cases of quartan malaria contracted after blood transfusion. Chin J Epidemiol 1982;3:294.

159. Vinetz JM, Li J, McCutchan TF, et al. *Plasmodium malariae* infection in an asymptomatic 74-year-old Greek woman with splenomegaly. N Engl J Med 1998;338:367–371.

160. White NJ. Why is it that antimalarial drug treatments do not always work? Ann Trop Med Parasitol 1998;92:449–458.

161. Guiguemde TR, Aouba A, Ouédraogo JB, et al. Ten-year surveillance of drug-resistant malaria in Burkina Faso (1982–1991). Am J Trop Med Hyg 1994;50:699–704.

162. Trape JF, Pison G, Preziosi MP, et al. Impact of chloroquine resistance on malaria mortality. C R Acad Sci Paris 1998;321:689–697.

163. Nwanyanwu OC, Ziba C, Kazembe P, et al. Efficacy of suphadoxine/pyrimethamine for *Plasmodium falciparum* malaria in Malawian children under five years of age. Trop Med Int Health 1996;1:231–235.

164. Ronn AM, Msangeni HA, Mhina J, et al. High level of resistance of *Plasmodium falciparum* to sulfadoxine-pyrimethamine in children in Tanzania. Trans R Soc Trop Med Hyg 1996;90:179–181.

165. Lobel HO, Varma JK, Miani M, et al. Monitoring for mefloquine-resistant *Plasmodium falciparum* in Africa: implications for travelers' health. Am J Trop Med Hyg 1998;59:129–132.

166. Mockenhaupt FP. Mefloquine resistance in *Plasmodium falciparum*. Parasitol Today 1995;11:248–253.

167. Cerutti C Jr, Durlacher RR, de Alencar FE, et al. In vivo efficacy of melfoquine for the treatment of falciparum malaria in Brazil. J Infect Dis 1999;180:2077–2080.

168. Noronha E, Alecrim MD, Romero GA, et al. RIII mefloquine resistance in children with falciparum malaria in Manaus, AM, Brazil. Rev Soc Bras Med Trop 2000;33:201–205.

169. Rieckmann KH, Davis DR, Hutton DC. *Plasmodium vivax* resistance to chloroquine? Lancet 1989;2:1183–1184.

170. Baird JK, Wiady I, Fryauff DJ, et al. In vivo resistance to chloroquine by *Plasmodium vivax* and *Plasmodium falciparum* at Nabire, Irian Jaya, Indonesia. Am J Trop Med Hyg 1997;56:627–631.

171. Fryauff DJ, Tuti S, Mardi A, et al. Chloroquine-resistant *Plasmodium vivax* in transmigration settlements of West Kalimantan, Indonesia. Am J Trop Med Hyg 1998;59:513–518.

172. Phillips EJ, Keystone JS, Kain KC. Failure of combined chloroquine and high-dose primaquine therapy for *Plasmodium vivax* malaria acquired in Guyana, South America. Clin Infect Dis 1996;23:1171–1173.

173. Signorini L, Matteelli A, Castelnuovo F, et al. Short report: primaquine-tolerant *Plasmodium vivax* in an Italian traveler from Guatemala. Am J Trop Med Hyg 1996;55:472–473.

174. Smoak BL, DeFraites RF, Magill AJ, et al. *Plasmodium vivax* infections in U.S. army troops: failure of primaquine to prevent relapse in studies from Somalia. Am J Trop Med Hyg 1997;56:231–234.

175. Peters W. Use of drug combinations. In: Peters W, Richards WHG. Antimalarial drugs II. Current antimalarials and new drug developments. Berlin: Springer-Verlag, 1984.

176. Fernex M, Mittelholzer ML, Reber R, et al. A drug combination to overcome and prevent development of drug resistance in malaria parasites. In: Boray JC, Martin PJ, Roush RT, editors. Round table conference: resistance of parasites to antiparasitic drugs. Paris: VIIth International Congress of Parasitology, 1990. p. 17–24.

177. Salako LA, Adio RA, Walker O, et al. Mefloquine-sulphadoxine-pyrimethamine (Fansimef®, Roche) in the prophylaxis of *Plasmodium falciparum* malaria: a double-blind, comparative, placebo-controlled study. Ann Trop Med Parasitol 1992;86:575–581.

178. Eamsila C, Singharaj P, Yooyen P, et al. Prevention of *Plasmodium falciparum* malaria by Fansimef® and Lariam® in the northeastern part of Thailand. Southeast Asian J Trop Med Public Health 1993;24:672–676.

179. White NJ. Combination treatment for falciparum prophylaxis. Lancet 1987; 21:680–681.

180. Watkins WM, Mosobo M. Treatment of *Plasmodium falciparum* malaria with pyrimethamine-sulfadoxine: selective pressure for resistance is a function of long elimination half-life. Trans R Soc Trop Med Hyg 1993;87:75–78.

181. Watkins W, Winstanley P. Chlorproguanil-dapsone (Lapdap) for uncomplicated falciparum malaria: theoretical basis and drug development. Liverpool: 2nd European Congress for Tropical Medicine; 1998. Abstract No.:376.

182. Nosten F, van Vugt M, Price R, et al. Effects of artesunate-mefloquine combination on incidence of *Plasmodium falciparum* malaria and mefloquine resistance in western Thailand: a prospective study. Lancet 2000:356:297–302.

183. Wongsrichanalai C, Thimasarn K, Sirichaisinthop J. Antimalarial drug combination policy: a caveat. Lancet 2000;355:2245–2247.

184. Hastings IM, D'Alessandro U. Modelling a predictable disaster: the rise and spread of drug-resistant malaria. Parasitol Today 2000;16:340–347.

185. Eisen DP, Saul A. Disappearance of pan-malarial antigen reactivity using the ICT malaria P.f./P.v™ kit parallels decline of patent parasitaemia as shown by microscopy. Trans R Soc Trop Med Hyg 2000;94:169–170.

186. Bottius E, Guanzirolli A, Trape JF, et al. Malaria: even more chronic in nature than previously thought: evidence for subpatent parasitaemia detectable by the polymerase chain reaction. Trans R Soc Trop Med Hyg 1996;90:15–19.

187. Wagner G, Kkoram K, McGuinness D, et al. High incidence of asymptomatic malaria infections in a birth cohort of children less than one year of age in Ghana, detected by multicopy gene polymerase chain reaction. Am J Trop Med Hyg 1998;59: 115–123.

188. May J, Mockenhaupt FP, Ademowo OG, et al. High rate of mixed and subpatent malarial infections in southwest Nigeria. Am J Trop Med Hyg 1999;61:339–343.

189. Snow RW, Omumbo JA, Lowe B, et al. Relation between severe malaria morbidity in children and level of *Plasmodium falciparum* transmission in Africa. Lancet 1997;349:1650–1654.

190. Anonymous. *Plasmodium falciparum*: a major health hazard to Africans and Asians returning home. Lancet 1985;ii:871–872.

191. El Hamad I, Matteelli A, Castelli F, et al. Malaria prevention in immigrants to malaria-free countries. Proceedings of the 6th Conference of the International Society of Travel Medicine; 1999 June 6–10; Montreal. Abstract No.: D05.

192. Bloland PB, Boriga DA, Ruebush TK, et al. Longitudinal cohort study of the epidemiology of malaria infections in an area of intense malaria transmission. II. Descriptive epidemiology of malaria infection and disease among children. Am J Trop Med Hyg 1999;60:641–648.

193. Genton B, Al-Yaman F, Beck HP, et al. The epidemiology of malaria in the Wosera area, East Sepik Province, Papua New Guinea, in preparation for vaccine trials. I. Malariometric indices and immunity. Ann Trop Med Parasitol 1995;89:359–376.

194. Zucker JR. Changing patterns of autochthonous malaria transmission in the United States: a review of recent outbreaks. Emerg Infect Dis 1996;2:37–43.

195. Singal M, Shaw PK, Lindsay RC, et al. An outbreak of introduced malaria in California possibly involving secondary transmission. Am J Trop Med Hyg 1977;26:1–9.

196. Centers for Disease Control. *Plasmodium vivax* malaria — San Diego county, California, 1986. MMWR Morb Mortal Wkly Rep 1986;35:679–681.

197. Centers for Disease Control. Mosquito-transmitted malaria — California and Florida, 1990. MMWR Morb Mortal Wkly Rep 1991;40:106–108.

198. Centers for Disease Control. Probable locally acquired mosquito-transmitted *Plasmodium vivax* infection — Georgia, 1996. MMWR Morb Mortal Wkly Rep 1997;46:264–267.

199. Centers for Disease Control. Mosquito-transmitted malaria — Michigan, 1995. MMWR Morb Mortal Wkly Rep 1996;45:398–400.

200. Brook JH, Genese CA, Bloland PB, et al. Brief report: malaria probably locally acquired in New Jersey. N Engl J Med 1994;331:22–23.

201. Centers for Disease Control. Probable locally acquired mosquito-transmitted *Plasmodium vivax* infection — Suffolk county, New York, 1999. MMWR Morb Mortal Wkly Rep 2000;49:495–498.

202. Centers for Disease Control. Local transmission of *Plasmodium vivax* malaria — Houston, Texas, 1994. MMWR Morb Mortal Wkly Rep 1995;44:295–301.

203. Cristau P, Alandry G, Melin R, et al. Paludisme à *Plasmodium vivax*. Rôle probable d'une contamination intra-hospitalière. Nouv Presse Méd 1978;7:3674.

204. Gentilini M, Danis M. Le paludisme autochtone. Méd Mal Infect 1981;11:356–362.

205. Baldari M, Tamburro A, Sabatinelli G, et al. Malaria in Maremma, Italy. Lancet 1998;351:1246–1247.

206. Sergiev VP, Baranova AM, Orlov VS, et al. Importation of malaria into the USSR from Afghanistan, 1981–89. Bull World Health Organ 1993;71:385–388.

207. Ollomo B, Karch S, Bureau P, et al. Lack of malaria parasite transmission between apes and humans in Gabon. Am J Trop Med Hyg 1997;56:440–445.

208. Deane LM. Simian malaria in Brazil. Mem Inst Oswaldo Cruz 1992;87 Suppl 3:1–20.

209. De Arruda M, Nardin EH, Nussenzweig RS, et al. Sero-epidemiological studies of malaria in Indian tribes and monkeys of the Amazon basin of Brazil. Am J Trop Med Hyg 1989;41:379–385.

210. De Arruda ME, Aragaki C, Gagliardi F, et al. A seroprevalence and descriptive epidemiological study of malaria among Indian tribes of the Amazon basin of Brazil. Ann Trop Med Parasitol 1996;90:135–143.

211. Desowitz RS. Who gave pinta to the Santa Maria? New York: W.W. Norton & Company, 1997.

212. Welch SG, McGregor IA, Williams K. The Duffy blood group and malaria prevalence in Gambian West Africans. Trans R Soc Trop Med Hyg 1977;27:664–670.

213. Fang XD, Kaslow DC, Adams JH, et al. Cloning of the *Plasmodium vivax* Duffy receptor. Mol Biochem Parasitol 1991;44:125–132.

214 Jarolim P, Palek J, Amato D, et al. Deletion in erythrocyte band 3 gene in malaria-resistant Southeast Asian ovalocytosis. Proc Natl Acad Sci U S A 1991;88:11022–11026.

215. Foo LC, Rekhraj V, Chiang GL, et al. Ovalocytosis protects against severe malaria parasitemia in the Malayan aborigines. Am J Trop Med Hyg 1992;47:271–275.

216. Genton B, Al-Yaman F, Mgone CS, et al. Ovalocytosis and cerebral malaria. Nature 1995;378:564–565.

217. Allen SJ, O'Donnell A, Alexander ND, et al. Prevention of cerebral malaria in children in Papua New Guinea by southeast Asian ovalocytosis band 3. Am J Trop Med Hyg 1999;60:1056–1060.
218. Le Hesran JY, Personne I, Personne P, et al. Longitudinal study of *Plasmodium falciparum* infection and immune responses in infants with or without the sickle cell trait. Int J Epidemiol 1999;28:793–798.
219. Stirnadel HA, Stockle M, Felger I, et al. Malaria infection and morbidity in infants in relation to genetic polymorphisms in Tanzania. Trop Med Int Health 1999;4:187–193.
220. Sokhna CS, Rogier C, Dieye A, et al. Host factors affecting the delay of reappearance of *Plasmodium falciparum* after radical treatment among a semi-immune population exposed to intense perennial transmission. Am J Trop Med Hyg 2000;62:266–270.
221. Ruwende C, Khoo SC, Snow RW, et al. Natural selection of hemi- and heterozygotes for G6PD deficiency in Africa by resistance to severe malaria. Nature 1995;376:246–249.
222. Kaneko A, Taleo G, Kalkoa M, et al. Malaria epidemiology, glucose 6-phosphate dehydrogenase deficiency and human settlement in the Vanuatu archipelago. Acta Trop 1998;70:285–302.
223. Verle P, Nhan DH, Tinh TT, et al. Glucose-6-phosphate dehydrogenase deficiency in northern Vietnam. Trop Med Int Health 2000;5:203–206.
224. Williams TN, Maitland K, Bennett S, et al. High incidence of malaria in α-thalassaemic children. Nature 1996;383:522–525.
225. Hill AVS, Allsopp EM, Kwiatkowski D, et al. Common West African HLA antigens are associated with protection from severe malaria. Nature 1991;352:595–600.
226. Beck HP, Felger I, Barker M, et al. Evience of HLA class II association with antibody response against the malaria vaccine SPF66 in a naturally exposed population. Am J Trop Med Hyg 1995;53:284–288.
227. Smith T, Felger I, Tanner M, et al. The epidemiology of multiple *Plasmodium falciparum* infections. 11. Premunition in *Plasmodium falciparum* infection: insight from the epidemiology of multiple infections. Trans R Soc Trop Med Hyg 1999;93 Suppl 1:S59–S64.
228. Mehlotra RK, Lorry K, Kastens W, et al. Random distribution of mixed species malaria infections in Papua New Guinea. Am J Trop Med Hyg 2000;62:225–231.
229. Mason DP, McKenzie FE, Bossert WH. The blood-stage dynamics of mixed *Plasmodium malariae-Plasmodium falciparum* infections. J Theor Biol 1999;198:549–566.
230. Redd SC, Bloland PB, Kazembe PN, et al. Usefulness of clinical case-definition in guiding therapy for African children with malaria or pneumonia. Lancet 1992;340:1140–1143.
231. O'Dempsey TJD, McArdle TF, Laurence BE, et al. Overlap in the clinical features of pneumonia and malaria in African children. Trans R Soc Trop Med Hyg 1993;87:662–665.
232. Rooth IB, Bjorkman A. Suppression of *Plasmodium falciparum* infections during concomitant measles or influenza but not during pertussis. Am J Trop Med Hyg 1992;47:675–681.
233. Wright PW, Wilbur GA, Ardill WD, et al. Initial clinical assessment of the comatose patient: cerebral malaria vs. meningitis. Pediatr Infect Dis J 1993;12:37–41.
234. Delley V, Bouvier P, Breslow N, et al. What does a single determination of malaria parasite density mean? A longitudinal survey in Mali. Trop Med Int Health 2000;5:404–412.

235. Roberts DR, Laughlin LL, Hsheih P, et al. DDT, global strategies, and a malaria control crisis in South America. Emerg Infect Dis 1997;3:295–302.

236. Stürchler D. How much malaria is there worldwide? Parasitol Today 1989;5:39–40.

237. Kroeger A, González M, Ordóñez-González J. Insecticide-treated materials for malaria control in Latin America: to use or not to use? Trans R Soc Trop Med Hyg 1999;93:565–570.

238. Lell B, Luckner D, Njavé M, et al. Randomised placebo-controlled study of atovaquone plus proguanil for malaria prophylaxis in children. Lancet 1998;351:709–713.

239. Beach RF, Ruebush TK, Sexton JD, et al. Effectiveness of permethrin-impregnated bed nets and curtains for malaria control in a holoendemic area of Western Kenya. Am J Trop Med Hyg 1993;49:290–300.

240. Shanks GD, Gordon DM, Klotz FW, et al. Efficacy and safety of atovaquone/proguanil as suppressive prophylaxis for *Plasmodium falciparum* malaria. Clin Infect Dis 1998;27:494–499.

241. Sukwa TY, Mulenga M, Chisdaka N, et al. A randomized, double-blind, placebo-controlled field trial to determine the efficacy and safety of Malarone™ (atovaquone/proguanil) for the prophylaxis of malaria in Zambia. Am J Trop Med Hyg 1999;60:521–525.

242. Urdaneta M, Prata A, Struchiner CJ, et al. Evaluation of SPf66 malaria vaccine efficacy in Brazil. Am J Trop Med Hyg 1998;58:378–385.

243. Roper MH, Carrion Torres RS, Cava Goicochea CG, et al. The epidemiology of malaria in an epidemic area of the Peruvian Amazon. Am J Trop Med Hyg 2000;62:247–256.

244. Fryauff DJ, Baird K, Purnomo, et al. Malaria in nonimmune population after extended chloroquine or primaquine prophylaxis. Am J Trop Med Hyg 1997;56:137–140.

245. Nosten F, Luxemburger C, Kyle DE, et al. Randomised double-blind placebo-controlled trial of SPf66 malaria vaccine in children in northwestern Thailand. Lancet 1996;348:701–707.

246. Eamsila C, Sasiprapha T, Sangkharomya S, et al. Randomized, double-blind, placebo controlled evaluation of monthly WR 238605 (tafenoquine) for prophylaxis of *Plasmodium falciparum* and *P. vivax* in Royal Thai Army soldiers [Abstract no. 845]. Am J Trop Med Hyg 1999;61 Suppl 3:502.

247. Carme B, Venturin C. Le paludisme dans les Amériques. Med Trop 1999;59:298–302.

248. Beaudoin RL. Life cycle I. The exoerythrocytic stages of malaria parasites in humans. In: López-Antuñano FJ, Schmunis G, editors. Diagnosis of malaria. Washington (DC): Pan American Health Organization, 1990.

249. Revel MP, Datry A, Raimond AS, et al. *Plasmodium falciparum* malaria after three years in a non-endemic area. Trans R Soc Trop Med Hyg 1988;82:832.

250. Krajden S, Panisko DM, Tobe B, et al. Prolonged infection with *Plasmodium falciparum* in a semi-immune patient. Trans R Soc Trop Med Hyg 1991;85:731–732.

251. Centers for Disease Control. Malaria surveillance—United States, 1995. MMWR Morb Mortal Wkly Rep 1999;48 Suppl 1:1–24.

252. Babiker HA, Abdel-Muhsin AMA, Ranford-Cartwright LC, et al. Characteristics of *Plasmodium falciparum* parasites that survive the lengthy dry season in eastern Sudan where malaria transmission is markedly seasonal. Am J Trop Med Hyg 1998;59:582–590.

253. Charmot G, Bricaire F, Bastin R. Paludisme à *Plasmodium ovale* en France. Nouv Presse Med 1979;8:35.

254. Garnham PCC. Hypnozoites and relapses in *Plasmodium vivax* and in vivax-like malaria. Trop Geogr Med 1988;40:187–195.

255. Ye YI, Xu ZG, Zhao X. Experimental observation on the incubation period and relapse pattern of *Plasmodium vivax* in Guangxi. Chin J Parasitol Parasitic Dis 1988;6:166–168.

256. Izri MA, Lortholary O, Guillevin L, et al. Accès palustre à *Plasmodium vivax* plus de cinq ans après un séjour à Meknès (Maroc). Bull Soc Pathol Exot 1994;87:189.

257. Kain KC, Keystone JS. Malaria in travelers. Epidemiology, disease, and prevention. Infect Dis Clin North Am 1998;12:267–284.

258. Newton NA, Schnepf GA, Wallace MR, et al. Malaria in US marines returning from Somalia. JAMA 1994;272:397–399.

259. World Health Organization. Severe falciparum malaria. Trans R Soc Trop Med Hyg 2000;94 Suppl 1:S1–S90.

260. Petersen E, Hogh B, Marbiah NT, et al. Clinical and parasitological studies on malaria in Liberian adults living under intense malaria transmission. Ann Trop Med Parasitol 1991;85:577–584.

261. Rougemont A, Breslow N, Brenner E, et al. Epidemiological basis for clinical diagnosis of childhood malaria in endemic zone in West Africa. Lancet 1991;338:1292–1295.

262. Rooth I, Björkman A. Fever episodes in a holoendemic malaria area of Tanzania: parasitological and clinical findings and diagnostic aspects related to malaria. Trans R Soc Trop Med Hyg 1992;86:479–482.

263. Armstrong Schellenberg JRM, Smith T, Alonso PL, et al. What is clinical malaria? Finding case definitions for field research in highly endemic areas. Parasitol Today 1994;10:439–442.

264. Genton B, Smith T, Baea K, et al. Malaria: how useful are clinical criteria for improving the diagnosis in a highly endemic area? Trans R Soc Trop Med Hyg 1994:88:537–541.

265. Gomes M, Espino FE, Abaquin J, et al. Symptomatic identification of malaria in the home and in the primary health care clinic. Bull World Health Organ 1994;72:383–390.

266. Smith T, Hurt N, Teuscher T, et al. Is fever a good sign for clinical malaria in surveys of endemic communities? Am J Trop Med Hyg 1995;52:306–310.

267. Rogier C, Commenges D, Trape JF. Evidence for an age-dependent pyrogenic threshold of *Plasmodium falciparum* parasitemia in highly endemic populations. Am J Trop Med Hyg 1996;54:613–619.

268. Bovier P, Rougemont A, Breslow N, et al. Seasonality and malaria in a West African village: does high parasite density predict fever incidence? Am J Epidemiol 1997;145:850–857.

269. Luxemburger C, Nosten F, Kyle DE, et al. Clinical features cannot predict a diagnosis of malaria or differentiate the infecting species in children living in an area of low transmission. Trans R Soc Trop Med Hyg 1998;92:45–49.

270. Olalaeye BO, Williams LA, D'Alessandro U, et al. Clinical predictors of malaria in Gambian children with fever or a history of fever. Trans R Soc Trop Med Hyg 1998;92:300–304.

271. Rogier C, Ly AB, Tall A, et al. *Plasmodium falciparum* clinical malaria in Dielmo, a holoendemic area in Senegal: no influence of acquired immunity on initial symptomatology and severity of malaria attacks. Am J Trop Med Hyg 1999;60:410–420.

272. Bojang KA, Obaro S, Morison LA, et al. A prospective evaluation of a clinical algo-rithm for the diagnosis of malaria in Gambian children. Trop Med Int Health 2000:5:231–236.

273. Cot M, Roisin A, Barro D, et al. Effect of chloroquine chemoprophylaxis during preg-nancy on birth weight: results of a randomized trial. Am J Trop Med Hyg 1992;46:21–27.

274. Nosten F, ter Kuile F, Maelankiri L, et al. Mefloquine prophylaxis prevents malaria during pregnancy: a double-blind, placebo-controlled study. J Infect Dis 1994;169:595–603.

275. White NJ, Krishna S. Treatment of malaria: some considerations and limitations of the current methods of assessment. Trans R Soc Trop Med Hyg 1989;83:767–777.

276. Hatz C, Abdulla S, Mull R, et al. Efficacy and safety of CGP 56697 (artemether and benflumetol) compared with chloroquine to treat acute falciparum malaria in Tan-zanian children aged 1–5 years. Trop Med Int Health 1998;3:498–504.

277. Boustos DG, Canfield CJ, Canete-Miguel E, et al. Atovaquone-proguanil compared with chloroquine and chloroquine-sulfadoxine-pyrimethamine for treatment of acute *Plasmodium falciparum* malaria in the Philippines. J Infect Dis 1999;179:1587–1590.

278. Looareesuwan S, Wilairatana P, Chalermarut K, et al. Efficacy and safety of ato-vaquone/proguanil compared with mefloquine for treatment of acute *Plasmodium falciparum* malaria in Thailand. Am J Trop Med Hyg 1999;60:526–532.

279. Van Vugt M, Wilairatana P, Gemperli B, et al. Efficacy of six doses of artemether-lume-fantrine (benflumethol) in multidrug-resistant *Plasmodium falciparum* malaria. Am J Trop Med Hyg 1999;60:936–492.

280a. Von Seidlein L, Milligan P, Pinder M, et al. Efficacy of artesunate plus pyrethamine-sulphadoxine for uncomplicated malaria in Gambian children: a double-blind, randomized, controlled trial. Lancet 2000;355:352–357.

280b. Najera JA, Hempel J. The burden of malaria. Geneva: World Health Organization, 1996; CTD/MAL/96.10:1–58.

281. Bojang KA, Obaro SK, D'Alessandro U, et al. An efficacy trial of the malaria vaccine SPf66 in Gambian infants—second year of follow-up. Vaccine 1998;16:62–67.

282. D'Alessandro U, Leach A, Drakeley C, et al. Efficacy trial of malaria vaccine SPf66 in Gambian infants. Lancet 1995;346:462–467.

283. Marbiah NT, Petersen E, David K, et al. A controlled trial of lambda- cyhalothrin-impregnated bed nets and/or dapsone/pyrimethamine for malaria control in Sier-ra Leone. Am J Trop Med Hyg 1998;58:1–6.

284. Lemnge MM, Msangeni HA, Ronn AM, et al. Maloprim® malaria prophylaxis in children living in a holoendemic vilage in north-eastern Tanzania. Trans R Soc Trop Med Hyg 1997;91:68–73.

285. Alonso PL, Smith T, Armstrong-Schellenberg JRM, et al. Randomised trial of efficacy of SPf66 vaccine against *Plasmodium falciparum* malaria in children in southern Tanzania. Lancet 1994;344:1175–1181.

286. Richards FO Jr, Klein RE, Flores RF, et al. Permethrin-impregnated bet nets for malar-ia control in northern Guatemala: epidemiologic impact and community accep-tance. Am J Trop Med Hyg 1993;49:410–418.

287. Kamol-Ratanakul P, Prasittisuk C. The effectiveness of permethrin-impregnated bed nets against malaria for migrant workers in eastern Thailand. Am J Trop Med Hyg 1992;47:305–309.

288. Brinkmann U, Brinkmann A. Malaria and health in Africa: the present situation and epidemiological trends. Trop Med Parasitol 1991;42:204–213.

289. Luxemburger C, Ricci F, Nosten F, et al. The epidemiology of severe malaria in an area of low transmission in Thailand. Trans R Soc Trop Med Hyg 1997;91:256–262.

290. Peters W. The global malaria problem and its military implications. Proceedings of the 27th International Congress of Military Medicine and Pharmacy; 1988; Interlaken, Switzerland. Abstract Vol. p. 1.

291. Pascal B, Baudon D, Keundjian A, et al. Epidémie de paludisme au cours d'une intervention militaro-humanitaire en Afrique. Med Trop 1997;57:253–255.

292. Steffen R, Behrens RH. Travellers' malaria. Parasitol Today 1992;8:61–66.

293. Steffen R, Fuchs E, Schildknecht J, et al. Mefloquine compared with other malaria chemoprophylactic regimens in tourists visiting East Africa. Lancet 1993;341:1299–1303.

294. World Health Organization. Management of severe malaria. A practical handbook. Geneva: World Health Organization, 2000.

295. Murray CJL, Lopez AD. The global burden of disease. Harvard School of Public Health, World Health Organization, and World Bank, 1996.

296. Molyneux ME, Taylor TE, Wirima JJ, et al. Clinical features and prognostic indicators in paediatric cerebral malaria: a study of 131 comatose Malawian children. QJM 1989;71:441–459.

297. Hien TT, Day NPJ, Phu NH, et al. A controlled trial of artemether or quinine in Vietnamese adults with severe falciparum malaria. N Engl J Med 1996;335:76–83.

298. Van Hensbroek MB, Onyiorah E, Jaffar S, et al. A trial of artemether or quinine in children with cerebral malaria. New Engl J Med 1996;335:69–75.

299. Zucker JR, Lackritz EM, Ruebush TK 2nd, et al. Childhood mortality during and after hospitalization in western Kenya: effect of malaria treatment regimens [published erratum appears in Am J Trop Med Hyg 1997;56:358]. Am J Trop Med Hyg 1996;55:655–660.

300. Alles HK, Mendis KN, Carter R. Malaria mortality rates in South Asia and in Africa: implications for malaria control. Parasitol Today 1998;14:369–375.

301. Van TH, Thanh CV, Kim AT. Severe malaria in a provincial hospital in Vietnam [letter]. Lancet 1990;2:1316.

302. Behrens RH, Curtis CF. Malaria in travellers: epidemiology and prevention. Br Med Bull 1993;49:363–381.

303. Sabatinelli G, D'Ancona F, Majori G, et al. Fatal malaria in Italian travelers. Trans R Soc Trop Med Hyg 1994;88:314.

304. Schöneberg I, Apitzsch L, Rasch G. Malaria-Erkrankungen und Sterbefälle in Deutschland 1993–1997. Gesundheitswesen 1998;60:755–761.

305. Snow RW, Craig M, Deichmann U, et al. Estimating mortality, morbidity and disability due to malaria among Africa's non-pregnant population. Bull World Health Organ 1999;77:624–640.

306. Arnold K, Tran TH, Nguyen TC, et al. A randomized comparative study of artemisinine (qinghaosu) suppositories and oral quinine in acute falciparum malaria. Trans R Soc Trop Med Hyg 1990;84:499–502.

307. Kidane G, Morrow RH. Teaching mothers to provide home treatment of malaria in Tigray, Ethiopia: a randomised trial. Lancet 2000;356:550–555.

308. Thomson MC, Connor SJ, Milligan PJM, et al. The ecology of malaria—as seen from Earth-observation satellites. Ann Trop Med Parasitol 1996;90:243–264.

309. Beck LR, Rodriquez MH, Dister SW, et al. Assessment of a remote sensing-based model for predicting malaria transmission risk in villages of Chiapas, Mexico. Am J Trop Med Hyg 1997;56:99–106.

310. Kleinschmidt I, Bagayoko M, Clarke GPY, et al. A spatial statistical approach to malaria mapping. Int J Epidemiol 2000;29:355–361.

311. Indaratna K, Hutubessy R, Chupraphawan S, et al. Application of geographical information systems to co-analysis of disease and economic resources: dengue and malaria in Thailand. Southeast Asian J Trop Med Public Health 1998;29:669–684.

312. Hu H, Singhasivanon P, Salazar NP, et al. Factors influencing malaria endemicity in Yunnan province, PR China (analysis of spatial pattern by GIS). Southeast Asian J Trop Med Public Health 1998;29:191–200.

SELECTED WEB SITES

http://www.who.int/ith/. World Health Organization (WHO) site for international travel, with information on malaria prevention.

http://www.who.int/rbm/. WHO roll-back-malaria effort.

http://www.who.int/tdr/. WHO research effort on tropical diseases (TDR), with numerous links.

http://www.who.int/wer. WHO global surveillance information (*Weekly Epidemiological Record*).

http://www.eurosurv.org. European surveillance information (*Eurosurveillance Weekly*).

http://www.dcd.gov/travel. Centers for Disease Control (CDC) site for international travel, with information on malaria prevention.

http://www.cdc.gov/epo/mmwr/mmwr.html. CDC surveillance information (*Morbidity and Mortality Weekly Report*).

Chapter 3

Geographic Distribution of Malaria at Traveler Destinations

Maia Funk-Baumann

ABSTRACT

This chapter outlines the risk of malaria in countries visited by travelers. There are various indices used to define the risk for travelers. Continental malaria risk and a list of malaria distribution of all countries presently harboring malaria follows, with data from the most reliable sources currently available. It was not possible to provide comparable risk data because the sources apply different methods to measure malaria risk. The data provided are reliable at the time of writing; however, there is potential for rapid change in a given geographic area. Risk estimation remains the result of consideration of the infectious agent and its resistance, vector and vector control, climate, sudden rainfalls, host economy, host profession, population genetics, and even wars and politics.

Key words: annual parasite index (API); circumsporozoite antibodies (CS); distribution; entomological inoculation rate (EIR); geography; incidence; infant conversion rate; malaria; prevalence; resistance; risk; Roll Back Malaria; spleen rate.

FACTORS INFLUENCING MALARIA DISTRIBUTION

Human malaria transmission and distribution are directly related to the interaction between the vector (anopheline mosquito), the parasite (*Plasmodium* species), and the human host; they are interdependent.[1] The presence of malaria requires appropriate climate and environment, host behavior, and genetics. Re-emergence is often linked to environmental and/or behavioral change[2] and low economic status.[3] Irrigation or dam projects change the environment; wars and unrest lead to retention of appropriate medical diagnosis and treatment.[4] Import of vectors might be an important fact in malaria distribution.[5] Recent studies based on predictive mathematic modeling of climate change have projected that the range of malaria transmission will expand to about 60% of the world's population in the near future.[6,7] Future malaria regions will largely be socioeconomically underdeveloped areas on the fringes of well-known infected areas.[8] Interaction with other diseases[9] and genetic disposition[10-12] may contribute to malaria susceptibility.[13,14]

Malaria has been recorded as far north as 64° N (Archangel, Russian Federation) and as far south as 32° S latitude (Córdoba, Argentina). Transmission occurs at altitudes of up to 2,800 m in equatorial regions, and global warming could raise the range of transmission to higher latitudes in the temperate regions and higher altitudes in the tropics.[15]

Factors influencing malaria distribution are interdependent.

The number of vectors are influenced by the following:

- Geography/climate/annual rainfall (continuous, permanent)[16-19]
- *Anopheles* species[20,21]
- Host density (population density)
- Socioeconomic status of the host population (housing conditions, water management, mosquito control)[22]
- Resistance to insecticides[23]

Susceptibility of the host is dependent on the following factors:

- Immunity grade (e.g., nonimmune, semi-immune), genetic factors[19,21,24-28]
- Health status[14,29]
- Pregnancy[30,31]
- Profession[32]
- Socioeconomic status (housing conditions, water management, mosquito control)[33-35]
- Infected-vector density[36-38]
- Infected-population density

Distribution of the parasite is dependent on the following:

- *Plasmodium* species and strain[19]
- Vector (*Anopheles* species)[5]
- Geography/climate/temperature[19]
- Resistance to antimalarials

CURRENT MALARIA DISTRIBUTION

More than 40% of the world's population lives in malaria-endemic regions. Malaria occurs now in almost half of the countries in the world, predominantly in poorer economic regions and in tropical climates. Annual global incidence is estimated to be 300 to 500 million cases. High malaria transmission occurs mostly in sub-Saharan Africa and parts of eastern Oceania. In 1999, it was estimated that 87% of malaria deaths occurred in areas with high transmission.[39] Areas of low to moderate transmission are found mostly in Asia and Latin America but also in parts of Africa such as the highlands and desert fringes.

Official reporting and case figures depend highly on government socioeconomic potential, the quality of medical facilities, and communication between facilities and government. Reporting systems require proper organization and financial resources. Many poor countries depend widely on nongovernmental health facilities with low budgets that often have a poor affiliation to reporting systems. Under-reporting in low economic countries is common and leads to unrealistic low incidence figures. Due to worldwide spread of parasites and intensification of their resistance to antimalarial drugs, malaria control has become increasingly necessary and costly. In the future, the new rapid malaria detection tests[40–42] will hopefully provide better and more rapid diagnosis in areas where malaria control has been insufficient.

DISTRIBUTION OF VARIOUS *PLASMODIUM* SPECIES

Plasmodium falciparum accounts for over 50% of malaria infections in most East Asian countries, over 90% in sub-Saharan Africa, and almost 100% in Hispaniola. *Plasmodium vivax* is rarely present in sub-Saharan West Africa, because many native Africans lack the Duffy blood group antigen that is necessary for parasite invasion of the erythrocytes. *P. vivax* and *P. falciparum* are present in Latin America, on the Indian subcontinent, in Southeast Asia, and in Oceania. *Plasmodium ovale* occurs mainly in Africa and Papua New Guinea. *Plasmodium malariae* is present in most areas but is rare (Table 3–1).

MALARIA RISK

Data regarding indices and rates of malaria risk appear in Table 3–2.[18,37,38,43–52] Endemic malaria is characterized by a constant incidence of cases over many (at least 3) successive years. Epidemic malaria is indicated by distinct and sharp rises of malaria cases in indigenous populations.

Characteristics of stable (endemic) malaria areas are as follows:

• Natural transmission: present for many years
• Incidence: constant and predictable
• Prevalence: stable
• Transmission: predictable and high
• Immunity: semi-immunity predominant
• Epidemics: none
• Are usually high-risk areas for nonimmune travelers

Table 3–1. **Distribution of Malaria Species**

Location	Presence of Plasmodium Species			
	P. falciparum	P. vivax	P. ovale	P. malariae
Africa				
North	–	(+)	–	–
Sub-Sahara	++	(+)	+	+
Asia				
India	+	++	(+)	(+)
Southeast Asia	++	+	(+)	(+)
Americas				
Central	+	++	(+)	(+)
Hispaniola	++	(+)	(+)	(+)
South of Costa Rica	+	++	(+)	+
Oceania				
Papua New Guinea	++	+	+	(+)
Vanuatu	++	+	+	(+)
Solomon Islands	++	+	+	(+)

++ = predominant; + = present; (+) = rarely present; – = absent.

Characteristics of unstable malaria areas are as follows:

• Natural transmission: varies from year to year
• Incidence: not constant
• Prevalence: not constant
• Transmission: medium to low
• Immunity: low or absent
• Epidemics: possible
• Are usually low-moderate-risk areas for nonimmune travelers

MAPS

For most Asian and South American countries, malaria control measures and reporting systems have led to reliable data on malaria distribution and resistance situations. In sub-Saharan Africa, these controls have never been established. However, since virtually nothing has changed the malaria situation of the sub-Saharan areas for many years, there are now possibilities for controlling and predicting data with the new technologies of malaria mapping.[39,46–51,53,54] Various satellites and geographic-based information systems give information (e.g., vegetation, temperature, climatic changes,[55] cloud densities, and population densities) for the development of malaria risk maps. There is hope to determine the most relevant data for predicting malaria transmission in Africa.

Table 3–2. **Indices, Rates, and Terms of Malaria Risk**

Index (Reference)	Diagnostic Method	Description
Malaria prevalence*	Clinical or microscopic	Number of infected people (e.g., per 1,000 persons) at a certain time
Malaria incidence*[43]	Clinical or microscopic	Number of new infections (e.g., per 1,000 persons)/ time (e.g., year) Incidence is equivalent to API if diagnosis is done microscopically
Annual parasite index (API)*	Microscopic	Number of new infections (e.g., per 1,000 persons)/ time (e.g., year) Good index for estimating malaria risk in indigenous people Not suitable for estimating risk in travelers, but may give indirect information on local malaria situation and risk
Spleen rate*	Clinical	Proportion of individuals in a certain age range (mostly 2–9) with enlarged spleen Good, but not highly evident, index for estimating malaria risk in indigenous people—these data give the figures for *endemicity grade* Not suitable for estimating risk in travelers, but may give indirect information on local malaria situation and risk
Infant conversion rate*	Microscopic	Fraction of parasite-negative infants becoming positive/time Good index for estimating malaria risk in indigenous people Not suitable for estimating risk in travelers, but may give indirect information on local malaria situation and risk
Circumsporozoite (CS) antibodies*[44,45]	—	ELISA testing of circulating antibodies to circumsporozoite antigen Testing of returned travelers gives good information on risk in the visited region Good index for estimating malaria risk in travelers
Entomological inoculation rate (EIR)[†37,38]	—	Daily number of infectious mosquito bites (sporozoite stage parasites) a person is exposed to in a certain time period, typically a year Good index for estimating malaria risk in indigenous people in a small area; suitable also for estimating travelers' risk Local variability may be high
Geographic information system (GIS)[‡ 18,46–52]	—	Computer programs that combine spatial and descriptive data for mapping and spatial analysis Good index for estimating malaria risk in indigenous people and travelers Local situations cannot be assessed Used to create MARA/ARMA maps (see "Maps")

ELISA = enzyme-linked immunosorbent assay; MARA/ARMA = mapping malaria risk in Africa/atlas du risque de la malarie en Afrique.
* Index related to malaria diagnosis in humans.
† Index related to exposure to malaria-carrying insects.
‡ Index related to geographic, climatic, and population-based data.

The Roll Back Malaria (RBM)[53,54] campaign has initiated various efforts for malaria control in Africa, and the MARA/ARMA (mapping malaria risk in Africa/atlas du risque de la malaria en Afrique)[51] organization has created maps with the available data (http://www.mrd.ac.za/mara). However, sudden climatic changes may result in epidemics that cannot be predicted, and wars, unforeseen migrations, and unrest can also falsify predictions.

The MARA/ARMA collaboration was initiated to provide an atlas of malaria for Africa through the use of a geographic information system (GIS), by integrating spatial malaria and environmental data sets, and producing maps of the distribution

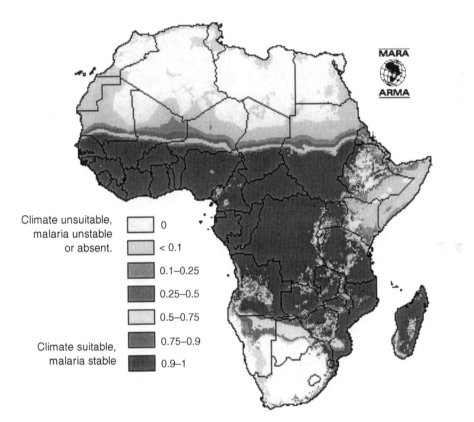

Figure 3–1. MARA/ARMA: malaria distribution in Africa. This map is a theoretic (although reasonably accurate) model based on available long-term climate data. It has a resolution of about 5 × 5 km. It shows the theoretic suitability of local climate and, therefore, the potential distribution of stable malaria transmission in the average year. Where climate is "suitable" (red = 1), malaria is likely *endemic* (hypo- , meso- , hyper- , or holoendemic). "Suitable" areas may have little or no malaria because of malaria control. Where climate is "unsuitable" (white = 0), malaria is likely *epidemic* or *absent.* Some "unsuitable" areas may actually have endemic malaria because of the presence of surface water in an area where there is little or no rain. In the marginally suitable areas (0.1–0.9), transmission may occur at steady but low levels (e.g., in eastern Africa) or in strongly seasonal cycles with great interannual variation (e.g., in western and southern Africa). For more detailed information, please see the MARA/ARMA technical report: http://www.mrc.ac.za/mara/trview_e.htm#Malaria%20Distribution%20Model. (Reproduced with permission from MARA/ARMA.)

(Figure 3–1), type, and severity of malaria. The initiative is noninstitutional and is run in the spirit of open collaboration with regional and international efforts.

MALARIA DISTRIBUTION IN VARIOUS CONTINENTS

Different reporting systems and case definitions and the lack of reporting consistency permit only limited comparison between different continents, countries, and areas.

Africa

Northern Africa has achieved malaria transmission control, and only a few cases, mostly imported, are occasionally seen in Morocco and Egypt. Seasonal malaria is present on the fringes of high-transmission areas.[56–59]

Sub-Saharan Africa experiences about 100 million cases each year, with 1 million deaths. In many rural parts of Africa, as many as 90% of deaths from malaria occur at home and are not registered in any formal way.[60] Modeled transmission maps[51] (available at http://www.mrd.ac.za/mara) for Africa have been created based on population and climate models (Figure 3–2, *A* to *C*).[48,61] These maps are applicable only to countries with stable conditions and that lack effective malaria control measures.

Most of the densely populated regions of Kenya are considered holoendemic areas with malaria existing up to altitude levels of 2,500 m. The map in Figure 3–2*A* does not show the facts of migration, climatic changes, local situations, drought areas, areas prone to heavy rainfalls, or refugee situations in the north along the Somalian border. Risk estimation for travelers has to be achieved by combining malaria maps, climate situations, news, politics, and malaria data from returned travelers. The maps for Tanzania and Ghana (see Figure 3–2, *B* and *C*) show only holoendemic high-risk areas.

The Americas

In 1992, countries in the Americas adopted the Global Malaria Control Strategy for early detection, treatment, and prevention.[62–64] In the following years, case detection rates among the population living in areas favorable for malaria transmission improved markedly.

The Americas categorize their malarious areas into low-, moderate-, and high-risk areas, according to level of exposure to malaria transmission (Table 3–3). Most countries report only laboratory-confirmed cases (annual parasite index [API]), which leads to under-reporting.

Malaria is present in 21 countries or areas of Latin America, whereas countries of the Caribbean and North America are malaria free. In 1999, the total population living in countries with malaria transmission was 472 million, and of these, 44.1% (208 million) lived in areas with actual transmission. One hundred thirty-one mil-

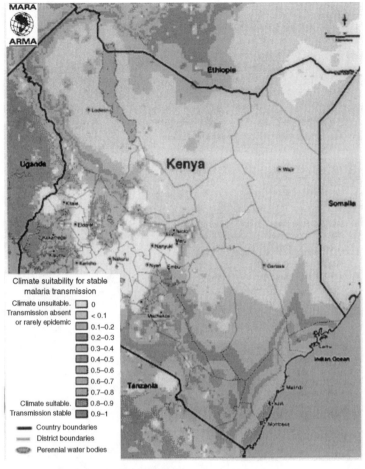

A

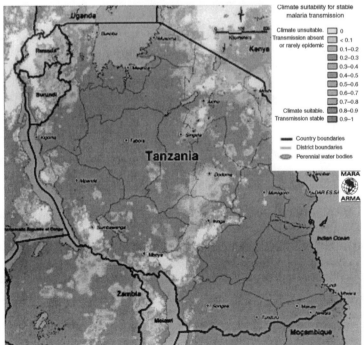

B

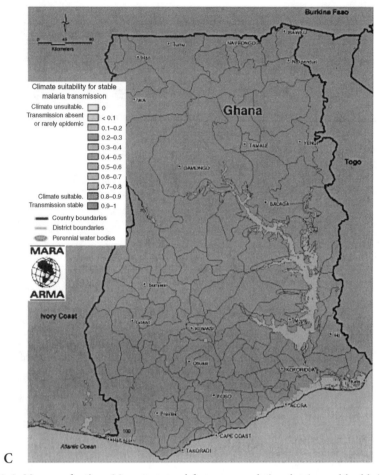

C

Figure 3–2. **Maps production:** Maps on natural features, population density, and health infrastruc-
tures prepared by the WHO/UNICEF Joint Program on Mapping for Public Health (Health Map). Maps
on malaria distribution in Africa produced by MARA/ARMA. Maps on malaria distribution elsewhere
produced by Health Map, based on International Travel and Health, WHO, 1998.
Sources Roads, rivers, lakes, national administrative boundaries, first-level subnational administrative
boundaries, and urbanized areas provided by African Data Sampler, World Resources Institute; digital
elevation by M.F. Hutchinson et al., Center for Resource and Environmental Studies, Australian
National University.
For more information on African Data Sampler, World Resource Institute, Washington, D.C.:
http://www.igc.org/wri/sdis/maps/ads/ads_idx.html.
For more information on the NCGIA, contact National Center for Geographic Information and
Analysis, State University of New York, U.S.A.
(Reproduced with the permission of MARA/ARMA. Copyright MARA/ARMA.)

lion people, more than half of the malaria-risk population, are located in areas with
low or very low risk. Of the population in the malaria-risk countries, 16.3% were
living in moderate- to high-risk areas, with APIs from 0.18 per 1,000 in El Salvador
to 1,000 per 1,000 in parts of Suriname and Guyana.[65]

Of all countries in the Americas, Brazil and the sub-Andean regions reported
the most malaria cases (50.5% and 32.3%, respectively); however, the highest APIs
were found in the northern South American states of French Guyana (API:

Table 3–3. **Risk Criteria in the Americas**

Country	Low Risk	Moderate Risk	High Risk
Brazil	API > 1, < 10	API > 10, < 50	API > 50, < 1,000
Other countries	≤ 1	≥ 1 ≤, 10	API ≥ 10

API = annual parasite index (new infections/1,000 persons/year).
Data from Pan American Health Oragnization/World Health Organiztion. Status of malaria programs in the Americas report (based on 1999 data). Washington: PAHO/WHO 2000.

331.69/1,000), Suriname (API: 309.76/1,000), and Guyana (API: 206.31/1,000), followed by Brazil's rain-forest (API: 118.8/1,000) and northern parts of Peru (API: 112.6/1,000). These regions must be considered high-risk areas for travelers to South America.

At greatest risk are those with malaria who do not have easy access to prompt diagnosis and treatment, that is, indigenous people and those who work in subsistence agriculture, mining, and logging. These population groups have increased lately. Bolivia, Brazil, Colombia, El Salvador, Guatemala, Honduras, Nicaragua, Panama, Peru, and Venezuela all have experienced significant advances in malaria control; however, reductions in health care budgets will make further improvements unlikely.

Asia and Oceania

Most countries in Asia and Oceania report only laboratory-confirmed cases, which leads to heavy under-reporting. China and Papua New Guinea also report clinical cases. The highest-risk areas are Papua New Guinea (Sepik River region) and some eastern parts of Indonesia. High-risk areas are also some border areas of Thailand, Cambodia, and Myanmar, as a result of population unrest, mining, logging, and civil wars. Multidrug resistance is well known, especially in Thailand and bordering countries. India has increasing malaria infection rates, and resistance is growing.

IMPACT OF MALARIA DISTRIBUTION ON TRAVELERS' MALARIA

Estimation of future travelers' malaria risk is derived from epidemiologic data of the countries to be visited and data originating from returned tourists with malaria (see Table 3–2).[66] In holoendemic areas, travelers' risk is usually high. Estimating the risk in nonholoendemic regions is difficult. Any one index may not give reliable information in areas prone to epidemics. Circumsporozoite index performed in returned travelers has been a reliable index so far.[44,45]

Malaria risk of the tourist traveling in malarious areas must be estimated by combining the given risks due to geography, personal behavior,[67–69] travel route, season, activities, travel style,[44] and compliance with antimalarial recommendations. The most important factor, however, remains the destination.[44] Geographic distribution of malaria transmission in local populations corresponds to the malaria risk of the traveler in the area. A traveler's susceptibility to the disease is that of a comparable nonimmune indigenous person.

Malaria risk for native people depends on malaria prevalence in their home area, their behavior, and their socioeconomic status.[70] Climate changes[6,7,71] and unknown factors may contribute to the appearance or re-appearance of malaria.[72] Areas with high mobility of people, such as areas with refugees,[73–75] areas of war,[76,77] and mining localities,[78–80] are more susceptible to malaria than other regions.

MALARIA DISTRIBUTION BY COUNTRY

Generally, if local climate is suitable, such as in tropical regions, malaria may exist at altitudes of up to 2,800 m. Limits are indicated in Table 3–4.[4,15,22,26,32,45,52,65,78,79,81–211]

Table 3–4. **Malaria Distribution and Risk by Country**

Country/Region	Distribution and Risk

Afghanistan	Malaria type: P.f.: ca.10% (in the S and Badakhshan); P.v.: 80–90%
	Malaria distribution and incidence: regional and seasonal: May–November (I = 12.18/1,000)
	Malaria risk and risk areas:
	  Low to moderate: all areas < 2,000 m
	  No malaria: mountains
	Resistance: P.f. resistant to chloroquine, sulfadoxine/pyrimethamine reported
	Remarks: many displaced people and refugee camps in war areas with possibly higher local incidence
	Literature: 81–84

Algeria	Malaria type: P.v.: 99%
	Malaria distribution: local. Most cases imported. 1997: 197 cases reported
	Malaria risk and risk areas:
	  Very low risk in remote areas in the SE: Ihrir, Dept. Ilizi, N of the Haggar mountains
	  No malaria: rest of the country
	Resistance: none reported
	Remarks: possibly most cases imported
	Literature: 82, 85

Angola	Malaria type: P.f.: 90%
	Malaria distribution and incidence: widespread (1995: I = 14/1,000)
	Malaria risk and risk areas:
	  High: ER: 0.9–1: most of the country. ER: 0.1–0.9: coastal dry regions up to Ambriz
	  Low: ER: < 0.1: Planalto mountains
	Resistance: P.f. resistant to chloroquine and sulfadoxine/pyrimethamine reported
	Remarks: coastal areas with epidemics
	Literature: 81, 82, 84, 86, 87

Argentina	Malaria type: 1999: P.v.: 100%
	Malaria distribution: local–regional. 1999: 174 cases reported
	Malaria risk and risk areas:
	  Low risk in the N: Salta and Jujuy provinces
	  Malaria free: rest of the country
	Resistance: none reported
	Remarks: mostly imported cases in Misiones. Heavy internal and international migration
	Literature: 15, 65, 81, 82, 88

Table continues until page 83

Country/Region	Distribution and Risk
Armenia	Malaria type: P.v. Malaria distribution and incidence: local. 1997: 567 indigenous cases (67% of cases reported) Malaria risk and risk areas: Masis district in the Ararat Valley (S of Yerevan) Remarks: no risk in common tourist areas Resistance: none reported Literature: 89, 90

Azerbaijan	Malaria type: P.v.: 100%
	Malaria distribution and incidence: regional (I = 1.3/1,000) and seasonal: June to September
	Malaria risk and risk areas:
	  Very low: rural lowland areas in the regions between Kura and Arax Rivers
	  Most affected regions: districts of Nakhichivan (10.4%), Imishli (14.6%), Fizuli (8.1%), Sabirabad (6.8%), Saatly (6%), Bejlagan (5.6%), and Bilasuvar (4.8%)
	  No malaria: rest of the country
	Resistance: reported to Delagil and Primaxin
	Literature: 81, 82, 91

Bangladesh	Malaria type: P.f.: 44%
	Malaria distribution and incidence: widespread. Regional and seasonal peaks (I = 0.6/1,000)
	Malaria risk and risk areas:
	  Moderate: regions bordering India (NE) and Myanmar (SE)
	  Low: rest of the country
	  No malaria: city of Dhaka
	Resistance: P.f. highly resistant to chloroquine (in the SE) and sulfadoxine/pyrimethamine reported
	Literature: 81, 82, 92

Belize	Malaria type: P.v.: 91%; P.f.: 9%
	Malaria distribution and incidence: widespread
	Malaria risk and risk areas:
	  Moderate–high: (API 11.18). Orange Walk and Corozal districts (50% of reported cases)
	  Lower risk in the rest of the country
	  Malaria free: Belize City
	Resistance: none reported
	Remarks: Cayo, Toledo, and Stann Creek states report the highest number of *P. falciparum* cases
	Literature: 65, 81, 82, 88

Benin	Malaria type: P.f.: 87% Malaria distribution and incidence: widespread (I = 115.9/1,000) Malaria risk and risk areas: High: ER = 0.9–1: whole country Resistance: P.f. resistant to chloroquine and sulfadoxine/pyrimethamine reported Remarks: risk also present in major cities Literature: 81, 82, 93–95

Bhutan	Malaria type: P.f.: 41%
	Malaria distribution and incidence: regional (I = 12.3/1,000)
	Malaria risk and risk areas:
	  Low: lowland districts in the S: Chirang, Gaylegphug, Samchi, Samdrupjongkhar, Shemgang
	  No malaria: Thimphu and high mountains
	Resistance: P.f. resistant to chloroquine and sulfadoxine/pyrimethamine reported
	Literature: 81, 82, 96

Bolivia	Malaria type: 1999: P.f.:15.1%; P.v.
	Malaria distribution and incidence: regional
	Malaria risk and risk areas:
	  High: Beni (Riberalta, API 239.05; Guayaramerin, API 147.04; Magdalena API: 59.56), lowland areas of Pando (API 81.02), Potosi (API 18.59), Tarjia, La Paz
	  Low: Cochabamba (E, NE), Sta. Cruz, (S, E), Chuquisaca (E)
	  No malaria: high mountains > 2,800 m
	Remarks: high risk predominantly in lowland areas. P.f. high in the departments of

Table continued

Country/Region	Distribution and Risk
	Riberalta, Pando, Guayaramerin; lower in Magdalena and la Paz Resistance: P.f. resistant to chloroquine and sulfadoxine/pyrimethamine reported mainly in Beni (Riberalta and Guayaramerin) Literature: 15, 65, 81, 82, 88

Botswana	Malaria type: P.f.: 95%
	Malaria distribution and incidence: regional and partly seasonal
	  (I =11.50/1,000)
	Malaria risk and risk areas:
	  High: ER = 0.9–1: international border areas: Kasane region, Ngamiland: N, NE,
	    Chobe. All year. ER = 0.8–0.9: Central Province (N, NW). Ngamiland (S):
	    November–June
	  Moderate: ER = 0.5–0.8: Central Province (N and E) Ngamiland (S): July–October
	  Low: ER <0.5: rest of the N half of the country
	  No malaria: ER = 0: S half of the country
	Resistance: P.f. resistant to chloroquine reported
	Remarks: seasonal transmission is dependent on rainfall, and season shift may be
	  possible
	Literature: 81, 82

Brazil	Malaria type: 1999: P.f.:18.8%; P.v.; P.m.
	Malaria distribution and incidence: regional. Very high risk (API ≥ 50) in 8 states.
	  High risk (API ≥10 ≤ 50) in 9 states
	Malaria risk and risk areas:
	  High: in areas with mining areas, rain forests with remote farms, intense internal
	    migration in parts of Rondonia (API 303.34), Amazonas (API 159.53), Roraima
	    (API 146.63), Acre (API 141.46), Parà (E, W) (API 135.55), Amapà (API 97.8),
	    Marañhao (API 95.42), Mato Grosso (API 62.82). Lower transmission intensity in
	    urban areas of Porto Velho, Boa Vista, Macapá, Manaus, Santarém, Maraba
	  Moderate in periurban areas or in heavy circulatory/migratory movement of people
	    to and from cities in parts of Amapà (API 44.8), Rondonia (API 40.4), Roraima
	    (API 20.99), Para (API 28.86), Marañhao (API 23.44), Tocantins (API 22.99),
	    Amazonas (API 21.02), Mato Grosso (API 18.4), Acre (API 17.47)
	  Low: rest of aforementioned regions and areas not predisposed to malaria
	    transmission
	  Malaria free: Belem, Manaus City, and rest of the country, especially E and NE coast,
	    Iguassu Falls
	Resistance: P.f. resistant to chloroquine and sulfadoxine/pyrimethamine common
	Remarks: most cases are reported in Amazonia, but with high variations in different
	  municipalities. Low overall incidence because only 12% of the population lives in
	  areas at risk for malaria. Many (95) Amazon municipalities have an API of 50/1,000,
	  which puts them at a high risk for malaria
	Literature: 65, 81, 82, 88, 97

Burkina Faso	Malaria type: P.f.: >85%
	Malaria distribution and incidence: widespread (1995: I=48/1,000)
	Malaria risk and risk areas:
	  High: ER = 0.9–1: whole country except extreme N
	  Moderate: ER = 0.5–0.9: extreme N
	Resistance: P.f. resistant to chloroquine reported
	Literature: 81, 82

Burundi	Malaria type: P.f.: >85%
	Malaria distribution and incidence: widespread (1995: I= 145/1,000)
	Malaria risk and risk areas:
	  High: ER = 0.9–1: W, SW, E, NE, Lake Tanganyika, and Lake Bangweulu
	  Moderate: ER = 0.5–0.9: E half of the country
	  Low: ER = < 0.1–0.5: high mountains
	Resistance: P.f. resistant to chloroquine, sulfadoxine/pyrimethamine, and cycloguanil
	  reported
	Remarks: low-risk areas might have higher risks due to heavy rainfalls, migration,
	  displaced people
	Literature: 81, 82, 98

Cambodia	Malaria type: P.f.: 90% Malaria distribution and incidence: widespread, with substantial regional differences (I=7.5/1,000)

Table continued

Country/Region	Distribution and Risk

	Malaria risk and risk areas:

Malaria risk and risk areas:
  High: international border areas of Koh Kong, Pursat, Prea Vihear, Stung Treng, Ratanakiri, Mondulkri
  Moderate: international border areas of Siem Reap, Kratie, Sihanouk Ville, Krong Kaep, Takeo
  Low: rest of the country, also tourist areas of Angkor Wat
  No malaria: city of Phnom Penh
Resistance: P.f. resistant to chloroquine, sulfadoxine/pyrimethamine, mefloquine, and quinine reported. High level of multidrug resistance in the western gem mining areas facing the international border with Thailand (Thailand province Trat and Ubon Ratchathani)
Remarks: multidrug resistance due to high migration rate in border areas, displaced people, refugee camps, and uncontrolled mining
Literature: 78, 82, 99–101

Cameroon
Malaria type: P.f.: > 85%
Malaria distribution and incidence: widespread (I = 46/1,000)
Malaria risk and risk areas:
  High: ER = 0.9–1: most of the country
  No malaria: Massif de l'Adamaoua in the W (high altitudes)
Resistance: P.f. multidrug resistance reported
Literature: 81, 82, 102–104

Cape Verde
Malaria type: no data
Malaria distribution and incidence: local–regional, seasonal. 1997: 20 cases reported
Malaria risk and risk areas:
  Very low risk in Sao Tiago Island, September–November
  No malaria: rest of the islands
Resistance: none reported
Remark: mostly imported cases
Literature: 81, 82, 105

Central African Republic
Malaria type: P.f.: >85%
Malaria distribution and incidence: widespread (1994: I = 24/1,000)
Malaria risk and risk areas: high: ER = 0.9–1: whole country
Resistance: P.f. resistant to chloroquine and sulfadoxine/pyrimethamine reported
Literature: 81, 82, 106

Chad
Malaria type: P.f.: >85%
Malaria distribution and incidence: widespread
Malaria risk and risk areas:
  High: most of the country (no ER data available)
  No malaria: extreme N (desert)
Resistance: P.f. resistant to chloroquine reported
Remarks: minimal data. High migration rates (nomadic lifestyles) might lead to some risk in generally malaria-free regions
Literature: 81, 82

China People's Republic
Malaria type: P.f.: S: >50%; P.v.: N: 100%; P.v.: central: >50%
Malaria distribution and incidence: patchy distribution, mostly in the S. Partly seasonal. 1997: 26,816 cases reported
Malaria risk and risk areas:
  Moderate: rural areas of Fujian, Guandong (incl. Hainan peninsula), Guangxi, Guizhou, Hunan, Jiangxi, Zheijiang, Yunnan, SE Tibet (border areas to India and Myanmar), throughout the year
  Low: north: rural areas S of Hebei, S of Liaoning, Shandong, Xinjjiang (Illi Valley bordering GUS), July–November
  Central: rural areas of Anhui, Henan, Hubei, Shaanxi (S); Shanghai Shi, Sichuan (E); May–December
  No malaria: most of the country, big cities
Resistance: P.f. resistant to chloroquine and sulfadoxine/pyrimethamine reported in Yunnan and Hainan
Remarks: no malaria in urban or densely populated plain areas; Hong Kong SAR: no malaria risk in urban and most rural areas; Macau SAR: no malaria risk
Literature: 78, 81, 82, 107

Table continued

Country/Region	Distribution and Risk

Colombia	Malaria type: 1999: P.f.: 37.98%; P.v. P.m.; La Guajira: P.f.: 80%
	Malaria distribution and incidence: widespread but patchy distribution
	Malaria risk and risk areas:
	  High: in areas with mining, migration, displacement, illegal crops in parts of
	    Amazonas lowlands (API 71.24), Guaviare (API 64.29), Bolivar (API 44.95),
	    Narina (API 44.86), Caqueta (API 24.36), Meta (S) (API 22.99), Choco (API
	    22.98), Valle (API 22.84), Antioquia (API 22.15), Putumayo (API 21.61), Vichada
	    (21.44), Cauca (API 15.72), Cordoba (API 15.12)
	  Low–moderate: lowlands and rural areas of Putumayo, Guaviare; Antioquia (N
	    half), Cordoba (S), Arauca (W), Magdalena (NE), La Guajira (SE), Vichada (W,
	    E), Guainia (valleys), Amazonas. Coastal areas in the provinces of Narino, Cauca,
	    Valle del Cauca (incl. Buenaventura), Atlantico (incl. Baraquilla)
	  No malaria: big cities, high mountains
	Resistance: P.f. resistant to chloroquine in Amazonia, Pacifico, and Uraba-Bajo Cauca
	  reported. Local multidrug resistance
	Literature: 15, 65, 81, 82, 88, 108

Comoros Islands	Malaria type: P.f.: 95% Malaria distribution and incidence: widespread (1996: I = 24/1,000) Malaria risk and risk areas: High: whole country Resistance: P.f. resistant to chloroquine reported Literature: 82, 109, 110
Congo Republic (Brazzaville)	Malaria type: P.f.: >90% Malaria distribution and incidence: widespread (I = 2/1,000) Malaria risk and risk areas: High: whole country (no ER data available) Resistance: P.f. resistant to chloroquine reported, multidrug resistance assumed Remarks: continuous war area, heavy under-reporting, and resistance to other antimalarials assumed Literature: 82, 109, 111, 112

Congo
Democratic
Republic,
formerly Zaïre
(Kinshasa)
	Malaria type: P.f.: >90%
	Malaria distribution and incidence: widespread
	Malaria risk and risk areas:
	  High: ER = 0.9–1: most of the country
	  Low–negligable: NE (mountains)
	Resistance: P.f. resistant to chloroquine and sulfadoxine/pyrimethamine reported
	Remarks: continuous war area, heavy under-reporting, and resistance to other
	  antimalarials assumed
	Literature: 82, 109

Costa Rica	Malaria type: P.v.: >99%
	Malaria distribution and incidence: regional
	Malaria risk and risk areas:
	  Moderate–high: border areas with heavy illegal migratory movements and/or high-
	    precipitation areas in parts of Canton los Chiles (Alajuela Province) (API 20.39),
	    Canton Matina (API 16.91), and Talamanca (Limón Province)
	  Low: in rural areas of Huetar Atlantica; Alejuela (N), Limon (central and S).
	  Very low risk: Atlantic coast and, to an even lesser extent, Pacific coast (Heredia,
	    Guanacaste)
	  No malaria: San José and central highlands
	Resistance: none reported
	Remarks: P.f.: mostly imported cases. Heavy illegal migration in border areas
	Literature: 15, 65, 82, 88, 109

Côte d'Ivoire	Malaria type: P.f.: 88% Malaria distribution and incidence: widespread (I=69/1,000) Malaria risk and risk areas: High: ER = 0.9–1: whole country Resistance: P.f. resistant to chloroquine and sulfadoxine/pyrimethamine reported Literature: 82, 109, 113
Djibouti	Malaria type: P.f.: 98% Malaria distribution and incidence: widespread (I=11/1,000) Malaria risk and risk areas: Moderate–high: most of the country (no ER data available) Resistance: P.f. resistant to chloroquine reported Literature: 82, 109, 114

Table continued

Country/Region	Distribution and Risk

Dominican Republic	Malaria type: P.f.: >99%
	Malaria distribution and incidence: widespread, patchy distribution. 1999: 678 cases reported
	Malaria risk and risk areas:
	  Moderate–high: in international migration areas or rice cultivation regions in Pepillo Salcedo (API 25.04), Castanuelas (API 21.28), Las Matas de Santa Cruz (API 12.34), Monte Cristi (API 11.98)
	  Low: eastern tourist areas
	  No malaria: big cities
	Resistance: none reported
	Remarks: higher risk in border communities and rice cultivation and large construction areas. Higher prevalence is closely related to fluctuations in the construction industry and migration
	Literature: 65, 82, 88, 109, 115–118

East Timor	Malaria type: P.f.: > 50% Malaria risk and risk areas: High: whole country Resistance: P.f. resistant to chloroquine and sulfadoxine/pyrimethamine reported Literature: 82

Ecuador	Malaria type: 1999: P.f.: 57.2%, up to 92%; coastal areas: P.f.: 16%; P.v.
	Malaria distribution and incidence: regional in lowlands
	Malaria risk and risk areas:
	  Moderate–high: due to climatic changes and heavy migration in parts of Loja (API 78.3), Cotopaxi (NW) (API 34.17), Manabi (coast and SW) (API 37.23), Bolivar (API 33.81), Esmeraldas (API 30.45), Sucumbios (API 29.12), Orellana (API 23.56), El Oro (API 20.64), Pichincha (API 13.81), Guayas (API 19.7), Los Rios
	  Low: Morona Santiago (except S)
	  No malaria: Zamora-Chinchipe, Canar, Azuay, Chimborazo, Quito (N, W), Imbabura, Carchi, Morona Santiago (S), Guayaquil
	Remarks: high migration rate
	Resistance: P.f. resistant to chloroquine reported in the Esmeralda province
	Literature: 15, 65, 82, 88, 109, 119

Egypt	Malaria type: P.v.: >99%
	Malaria distribution and incidence: local and seasonal. 1997: 11 cases reported. No cases reported since 1998
	Malaria risk and risk areas:
	  Low: very low risk in the rural El Faiyum governorate, June–October
	  No malaria: rest of the country
	Resistance: none reported
	Literature: 82, 109

El Salvador	Malaria type: P.v.: 99%; P.f.: < 1%
	Malaria distribution and incidence: widespread, patchy. 1999: 4,754 cases reported
	Malaria risk and risk areas:
	  Low: API 1999 = 0.18. Santa Ana province and N. Rural areas scattered throughout the country
	  No malaria: Pacific coast
	Resistance: none reported
	Literature: 65, 82, 88, 109

Equatorial Guinea	Malaria type: P.f.: >85% Malaria distribution and incidence: (1995: I=30/1,000) Malaria risk and risk areas: High: whole country (no ER data available) Resistance: P.f. resistant to chloroquine and sulfadoxine/pyrimethamine reported Literature: 82, 109

Eritrea	Malaria type: P.f.: >85%
	Malaria distribution and incidence: regional in lowlands (1995: I = 22/1,000)
	Malaria risk and risk areas:
	  High: ER = 0.9–1: NW
	  Moderate: ER = 0.6–0.9: central regions
	  Low–moderate: rest of the country
	  No malaria: Asmara, high altitudes >2,200 m
	Resistance: P.f. resistant to chloroquine and sulfadoxine/pyrimethamine reported

Table continued

Country/Region	Distribution and Risk
	Remarks: high migration rate, refugee camps, and many displaced people. Heavy under-reporting and higher incidence assumed. Nonstable transmission areas are prone to epidemics, especially in war regions Literature: 82, 109, 120

Ethiopia	Malaria type: P.f.: >80%; P.v.: >10%
	Malaria distribution and incidence: regional (I = 6/1,000)
	Malaria risk and risk areas:
	  High: whole country (lowlands). ER = 0.9–1: western parts and eastern lowlands
	  Low–moderate: ER = 0.1–0.9 rest of the non-high-altitude areas
	  No malaria: Addis Ababa, high mountains >2,000 m
	Resistance: P.f. highly resistant to chloroquine reported
	Remarks: high migration rate, refugee camps, and displaced people. Heavy under-reporting and higher incidence assumed
	Literature: 15, 22, 26, 82, 109, 120, 121

French Guiana	Malaria type: 1999: P.f.: 85.3%; P.v.; P.m.
	Malaria distribution and incidence: widespread in all 5 regions (API 28.53)
	Malaria risk and risk areas: all regions
	  High: Moroni (API 297.7) and Oyapock (API 110.7) river valleys (gold mining areas)
	  Low–moderate: Arriere pays (API 9.13), Littoral (API 5.76), Cayenne (API 4.23)
	  No malaria: big cities
	Resistance: P.f. resistant to chloroquine, quinine, halofantrine reported
	Literature: 65, 82, 88, 109, 122

Gabon	Malaria type: P.f.: 95% Malaria distribution and incidence: widespread (I = 31/1,000) Malaria risk and risk areas: High: whole country (no ER data available) Resistance: P.f. resistant to chloroquine and sulfadoxine/pyrimethamine reported Literature: 82, 109, 123
Gambia	Malaria type: P.f.: >85% Malaria distribution and incidence: widespread (I = 276/1,000) Malaria risk and risk areas: High: whole country (no ER data available) Resistance: P.f. resistant to chloroquine, sulfadoxine/pyrimethamine, and cycloguanil reported Literature: 82, 109, 124, 125

Georgia	Malaria type: P.v.: 100%
	Malaria distribution and incidence: focal and seasonal, June–October
	Malaria risk and risk areas:
	  Low: very low risk in the SE, at international border areas with Afghanistan
	  No malaria: rest of the country
	Resistance: none reported
	Remarks: in war areas: many displaced people and possibly higher risk
	Literature: 82, 109, 126

Ghana	Malaria type: P.f.: >85% Malaria distribution and incidence: widespread (I = 124/1,000) Malaria risk and risk areas: High: ER = 0.9–1: most of the country Resistance: P.f. resistant to chloroquine and sulfadoxine/pyrimethamine reported Literature: 82, 109, 124, 127

Guatemala	Malaria type: P.f.: 5%; P.v.: 95%
	Malaria distribution and incidence: regional
	Malaria risk and risk areas:
	  Moderate–high: Coban Alta Verapaz (API 67.22), Baja Verapaz, Petén sur Occidente (API 64.01), Petèn sur Oriente (API 45.8), Petèn Norte (API 19.4), San Marcos (API 10.53), Ixcan
	  Low: Esquintla, Huehuetenango, Izabal, Quichè (N), Retalhuleu, Suchitepequez, Zacapa. Very low risk in the rest of the country
	  No malaria: central highland high altitudes (>1,500 m)
	Remarks: high migration rate
	Resistance: P.v. resistant to primaquine reported
	Literature: 65, 82, 88, 109, 128, 129

Table continued

Country/Region	Distribution and Risk
Guinea-Bissau	Malaria type: P.f.: 90% Malaria distribution and incidence: widespread (1993: I = 144/1,000) Malaria risk and risk areas: High: ER = 0.9–1: whole country Resistance: P.f. resistant to chloroquine reported Literature: 82, 109, 130
Republic of Guinea	Malaria type: P.f.: 92% Malaria distribution and incidence: widespread (1997: I = 116/1,000) Malaria risk and risk areas: High: whole country (no ER data available) Resistance: P.f. resistant to chloroquine reported; P.v. resistant to chloroquine reported Literature: 82, 109, 124

Guyana	Malaria type: 1999: P.f.: 59.2%; P.v.; P.m.
	Malaria distribution and incidence: widespread
	Malaria risk and risk areas:
	  High: in areas with lack of appropriate transportation, in mining and logging areas, in populations showing low compliance with drug regimens, in poor housing conditions. Region 8 (Potaro-Siparuni) (API 1,201.56), Region 1 (Barima-Waini) (API 289.51), Region 9 (Upper Takutu–Upper Essequibo) (API 200.58), Region 7 (Cuyuni-Mazaruni) (API 187.35)
	  Low–moderate: S, SW of Region 7; W of Region 8. Very low risk in the E of Region 8
	  No malaria: coastal cities
	Resistance: P.f. resistant to chloroquine reported. P.v. resistant to chloroquine reported
	Remarks: gold mining and logging areas mostly affected. For more data, contact Dr. L. Validum, Malaria Control Service, Ministry of Health, Guyana
	Literature: 65, 82, 88, 109, 131

Haiti	Malaria type: P.f.: >85%
	Malaria distribution and incidence: widespread
	Malaria risk and risk areas:
	  Moderate–high: forested areas of Chantal, Gros Morne, Hinche, Jacmel, Maissade
	  Low: rest of the country
	Remarks: no recent data available
	Resistance: P.f. resistant to chloroquine reported
	Literature: 65, 82, 109, 124, 127

Honduras	Malaria type: P.v.; P.f.: 3–21%
	Malaria distribution and incidence: widespread, increasing
	Malaria risk and risk areas:
	  Moderate–high: swampy regions in the E (Mosquilia); Region VIII (API 41.05), Region VI (API 28.92), Region VII (API 21.20)
	  Low–moderate: E half of the country; Region III (API 2.83). Lower risk: W half of the country. Very low risk: extreme W and Tegucigalpa area
	Resistance: none reported
	Remarks: P.f. risk highest in Region VI in the NW, including Islas de Bahia
	Literature: 65, 82, 88, 109, 132

India	Malaria type: P.f.: 30–35%. N < S.
	Malaria distribution and incidence: widespread, but patchy risk (I = 2.76/1,000)
	Malaria risk and risk areas:
	  Moderate: all areas excluding N (mountains) and S
	  Low: S
	  No malaria: >2,000 m (Himachal Pradesh, Jammu and Kashmir, and Sikkim); extreme S.
	Resistance: P.f. highly resistant to chloroquine, sulfadoxine/pyrimethamine, and amodiaquine reported. Multidrug-resistant P.f. assumed at international border to Myanmar. P.v. resistant to chloroquine reported
	Remarks: frequent epidemics due to heavy rainfalls
	Literature: 4, 15, 82, 109, 133–137

Indonesia	Malaria type: P.f.: 66%
	Malaria distribution and incidence: widespread (1997: I = 0.8/1,000)
	Malaria risk and risk areas:
	  High: Irian Jaya, rural areas of Flores, Timor, Sumba, Sumbawa, and small islands in the E
	  Moderate: Nias Island, Java (central and Yogyakarta province), rural areas of the Moluccas

Table continued

Country/Region	Distribution and Risk

| | Low: Sumatra and Kalimantan, Lombok (Senggigi beach), Sulawesi, Bali, Java (rest of the island), Manado (city only), Jakarta, Bandung, Yogyakarta, Surabaya, Medan, Palembang, Ujungpandang |

Low: Sumatra and Kalimantan, Lombok (Senggigi beach), Sulawesi, Bali, Java (rest of the island), Manado (city only), Jakarta, Bandung, Yogyakarta, Surabaya, Medan, Palembang, Ujungpandang
No malaria: big cities and tourist resorts in Java, Bali
Resistance: P.f. resistant to chloroquine and sulfadoxine/pyrimethamine reported and other assumed; P.v. resistant to chloroquine reported
Remarks: reporting of the small islands and remote areas is poor. Incidence figures are highly misleading
Literature: personal communication, 82, 109, 138–143

Iran
Malaria type: P.f.: >20%
Malaria distribution and incidence: regional and seasonal
Malaria risk and risk areas:
Low: March–November: highest risk in rural areas of tropical part of the SE (Sistan-Baluchistan, Hormozgan, S Kerman). Lower risk and exclusively P.v. north of the Zagros Mountains and in the S and SW during summer months
No malaria: big cities and mountains (central and N)
Resistance: P.f. resistant to chloroquine and sulfadoxine/pyrimethamine reported at international border areas with Afghanistan and Pakistan
Literature: 82, 109, 144, 145

Iraq
Malaria type: P.f.: >1%
Malaria distribution and incidence: regional and seasonal (I = 0.64/1,000)
Malaria risk and risk areas:
Low: May–November. NE <1,500 m. Regions of Duhok, Erbil, Ninawa, Sulaymaniyah, Ta'mim provinces, including cities. E border to Iran, including the city of Basra
No malaria: city of Baghdad
Resistance: P.f. resistant to chloroquine reported
Literature: 82, 84, 109, 146

Kenya
Malaria type: P.f.: >85%
Malaria distribution and incidence: widespread. 1995: I = 152/1,000
Malaria risk and risk areas:
High: ER = 0.9–1: most coastal areas, S, and SW; game parks: Tsavo, South Kitui, Ngai-Ndethya, West Chyulu, Amboseli, Kora, Rahole, Bisanadi, Meru
Moderate–high: game parks: Turkana, Aberdare, Hell's Gate
Low–moderate: game parks: Mt. Elgon, Masai Mara, Lake Nakuru, Mt. Kenya. Areas prone to epidemics
No malaria: city of Nairobi and high mountains
Resistance: P.f. resistant to chloroquine and sulfadoxine/pyrimethamine reported
Remarks: tourism mostly in high-risk areas. Intensive migration has changed the transmission pattern. ER index applicable with caution. Highland malaria epidemics reported
Literature: 15, 45, 82, 109, 147

Korea, N and S
Malaria type: P.v.
Malaria distribution and incidence: local–regional
Malaria risk and risk areas:
Very low risk in the N Kyonggi-do and NW Kangwon-do province of S Korea; Bordering areas to N Korea (demilitarized zones); N Korea: low risk in neighboring areas to S Korea assumed
No malaria: rest of the countries
Resistance: none reported
Literature: 82, 109, 121, 148, 149

Laos
Malaria type: P.f.: 97%
Malaria distribution and incidence: widespread (I = 11.2/1,000)
Malaria risk and risk areas:
Low–moderate: whole country
No malaria: city of Vientiane
Resistance: P.f. highly resistant to chloroquine, sulfadoxine/pyrimethamine reported; mefloquine-resistant P.f. assumed in the SW (facing Ubon Ratchathani in Thailand)
Literature: 79, 82, 100, 109, 150–152

Liberia
Malaria type: P.f.: >90%
Malaria distribution and incidence: widespread. I: no data

Table continued

Country/Region	Distribution and Risk

Malaria risk and risk areas: High: ER = 0.9–1: whole country
Resistance: P.f. highly resistant to chloroquine, resistant to
   sulfadoxine/pyrimethamine and cycloguanil reported
Literature: 82, 109, 124

Madagascar
Malaria type: P.f.: >85%
Malaria distribution and incidence: widespread. I: no data
Malaria risk and risk areas:
   High: ER = 0.9–1: most of the country
   No malaria: Ankaratra mountain, high altitudes
Resistance: P.f. resistant to chloroquine reported
Literature: 15, 82, 109, 153–155

Malawi
Malaria type: P.f.: >90%
Malaria distribution and incidence: widespread (1994: I = 460/1,000)
Malaria risk and risk areas: widespread
   High: ER = 0.9–1: most of the country
   No malaria: Nyika plateau in the N
Resistance: P.f. highly resistant to chloroquine and resistant to
   sulfadoxine/pyrimethamine reported
Literature: 82, 109, 156, 157

Malaysia
Malaria type: P.f.: 70%; P.f.: 80% in Sabah
Malaria distribution and incidence: focal in the deep hinterlands and Sabah (I =
   1.2/1,000)
Malaria risk and risk areas:
   Moderate: rural areas of Sabah (Borneo: N) including coast
   Low: deep hinterlands of peninsular Malaysia (mountainous interior of Kelantan,
     Pahang, Perak provinces) and Sarawak
   No malaria: peninsular Malaysia: coast, cities; coast of Sarawak
Resistance: P.f. resistant to chloroquine and sulfadoxine/pyrimethamine reported
Literature: 32, 82, 109, 158, 159

Mali
Malaria type: P.f.: >85%
Malaria distribution and incidence: widespread (1997: I = 37/1,000)
Malaria risk and risk areas:
   High: ER = 0.9–1: Kayes, Koulikoro Segou, Sikasso, Mopti
   Moderate: ER = 0.1–0.9: most of the rest of the country (center and N of Timbuktu,
     Gao, Kidal). Areas prone to epidemics
   No malaria: desert in the N (El Khnachich)
Resistance: P.f. resistant to chloroquine, sulfadoxine/pyrimethamine, and cycloguanil
   reported
Remarks: high migration rates (nomadic lifestyles) might lead to high risk in
   medium-risk areas and some risk in generally malaria-free regions
Literature: 82, 109, 124

Mauritania
Malaria type: P.f.: >85%
Malaria distribution and incidence: regional and partly seasonal (1995: I = 87/1,000)
Malaria risk and risk areas:
   High: ER = 0.9–1: provinces of Trarza (S), Brakna, Gorgol, Assaba, Hodh el Gharbi,
     Guidimaka, Hodh ech Chargui (S), Tagant (S)
   Moderate: ER = 0.5–0.9: Hodh ech Chargui (central), Trarza (NE), Tagant (N);
     seasonal: July–October in Adrar (W half) and Inchiri
   Low: Hodh ech Chargui (N), Dakhlet Nouadhibou; seasonal: November–June in
     Adrar (W half) and Inchiri
   No malaria: NE (Tiris Zemmour), Adrar (NE)
Resistance: P.f. resistant to chloroquine reported
Remarks: high migration rates (nomadic lifestyles) might lead to high risk in
   medium-risk areas and some risk in generally malaria-free regions. Nonstable risk
   areas prone to epidemics
Literature: 82, 109, 124

Mauritius
Malaria type: P.v.; P.f.: 0%
Malaria distribution and incidence: local
Malaria risk and risk areas: very low risk
   No malaria: Rodriguez Island
Literature: 82, 160, 161

Table continued

Country/Region	Distribution and Risk
Mayotte	Malaria type: P.f.: 95% Malaria distribution and incidence: widespread Malaria risk and risk areas: High: whole country (no ER data available) Resistance: P.f. resistant to chloroquine reported Literature: 82, 109, 110, 162

Mexico	Malaria type: P.f.: 1%, international border areas of Chiapas, Tabasco; P.v.: rest of the
	  country
	Malaria distribution and incidence: regional and partly seasonal. 1999: API < 1
	Malaria risk and risk areas:
	  Low: rural areas only. Highest risk in Oaxaca (API 0.97), Quintana Roo (API 0.55),
	    Chiapas (API 0.25), Tabasco (API 0.17), Sinaloa (API 0.15). Lower risk (API < 0.1)
	    in Guerrero, Michoacàn, and Campeche. Minimal risk in lowland areas in the N,
	    NW, and Cancun
	  No malaria: rest of the country (incl. Baja California) and most big cities
	Resistance: none reported
	Literature: 65, 82, 88, 109

Morocco	Malaria type: P.v.; P.f.: <1%
	Malaria distribution and incidence: local and seasonal. 1997: 125 cases reported
	Malaria risk and risk areas:
	  Very low in remote areas of the Khourigba Province
	  No malaria: rest of the country
	Resistance: P.f. resistant to chloroquine reported
	Remarks: most cases imported
	Literature: 82, 109, 163

Mozambique	Malaria type: P.f.: 95% Malaria distribution and incidence: widespread. I = no data Malaria risk and risk areas: High: ER = 0.9–1: whole country Resistance: P.f. highly resistant to chloroquine and resistant to sulfadoxine/pyrimethamine reported Literature: 82, 109

Myanmar (Burma)	Malaria type: P.f.: 85%
	Malaria distribution and incidence: widespread (1997: I = 2.5/1,000)
	Malaria risk and risk areas:
	  High–moderate (1998: I > 15–20/1,000): rural areas in the border provinces toward
	    Thailand (Kayah, Kayin), India (Kachin and Sagaing), Laos/China (Shan: E)
	  Low–moderate: rural areas of the rest of the country
	  No malaria: cities of Yangon and Mandalay
	Resistance: P.f. resistant to chloroquine, sulfadoxine/pyrimethamine, quinine, and
	  mefloquine reported. High level of multidrug resistance in the eastern gem mining
	  areas (eastern part of Shan state) facing the international border with Thailand
	  (Thailand provinces Tak, Mae Hong Son, Kanchanaburi, Ranong). P.v. resistant to
	  choloroquine reported
	Remarks: multidrug resistance due to high migration rate in border areas, displaced
	  people, refugee camps, and uncontrolled mining
	Literature: 78, 79, 82, 109, 164

Namibia	Malaria type: P.f.: 90%
	Malaria distribution and incidence: regional (I = 262/1,000) and partly seasonal
	Malaria risk and risk areas:
	  High: ER = 0.9–1: NE—all year in Ovamboland: Kunene valley, Caprivi Strip,
	    Okavango valley; seasonal: November–June: Etosha Pan
	  Moderate: ER = 0.5–0.9: July to October: Otjozondjupa, Omaheke provinces
	  Low: ER ≤ 0.1: very low risk in the rest of N half of the country
	  No malaria: desert and coast
	Resistance: P.f. resistant to chloroquine reported
	Literature: 82, 109, 165

Nepal	Malaria type: P.f.: 12%
	Malaria distribution and incidence: regional in the S
	Malaria risk and risk areas:
	  Moderate: rural areas of the Therai districts; S of the provinces of Mahakali, Seti, Bheri,
	    Rapti, Lumbini, Narayani (Chitwan Natl. Park), Janakpur, Sagarmatha, Kosi, Mehi

Table continued

Country/Region	Distribution and Risk
	Low: other non-high-altitude areas < 2,000 m No malaria: high altitudes (> 2,000 m), Kathmandu; provinces of Karnali (Rara Natl. Park), Dhaulagiri, Ghandaki (N), Bagmati (Langtang Natl. Park), Sagarmatha Natl. Park Resistance: P.f. resistant to chloroquine and sulfadoxine/pyrimethamine reported Literature: 15, 82, 109, 166

Nicaragua	Malaria type: P.v.: 95.6%; P.f.: 4.41% (1995)
	Malaria distribution and incidence: regional
	Malaria risk and risk areas:
	  High: in areas with internal migration, inaccessibility, and inadequate drug supply: rural areas of Rio San Juan (API 25.64), R.A.A.N (API 21.97), Nuevo Segovia (API 21.3), Chinandega (API 19.0), R.A.A.S. (API 15.81), Jinotega (API 13.77), Granada (API 11.39)
	  Very low risk in the rest of the country
	Resistance: P.f. resistant to chloroquine reported
	Remarks: 25% of cases from the Managua region. Increased rainfalls led to the formation of huge swamps in Managua's coastal areas
	Literature: 65, 82, 88, 109

Niger	Malaria type: P.f. predominant, no data
	Malaria distribution and incidence: no data
	Malaria risk and risk areas:
	  High: ER = 0.9–1: most parts of the country, especially provinces of Niamey, Dosso, Tahoua, Maradi, Zinder, Agadez (S)
	  No malaria: provinces of Diffa (N), Agadez (N)
	Resistance: P.f. resistant to chloroquine reported
	Remarks: high migration rates (nomadic lifestyles) might lead to high risk in medium-risk areas and some risk in generally malaria-free regions
	Literature: 82, 109

Nigeria	Malaria type: P.f.: >85% Malaria distribution and incidence: widespread (I = 6/1,000) Malaria risk and risk areas: High: ER = 0.9–1: whole country Resistance: P.f. resistant to chloroquine and sulfadoxine/pyrimethamine reported Remarks: civil war, displaced people, and migration may lead to heavy under-reporting Literature: 82, 109, 167–169

Oman	Malaria type: P.f.: >70%
	Malaria distribution and incidence: regional (1997: I = 0.46/1,000)
	Malaria risk and risk areas:
	  Moderate: rural remote areas of the N: Batinah (N) and Musandam
	  No malaria: rest of the country
	Resistance: P.f. resistant to chloroquine reported
	Remarks: high migration rates (nomadic lifestyles) might lead to some risk in generally malaria-free regions
	Literature: 82, 109, 170

Pakistan	Malaria type: P.f.: 46%
	Malaria distribution and incidence: regional (1997: I = 0.6/1,000)
	Malaria risk and risk areas:
	  Low: nonmountainous regions, incl. cities; refugee camps
	  No malaria: >2,000 m
	Resistance: P.f. resistant to chloroquine and sulfadoxine/pyrimethamine reported
	Literature: 15, 82, 109, 171

Panama	Malaria type: P.f.: 13%; P.v.: 87%
	Malaria distribution and incidence: regional. 1997: 505 cases reported
	Malaria risk and risk areas:
	  Low: rural areas of the provinces of Darien, San Blas; Bocas del Toro, Veraguas (N); Chiriui (SW), Panama (SE)
	  No malaria: Panama, Colon; Panama Canal zone, central highlands
	Resistance: P.f. resistant to chloroquine reported in the provinces Darien and San Blas
	Remarks: 85% of cases from the areas bordering Colombia and Costa Rica
	Literature: 65, 82, 88, 109

Table continued

Country/Region	Distribution and Risk
Papua New Guinea	Malaria type: P.f.: >80%; P.v.; P.m. Malaria distribution and incidence: widespread Malaria risk and risk areas: High: whole country <1,800 m Resistance: P.f. multidrug resistance reported; P.v. chloroquine resistance reported Remarks: highest risk in the E Sepik region Literature: 82, 109, 172–174

Paraguay	Malaria type: 1999: P.v.: 100%
	Malaria distribution and incidence: regional–local
	Malaria risk and risk areas:
	  Low–moderate: Canendiyu (API 9.32), Caaguazu (API 6.91), Alto Parana (API 5.41)
	  No malaria: rest of the country, Iguassu Falls
	Resistance: P.f. chloroquine resistance reported
	Remarks: 90% of cases from Caauazu, Canendiyu, and Alto Parana bordering Brazil; rest of cases in provinces bordering the aforementioned provinces
	Literature: 65, 82, 88, 109

Peru	Malaria type: 1999: P.f.: 40.3%; P.v.; P.m.
	Malaria distribution and incidence: regional and partly seasonal
	Malaria risk and risk areas:
	  Moderate: lowland jungles of the Health Departments: Tumbes (API 112.60), Ayacucho (API 61.42), Loreto (incl. Iquitos) (API 56.25), Lambayeche (API 53.76), Piura I (API 53.3), Piura II (API 50.28), Junin (API 34.52), Cuzco (API 33.7), San Martin (N) (API 26.2), Madre de Dios (API 17.66), Ucayali (API 14.98), Jaen-bagua (API 12.72)
	  Low: Pasco, Huanaquo; NE coast: La Libertad, Cajamarcha (N); central and northeastern mountainous jungle regions: Luciano Castillo, San Martin, Amazonas, Apurimac
	  No malaria: Lima, Cuzco (City), Machu Picchu, Puno, Ayacucho, and Huancayo
	Resistance: P.f. highly chloroquine resistant and sulfadoxine/pyrimethamine resistant reported
	Remarks: most of the cases from the tropical and irrigated desert areas at the northern coast, northeastern and southeastern mountainous jungle regions, and lowlands or Amazon jungle. Internal migration and new irrigation projects create higher risks. Most P.f. infections from Tumbes, Piura II, Lambayeche, Piura I, and Loreto
	Literature: 15, 65, 82, 88, 109, 175

Philippines	Malaria type: P.f.: 74%
	Malaria distribution and incidence: widespread, patchy (I=0.57/1,000)
	Malaria risk and risk areas:
	  Low–moderate: Mindanao (E), Mindoro, Palawan, Sulu Archipelago, Luzon (N, SE)
	  Low: rest of the country
	  No malaria: city of Manila; Bohol, Catanduanes, Cebu; plains of the islands of Negros and Panay
	Resistance: P.f. chloroquine resistance reported
	Literature: 82, 109, 176

Russian Federation	Malaria type: P.v.; (P.f. imported) Malaria distribution and incidence: local outbreaks Malaria risk and risk areas: Very low: southern border areas, Moscow region, and Dagestan Resistance: none reported Literature: 177, 178
Rwanda	Malaria type: P.f.: 90% Malaria distribution and incidence: widespread (I=153/1,000) Malaria risk and risk areas: High: ER = 0.9–1: most of the country Resistance: P.f. highly chloroquine resistant and sulfadoxine/pyrimethamine resistant reported Literature: 82, 109, 179
Sahara	Malaria type: no data Malaria distribution and incidence: no data Malaria risk and risk areas: no data Resistance: no data Remarks: no data available Literature: 180

Table continued

Country/Region	Distribution and Risk
São Tomé and Principe	Malaria type: P.f.: >90% Malaria distribution and incidence: widespread Malaria risk and risk areas: High: whole country (no ER data available) Resistance: P.f. chloroquine resistance reported Remarks: no data on incidence available since 1989 Literature: 82, 109, 181

Saudi Arabia	Malaria type: P.f.: 80%
	Malaria distribution and incidence: regional
	Malaria risk and risk and incidence:
	  Low: rural areas of western provinces
	  No malaria: urban areas of Jiddah, Al Medina, Makkah, and Taïf; desert: E, N, central provinces, and mountainous areas of the S (Asir Province)
	Resistance: P.f. chloroquine resistance reported
	Remarks: no malaria risk for Muslim pilgrims going for Hajj or Umra and staying only in holy sites
	Literature: 82, 109, 182

Senegal	Malaria type: P.f.: >85% Malaria distribution and incidence: widespread (1995: I = 76/1,000) Malaria risk and risk areas: High: whole country (no ER data available) Resistance: P.f. multidrug resistance reported Remarks: less risk from January–June in central western parts of the country Literature: 82, 109, 183–185
Sierra Leone	Malaria type: P.f.: 61–85% Malaria distribution and incidence: widespread. No data on incidence Malaria risk and risk areas: High: whole country (no ER data available) Resistance: P.f. chloroquine resistance reported, and resistance to other malaria drugs assumed Remarks: civil war, displaced people, and migration may create higher risk of malaria and higher grades of resistance Literature: 82, 109, 124, 185

Solomon Islands	Malaria type: P.f.: 52%; P.v.: 29% (Guadalcanal Island)
	Malaria distribution and incidence: widespread (1997: I = 170.3/1,000)
	Malaria risk and risk areas:
	  High: most of the country
	  No malaria: some remote eastern and southern outlying islets
	Resistance: P.f. chloroquine and sulfadoxine/pyrimethamine resistance reported
	Literature: 82, 109, 186, 187

Somalia	Malaria type: P.f.: 95%
	Malaria distribution and incidence: widespread
	Malaria risk and risk areas:
	  High: ER = 0.9–1: NW
	  Moderate: ER = 0.1–0.9: rest of the country
	Resistance: P.f. resistant to chloroquine, sulfadoxine/pyrimethamine, mefloquine, and doxycycline reported; P.v. primaquine resistance reported
	Remarks: ER index not applicable. Civil war and famine have resulted in many displaced people and migration. Local outbreaks common
	Literature: 82, 109, 188, 189

South Africa	Malaria type: P.f.: 90%
	Malaria distribution and incidence: regional and partly seasonal (1996: I = 0.7/1,000)
	Malaria risk and risk areas: (no ER data available)
	  High: October–May: Mpumalanga province (N and E), border areas of the northern and NW provinces; game parks: Kruger Natl. Park, Sabie-Sand, Klaserie, Sharalumi, Timbavati, Thornybush, Manyeleli, Ndumu, Tembe
	  Moderate: October–May: KwaZulu and game parks: Kosi Bay, Mkuze, Sodwana, False Bay, Fanies Island. June–September: aforementioned high-risk areas
	  Low: areas bordering Mpumalanga and northern province to the S and W; KwaZulu S to the Tugela River and coast; game parks: Tshipese, Hans Merensky, Groot-Letaba, Blyderivierpoort, Hluhluwe, Umfolozi. June–September: aforementioned moderate-risk areas
	  No malaria: rest of the country; game parks: Pilanesberg, Itala
	Resistance: P.f. chloroquine and sulfadoxine/pyrimethamine resistance reported

Table continued

Country/Region	Distribution and Risk
	Remarks: climatic changes, heavy rainfalls, and migration in international border areas may create higher malaria risk Literature: 82, 109, 190–192

Sri Lanka	Malaria type: P.f.: 22%
	Malaria distribution and incidence: widespread. 1997: I = 11.8/1,000
	Malaria risk and risk areas:
	  Low–moderate: most of the country
	  No malaria: districts of Colombo, Nujwara Eliya, Kalutara
	Resistance: P.f. chloroquine and sulfadoxine/pyrimethamine resistance reported
	Remarks: due to civil war, higher risks and more resistance locally possible because of displaced people and refugees
	Literature: 82, 109, 193

Sudan	Malaria type: P.f.: >95%
	Malaria distribution and incidence: widespread
	Malaria risk and risk areas: (no ER data available)
	  High: most of the country
	  Low–moderate: N and Red Sea coast
	  No malaria: desert
	Resistance: P.f. highly resistant to chloroquine and resistant to sulfadoxine/pyrimethamine reported
	Remarks: higher risks and additional resistance possible due to civil war, famine, and displaced people
	Literature: 82, 109, 194

Suriname	Malaria type: 1999: P.f.: 83.5%; P.v.; P.m.
	Malaria distribution and incidence: widespread
	Malaria risk and risk areas:
	  High: SE: Sipaliwini district with provinces of Marowijne (S) (API 1,265.89), Tapanahoni (API 380.7), Upper Suriname (API 65.51), Upper Saramacca (API 249.8); Brokopondo district (S) (API 55.58); international border areas in the S of Nickerie province (claimed by Suriname and Guyana)
	  Moderate: Nickerie province: N and S of the lakes; Brokopondo province: N of Prof. van Blommestein Meer; provinces of Commewijine (S) and Marowijine (N)
	  Low: some coastal areas to the W; provinces of Nickerie (S) and Coronie
	  Very low: Paramaribo and E coast
	Resistance: P.f. resistant to chloroquine, sulfadoxine/pyrimethamine, and quinine reported
	Literature: 65, 82, 88, 109, 195

Swaziland	Malaria type: P.f.: >90%
	Malaria distribution and incidence: regional
	Malaria risk and risk areas:
	  High: lowlands in the E and N; Big Bend, Tshaneni, Mhlume, Simunye
	  No malaria: highlands (W half of the country)
	Resistance: P.f. highly chloroquine resistant reported
	Remarks: Higher risk from October–June
	Literature: 82, 109

Syria	Malaria type: P.v.: 100%
	Malaria distribution and incidence: local and seasonal
	Malaria risk and risk areas:
	  Low: very low from May–October: only rural areas in the NE at international borders beside Turkey and Iraq: provinces of Halab and Al Hasakah
	  No malaria: rest of the country, including frequently visited archaeological sites
	Resistance: none reported
	Literature: 82, 84, 109, 196

Tajikistan	Malaria type: P.f.: 9%; P.v.
	Malaria distribution and incidence: local–regional and seasonal
	Malaria risk and risk areas:
	  Low: very low risk from June–October: international border areas in the S (Kathlon) beside Afghanistan. Most-affected regions: Khatlon (85.3%), Dushanbe (10.5%), Gorno-Badakhshan (3.5%), and Leninabad (0.7%)
	  No malaria: rest of the country

Table continued

Country/Region	Distribution and Risk
	Resistance: P.f. chloroquine resistance suspected Literature: 82, 89, 109

Tanzania	Malaria type: P.f.: >85%
	Malaria distribution and incidence: widespread (1997: I = 36/1,000)
	Malaria risk and risk areas:
	  High: ER = 0.9–1: most of the country; game parks: Serengeti, Ngorongoro, Rungwa, Ruaha, Selous, Mkomazi, Ugalla River, Maswa, Biharamulo, Katawi, Tarangire, Arusha, Mikumi, Mt. Meru (lower parts), Kilimanjaro (lower parts), Lake Manyara, Masai Mara, Mahale
	  No malaria: high mountains
	Resistance: P.f. highly chloroquine resistant and sulfadoxine/pyrimethamine resistant reported
	Literature: 45, 82, 109, 197

Thailand	Malaria type: P.f.: 56%
	Malaria distribution and incidence: regional. (1997: I = 1.6/1,000)
	Malaria risk and risk areas:
	  High–moderate: 1998: I = > 15 to > 20/1,000; international border areas of the provinces Tak, Trat, Surat Thani, Kanchanaburi, Yala
	  Moderate: 1998: I = 10–15/1,000; international border areas of the provinces Chantaburi, Mae Hong Son, Nakhon Si Thammarat, Prachuap Khiri Khan, Krabi, Sa Kaeo
	  Low: 1998: I < 10/1,000; rest of the country, inland areas
	  No malaria: Bangkok, Chiang Mai, Songhkla, resort areas of Pattaya, Phuket, Samui
	Resistance: P.f. resistant to chloroquine, sulfadoxine/pyrimethamine, mefloquine, artesunate, and quinine reported. High multidrug resistance in the gem mining areas at the international border beside Myanmar and Cambodia
	Remarks: multidrug resistance due to high migration rates in border areas, displaced people, refugee camps, and uncontrolled mining.
	Literature: 78, 79, 82, 109, 198, 199

Togo	Malaria type: P.f.: >85% Malaria distribution and incidence: widespread (1994: I = 78/1,000) Malaria risk and risk areas: (no ER data available) High: whole country Resistance: P.f. chloroquine resistance reported Literature: 82, 109
Trinidad and Tobago	Malaria type: 1999: P.m. Malaria distribution and incidence: local—cases in the Nariva and Mayaro area of Trinidad 1994–1995 Malaria risk and risk areas: very low risk on Trinidad island (SE): Nariva and Mayaro provinces Resistance: none reported Literature: 200

Turkey	Malaria type: P.v.
	Malaria distribution and incidence: regional and seasonal. 1997: 35,456 cases reported
	Malaria risk and risk areas:
	  Low–moderate: March–November: 87.1% of cases in SE Anatolia: Batman, Diyarbakir, Mardin, Mus, Sanliurfa, Sirnak, Siirt. Regions of the big dam projects
	  Low: March–November: Adana area (8.7% of cases), Cukurova, and Amicova plains
	  No malaria: rest of the country, including most tourist areas
	Resistance: none reported
	Remarks: migration and irrigation projects might change malaria risk
	Literature: 82, 84, 89, 109, 201

Turkmenistan	Malaria type: P.v.
	Malaria distribution and incidence: regional and seasonal (1998: 115 indigenous cases)
	Malaria risk and risk areas:
	  Low: June–October: very low risk in the SE: Kushka district (90%) and international border areas
	  No malaria: rest of the country
	Resistance: none reported
	Literature: 89

Table continued

Country/Region	Distribution and Risk

Uganda	Malaria type: P.f.: >85%
	Malaria distribution and incidence: widespread
	Malaria risk and risk areas:
	  High: ER=0.9–1: most of the country, including game parks
	  No malaria: high mountains
	Resistance: P.f. chloroquine resistance reported; sulfadoxine/pyrimethamine and other resistance suspected
	Remarks: refugees and displaced people from bordering countries might cause changes in local malaria risks and resistance
	Literature: 82, 109, 202–204

United Arab Emirates	Malaria type: P.f.: 23%
	Malaria distribution and incidence: regional. 1997: 99 cases reported
	Malaria risk and risk areas:
	  Low: very low risk in the northern Emirates bordering Oman (Musandam province)
	  No malaria: rest of the country
	Resistance: none reported
	Remarks: most cases imported
	Literature: 82, 109, 205

Uzbekistan	Malaria type: P.v. (P.f. imported) Malaria distribution and incidence: regional and seasonal (mostly June–Sept.) Malaria risk and risk areas: border areas to Tajikistan, Azerbaijan, Afghanistan. Most imported cases in the Surkhandarin region, bordering Afghanistan and Tajikistan Resistance: none reported Remarks: most cases imported Literature: 206

Vanuatu	Malaria type: P.f.: 62%
	Malaria distribution and incidence: widespread (API 2000: ca. 18)
	Malaria risk and risk areas:
	  Moderate–low: most of the country. 1999: highest API in Sanma Province (API 53.71), lowest in Tafein (API 1.13)
	  No malaria: Port-Vila
	Resistance: P.f. highly chloroquine resistant and sulfadoxine/pyrimethamine resistant reported; P.v. chloroquine resistance reported
	Literature: 82, 109, 207

Venezuela	Malaria type: 1999: P.f.: 18.5%, P.v.; P.m.
	Malaria distribution and incidence: regional
	Malaria risk and risk areas:
	  High: Amazonas (lowlands) (API 47.68)
	  Moderate: Sucre (API 8.46), Bolivar (API 5.68)
	  Low: rural areas in all international border areas; Amacuro (W); Monagas (SE); inner border areas of Tachira/Barinas/Apure.
	  Very low: rural areas in Apure (E); Amacuro (rest of the state and coast)
	  No malaria: coastal areas to the W, Caracas, and big cities
	Resistance: P.f. chloroquine resistance reported
	Literature: 52, 65, 82, 109, 208

Vietnam	Malaria type: P.f.: 60 to > 90%
	Malaria distribution and incidence: widespread (1998: I=1–10/1,000)
	Malaria risk and risk areas:
	  Moderate–high: southern provinces of Ca Mau and Bac Lieu and the highland areas S of 18° N < 1,500 m
	  Low–moderate: extreme S and some rural international borders areas to Cambodia, Laos (S). Lower risk in the rest of the country
	  No malaria: big cities, Red River delta, coastal plains north of Nha Trang, coastal parts of the Mekong delta
	Resistance: P.f. highly chloroquine resistant and sulfadoxine/pyrimethamine resistant reported
	Literature: 52, 79, 82, 100, 109, 209

Yemen	Malaria type: P.f.: 95% Malaria distribution and incidence: widespread Malaria risk and risk areas: High: Sokotra Island (Sokotra: 1996–1997: spleen rate, ages 2–9: 72.1%)

Table continued

Country/Region	Distribution and Risk
	Low–moderate: mainland Yemen No malaria: San'a; >2,000 m Resistance: P.f. chloroquine resistance reported Literature: 82, 84, 109
Zambia	Malaria type: P.f.: 90% Malaria distribution and incidence: widespread (1996: I=340/1,000) Malaria risk and risk areas: High: ER = 0.9–1: most of the country and all game parks Resistance: P.f. chloroquine and sulfadoxine/pyrimethamine resistance reported Literature: 82, 109, 210

Zimbabwe	Malaria type: P.f.: 97%
	Malaria distribution and incidence: widespread (1995: I=29/1,000)
	Malaria risk and risk areas:
	  High: ER=0.9–1: most of the country and all game parks
	  Low: very low risk in Bulawayo, Harare, and highlands
	Resistance: P.f. chloroquine resistance reported
	Remarks: Harare and Bulawayo have negligible risk
	Literature: 82, 109, 211

I=incidence-based data. (Malaria-risk areas are provided by the countries. In very-low-incidence areas, no incidence rate is indicated. Generally, incidence figures are low due to under-reporting. Most data is from 1997.)[43,81] API=annual parasite index /1,000 (data for the Americas is from 1999.)[65] ER = environmental risk-based data (0 = climate not suitable; <0.1–0.8 = transmission absent or rarely epidemic; 0.8–0.9 = climate suitable; 0.9–1 = transmission stable); () = possible under-reporting or unrealistic data due to high variations of regional malaria; P.f. = *Plasmodium falciparum*; P.v. = *P. vivax*; P.m. = *P. malariae*; P.o. = *P. ovale*; N = north; S = south; W = west; E = east; NE = northeast; NW = northwest; SE = southeast; SW = southwest.

REFERENCES

1. Mackinnon MJ, Gunawardena DM, Rajakaruna J, et al. Quantifying genetic and non-genetic contributions to malarial infection in a Sri Lankan population. Proc Natl Acad Sci U S A 2000;97:12661–12666.
2. Wilson ME. Infectious diseases: an ecological perspective [published erratum appears in BMJ 1996;312:220]. BMJ 1995;311:1681–1684.
3. Castilla RE, Sawyer DO. Malaria rates and fate: a socioeconomic study of malaria in Brazil. Soc Sci Med 1993;37:1137–1145.
4. Sharma VP. Re-emergence of malaria in India. Indian J Med Res 1996;103:26–45.
5. Packard RM, Gadehla P. A land filled with mosquitoes: Fred L. Soper, the Rockefeller Foundation, and the *Anopheles gambiae* invasion of Brazil. Med Anthropol 1997;17:215–238.
6. Martens WJ. Climate change and malaria: exploring the risks. Med War 1995;11:202–213.
7. Martens WJ, Niessen LW, Rotmans J, et al. Potential impact of global climate change on malaria risk. Environ Health Perspect 1995;103:458–464.
8. Sawyer D. Economic and social consequences of malaria in new colonization projects in Brazil. Soc Sci Med 1993;37:1131–1136.
9. McNicholl JM, Downer MV, Udhayakumar V, et al. Host-pathogen interactions in emerging and re-emerging infectious diseases: a genomic perspective of tuberculosis, malaria, human immunodeficiency virus infection, hepatitis B, and cholera. Annu Rev Public Health 2000;21:15–46.
10. Hill AV. Genetic susceptibility to malaria and other infectious diseases: from the MHC to the whole genome. Parasitology 1996;112:S75–S84.

11. Mason SJ, Miller LH, Shiroishi T, et al. The Duffy blood group determinants: their role in the susceptibility of human and animal erythrocytes to *Plasmodium knowlesi* malaria. Br J Haematol 1977;36:327–335.

12. Hill AV, Allsopp CE, Kwiatkowski D, et al. Common west African HLA antigens are associated with protection from severe malaria. Nature 1991;352:595–600.

13. Tswana SA, Nystrom L, Moyo SR, et al. The relationship between malaria and HIV. Cent Afr J Med 1999;45:43–45.

14. French N, Gilks CF. Royal Society of Tropical Medicine and Hygiene meeting at Manson House, London, 18 March 1999. Fresh from the field: some controversies in tropical medicine and hygiene. HIV and malaria, do they interact? Trans R Soc Trop Med Hyg 2000;94:233–237.

15. Reiter P. Global-warming and vector-borne disease in temperate regions and at high altitude [letter]. Lancet 1998;351:839–840.

16. Thomas CJ, Lindsay SW. Local-scale variation in malaria infection amongst rural Gambian children estimated by satellite remote sensing. Trans R Soc Trop Med Hyg 2000;94:159–163.

17. Reiter P. Malaria and global warming in perspective?[letter]. Emerg Infect Dis 2000;6:438–439.

18. Coetzee M, Craig M, le Sueur D. Distribution of African malaria mosquitoes belonging to the *Anopheles gambiae* complex. Parasitol Today 2000;16:74–77.

19. Gilles HM. Epidemiology of malaria. In: Warrell HMGDA, editor. Bruce-Chwatt's essential malariology. London:Edward Arnold, 1993.

20. Grillet ME. Factors associated with distribution of *Anopheles aquasalis* and *Anopheles oswaldoi* (Diptera: Culicidae) in a malarious area, northeastern Venezuela. J Med Entomol 2000;37:231–238.

21. Mouchet J. [Vectors and environmental factors in malaria]. Transfus Clin Biol 1999;6:35–43.

22. Nigatu W, Abebe M, Dejene A. *Plasmodium vivax* and *P. falciparum* epidemiology in Gambella, south-west Ethiopia. Trop Med Parasitol 1992;43:181–185.

23. Hargreaves K, Koekemoer LL, Brooke BD, et al. *Anopheles funestus* resistant to pyrethroid insecticides in South Africa. Med Vet Entomol 2000;14:181–189.

24. Lensen A, Mulder L, Tchuinkam T, et al. Mechanisms that reduce transmission of *Plasmodium falciparum* malaria in semiimmune and nonimmune persons. J Infect Dis 1998;177:1358–1363.

25. Hadis M, Lulu M, Makonnen Y, Asfaw T. Host choice by indoor-resting *Anopheles arabiensis* in Ethiopia. Trans R Soc Trop Med Hyg 1997;91:376–378.

26. Mathews HM, Armstrong JC. Duffy blood types and vivax malaria in Ethiopia. Am J Trop Med Hyg 1981;30:299–303.

27. Friedman MJ. Erythrocytic mechanism of sickle cell resistance to malaria. Proc Natl Acad Sci U S A 1978;75:1994–1997.

28. Lell B, May J, Schmidt-Ott RJ, et al. The role of red blood cell polymorphisms in resistance and susceptibility to malaria. Clin Infect Dis 1999;28:794–799.

29. Verhoeff FH, Brabin BJ, Hart CA, et al. Increased prevalence of malaria in HIV-infected pregnant women and its implications for malaria control. Trop Med Int Health 1999;4:5–12.

30. Dobson R. Mosquitoes prefer pregnant women. BMJ 2000;320:1558A.

31. Lindsay S, Ansell J, Selman C, et al. Effect of pregnancy on exposure to malaria mosquitoes [letter]. Lancet 2000;355:1972.

32. Rahman WA, Adanan CR, Abu Hassan A. A study on some aspects of the epidemiology of malaria in an endemic district in northern peninsular Malaysia near Thailand border. Southeast Asian J Trop Med Public Health 1998;29:537–540.

33. van der Hoek W, Konradsen F, Dijkstra DS, et al. Risk factors for malaria: a microepidemiological study in a village in Sri Lanka. Trans R Soc Trop Med Hyg 1998;92:265–269.

34. Snow RW, Peshu N, Forster D, et al. Environmental and entomological risk factors for the development of clinical malaria among children on the Kenyan coast. Trans R Soc Trop Med Hyg 1998;92:381–385.

35. Htay A, Minn S, Thaung S, et al. Well-breeding *Anopheles dirus* and their role in malaria transmission in Myanmar. Southeast Asian J Trop Med Public Health 1999;30:447–453.

36. Lindblade KA, Walker ED, Wilson ML. Early warning of malaria epidemics in African highlands using *Anopheles* (Diptera: Culicidae) indoor resting density. J Med Entomol 2000;37:664–674.

37. Hay SI, Rogers DJ, Toomer JF, Snow RW. Annual *Plasmodium falciparum* entomological inoculation rates (EIR) across Africa: literature survey, Internet access and review. Trans R Soc Trop Med Hyg 2000;94:113–127.

38. Beier JC, Killeen GF, Githure JI. Short report: entomologic inoculation rates and *Plasmodium falciparum* malaria prevalence in Africa. Am J Trop Med Hyg 1999;61:109–113.

39. World Health Organization. Malaria diagnosis. New perspectives. WHO/RBM. Geneva: WHO, 2000.

40. Singh N, Valecha N. Evaluation of a rapid diagnostic test, 'Determine malaria pf', in epidemic-prone, forest villages of central India (Madhya Pradesh). Ann Trop Med Parasitol 2000;94:421–427.

41. Thepsamarn P, Prayoollawongsa N, Puksupa P, et al. The ICT Malaria Pf: a simple, rapid dipstick test for the diagnosis of *Plasmodium falciparum* malaria at the Thai-Myanmar border. Southeast Asian J Trop Med Public Health 1997;28:723–726.

42. Palmer CJ, Lindo JF, Klaskala WI, et al. Evaluation of the OptiMAL test for rapid diagnosis of *Plasmodium vivax* and *Plasmodium falciparum* malaria. J Clin Microbiol 1998;36:203–206.

43. Malaria, 1982–1997. Wkly Epidemiol Rec 1999;74:265–270.

44. Jelinek T, Nothdurft HD. [Determination of actual risk factors for malaria infection for travelers by means of measurement of circumsporozoite antibodies]. Wien Med Wochenschr 1997;147:471–474.

45. Nothdurft HD, Jelinek T, Bluml A, et al. Seroconversion to circumsporozoite antigen of *Plasmodium falciparum* demonstrates a high risk of malaria transmission in travelers to East Africa. Clin Infect Dis 1999;28:641–642.

46. Patz JA, Strzepek K, Lele S, et al. Predicting key malaria transmission factors, biting and entomological inoculation rates, using modelled soil moisture in Kenya. Trop Med Int Health 1998;3:818–827.

47. Hay SI, Snow RW, Rogers DJ. Predicting malaria seasons in Kenya using multitemporal meteorological satellite sensor data. Trans R Soc Trop Med Hyg 1998;92:12–20.

48. Snow RW, Craig MH, Deichmann U, le Sueur D. A preliminary continental risk map for malaria mortality among African children. Parasitol Today 1999;15:99–104.

49. Craig MH, Snow RW, le Sueur D. A climate-based distribution model of malaria transmission in sub-Saharan Africa. Parasitol Today 1999;15:105–111.

50. Omumbo J, Ouma J, Rapuoda B, et al. Mapping malaria transmission intensity using geographical information systems (GIS): an example from Kenya [published erratum appears in Ann Trop Med Parasitol 1998;92:351]. Ann Trop Med Parasitol 1998;92:7–21.

51. MARA/ARMA. Towards an atlas of malaria risk in Africa. Durban: Republic of South Africa, 1998.

52. Barrera R, Grillet ME, Rangel Y, et al. Temporal and spatial patterns of malaria reinfection in northeastern Venezuela. Am J Trop Med Hyg 1999;61:784–790.

53. Nabarro DN, Tayler EM. The "Roll Back Malaria" campaign. Science 1998;280:2067–2068.

54. Nabarro D. Roll Back Malaria. Parassitologia 1999;41:501–504.

55. Connor SJ, Thomson MC, Molyneux DH. Forecasting and prevention of epidemic malaria: new perspectives on an old problem. Parassitologia 1999;41:439–448.

56. Elhassan IM, Hviid L, Jakobsen PH, et al. High proportion of subclinical *Plasmodium falciparum* infections in an area of seasonal and unstable malaria in Sudan. Am J Trop Med Hyg 1995;53:78–83.

57. Theander TG. Unstable malaria in Sudan: the influence of the dry season. Malaria in areas of unstable and seasonal transmission. Lessons from Daraweesh. Trans R Soc Trop Med Hyg 1998;92:589–592.

58. Ramsdale CD, de Zulueta J. Anophelism in the Algerian Sahara and some implications of the construction of a trans-Saharan highway. J Trop Med Hyg 1983;86:51–58.

59. Monjour L, Richard-Lenoble D, Palminteri R, et al. A sero-epidemiological survey of malaria in desert and semidesert regions of Mauritania. Ann Trop Med Parasitol 1984;78:71–73.

60. Greenwood B. Malaria mortality and morbidity in Africa [editorial; comment]. Bull World Health Organ 1999;77:617–618.

61. Connor SJ, Thomson MC, Flasse SP, Perryman AH. Environmental information systems in malaria risk mapping and epidemic forecasting. Disasters 1998;22:39–56.

62. Global malaria control. WHO malaria unit. Bull World Health Organ 1993;71:281–284.

63. Implementation of the global malaria control strategy. Report of a WHO study group on the implementation of the Global Plan of Action for Malaria Control 1993–2000. World Health Organ Tech Rep Ser 1993;839:1–57.

64. Global malaria control strategy. Bull Pan Am Health Organ 1993;27:280–283.

65. Pan American Health Organization/World Health Organization. Status of malaria programs in the Americas report (based on 1999 data). Washington:Pan American Sanitary Bureau, 2000.

66. Muentener P, Schlagenhauf P, Steffen R. Imported malaria (1985–95): trends and perspectives. Bull World Health Organ 1999;77:560–566.

67. Lengeler C. Insecticide-treated bednets and curtains for preventing malaria. Cochrane Database Syst Rev 2000:2.

68. Lengeler C, Armstrong-Schellenberg J, D'Alessandro U, et al. Relative versus absolute risk of dying reduction after using insecticide-treated nets for malaria control in Africa. Trop Med Int Health 1998;3:286–290.

69. Nevill CG, Some ES, Mung'ala VO, et al. Insecticide-treated bednets reduce mortality and severe morbidity from malaria among children on the Kenyan coast. Trop Med Int Health 1996;1:139–146.

70. Ghebreyesus TA, Haile M, Witten KH, et al. Household risk factors for malaria among children in the Ethiopian highlands. Trans R Soc Trop Med Hyg 2000;94:17–21.
71. Bouma MJ, Dye C, van der Kaay HJ. Falciparum malaria and climate change in the northwest frontier province of Pakistan. Am J Trop Med Hyg 1996;55:131–137.
72. Ning X, Qin L, Jinchuan Y, et al. Surveillance of risk factors from imported cases of falciparum malaria in Sichuan, China. Southeast Asian J Trop Med Public Health 1999;30:235–239.
73. Miller JM, Boyd HA, Ostrowski SR, et al. Malaria, intestinal parasites, and schistoso-miasis among Barawan Somali refugees resettling to the United States: a strategy to reduce morbidity and decrease the risk of imported infections. Am J Trop Med Hyg 2000;62:115–121.
74. Crowe S. Malaria outbreak hits refugees in Tanzania [news]. Lancet 1997;350:41.
75. Suleman M. Malaria in Afghan refugees in Pakistan. Trans R Soc Trop Med Hyg 1988;82:44–47.
76. Packard RM. 'No other logical choice': global malaria eradication and the politics of international health in the post-war era. Parassitologia 1998;40:217–229.
77. Garfield RM, Prado E, Gates JR, Vermund SH. Malaria in Nicaragua: community-based control efforts and the impact of war. Int J Epidemiol 1989;18:434–439.
78. Singhasivanon P. Mekong malaria. Malaria, multi-drug resistance and economic development in the greater Mekong subregion of Southeast Asia. Southeast Asian J Trop Med Public Health 1999;30:i–iv, 1–101.
79. Malaria, multi-drug resistance and economic development in the greater Mekong subregion of Southeast Asia. Southeast Asian J Trop Med Public Health 1999;30.
80. de Andrade AL, Martelli CM, Oliveira RM, et al. High prevalence of asymptomatic malaria in gold mining areas in Brazil [letter]. Clin Infect Dis 1995;20:475.
81. World Health Organization. Roll Back Malaria—country profiles. Geneva: WHO, 2000. Available from: http://mosquito.who.int/cgi-bin/rbm/country profile.
82. World Health Organization. International travel and health. Geneva:WHO, 2001.
83. Mustafa KS. [The malaria situation in Afghanistan]. Med Parazitol (Mosk) 2000:17–19.
84. Beljaev AE. [The malaria situation in the WHO eastern Mediterranean region]. Med Parazitol (Mosk) 2000:12–15.
85. Bouratbine A, Chahed MK, Aoun K, et al. [Imported malaria in Tunisia]. Bull Soc Pathol Exot 1998;91:203–207.
86. Suleimanov SD. [Drug-resistant tropical malaria in Angola]. Med Parazitol (Mosk) 1994:8–10.
87. Kyronseppa H, Lumio J, Ukkonen R, Pettersson T. Chloroquine-resistant malaria from Angola [letter]. Lancet 1984;1:1244.
88. World Health Organization/PAHO. Health in the Americas 1998. Epidemiol Bull 1998;19:1–6.
89. Sabatinelli G. [The malaria situation in the WHO European region]. Med Parazitol (Mosk) 2000:4–8.
90. Epidemic malaria transmission—Armenia, 1997. MMWR Morb Mortal Wkly Rep 1998;47:526–528.
91. Tuinov VA, Tuinov SV, Davydovskaia TM. [Clinico-epidemiological analysis of imported malaria in Donetsk region (1979–1997)]. Ter Arkh 1998;70:43–45.
92. Rosenberg R, Maheswary NP. Forest malaria in Bangladesh. I. Parasitology. Am J Trop Med Hyg 1982;31:175–182.

93. International Association for Medical Assistance to Travellers. World malaria risk chart. Guelph, Ontario:IAMAT, 2000.

94. Gbary AR, Guiguemde TR, Ouedraogo JB. [Emergence of chloroquine-resistant malaria in West Africa: the case of Sokode (Togo)]. Trop Med Parasitol 1988;39:142–144.

95. Ibhanesebhor SE, Otobo ES, Ladipo OA. Prevalence of malaria parasitaemia in transfused donor blood in Benin City, Nigeria. Ann Trop Paediatr 1996;16:93–95.

96. Rajagopal R. Studies on malaria in Bhutan. J Commun Dis 1985;17:278–286.

97. Milliken W. Malaria and antimalarial plants in Roraima, Brazil. Trop Doct 1997;27:20–25.

98. Coosemans MH, Barutwanayo M, Onori E, et al. Double-blind study to assess the efficacy of chlorproguanil given alone or in combination with chloroquine for malaria chemoprophylaxis in an area with *Plasmodium falciparum* resistance to chloroquine, pyrimethamine and cycloguanil. Trans R Soc Trop Med Hyg 1987;81:151–156.

99. Wernsdorfer WH, Chongsuphajaisiddhi T, Salazar NP. A symposium on containment of mefloquine-resistant falciparum malaria in Southeast Asia with special reference to border malaria. Southeast Asian J Trop Med Public Health 1994;25:11–18.

100. Regional malaria control programme in Cambodia, Laos and Vietnam. 2000:1996–1998. Available from: URL: http://mekong-malaria.org.

101. Mey BD. Malaria in Cambodia. Mekong Malaria Forum 1999;2.

102. Basco LK, Ringwald P. Molecular epidemiology of malaria in Yaounde, Cameroon IV. Evolution of pyrimethamine resistance between 1994 and 1998. Am J Trop Med Hyg 1999;61:802–806.

103. Ringwald P, Basco LK. Comparison of in vivo and in vitro tests of resistance in patients treated with chloroquine in Yaounde, Cameroon. Bull World Health Organ 1999;77:34–43.

104. Brasseur P, Kouamouo J, Moyou-Somo R, Druilhe P. Multi-drug resistant falciparum malaria in Cameroon in 1987–1988. II. Mefloquine resistance confirmed in vivo and in vitro and its correlation with quinine resistance. Am J Trop Med Hyg 1992;46:8–14.

105. Sixl W, Sixl-Voigt B. Serological screenings of various infectious diseases on the Cape Verde Islands (West Africa). J Hyg Epidemiol Microbiol Immunol 1987;31:469–471.

106. Darie H, Reyle Y, Hovette P, Touze JE. [Current aspects of malaria in expatriates in the Central African Republic]. Med Trop (Mars) 1991;51:441–444.

107. Xu J, Liu H. Border malaria in Yunnan, China. Southeast Asian J Trop Med Public Health 1997;28:456–259.

108. Restrepo M, Botero D, Marquez RE, et al. A clinical trial with halofantrine on patients with falciparum malaria in Colombia. Bull World Health Organ 1996;74:591–597.

109. World Health Organization. Roll Back Malaria—a global partnership. WHO, 2000.

110. Ouledi A. [Epidemiology and control of malaria in the Federal Islamic Republic of Comoros]. Sante 1995;5:368–371.

111. Chandenier J, Ndounga M, Carme B, et al. [Drug sensitivity of *Plasmodium falciparum* in vivo and in vitro in Brazzaville (Congo)]. Sante 1995;5:25–29.

112. Carme B, Hayette MP, Mbitsi A, et al. [*Plasmodium falciparum* index and level of parasitemia: diagnostic and prognostic value in the Congo]. Ann Soc Belg Med Trop 1995;75:33–41.

113. Sossouhounto RT, Soro BN, Coulibaly A, et al. Mefloquine in the prophylaxis of *P. falciparum* malaria. J Travel Med 1995;2:221–224.

114. Fox E, Abbate EA, Leef M, et al. [Malaria in the Djibouti Republic. Results of a serologic survey in Ambouli]. Med Trop (Mars) 1989;49:159–160.

115. Greenaway CA, MacLean JD. Malaria in tourists to the Dominican Republic. Can Dis Wkly Rep 1990;16:227–229.

116. Schilthuis HJ, Overbosch D. [Increase of malaria in the Dominican Republic]. Ned Tijdschr Geneeskd 2000;144:385–386.

117. Jelinek T, Grobusch M, Harms-Zwingenberger G, et al. Falciparum malaria in European tourists to the Dominican Republic. Emerg Infect Dis 2000;6:537–538.

118. 3rd update on malaria in the Dominican Republic. Vol. 2000, 2000. Available from: URL: http://www.hc-sc.gc.ca/hpb/lcdc/ash/mdr1224e.html.

119. San Sebastian M, Jativa R, Goicolea I. Epidemiology of malaria in the Amazon basin of Ecuador. Rev Panam Salud Publica 2000;7:24–28.

120. Alene GD, Bennett S. Chloroquine resistance of *Plasmodium falciparum* malaria in Ethiopia and Eritrea. Trop Med Int Health 1996;1:810–815.

121. Schwartz E, Sidi Y. New aspects of malaria imported from Ethiopia. Clin Infect Dis 1998;26:1089–1091.

122. Carme B, Venturin C. [Malaria in the Americas]. Med Trop 1999;59:298–302.

123. Deloron P, Mayombo J, Le Cardinal A, et al. Sulfadoxine-pyrimethamine for the treatment of *Plasmodium falciparum* malaria in Gabonese children. Trans R Soc Trop Med Hyg 2000;94:188–190.

124. Durand R, di Piazza JP, Longuet C, et al. Increased incidence of cycloguanil resistance in malaria cases entering France from Africa, determined as point mutations in the parasites' dihydrofolate-reductase genes. Ann Trop Med Parasitol 1999;93:25–30.

125. Menon A, Otoo LN, Herbage EA, Greenwood BM. A national survey of the prevalence of chloroquine resistant *Plasmodium falciparum* malaria in The Gambia. Trans R Soc Trop Med Hyg 1990;84:638–640.

126. Imnadze P. [Malaria in Georgia]. Med Parazitol (Mosk) 2000:19–20.

127. Nguyen C, Gregson D, Mouldey P, Keystone JS. Falciparum malaria resistant to chloroquine, quinine and Fansidar in a non-immune patient infected in Ghana. Trans R Soc Trop Med Hyg 1989;83:485–486.

128. Signorini L, Matteelli A, Castelnuovo F, et al. Short report: primaquine-tolerant *Plasmodium vivax* in an Italian traveler from Guatemala. Am J Trop Med Hyg 1996;55:472–473.

129. Gascon J, Gomez Arce JE, Menendez C, et al. Poor response to primaquine in two cases of *Plasmodium vivax* malaria from Guatemala. Trop Geogr Med 1994;46:32–33.

130. Lefait JF, Lefait-Robin R. [Malaria at the medical center of the mission of French cooperation in Bissao]. Med Trop 1998;58:98–102.

131. Barrett JP, Behrens RH. Prophylaxis failure against vivax malaria in Guyana, South America. J Travel Med 1996;3:60–61.

132. Palmer CJ, Makler M, Klaskala WI, et al. Increased prevalence of *Plasmodium falciparum* malaria in Honduras, Central America. Rev Panam Salud Publica 1998;4:40–42.

133. Sharma VP. Current scenario of malaria in India. Parassitologia 1999;41:349–353.

134. Van den Abbeele K, Van den Enden E, Van den Ende J. Combined chloroquine and primaquine resistant *Plasmodium vivax* malaria in a patient returning from India. Ann Soc Belg Med Trop 1995;75:73–74.

135. Dua VK, Kar PK, Sharma VP. Chloroquine resistant *Plasmodium vivax* malaria in India. Trop Med Int Health 1996;1:816–819.

136. Singh RK. Emergence of chloroquine-resistant vivax malaria in south Bihar (India). Trans R Soc Trop Med Hyg 2000;94:327.

137. Gupta R. Correlation of rainfall with upsurge of malaria in Rajasthan. J Assoc Physicians India 1996;44:385–389.

138. Pribadi W, Sutanto I, Atmosoedjono S, et al. Malaria situation in several villages around Timika, south central Irian Jaya, Indonesia. Southeast Asian J Trop Med Public Health 1998;29:228–235.

139. Fryauff DJ, Soekartono, Tuti S, et al. Survey of resistance in vivo to chloroquine of *Plasmodium falciparum* and *P. vivax* in North Sulawesi, Indonesia. Trans R Soc Trop Med Hyg 1998;92:82–83.

140. Fryauff DJ, Tuti S, Mardi A, et al. Chloroquine-resistant *Plasmodium vivax* in transmigration settlements of West Kalimantan, Indonesia. Am J Trop Med Hyg 1998;59:513–518.

141. The Working Group for Malaria Prophylaxis. [Malaria prophylaxis; advice for the individual traveller]. Ned Tijdschr Geneeskd 1998;142:912–914.

142. Arbani PR. Malaria control program in Indonesia. Southeast Asian J Trop Med Public Health 1992;23 Suppl 4:29–38.

143. Anthony RL, Bangs MJ, Hamzah N, et al. Heightened transmission of stable malaria in an isolated population in the highlands of Irian Jaya, Indonesia. Am J Trop Med Hyg 1992;47:346–356.

144. Arshi S, Barough MR, Zareh M. [The malaria situation in the Islamic Republic of Iran]. Med Parazitol (Mosk) 2000:21.

145. Manouchehri AV, Zaim M, Emadi AM. A review of malaria in Iran, 1975–90. J Am Mosq Control Assoc 1992;8:381–385.

146. Centers for Disease Control. Health information for international travel. Atlanta (GA): CDC, 1999–2000.

147. Malakooti MA, Biomndo K, Shanks GD. Reemergence of epidemic malaria in the highlands of western Kenya. Emerg Infect Dis 1998;4:671–676.

148. Strickman D, Miller ME, Kim HC, Lee KW. Mosquito surveillance in the Demilitarized Zone, Republic of Korea, during an outbreak of *Plasmodium vivax* malaria in 1996 and 1997. J Am Mosq Control Assoc 2000; 16:100–113.

149. Ree HI. Unstable vivax malaria in Korea. Korean J Parasitol 2000;38:119–138.

150. Anothay O, Pongvongsa T. Childhood malaria in the Lao People's Democratic Republic. Bull World Health Organ 1998;76:29–34.

151. Kobayashi J, Vannachone B, Sato Y, et al. An epidemiological study on *Opisthorchis viverrini* infection in Lao villages. Southeast Asian J Trop Med Public Health 2000;31:128–132.

152. Kobayashi J, Vannachone B, Sato Y, et al. Current status of malaria infection in a southeastern province of Lao PDR. Southeast Asian J Trop Med Public Health 1998;29:236–241.

153. Albonico M, De Giorgi F, Razanakolona J, et al. Control of epidemic malaria on the highlands of Madagascar. Parassitologia 1999;41:373–376.

154. Laventure S, Mouchet J, Blanchy S, et al. [Rice: source of life and death on the plateaux of Madagascar]. Sante 1996;6:79–86.

155. Mouchet J, Blanchy S. [Particularities and stratification of malaria in Madagascar]. Sante 1995;5:386–388.

156. Ager A. Perception of risk for malaria and schistosomiasis in rural Malawi. Trop Med Parasitol 1992;43:234–238.

157. Verhoeff FH, Brabin BJ, Masache P, et al. Parasitological and haematological responses to treatment of *Plasmodium falciparum* malaria with sulphadoxine-pyrimethamine in southern Malawi. Ann Trop Med Parasitol 1997;91:133–140.

158. Mak JW, Jegathesan M, Lim PK, et al. Epidemiology and control of malaria in Malaysia. Southeast Asian J Trop Med Public Health 1992;23:572–577.

159. Comm SA, Noorhidayah I, Osman A. [Seasonal migration: a case control study of malaria prevention in Sabah]. Med J Malaysia 1999;54:200–209.

160. Julvez J. [History of insular malaria in the southwestern Indian Ocean: an eco-epidemiologic approach]. Sante 1995;5:353–358.

161. Bruce-Chwatt LJ, Bruce-Chwatt JM. Malaria in Mauritius—as dead as the dodo. Bull N Y Acad Med 1974;50:1069–1080.

162. el-Amine Ali Halidi M. [Malaria in Mayotte: past, present and future]. Sante 1995;5:362–367.

163. Malaria. Retrospective and current situation. Wkly Epidemiol Rec 1992;67:60–63.

164. Wernsdorfer WH. Epidemiology of drug resistance in malaria. Acta Trop 1994;56:143–156.

165. Sharp BL, Freese JA. Chloroquine-resistant *Plasmodium falciparum* malaria in the Kavango region of Namibia. S Afr Med J 1990;78:322–323.

166. Sakai Y, Kobayashi S, Shibata H, et al. Molecular analysis of alpha-thalassemia in Nepal: correlation with malaria endemicity. J Hum Genet 2000;45:127–132.

167. Ezedinachi E. In vivo efficacy of chloroquine, halofantrine, pyrimethamine-sulfadoxine and qinghaosu (artesunate) in the treatment of malaria in Calabar, Nigeria. Cent Afr J Med 1996;42:109–111.

168. Sowunmi A, Oduola AM. Comparative efficacy of chloroquine/chlorpheniramine combination and mefloquine for the treatment of chloroquine-resistant *Plasmodium falciparum* malaria in Nigerian children. Trans R Soc Trop Med Hyg 1997;91:689–693.

169. Ezedinachi EN, Ekanem OJ, Chukwuani CM, et al. Efficacy and tolerability of a low-dose mefloquine-sulfadoxine-pyrimethamine combination compared with chloroquine in the treatment of acute malaria infection in a population with multiple drug-resistant *Plasmodium falciparum*. Am J Trop Med Hyg 1999;61:114–119.

170. Scrimgeour EM, Mehta FR, Suleiman AJ. Infectious and tropical diseases in Oman: a review. Am J Trop Med Hyg 1999;61:920–925.

171. Shah I, Rowland M, Mehmood P, et al. Chloroquine resistance in Pakistan and the upsurge of falciparum malaria in Pakistani and Afghan refugee populations. Ann Trop Med Parasitol 1997;91:591–602.

172. Murphy GS, Basri H, Purnomo, et al. Vivax malaria resistant to treatment and prophylaxis with chloroquine. Lancet 1993;341:96–100.

173. Genton B, al-Yaman F, Beck HP, et al. The epidemiology of malaria in the Wosera area, East Sepik Province, Papua New Guinea, in preparation for vaccine trials. I. Malariometric indices and immunity. Ann Trop Med Parasitol 1995;89:359–376.

174. Hii J, Dyke T, Dagoro H, Sanders RC. Health impact assessments of malaria and Ross River virus infection in the Southern Highlands Province of Papua New Guinea. P N G Med J 1997;40:14–25.

175. Aramburu Guarda J, Ramal Asayag C, Witzig R. Malaria reemergence in the Peruvian Amazon region. Emerg Infect Dis 1999;5:209–215.

176. Asinas CY. Current status of malaria and control activities in the Philippines. Southeast Asian J Trop Med Public Health 1992;23 Suppl 4:55–59.

177. Sergiev VP, Baranova AM, Artem'ev MM, et al. [Local cases of tropical and tertian malaria in Moscow Province]. Med Parazitol (Mosk) 2000:34–36.

178. Baranova AM, Sergiev VP. [The malaria situation in the Russian Federation (1997–1999)]. Med Parazitol (Mosk) 2000:22–5.

179. Wolday D, Kibreab T, Bukenya D, Hodes R. Sensitivity of *Plasmodium falciparum* in vivo to chloroquine and pyrimethamine-sulfadoxine in Rwandan patients in a refugee camp in Zaire. Trans R Soc Trop Med Hyg 1995;89:654–656.

180. Myrvang B, Godal T. [WHO's malaria program Roll Back Malaria]. Tidsskr Nor Laegeforen 2000;120:1661–1664.

181. Pinto J, Sousa CA, Gil V, et al. Malaria in São Tomé and Principe: parasite prevalences and vector densities. Acta Trop 2000;76:185–193.

182. Kinsara AJ, Abdelaal MA, Jeje OM, Osoba AO. Chloroquine-resistant *Plasmodium falciparum* malaria: report of two locally acquired infections in Saudi Arabia. Am J Trop Med Hyg 1997;56:573–575.

183. Botella de Maglia J, Valls Ferrer JM, Martinez Paz ML, Espacio Casanovas A. [*Plasmodium falciparum* resistant to sulfadoxine/pyrimethamine in Senegal]. Ann Med Interna 1991;8:79–81.

184. Pradines B, Rogier C, Fusai T, et al. [In vitro sensitivity of 85 *Plasmodium falciparum* isolates in the Fatick region, Senegal]. Med Trop 1996;56:141–145.

185. Barnish G, Maude GH, Bockarie MJ, et al. The epidemiology of malaria in southern Sierra Leone. Parassitologia 1993;35 Suppl:1–4.

186. Mizushima Y, Kato H, Ohmae H, et al. Prevalence of malaria and its relationship to anemia, blood glucose levels, and serum somatomedin c (IGF-1) levels in the Solomon Islands. Acta Trop 1994;58:207–220.

187. Isaacs RD, Ellis-Pegler RB. *Plasmodium falciparum* RI resistance to quinine and sulphadoxine-pyrimethamine in the Solomon Islands [letter]. Med J Aust 1987;146:449–450.

188. Smoak BL, DeFraites RF, Magill AJ, et al. *Plasmodium vivax* infections in U.S. Army troops: failure of primaquine to prevent relapse in studies from Somalia. Am J Trop Med Hyg 1997;56:231–234.

189. Wallace MR, Sharp TW, Smoak B, et al. Malaria among United States troops in Somalia. Am J Med 1996;100:49–55.

190. Waner S. Health risks of travelers in South Africa. J Travel Med 1999;6:199–203.

191. Durrheim DN, Braack LE, Waner S, Gammon S. Risk of malaria in visitors to the Kruger National Park, South Africa. J Travel Med 1998;5:173–177.

192. Kruger P, Durrheim DN, Hansford CF. Increasing chloroquine resistance—the Mpumalanga Lowveld story, 1990–1995 [letter]. S Afr Med J 1996;86:280–281.

193. Handunnetti SM, Jayasinghe S, Pathirana PP, et al. Sulphadoxine-pyrimethamine and chloroquine resistant *Plasmodium falciparum* infection in Sri Lanka. Ceylon Med J 1994;39:45–46.

194. Arnot D. Unstable malaria in Sudan: the influence of the dry season. Clone multiplicity of *Plasmodium falciparum* infections in individuals exposed to variable levels of disease transmission. Trans R Soc Trop Med Hyg 1998;92:580–585.

195. Raccurt CP. [Malaria, *Anopheles*, the anti-malaria campaign in French Guyana: between dogmatism and judgment]. Med Trop 1997;57:401–406.

196. Fouad FM. [The malaria situation in the Syrian Arab Republic]. Med Parazitol (Mosk) 2000:25.
197. Gorissen E, Ashruf G, Lamboo M, et al. In vivo efficacy study of amodiaquine and sulfadoxine/pyrimethamine in Kibwezi, Kenya and Kigoma, Tanzania. Trop Med Int Health 2000;5:459–463.
198. Thimasarn K, Jatapadma S, Vijaykadga S, et al. Epidemiology of malaria in Thailand. J Travel Med 1995;2:59–65.
199. Chareonviriyaphap T, Bangs JJ, Supaporn R. Status of malaria in Thailand. Southeast Asian J Trop Med Public Health 2000;31.
200. Chadee DD, Beier JC, Doon R. Re-emergence of *Plasmodium malariae* in Trinidad, West Indies. Ann Trop Med Parasitol 1999;93:467–475.
201. Tabuk TC, Ulger S. [The malaria situation in Turkey]. Med Parazitol (Mosk) 2000:26–27.
202. Mouchet J. [Origin of malaria epidemics on the plateaus of Madagascar and the mountains of East and South Africa]. Bull Soc Pathol Exot 1998;91:64–66.
203. Ndyomugyenyi R, Magnussen P. In vivo sensitivity of *Plasmodium falciparum* to chloroquine and sulfadoxine-pyrimethamine among schoolchildren in rural Uganda: a comparison between 1995 and 1998. Acta Trop 2000;76:265–270.
204. Mutanda LN. Assessment of drug resistance to the malaria parasite in residents of Kampala, Uganda. East Afr Med J 1999;76:421–424.
205. Dar FK, Bayoumi R, al Karmi T, et al. Status of imported malaria in a control zone of the United Arab Emirates bordering an area of unstable malaria. Trans R Soc Trop Med Hyg 1993;87:617–619.
206. Razakov Sh A. [The epidemic situation with malaria in Uzbekistan]. Med Parazitol (Mosk) 2000:32–34.
207. Kriechbaum AJ, Baker MG. The epidemiology of imported malaria in New Zealand 1980–92. N Z Med J 1996;109:405–407.
208. Bouma MJ, Dye C. Cycles of malaria associated with El Niño in Venezuela. JAMA 1997;278:1772–1774.
209. Nguyen VH. Remarks on malaria control in Vietnam. Mekong Malaria Forum 1999;2.
210. Williams HA, Kachur SP, Nalwamba NC, et al. A community perspective on the efficacy of malaria treatment options for children in Lundazi district, Zambia. Trop Med Int Health 1999;4:641–652.
211. Makono R, Sibanda S. Review of the prevalence of malaria in Zimbabwe with specific reference to parasite drug resistance (1984–96). Trans R Soc Trop Med Hyg 1999;93:449–452.

Chapter 4

EVIDENCE OF MALARIA EXPOSURE IN TRAVELERS

Tomas Jelinek

ABSTRACT

Evidence of exposure to *Plasmodium falciparum* in travelers can be obtained by detection of anticircumsporozoite antibodies. As their detection indicates plasmodial infection but not necessarily development of disease, they have been shown to be reliable indicators of transmission to nonimmune tourists. Results of a series of studies that have been done among travelers to malarious areas suggest a much higher incidence of infection than previously estimated by extrapolation of data from symptomatic travelers. For high-risk areas, these results emphasize the importance of adequate malaria chemoprophylaxis in nonimmune travelers. Using the described method, estimates of the true infection rate of malaria in travelers can be derived for certain areas, and ultimately, a worldwide mapping of risk areas for travelers could be achieved.

Key words: circumsporozoite antibodies; malaria diagnosis; malaria epidemiology.

INTRODUCTION

The first antigens presented to the immune system of a human host who is infected with malaria parasites are the surface antigens of plasmodial sporozoites. These plasmodial stages are abundant in the salivary glands of the anophelide vector: every infected mosquito carries 10,000 to 20,000 sporozoites. During the infective bite, only a few parasites enter the host: experimental studies have shown that only 10 to 20 sporozoites are injected per mosquito bite. For a very limited amount of time (minutes to a few hours), the immune system of the infected host has the possibility to produce protective antibodies before the parasites are taken up into liver cells and are transformed to the merozoite stage, the form seen in slides of blood taken from malaria patients. Therefore, the detection of significant titers of circumsporozoite antibodies in a person indicates the mere fact of malaria infection, not necessarily the development of disease. Nonimmune individuals traveling to endemic areas under protection of adequate malaria chemoprophylaxis may very well suffer one or several infective mosquito bites without any manifestation of disease. Although the clinical manifestation of malaria is blocked effectively by prophylactic drugs in such persons, an antibody response is still provoked by the passage of infective sporozoites through the blood stream into hepatocytes. Detection of one type of specific antibody may well be a tool to retrospectively demonstrate the efficacy of chemoprophylaxis to individual travelers. More important, a mapping of the risks of malarial infection for travelers in different endemic areas may be possible by the detection of this immune response, thus making it possible to determine indications for malaria chemoprophylaxis in specific areas. There are only very limited data available concerning the incidence of malaria infection among international travelers to malarious areas since most travelers are advised to practice appropriate prophylactic measures. Therefore, risk estimates for malaria infection among travelers are usually derived from transmission rates in semi-immune populations and semiquantitative reports about infections in unprotected tourists. On the basis of these data, the risk for malaria infection for unprotected travelers to West and East Africa has been estimated to be around 1.2% per month.[1] The recommendations for prophylactic measures against malaria infection for travel to malarious areas are based in part on such estimates, depending on the anticipated infection rate and on data about drug resistance in *Plasmodium falciparum*. Generally, precautions to avoid mosquito bites and strict intake of antimalarials assumed to be effective against *P. falciparum* are emphasized.[2]

CIRCUMSPOROZOITE ANTIBODIES

Host immune response during that very early stage of plasmodial infection is primarily humoral. Antibodies to sporozoites of *Plasmodium* spp are directed against a main surface antigen, the circumsporozoite (CS) protein. The immunodominant epitope of the *Plasmodium falciparum* CS protein consists of highly conserved tandem repeats of amino acids (asparagine-alanine-asparagine-proline [Asn-Ala-Asn-Pro] = NANP).[3] Several NANP repeats of variable length have been synthesized, using either chemical[3] or recombinant deoxyribonucleic acid (DNA) techniques,[4] and a variety of immunoassays have been tested to detect humoral immunity to *P. falciparum* sporozoites.[3,5] In individuals living in endemic areas, prevalence and levels of sporozoite antibodies have been shown to correlate with the entomological inoculation rate assessed at the same time for the same area, and the development of detectable titers in a given population has been used as a reliable indicator of transmission in endemic areas.[6-9] Seroconversion rates of 60% to *Plasmodium vivax*–specific CS antibodies have been found in patients suffering from vivax malaria for the first time.[10,11]

The immune system of a nonimmune traveler is completely ignorant of the antigens with which it is confronted at the moment of infection with *Plasmodium falciparum* sporozoites. Given the brief time frame sporozoites are circulating before absoption in hepatozytes, the question of whether (and how fast) a measurable reaction develops in the human host remains unsolved. Yet, knowledge of this process may be essential for developing infection-blocking vaccines and (more in the scope of this chapter) for interpreting any test detecting anti-CS antibodies. In an attempt to get information on the latter question, the usefulness of an enzyme-linked immunosorbent assay (ELISA) test system for the detection of CS antibodies in nonimmune patients was evaluated after one episode of malaria infection, and the outcome was compared to that of the detection of antimerozoite antibodies.[12] In one study, three different panels of sera from nonimmune patients who presented to an outpatient clinic were investigated. The first group consisted of 156 specimens from 98 patients with *P. falciparum* malaria. The second group was formed by 76 specimens derived from 64 patients with vivax malaria. The third panel contained sera of 32 patients who had not been to malarious areas previous-

Table 4–1. *Plasmodium falciparum* Sporozoite and Merozoite Antibodies in Nonimmune Patients with Falciparum Malaria*

Time Period (days)[†]		Sporozoite Antibodies (ELISA)		Merozoite Antibodies (IFAT)		Both Tests	
		Positive [‡]	Negative	Positive [§]	Negative	Positive	Negative
0–7							
	Number of patients	28	49	38	39	40	37
	%	36.4	63.6	49.4	50.6	51.9	48.1
	GMT	20.3	2.1	811.8	2.4	—	—
	95% CI	(14.0–25.8)	(1.6–3.2)	(399.3–1,224.3)	(0–8.1)	—	—
8–90							
	Number of patients	24	19	34	9	41	2
	%	55.8	44.2	79.1	20.9	95.3	4.7
	GMT	27.1	1.9	477.7	10.7	—	—
	95% CI	(2.6–51.6)	(0.3–3.5)	(177.8–777.6)	(0–27.7)	—	—
91+							
	Number of patients	14	22	12	24	16	20
	%	38.9	61.1	33.3	66.7	44.4	55.6
	GMT	13.7	2	458.7	4	—	—
	95% CI	(8.1–19.3)	(0.9–3.1)	(134.3–783.1)	(0–9.4)	—	—

GMT = geometric mean titer; ELISA = enzyme-linked immunosorbent assay; IFAT = immunofluorescence assur test.
* 156 specimens derived from 98 patients.
† After onset of symptoms.
‡ Positive defined as antibody level ≥ 6.25 international ELISA units (IEU).
§ Positive defined as antibody titer ≥ 1:64.
Reprinted with permission from Jelinek T, Nothdurft HD, Löscher T. Evaluation of sporozoite antibody testing as a seroepidemiological method for the retrospective diagnosis of malaria in non-immune travelers. Trop Med Parasitol 1995;46:154–157.

ly. Results are shown in Table 4–1. While the sensitivity was found to be rather low (55.8%) during a period of 8 to 90 days after the onset of symptoms, specificity was assessed at 100%. Therefore, although lacking high sensitivity, this test appears to be a useful and very specific tool for the assessment of the risk of malaria infection in endemic areas; at the very least, it can provide an estimate of the lower limit of risk for malaria infection. Another result of this study was a significant difference between CS-positive and CS-negative patients in terms of time exposure: the mean value was 30.9 days (95% confidence interval [CI]: 25.7 to 36.2 days) for patients who tested positively and 19.6 days (95% CI: 15.1 to 24.1 days) for patients who tested negatively. A clear correlation between time of travel and the level of CS antibodies was also shown in a later study among nonfebrile returnees from East Africa (Figure 4–1). Thus, duration of exposure seems to play an important role in the development of CS antibodies. This fact may limit the possibilities of antibody detection in short-term travelers considerably.

STUDIES IN TRAVELERS

Equipped with published experience on sensitivity and specificity of anti-CS-antibody detection and with data from studies in endemic areas, a small number of studies of travelers has been conducted. In a study of 222 nonfebrile returnees from sub-Saharan Africa, serum specimens from 47 patients (21.2%) were found to be positive, and 175 specimens (78.8%) were negative (see Table 4–2). In that study

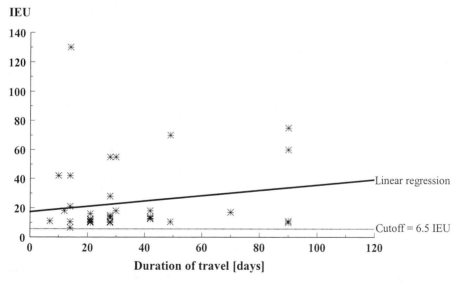

Figure 4–1. Correlation of duration of travel and international ELISA units (IEU) in patients with antibodies to circumsporozoite antigen of *Plasmodium falciparum* (n = 47). Linear regression data: $R^2 = 0.0275$, b = 0.18, a = 17.35. (Adapted from Jelinek T, Löscher T, Nothdurft HD. High prevalence of antibodies against circumsporozoite antigen of *Plasmodium falciparum* without development of symptomatic malaria in travelers to sub-Saharan Africa. J Infect Dis 1996;174:1376–1379.)

Table 4–2. Detection of Antibodies against Circumsporozoite Antigen of *Plasmodium falciparum**

Characteristic	Antibody-Positive Travelers (%) n = 47	Antibody-Negative Travelers (%) n = 175
Male	21 (44.7)	83 (47.4)
Female	26 (55.3)	92 (52.6)
Age (mean years)	38	36
Destination		
West Africa	16 (34)	56 (32)
East Africa	27 (57.5)	97 (55.4)
Southern Africa	4 (8.5)	22 (12.6)
Duration of journey (median days)	29	27
Symptom		
Diarrhea	41 (87.2)	125 (71.4)
Skin problems	3 (6.4)	33 (18.9)
Other	3 (6.4)	17 (9.7)
Type of travel		
Package-tour tourist	8 (17)	134 (76.6)
Individual traveler	39 (83)	41 (23.4)

*In 222 travelers to sub-Saharan Africa without symptomatic malaria: comparison of characteristics in negative and positive individuals.

Data adapted from Jelinek T, Löscher T, Nothdurft HD. High prevalence of antibodies against circumsporozoite antigen of *Plasmodium falciparum* without development of symptomatic malaria in travelers to sub-Saharan Africa. J Infect Dis 1996;174;1376–1379.

group, no significant differences were detected in regard to sex, age, destination and duration of journey, or symptoms on presentation between patients testing positive or negative for CS antibodies. However, although no significant findings were obtained for symptoms on return ($p = .07$), it was apparent that patients with CS antibodies presented somewhat more frequently with diarrhea than did travelers without CS antibodies. This finding might indicate greater exposure to disease in this group, possibly through behavioral differences. That suspicion was somewhat underlined by another, more significant finding: there was a considerable difference in regard to the type of travel between seropositive and seronegative patients; only 8 of 47 CS-positive patients (17%) traveled on a package tour whereas 134 of 175 CS-negative patients (76.6%) did so ($p < .001$). Thirty-nine of 80 individual travelers (48.8%) had contact with malaria parasites whereas this was true for only 8 of 142 package-tour tourists (5.6%) (see Table 4–2). The risk of malaria infection was therefore 8.7 times greater for individual tourists than for travelers on a package tour. Judging from the results of this investigation, individual travelers appear to be at a significantly greater risk of exposure to malaria than package-tour tourists, possibly because individual tourists travel and sleep under more casual circumstances than package-tour tourists.

In an investigation of a Danish school class that traveled to East Africa for 1 month under fairly simple conditions, an astounding 80% of students were found to be seropositive for CS antibodies after their return.[13] Three of those 18 travelers had febrile episodes during their travel and treated themselves with therapeutic doses of mefloquine. Subsequently, malaria was confirmed in 2 of those 3 patients by the additional detection of merozoite antibodies. Less dramatic, an investigation among 548 Dutch short-term travelers to malarious areas yielded an outcome of 7 (1.3%) CS antibody–positive patients on return.[14] More elaborate in design, this study looked for seroconversion rates for travelers, thus bypassing possible problems with cross-reactions (the test kit used for antibody detection had not been evaluated previously for travelers) and selection bias. Estimated incidence rates for *Plasmodium falciparum* infection per 1,000 person-months of travel were assessed at 16.9 (95% CI: 8 to 31) for all destinations and at 91.6 (95% CI: 33 to 200) for West Africa. Obviously, the power of this survey was hampered by the previously demonstrated decreased sensitivity of CS-antibody assays in short-term travelers (Figure 4–2), which would leave antigen contacts of a significant number of study participants undiagnosed.

Probably the closest estimate of the true incidence of *P. falciparum* infection was given by another study that investigated seroconversion rates in travelers.[15] Here, 262 travelers were recruited before departure to East Africa. To form a homogeneous study group, inclusion criteria allowed only for tourists who traveled for a hotel stay at the coast (with an optional venture inland). An addditonal 310 volunteers who did not travel to malarious areas were selected as a control group. To prevent clini-

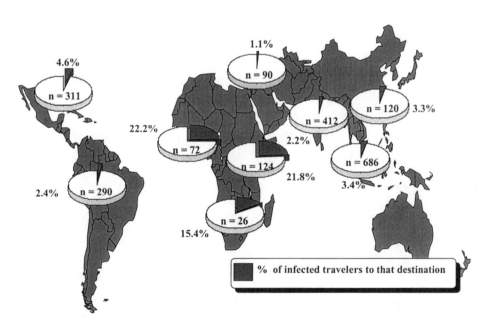

Figure 4–2. Preliminary mapping of risks of *Plasmodium falciparum* infection for travelers (based on data from 2,131 travelers). (Reprinted with permission from Jelinek T, Blüml A, Löscher T, Nothdurft H. Assessing the incidence of infection with *Plasmodium falciparum* among international travelers. Am J Trop Med Hyg 1998;59:35–37.)

cal episodes of malaria, all travelers were subjected to chemoprophylaxis with either mefloquine or chloroquine/proguanil. Serum samples were drawn before departure and after return from the journey. In this study, 4.96% of the travelers developed a serologic response to CS antigen during their journey (Table 4–3). This proportion is considerably higher than the previously estimated infection rate of 2% to 3% for average travelers to West and East Africa[1] but not as high as the rate of 21.2% for positive reactions to CS antigen that was found among 222 patients in a study mentioned earlier.[16] Considering the previously demonstrated low sensitivity of the ELISA used in this investigation, at least one-third of all infected persons remain undetected by this test. In terms of specificity, no specimen of the malaria-negative control group proved to be positive for CS antibodies, again confirming a high specificity concerning the diagnosis of *Plasmodium* parasite infection by this method. Therefore, the actual infection rate was probably considerably higher than the rate of positive antibody responses to CS antigen that could be measured in this study. There were no significant detectable differences in regard to sex, age, destination and duration of journey, travel circumstance (package-tour tourist versus individual traveler), or compliance with malaria prophylaxis. On first sight, the lack of difference in positive samples among package-tour tourists and individual travelers does not correspond to earlier findings (see Table 4–2). However, this is most likely explained by the inclusion criteria used in this study, which were designed to select as homogeneous a population of travelers as possible and which therefore ensured the exclusion of the bulk of individual travelers to East Africa. Neither lapses in compliance with chemoprophylaxis nor the lack of prophylaxis against exposure to mosquito bites represented a significant risk for the development of CS antibodies ($p = .24$ and $.83$, respectively). Although the occurrence of travel-related illness during or after the journey was not a significant risk ($p = .07$), it was apparent that patients with CS antibodies complained somewhat more frequently about diarrhea, nausea, or flulike symptoms than travelers without CS antibodies. As in previous studies on this subject, this finding might indicate a greater exposure to disease in general in that group, possibly through behavioral differences.

Table 4–3. Seroconversion of Circumsporozoite Antibodies in Travelers to Kenya

	CS Positive * (%)	CS Negative* (%)
Travelers (n = 262)		
Before travel	0 (0)	262 (100)
After travel	13 (4.96)	249 (95.04)
Controls (n = 310)	0 (0)	310 (100)

CS = circumsporozoite.
* > 6.25 international ELISA units (IEU) in enzyme-linked immunosorbent assay (ELISA).
Reprinted with permission of Nothdurft H, Jelinek T, Blüml A, et al. Seroconversion to circumsporozoite antigen of *Plasmodium falciparum* demonstrates a high risk for malaria infection among travelers to East Africa. Clin Infect Dis 1999;28:641–642.

The attempt to assess the incidence of *P. falciparum* infection in travelers on a more international scale was made by a large study among 2,131 German travelers.[17] Out of those, 4.9% had significant antibody titers against the CS antigen of *P. falciparum* after their journey to an area endemic for malaria (Table 4–4). Not surprisingly, a significantly above-average risk for malaria infection was detected among travelers to sub-Saharan Africa (East Africa, risk ratio [RR] = 4.5, $p < .001$; West Africa, RR = 4.5, $p < .001$; and southern Africa, RR = 3.2, $p = .015$). Notwithstanding the destination, the percentage of patients with a positive antibody response to CS antigen tended to be considerably higher than previous risk estimates (see Table 4–4).[1] Areas with a comparatively low risk of malaria infection but not necessarily significant differences between positive and negative travelers were Central America (RR = 0.86, $p < .001$), the Indian subcontinent (RR = 0.45, $p = .015$), South America (RR = 0.49, $p = .091$), East Asia (RR = 0.68, $p = .441$), West Asia (RR = 0.24, $p = .099$), and Southeast Asia (RR = 0.69, $p = .094$). As in most previous studies, patients with CS antibodies did present somewhat more frequently with diarrhea than travelers without diarrhea. Again, this finding might indicate a greater exposure to disease in general in this group, possibly through behavioral differences that were not registered in detail at admission.

LESSONS LEARNED AND FUTURE APPLICATIONS

What are the lessons learned from these studies? First of all, testing for CS antibodies in nonimmune travelers can detect a clinically inapparent *P. falciparum*

Table 4–4. Antibody Reactions to Circumsporozoite Antigen of *Plasmodium falciparum* among International Travelers: Geographic Distribution and Risk Ratio

Geographic Area	All Travelers (N = 2,131)	Positive* Travelers (n = 104)	% of Seropositive Travelers to All Travelers to Area	Risk Ratio†
Central America	311	13	4.2	0.86
South America	290	7	2.4	0.49
East Asia	120	4	3.3	0.68
Indian subcontinent	412	9	2.2	0.45
West Asia	90	1	1.1	0.24
Southeast Asia	686	23	3.4	0.69
Southern Africa	26	4	15.4	3.2
East Africa	124	27	21.8	4.5
West Africa	72	16	22.2	4.5

* Defined as circumsporozoite (CS) antibody titer > 6.25 international ELISA units (IEU).
† Risk ratio (RR) calculated as risk to travel to a certain destination over risk to become seropositive there (RR = 1.0: average risk for seropositivity for all travelers).
Reprinted with permission from Jelinek T, Blüml A, Löscher T, Nothdurft H. Assessing the incidence of infection with *Plasmodium falciparum* among international travelers. Am J Trop Med Hyg 1998;59:35–37.

infection with high specificity. The low sensitivity of the method is deplorable but may not be overcome by future technical modifications since it is quite likely that a sizable percentage of infected individuals fail to develop a measurable antibody response to CS antigen. However, regardless of its limited sensitivity, this method has the potential to become a valuable tool for determining the efficacy of malaria prevention measures and for approximately measuring the efficacy of malaria chemoprophylaxis in travelers.

Studies on the seroconversion of CS antibodies have begun to change our picture of malaria risks for travelers. With this method of measurement of CS antibodies at hand, it is simply not good enough to use extrapolations of malaria endemicity in indigenous populations for recommending chemoprophylactic measures to travelers. With this method, the screening of symptomatic and asymptomatic travelers to malarious areas could produce reliable data regarding lower estimates of malaria risks in tourists and therefore the true necessity of malaria chemoprophylaxis in various endemic areas. Initial attempts in that direction have been made (see Figure 4–2). Results show higher-than-expected risks for most parts of sub-Saharan Africa, for individual travelers (see Table 4–2), and for travelers who acquire other diseases during their journey. Ultimately, a much better understanding of risk areas and behavior for travelers may become possible by creating a constantly updated mapping of travelers' routes through malarious areas. As that approach needs input from a large number of travelers to many different destinations, it can be carried out only by a large network of collaborating travel clinics.

REFERENCES

1. Steffen R, Fuchs E, Schildknecht J, et al. Mefloquine compared with other malaria chemoprophylactic regimens in tourists visiting East Africa. Lancet 1993;341:1299–1303.
2. International travel and health. Geneva: World Health Organisation, 1995.
3. Zavala F, Tam JP, Hollingdale MR, et al. Rationale for development of a synthetic vaccine against *Plasmodium falciparum* malaria. Science 1985;228:1436–1440.
4. Young JF, Hockmeyer WT, Gross M, et al. Expression of *Plasmodium falciparum* circumsporozoite proteins in *Escherichia coli* for potential use in a human malaria vaccine. Science 1985;228:958–962.
5. Esposito F, Fabrizi P, Provvedi A, et al. Evaluation of an ELISA kit for epidemiological detection of antibodies to *Plasmodium falciparum* sporozoites in human sera and bloodspot eluates. Acta Trop 1990;47:1–10.
6. Esposito F, Lombardi S, Modiano D, et al. Prevalence and levels of antibodies to the circumsporozoite protein of *Plasmodium falciparum* in an endemic area and their relationship to the resistance against malaria infection. Trans R Soc Trop Med Hyg 1988;32:827–832.
7. Druilhe P, Pradier O, Marc JP, et al. Levels of antibodies to *Plasmodium falciparum* sporozoite surface antigens reflect malaria transmission rates and are persistent in the absence of reinfection. Infect Immun 1986;53:393–397.

8. Del Giudice G, Engers HD, Tougne C, et al. Antibodies to the repetitive epitope of *Plasmodium falciparum* circumsporozoite protein in a rural Tanzanian community: a longitudinal study of 132 children. Am J Trop Med Hyg 1987;36:203–212.

9. Webster HK, Gingrich JB, Wongsrichalai C, et al. Circumsporozoite antibody as a serological marker of *Plasmodium falciparum* transmission. Am J Trop Med Hyg 1992;47:489–497.

10. Fonte CJ, Bathurst I, Krettli AU. *Plasmodium vivax* antibodies in individuals exposed during a single malaria outbreak in a non-endemic area. Am J Trop Med Hyg 1991;42:28–35.

11. Kremsner PG, Neifer S, Zotter GM, et al. Prevalence and level of antibodies to the circumsporozoite proteins of human malaria parasites, including a variant of *Plasmodium vivax*, in the population of two epidemiologically distinct areas in the state of Acre, Brazil. Trans R Soc Trop Med Hyg 1994;86:23–27.

12. Jelinek T, Nothdurft HD, Löscher T. Evaluation of sporozoite antibody testing as a seroepidemiological method for the retrospective diagnosis of malaria in non-immune travelers. Trop Med Parasitol 1995;46:154–157.

13. Molle I, Petersen E, Buhl M. Retrospective evaluation of exposure to *P. falciparum* using antibodies to circumsporozoite protein and to cultured *P. falciparum* antigens. Scand J Infect Dis 1999;31:69–71.

14. Cobelens F, Verhave J, Leentvar-Kuijpers A, Kager P. Testing for anti-circumsporozoite and anti-blood-stage antibodies for epidemiologic assessment of *Plasmodium falciparum* infection in travelers. Am J Trop Med Hyg 1998;58:75–80.

15. Nothdurft H, Jelinek T, Blüml A, et al. Seroconversion to circumsporozoite antigen of *Plasmodium falciparum* demonstrates a high risk for malaria infection among travellers to East Africa. Clin Infect Dis 1999;28:641–642.

16. Jelinek T, Löscher T, Nothdurft HD. High prevalence of antibodies against circumsporozoite antigen of *Plasmodium falciparum* without development of symptomatic malaria in travellers to sub-Saharan Africa. J Infect Dis 1996;174:1376–1379.

17. Jelinek T, Blüml A, Löscher T, Nothdurft H. Assessing the incidence of infection with *Plasmodium falciparum* among international travelers. Am J Trop Med Hyg 1998;59:35–37.

Chapter 5

THE PARASITE

David C. Warhurst

BIOLOGY

Malaria is a mosquito-transmitted parasitic disease caused by *Plasmodium* spp., which are microscopic protozoa of the phylum Apicomplexa.[1] Apicomplexa are predominantly intracellular parasites, whose invasive stages involve organelles used for active cellular invasion grouped in a so-called apical complex (apical ring, conoid, rhoptries, and micronemes). They are characterized by haploid asexual multiplication stages (schizonts or meronts), which give rise to immature sexual stages (gametocytes) developing into male and female gametes whose fusion results in a diploid zygote; this zygote undergoes meiosis, and the resultant haploid stages further multiply to proliferate the asexual generation.

Plasmodium belongs to the suborder Haemosporina, which includes vector-borne genera found in tissues and blood. *Hepatocystis, Leucocytozoon,* and *Haemoproteus*[2] have nonmultiplying blood stages, which are used to infect the vector. In contrast, *Plasmodium* undergoes repeated cycles of multiplication in erythrocytes (blood schizogony), a process which is responsible for all the disease processes in mammals. During intraerythrocytic growth, the developing schizont digests up to 70% of the hemoglobin content.[3] The residual soluble toxic product of hemoglobin digestion, hemin (ferriprotoporphyrin IX), is converted to insoluble crystals of malaria pigment (hemozoin),[4] characteristic of the blood stage of malaria parasites.

Of the four species found in man, *Plasmodium falciparum* is the most pathogenic. About five million years ago, it is believed to have separated from malarias of other large apes in Africa; it subsequently spread to the rest of the Old World with human migration.[5] Evidence from hemoglobinopathies and other blood disorders associated with resistance to malaria suggests that the infection was introduced into the Americas from Africa in the post-Columbian era.[6]

Life Cycle and Relevant Epidemiologic Factors

Between dusk and dawn, the feeding female *Anopheles* mosquito injects approximately 20 to 200 sporozoites into the blood stream; some enter hepatocytes in the liver within 30 minutes. The intrinsic cycle in man (Figure 5–1) has one asexual multiplication stage (tissue schizogony) in the hepatocyte, which gives rise to thousands of infective merozoites, within 5.5 to 7 days in *P. falciparum* and within 30

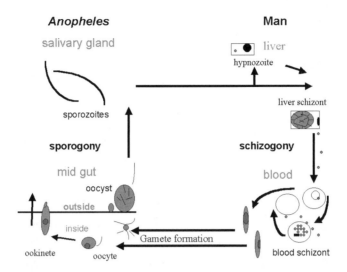

Figure 5–1. Life cycle of malaria parasites infecting man. Reactivated dormant liver stages (hypnozoites) are responsible for relapses in *P. vivax* and *P. ovale*. (See Color Plates)

days in the other species. These invade red blood cells (RBCs) to set up a series of asexual multiplication cycles of blood schizogony. Growth and division of the parasite within the RBC produces 8 to 24 infective merozoites, followed by bursting of the RBC and infection of fresh RBCs by the merozoites. This cycle takes 48 hours in *P. vivax*, *P. falciparum*, and *P. ovale* (tertian malarias) and 72 hours in *P. malariae* (quartan malaria). The completion of the cycle and release of merozoites generally coincides with a fever, associated with the release of tumor necrosis factor (TNF) by the lymphoid system in response to released antigens.[7] In many *P. falciparum* infections, the presence of several broods of parasites leads to daily fever (subtertian or quotidian fever). Some blood merozoites will develop into the potential sexual gametes, the gametocytes. Fifteen days or more need to elapse after the infective bite before mature mosquito-infective gametocytes are present in the blood. When the vector, a suitable fertilized female *Anopheles* mosquito, takes a blood meal containing gametocytes from a carrier, the extrinsic cycle of sporogony begins. The female and male sexual stages (macro- and microgametes) develop within minutes in her stomach, and sexual fusion occurs to produce a motile diploid zygote (ookinete), which penetrates and encysts on the outside of the stomach, bathed in the hemocoelom fluid, as an oocyst. The developing oocyst first divides meiotically with recombination and then mitotically to give infective sporozoites, which accumulate in the salivary gland about 12 to 30 days after the infective meal and are injected into the new human host when the mosquito bites again. The rate of development of the parasites in the mosquito is positively correlated to temperature, with maturity in 30 days at 16°C for *P. vivax* and 20°C for *P. falciparum*. The balance between this and survival of infected mosquitoes (usually much less than 30 days) determines quantitative differences in the potential for transmission of different malaria species between and within different climatic zones.

The importance of an anopheline species as a malaria vector depends on its *susceptibility* to infection, the *longevity* of the fertilized females, the *number* of mosquitoes available in the transmission season, and the *probability* that they will feed on man. The number of mated females ready to bite will depend on the rate of maturation of the larvae in water, which is temperature dependent. The breeding of mosquitoes demands standing or, in some species, very slow-moving water. For some species, large stagnant areas such as paddy fields, tree holes or the leaf bases of plants, or slower running water at the edges of streams with thick edging vegetation are sufficient. Clearance of stream-side vegetation sometimes has an impact on transmission. Some mosquito species prefer fresh water for breeding; others prefer brackish water. Although the availability of water is essential for larval growth, heavy rain can wash away and damage larvae. Little biting takes place at relative humidities below 52%. Otherwise, the biting habits of different anopheline species vary widely. Some will preferentially bite humans (anthropophagic), while others prefer domestic or farm animals (zoophagic). Availability of the animal or human is important. The fertilized females may rest in human (endophilic) habitations or prefer to rest in woodland or other external (exophilic) areas. These factors may determine the usefulness of precautions (e.g., house spraying with insecticides) and the population groups at risk (e.g., persons at home or those visiting forested areas at night).

The human population is the only significant reservoir of malaria infection. While between 1 in 40 and 1 in 400 female gametocytes of *P. falciparum* from a blood meal becomes an oocyst[8] (which will have ~4,000 sporozoites in 9 to 10 days), only 100 to 1,000 sporozoites reach the salivary glands, and during the blood meal, often only a few of these are injected. Losses that occur in the delivery of the sporozoite to the hepatocyte are compensated for since one pre-erythrocytic stage may give rise to between 10,000 and 30,000 merozoites, and further multiplication takes place in the blood cycle of *P. falciparum* at a rate of at least 16 replications per 48 hours before immune attack reduces the numbers of the multiplying blood stages or death supervenes. From an evolutionary point of view, multiplication in the human host is aimed at maximizing the production of gametocytes; these are responsible for producing the next sexual cycle. In highly endemic regions, a balance is achieved that maximizes the transmission of the organism and minimizes the mortality of the host, by coadaptation of both. In areas with lower endemicity, epidemics occur in which the case-fatality rate may be 50% or more. It is clearly disadvantageous to the parasite if large numbers of the host die, because the maintenance of the parasite in dry or cold seasons, which are mosquito free, depends entirely on the persistence of the intrinsic cycle in the human host.

In *P. falciparum* (malignant tertian malaria) and *P. malariae* (quartan malaria), all sporozoites successfully infecting the liver develop without delay to give rise to a blood infection. In the absence of mosquito transmission, the intrinsic cycle is maintained by continued multiplication of the blood stages, suppressed, but not completely eliminated, by the immune response. Low-level asymptomatic infections of *P. malariae* have long been recognized to persist for more than 50 years, often being detected through subinoculation in blood or organ donations or by exacerbation of the parasitemia following splenectomy. For *P. falciparum*, the blood usually is reported to become clear of infection 6 to 18 months after natural recovery, but the malaria eradication program in the 1960s revealed that blood infection can occasionally persist for up to 3 years. Recently, application of the polymerase chain reaction in endemic sites with long dry seasons demonstrated that persistent low-level parasitemias composed of several clones are a common and important feature of malaria epidemiology. In the United Kingdom, blood taken from a donor with sickle cell trait who had carried the parasite for 3 years recently caused a fatal transfusion infection. Persistence of the intrinsic cycle in "benign tertian" *P. vivax* and *P. ovale*, which are apparently completely cleared from the blood soon after symptomatic recovery, is due to periodic release of liver merozoites from pre-erythrocytic schizonts, newly developed from "reawakened" hypnozoites. These dormant stages developed from a proportion of the inoculated sporozoites that did not develop immediately into pre-erythrocytic schizonts. These hypnozoites[9] may persist in the liver for several months to 5 years before undergoing schizogony and giving rise to blood stages and symptomatic malaria. In *P. vivax*, geographically delimited strains were recognized early, and, depending on the length of the winter period (in temperate zones) or the dry season (in tropical areas), the proportion of sporozoites destined to become hypnozoites can range from low levels to 100%. In the latter case, seen in strains termed *P. vivax hibernans* from northern Russia, the incubation period for the disease was found to be more than 1 year.

Since the malaria cycle depends so much on climatic variables, it is not surprising that in areas of seasonal malaria liable to epidemic outbreaks (such as higher-altitude regions of endemic zones), they occur relatively sporadically. There may be a periodicity of 5 to 8 years, which seems to be related globally to El Niño/southern oscillation events, detectable by observing climatic variables in the Gulf of Mexico.

For an infection to spread, at least one new infection must develop from each case ($R_0 \cong 1$, where R_0 is the basic reproduction rate). In highly endemic areas (> 50% prevalence of infection), transmission is relatively continuous (stable malaria), and the $R_0 \cong 1,000$. Control interventions in such areas that change the R_0 from, for example, 1,000 to 100, have practically no effect on malaria prevalence. In a region where malaria transmission is seasonal and $R_0 \cong 10$, an intervention that reduces R_0 to 1 will have a marked effect on prevalence. This is explained by a curve that relates prevalence to R_0 (Ross/Macdonald model equation).[1]

Unstable malaria is easier to control than stable malaria; from the 1930s to 1960, with the aid of marsh drainage, DDT, and chloroquine, the disease was eradicated from the Mediterranean region, the southern states of North America, and some islands.

Biochemical Features

The haploid genome of the human parasite *Plasmodium falciparum*, currently being sequenced, comprises 14 chromosomes containing 27 megabase pairs of deoxyribonucleic acid (DNA) in the haploid condition. The organism also has a mitochondrial (6.8 Kbp) and an apicoplast (35.5 Kbp) genome. The inheritance of alleles on genes, such as *CyB* coding for cytochrome-b in the linear mitochondrial genome is cytoplasmic and maternal, as in other sexually reproducing organisms with mitochondria.[10] The mitochondrion in blood stages of mammalian malarias has a functional electron transport chain, linked to synthesis of pyrimidines, using oxygen as terminal acceptor, but the Krebs cycle enzymes are only expressed in the mosquito stages. One of the essential functions of the apicoplast, which has a circular genome related to that of chloroplasts, is apparently type II synthesis of fatty acid substrates not available from the host.[11,12]

MODES OF ACTION OF ANTIMALARIAL DRUGS AND THE MECHANISMS AND DEVELOPMENT OF RESISTANCE

Antimalarial drugs fall into four main classes: blood schizonticides acting only on the hemoglobin-digesting cycle in the RBC; the antifolates, which attack tetrahydrofolate synthesis in all the growing stages; the antimitochondrials affecting synthesis and electron transport in the mitochondrion; and the 8-aminoquinolines, which interfere with redox processes in general and are probably effective also through the mitochondria. Resistance to blood schizonticides is achieved by modification of a membrane transport protein(s) that controls drug access and efflux. Easily developed resistance to antifolates and antimitochondrials depends on changed residues in target enzymes. The judicious use of drug combinations can help to avoid development of resistance and combat resistant infections, but new drugs are urgently needed.

Blood Schizonticides

When chloroquine, a cheap and safe drug, was introduced for *P. falciparum* treatment in the early 1950s, it was thought that the treatment, together with DDT for mosquito control, might result in global eradication of tropical malaria. Chloroquine is easily and rapidly absorbed and attacks the dividing stages in the blood that are responsible for malaria symptoms and pathology. Its toxicity is lower than that of the similar drug quinine; thus, it largely replaced quinine for treatment. In addition, chloroquine is a valuable preventative (suppressive prophylactic medicine). The site of action of blood schizonticides such as chloroquine, amodiaquine

(4-aminoquinolines), quinine, and the newer drugs mefloquine, and halofantrine and lumefantrine (arylaminoalcohols) is within the lysosome[13,14] of the blood-stage parasite, where they complex with hemin[15] and prevent its conversion to a nontoxic malaria pigment, hemozoin (mammalian cells which digest hemoglobin are able to detoxify hemin by ring breakage to give easily excreted bile pigments). Free radicals generated by the iron of hemin damage the parasite lysosome enzymes and membrane[16] and cause damage elsewhere in the cell. A new group of endoperoxide blood schizonticides (artemisinin, arteether, artemether, artesunate) based on the traditional Chinese herb qinghao, *Artemisia annua*, also act within the lysosome by reacting with heme (ferroprotoporphyrin IX), resulting in free radicals that alkylate vital proteins.[17]

Resistance

Following the appearance of chloroquine-resistant cases in Southeast Asia and South America around 1960,[18] quinine proved to be effective against the *P. falciparum* strains involved and was re-introduced there for therapy. Chloroquine resistance spread from the original foci and reached East Africa in 1978 and West Africa in 1985. Currently, strains resistant to chloroquine are reported throughout the tropics, but they have not reached Central America or North Africa. In parts of West Africa, where 20% or more of infections are resistant, the risk of malaria death among children is estimated to be 2 to 5 times higher than it was before resistance occurred.[19] Nevertheless, chloroquine is still the first-line antimalarial drug in most of Africa because of its low cost and availability, and also because widespread partial immunity in symptomatic older children and adults enhances the effect of the drug. When parasite breakthroughs occur in > 30% of treatments, as in parts of East and central Africa, change to another first-line treatment (usually an antifolate combination similar in price) is recommended; quinine remains the treatment for severe disease.

Mechanism of Resistance. It is believed that resistance prevents access of chloroquine to the digestive process within the lysosome, since the target for the drug, hemin, cannot be changed. This is achieved by reducing drug uptake by alterations in at least two proteins, one of which, PGH-1, belongs to the transmembrane multiple-drug-resistance (MDR) type and is specified by the gene *Pfmdr1* on chromosome 5. In addition, the gene *Pfcrt*, which specifies the transmembrane chloroquine-resistance transporter Pfcrt (Figure 5–2), is involved. This is located in the same region of chromosome 7 as gene *cg-2*,[20] which was earlier thought to be the crucial locus.[21] The Lys-76-Thr allele of *Pfcrt* is reported as predictive for chloroquine resistance in laboratory isolates from Africa, South America, and Asia[22] and in a field study in Mali.[23] Mutated *Pfcrt* allows the parasite to persist in chloroquine concentrations that kill sensitive parasites. Higher levels of resistance are apparently associated with mutation in *Pfmdr1* on a background of mutated *Pfcrt*[24]

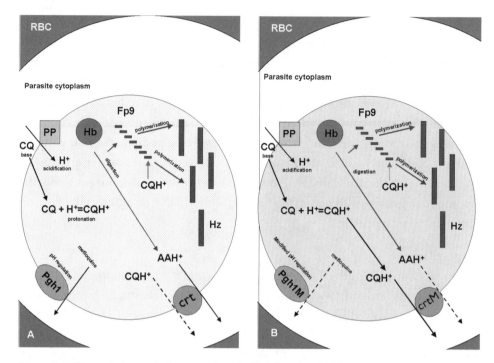

Figure 5–2. The malaria parasite lysosome in red cells infected with chloroquine-sensitive (Figure 2A) and -resistant (Figure 2B) *Plasmodium falciparum* parasites, and the different effects of chloroquine.[44]
A, Chloroquine-sensitive. The proton (H[+]) pump (PP) acidifies the lysosome contents (pH 5-6). This process is probably regulated by transmembrane protein Pgh1 releasing anions (?Cl[-]) into the lysosome to optimize transmembrane charge difference. Protein Pgh1 also functions (as a drug-exporter?) in resistance to mefloquine and artemisinin. Positively charged amino acids or short positively charged peptides (AAH[+]) are released during hemoglobin (Hb) digestion, together with toxic ferriprotoporphyrin IX (hemin: Fp9). Fp9 is detoxified by dimerization to insoluble β-hematin (hemozoin: Hz). It is likely that AAH[+] are exported to the cytoplasm on transmembrane protein Pfcrt (crt). Chloroquine base (CQ) from the cytoplasm (pH 7.4) dissolves in the lysosome membrane and enters the acidic contents, undergoing protonation to CQH[+], which is insoluble in membrane and becomes concentrated. CQH[+] binds to Fp9 and inhibits polymerization, leading to accumulation of Fp9, causing membrane damage. It is probable that Pfcrt has a limited affinity for CQH[+] and carries out some export of the drug in sensitive parasites.
B, Parasite with chloroquine-resistance-related amino acid changes in Pfcrt and Pgh1. The mutated Pfcrt (crtM) probably has increased affinity for CQH[+] and carries out significant export of the drug, enabling Fp9 polymerization to proceed normally. Concomitantly, the crtM would have a reduced affinity for AAH[+], which may lead to reduced efficiency for export of AAH[+] and, in the absence of drug, accumulation of more protons (H[+]) in the lysosome. Complementary mutation (reduced efficiency?) of Pgh1 (Pgh1M) may partially prevent this proton accumulation, increasing the fitness of the parasites with Pfcrt and Pgh1 mutated. The mutation in Pgh1 also increases sensitivity of the parasite to mefloquine and artemisinin, probably due to partial inactivation of its export function for these drugs. When Pgh1 is overexpressed, as is seen in Southeast Asia, innate resistance to hydrophobic drugs like mefloquine and artemisinin is enhanced, as expected. Resistance to chloroquine in such circumstances is still dependent on mutated *Pfcrt*. There is more variation, causing amino acid changes, among *Pfcrt* genotypes of chloroquine-resistant clones than in chloroquine-sensitive clones, and some of these variations seem to be geographically localized. These additional mutations probably serve to compensate to a greater or lesser extent for loss of function of Pfcrt following the Lys-76-Thr change. A change which accompanies Lys-76-Thr in all geographic locations examined so far (Ala-220-Ser) is in transmembrane domain 6, which would be directly opposite and at approximately the same level as residue 76 of transmembrane domain 1 in a membrane-pore model. (See Color Plates)

(see Figure 5–2, *A* and *B*). Resistance to quinine appears, however, to be related to mutations in *Pfmdr1* alone.[25] This accounts for the uncertain association of quinine resistance with chloroquine resistance observed in the field. Resistance to mefloquine is associated with the wild-type *Pfmdr1* gene;[26] amplification may be involved, and the mechanism appears also to be the control of drug passage through membranes, possibly by exporting the drug. The requirement for a wild-type (not mutated) protein here may account for the reciprocal mefloquine/chloroquine sensitivity often noticed,[27] particularly where *Pfmdr1* is not amplified. Although resistance to artemisinin derivatives is not yet clinically important, resistance in vitro apparently depends on the same mechanism as does mefloquine.

Artemisinin and related drugs, although rapidly effective in the treatment of chloroquine-resistant falciparum malaria, often fail to clear the parasites completely and need to be followed up with, for example, mefloquine. Lumefantrine, a drug similar to mefloquine and with similar resistance determinants, has been combined with artemether (coartemether) for oral treatment. This combination is particularly effective in Africa and is better tolerated than quinine. Because there is evidence that artemisinin derivatives suppress the formation of gametocytes by attacking the ring stages,[28] thereby reducing the chance of transmission of the infection, and because these agents have a very rapid effect, the World Health Organization is now encouraging wider trial of endoperoxide drugs in Africa, in combination[29] with other treatments. Care must be taken to control for antagonism by antifolates on artemisinins, an effect noted in rodent malaria studies[30] and in vitro.[31] In parts of Southeast Asia, the development of significant resistance to antifolates and the blood schizonticides quinine and mefloquine has necessitated the use of artemisinin derivatives with mefloquine,[32] a combination supported by observations of potentiation in rodent studies.

Antifolates

Antifolates (Figures 5–3, 5–4, and 5–5) are widely used in potentiating combinations (e.g., sulfadoxine/pyrimethamine [S/P]) as a second-line treatment in chloroquine resistance. They are classified as type 1: poorly active alone—sulfonamides and sulfones, which compete with *p*-aminobenzoic acid for the enzyme dihydropteroate synthase (DHPS); and type 2: pyrimethamine, cycloguanil (pro-drug proguanil), chlorcycloguanil (pro-drug chlorproguanil), and trimethoprim, which compete with dihydrofolate for the enzyme dihydrofolate reductase (DHFR). They attack the synthetic pathway to tetrahydrofolate, essential for DNA synthesis (see Figure 5–3). This means that they are effective against all the growing stages of the parasite: on the pre-erythrocytic schizonts in the liver (causal prophylactic effect), on the blood schizonts, and, through ingestion with the blood meal, on the growing oocysts in the mosquito vector (sporonticidal effect). This is a much broader range of activity than that seen for the blood schizonticides.

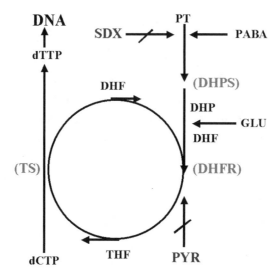

Figure 5–3. The role of the folate pathway in the supply of deoxythymidylate (dTTP) for DNA synthesis. Pteridine (PT) is combined with *p*-aminobenzoic acid (PABA) by the enzyme dihydropteroate synthase (DHPS) to give dihydropteroate (DHP) that is then joined to glutamic acid (GLU) to give dihydrofolate (DHF). This process is then reduced to tetrahydrofolate (THF) by dihydrofolate reductase (DHFR) releasing anions. THF acquires a methyl group from serine (enzyme serine hydroxymethyl transferase) that is transferred to deoxycytidylate (dCTP) by the enzymatic action of thymidylate synthase (TS), producing dTTP and regenerating DHF. Sulfonamides and sulfones (such as sulfadoxine [SDX]) block the pathway by mimicking PABA while dihydrofolate reductase inhibitors (such as pyrimethamine [PYR]) mimic DHF and block synthesis of THF. (See Color Plates)

Resistance

Resistance develops easily to both types of antifolates through point mutations in the *dhps* or *dhfr* genes[33] (see Figures 5–4 and 5–5), and now they are rarely used separately. Type 1/type 2 combinations (e.g., S/P) are active against *P. falciparum* strains resistant to either type, but one point mutation in each gene can allow resistance to the combination. In the case of S/P, used in highly endemic areas, significant resistance appears to develop within 3 years. The sulfone dapsone, with chlorproguanil, has shown encouraging results as a treatment for S/P-resistant malaria.

Antimitochondrials

Although artemisinin derivatives and the 8-aminoquinolines cause mitochondrial swelling in malaria parasites, this organelle is not currently regarded as their main target. Certain antibiotics affecting bacterial protein synthesis, such as tetracyclines (e.g., doxycycline), have a marked but slow-developing effect on malaria infections. They probably inhibit synthesis of protein on the bacterial-type ribosomes of the mitochondria.[34] These antibiotics are used to follow up quinine treatment of quinine-refractory strains of *P. falciparum* as an alternative to sulfadoxine/pyrimethamine. Doxycycline is finding favor as an alternative prophylactic drug when mefloquine and chloroquine/proguanil are not acceptable.[35] Atovaquone is a naphthoquinone whose

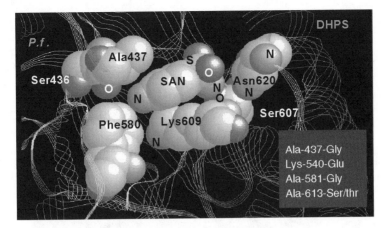

Figure 5–4. Sulfonamide drug (sulfanilamide [SAN]) in the PABA-binding pocket of *P. falciparum* DHPS modeled[45] on that of *Escherichia coli*.[46] Nitrogen (blue) and oxygen (red) atoms of the drug are held by H-bonds from oxygen of Ser-436 and Ser-607, and (probably) nitrogen of Asn-620. Phe-580, Pro-438 (not illustrated), the side chains of Ala-437, Asn-620, and Lys-609 line the pocket and hold the drug by hydrophobic attraction. (Carbon atoms are colored gray and form the framework of the structures, sulfur is yellow, and hydrogen atoms are omitted.)
Changes leading to resistance (weaker drug binding):
1. Replacement of Ala-437 by the smaller Gly-437 reduces the tight fit of the drug in the pocket.
2. Replacement of Lys-540 (not illustrated) by Glu-540. The loop bearing this residue holds Phe-580 in position for optimal interaction with the drug.
3. Change of Ala-581 to the smaller Gly-581. This residue is adjacent to the important hydrophobic amino acid Phe-580.
4. Change of Ala-613 to Ser-613 or Thr-613. The increase in bulk of this residue alters the orientation of the α-helix, thereby affecting drug binding to Ser-607 and Lys-609.
In Kenya and Tanzania, the predominant mutations seen in sulfadoxine resistance have been Gly-437 and Glu-540. (See Color Plates)

mode of action[36] is specific to the mitochondrial ubiquinone-linked electron transport chain of apicomplexan protozoa. It inhibits mitochondrial function by mimicking coenzyme Q_8, blocking electron transport through the cytochrome b-c_1 complex. Point mutations in the *Cy-B* gene sequence on the mitochondrial genome, such as (Met-133-Ile) (Figure 5–6), are associated with resistance.[37]

Resistance

Resistance develops easily, and atovaquone is used for treatment in potentiating combination with proguanil [38,39] as Malarone (Glaxo Wellcome). It is effective in uncomplicated falciparum malaria resistant to chloroquine and antifolates. This combination has causal prophylactic and sporonticidal effects but is unlikely to affect *P. vivax* liver hypnozoites or mature *P. falciparum* gametocytes. Other antibiotics in development affect the apicoplast[40] (see above).

8-Aminoquinolines

Primaquine and etaquine (tafenoquine) act through redox-active quinone metabolites, are selectively toxic to the pre-erythrocytic stages in the liver (causal prophy-

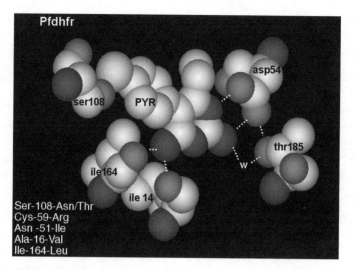

Figure 5–5. Pyrimethamine (PYR) in the DHF-binding pocket of *P. falciparum* DHFR modeled[47] on that of *Lactobacillus casei.*[48] Carbon atoms (light blue) form the framework of the structures. Nitrogen atoms (dark blue) of the drug (PYR) are held by H-bonds (dashed lines) from oxygen atoms (red) of Asp-54, Ile-164, and Ile-14. Ser-108 protrudes into the binding pocket and holds the chlorine atom (green) of the drug in place by hydrophobic attraction. Similarly, Ala-16 (not illustrated) holds the drug in place by hydrophobic attraction in the region of the important binding contacts with Asp-54 (hydrogens are omitted).

Changes leading to resistance (weaker drug binding):

1. Replacement of Ser-108 by the more bulky Asn- or Thr-108.
2. Replacement of amino acid Asn-51 by Ile-51 and/or Cys-59 by Arg-59 changes the orientation of the α-helix containing Asp-54 with respect to the drug.
3. Replacement of Ile-164 by the more bulky Leu-164.
4. Change of Ala-16 (not illustrated) to the more bulky Val-16. This alters the orientation of the drug-binding interaction with Asp-54.

In Africa, the predominant mutations observed in pyrimethamine resistance have been Asn-108, Ile-151, and Arg-59. (See Color Plates)

laxis), and are the only drugs that kill hypnozoites, thus allowing radical cure of relapsing *P. vivax* and *P. ovale.* They also kill the mature gametocytes of *P. falciparum* that infect the mosquito vector (i.e., they show tissue schizonticidal, hypnozoiticidal, and gametocidal effects). The effect of primaquine on blood stages, apart from killing gametocytes, is weak at nontoxic doses, but etaquine[41] has appreciable blood schizonticidal activity, which is apparently associated with binding to hemin.

Resistance

Currently, resistance is not a problem. 8-Aminoquinolines must be applied cautiously in populations carrying glucose-6-phosphate dehydrogenase deficiencies.

CLASSES OF ANTIMALARIAL DRUGS

Drug examples are in square brackets, thus [...]. Pro-drugs (drugs converted in the body to active metabolites) are in round brackets, thus (...).

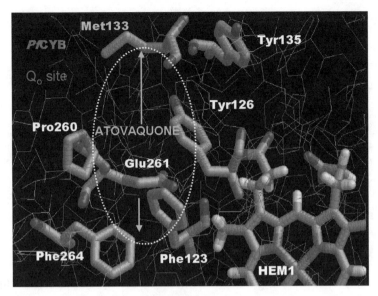

Figure 5–6. Binding site of atovaquone (dotted line shows outline of drug) in the Q_o ubiquinone site of cytochrome-*b* of *P. falciparum* modeled on the crystal structure of the bovine enzyme. The drug is held by hydrophobic attraction by Pro-260, Phe-264, Phe-123, Tyr-126, and Met-133. The primary mutation in resistance development appears to be a change from Met-133 to the more bulky Ile-133. HEM-1 = one of two intramembrane heme molecules associated with cytochrome-b. (See Color Plates)

- **Blood schizonticides.** These include 4-aminoquinolines [chloroquine, desethylamodiaquine (amodiaquine)]; natural [quinine] and synthetic aryl-aminoalcohols [mefloquine, halofantrine, and lumefantrine]; artemisinin derivatives [artemisinin, arteether, artemether, and artesunate]; and other endoperoxides [arteflene].

- **Antifolates.** These include sulfonamides [sulfadoxine, sulfamethoxazole]; sulfones [dapsone]; and the dihydrofolate reductase inhibitors [pyrimethamine, trimethoprim, cycloguanil (proguanil), and chlorcycloguanil (chlorproguanil)]. An experimental drug [WR99210 (PS15)] has similarities to trimethoprim and cycloguanil.

- **Antimitochondrials.** These include redox agents [atovaquone, proguanil, quinone metabolite of (primaquine), and quinone metabolite of (etaquine)] and bacterial protein synthesis inhibitors [tetracycline, doxycycline, azithromycin, clindamycin].

- **New drugs in development.** These include inhibitors of phospholipid synthesis, inhibitors of proteases,[42] and agents interfering with the function of the plastid or apicoplast.[43]

PARASITE STAGES ACTED ON BY DRUGS

[Drugs converted to active metabolites by the host are in round brackets, thus, (…).]

- **Sporozoite.** None.

- **Hypnozoite–anti-relapse activity.** (Primaquine) and (etaquine).

- **Pre-erythrocytic schizont–causal prophylactic activity.** Atovaquone, proguanil, (primaquine), (etaquine), pyrimethamine, (proguanil), (chlor-proguanil), and (PS15). The role of sulfonamides and sulfones is uncertain in man although they are active in experimental animals.

- **Blood schizont cycle.** Chloroquine, (amodiaquine), quinine, mefloquine, halo-fantrine, lumefantrine, artemisinins and other endoperoxides, (primaquine), (etaquine), pyrimethamine, (proguanil), (chlorproguanil), proguanil, ato-vaquone, sulfonamides, and sulfones.

- **Gametocyte (immature).** The same as for the blood schizont cycle.

- **Gametocyte (mature *P. falciparum*).** (Primaquine) and (etaquine).

- **Maturing ookinete and growing oocyst in the mosquito.** Sporonticidal activ-ity: pyrimethamine, (proguanil), (chlorproguanil), (PS15), sulfonamides, and sulfones carried over with the blood meal.

REFERENCES

1. Gilles HM, Warrell, DA, editors. Bruce-Chwatt's essential malariology. London: Arnold, 1993.
2. Garnham PCC. Malaria parasites and other haemosporidia. Oxford: Blackwell, 1966.
3. Eggleson KK, Duffin KL, Goldberg DE. Identification and characterization of Fal-cilysin, a metallopeptidase involved in hemoglobulin catabolism within the malar-ia parasite *Plasmodium falciparum*. J Biol Chem 1999;274:32411–32417.
4. Pagola S, Stephens PW, Bohle DS, et al. The structure of malaria pigment β-haematin. Nature 2000;404:307–310.
5. Escalante AA, Freeland DE, Collins WE, Lal AA. The evolution of primate malaria par-asites based on the gene encoding cytochrome *b* from the linear mitochondrial genome. Proc Natl Acad Sci U S A 1998;95:8124–8129.
6. Cavalli-Sforza LL, Menozzi P, Piazza A. The history and geography of human genes. Chichester, U.K.: Princeton University Press, 1994.
7. Kwiatkowski D, Cannon JG, Manogue KR, et al. Tumor necrosis factor production in falciparum malaria and its association with schizont rupture. Clin Exp Immunol 1989;77:361–366.
8. Ponnudurai R, Meuwissen JH, Leuwenberg AD, et al. The production of mature game-tocytes of *Plasmodium falciparum* in continuous cultures of different isolates infec-tive to mosquitoes. Trans R Soc Trop Med Hyg 1982;76:242–280.
9. Krotoski WA, Garnham PCC, Bray RS, et al. Observations on early and late post sporo-zoite tissue stages in human malaria. The discovery of a new latent form of *P. cynomolgi*. Am J Trop Med Hyg 1982;31:24–35.
10. Creasey AM, Ranford-Cartwright LC, Moore DJ, et al. Uniparental inheritance of the mitochondrial gene cytochrome b in *Plasmodium falciparum*. Curr Genet 1993;23:360–364.

11. Waller RE, Keeling PJ, Donald RG, et al. Nuclear encoded proteins target to the plastid in *Toxoplasma gondii* and *Plasmodium falciparum*. Proc Natl Acad Sci U S A 1998;95:12352–12357.

12. Surolia N, Surolia A. Triclosan offers protection against blood stages of malaria by inhibiting enoyl-ACP reductase of *Plasmodium falciparum*. Nat Med 2001;7:167–173.

13. Warhurst DC, Hockley DJ. Mode of action of chloroquine on *Plasmodium berghei* and *P. cynomolgi*. Nature 1967;214:935–936.

14. Homewood CA, Warhurst DC, Peters W, Baggaley VC. Lysosomes, pH and the antimalarial action of chloroquine. Nature 1972;235:50–52.

15. Chou AC, Chevli R, Fitch CD. Ferriprotoporphyrin IX fulfils the criteria for identification as the chloroquine receptor of malaria parasites. Biochemistry 1980;19:1543–1549.

16. Bray P, Mungthin M, Ridley RG, Ward SA. Access to haematin: the basis of chloroquine-resistance. Mol Pharmacol 1998;54:170–179.

17. Meshnick SR, Taylor TE, Kamchongwongpaisan S. Artemisinin and the antimalarial endoperoxides: from herbal remedy to targeted chemotherapy. Microbiol Rev 1996;60:301–315.

18. Peters W. Chemotherapy and drug resistance in malaria. London: Academic Press, 1987.

19. Trape JF, Pison G, Preziosi MP, et al. Impact of chloroquine-resistance on malaria mortality. C R Acad Sci III 1998;321:689–697.

20. Adagu IS, Warhurst DC. Association of *cg2* and *Pfmdr 1* genotype with chloroquine resistance in field samples of *Plasmodium falciparum* from Nigeria. Parasitology 1999;119:343–348.

21. Fidock DA, Nomura T, Cooper RA, et al. Allelic modifications of the cg2 and cg1 genes do not alter the chloroquine response of drug-resustant *Plasmodium falciparum*. Mol Biochem Parasitol 2000;110:1–10.

22. Fidock DA, Nomura T, Talley AK, et al. Mutations in the *P. falciparum* lysosome transmembrane protein PfCRT and evidence for their role in chloroquine-resistance. Mol Cell 2000;6:861–871.

23. Djimde A, Doumbo OK, Cortese JF, et al. A molecular marker for chloroquine-resistant falciparum malaria. N Engl J Med 2001;344:257–263.

24. Warhurst DC. A molecular marker for chloroquine-resistant malaria. N Engl J Med 2001;344:299–302.

25. Reed MB, Saliba KJ, Caruana SR, et al. Pgh 1 modulates sensitivity and resistance to multiple antimalarials in *Plasmodium falciparum*. Nature 2000;403:906–909.

26. Duraisingh MT, Roper C, Walliker D, Warhurst DC. Increased sensitivity to the antimalarials mefloquine and artemisinin is conferred by mutations in the *Pfmdr 1* gene of *Plasmodium falciparum*. Mol Microbiol 2000;36:955–961.

27. Burchard GD, Horstmann RD, Wernsdorfer WH, Dietrick M. *Plasmodium falciparum* malaria: resistance to chloroquine, but sensitivity to mefloquine in the Gabon. A prospective in-vitro study. Trop Med Parasitol 1984;35:1–4.

28. von Seidlein L, Bojang K, Jones P, et al. A randomized controlled trial of artemether/benflumetol, a new antimalarial and pyrimethamine/sulfadoxine in the treatment of uncomplicated falciparum malaria in African children. Am J Trop Med Hyg 1998;58:638–644.

29. White NJ. Preventing antimalarial drug resistance through combinations. Drug Resist Updates 1998;1:3–9.

30. Chawira AN, Warhurst DC, Robinson BL, Peters W. The effect of combinations of qinghaosu (Artemisinin) with standard antimalarial drugs in the suppressive treatment of malaria in mice. Trans R Soc Trop Med Hyg 1987;81:554–558.

31. Fivelman QL, Walden JC, Smith PJ, et al. The effect of artesunate combined with standard antimalarials against chloroquine-sensitive and chloroquine-resistant strains of *Plasmodium falciparum* in vitro. Trans R Soc Trop Med Hyg 1999;93:429–432.

32. Price RN, Nosten F, Luxemburger C, et al. Artesunate versus artemether in combination with mefloquine for the treatment of multidrug-resistant falciparum malaria. Trans R Soc Trop Med Hyg 1995;89:523–527.

33. Warhurst DC. Drug resistance in *Plasmodium falciparum* malaria. Infection 1999;27 Suppl 2:S55–S58.

34. Kiatfuengfoo R, Suthiphogchai T, Prapunwattana P, Yuthavong Y. Mitochondria as the site of action of tetracycline on *Plasmodium falciparum*. Mol Biochem Parasitol 1989;34:109–115.

35. Bradley DJ, Warhurst DC. Guidelines for the prevention of malaria in travelers from the United Kingdom. Commun Dis Rep Rev 1997;10:138–151.

36. Srivastava IK, Rottenberg H, Vaidya AB. Atovaquone, a broad spectrum antiparasitic drug, collapses mitochondrial membrane potential in a malaria parasite. J Biol Chem 1997;272:3961–3966.

37. Korsinczky M, Chen N, Kotecka B, et al. Mutations in *Plasmodium falciparum* cytochrome b that are associated with atovaquone resistance are located at a putative drug-binding site. Antimicrob Agents Chemother 2000;44:2100–2108.

38. Looareesuwan S, Viravan S, Webster HK, et al. Clinical studies of atovaquone, alone or in combination with other antimalarial drugs, for the treatment of acute uncomplicated malaria in Thailand. Am J Trop Med Hyg 1996;54:62–66.

39. Murphy AD, Lang-Unnasch N. Alternative oxidase inhibitors potentiate the activity of atovaquone against *Plasmodium falciparum*. Antimicrob Agents Chemother 1999;43:651–654.

40. Waller RF, Reed MB, Cowman AF, McFadden GI. Protein trafficking to the plastid of *Plasmodium falciparum* is via the secretory pathway. EMBO J 2000;19:1794–1802.

41. Brueckner RP, Coster T, Wesche DL, et al. Prophylaxis of *Plasmodium falciparum* infection in a human challenge model with WR 238605, a new 8-aminoquinoline antimalarial. Antimicrob Agents Chemother 1998;42:1293–1294.

42. Olson JE, Lee GK, Semenov A, Rosenthal PJ. Antimalarial effects in mice of orally administered peptidyl cysteine protease inhibitors. Bioorg Med Chem 1999;7:633–638.

43. Beeson JG, Winstanley PA, McFadden GI, Brown GV. New agents to combat malaria. Nat Med 2001;7:149–150.

44. Warhurst DC. A molecular marker for chloroquine-resistant falciparum malaria [editorial]. N Engl J Med 2001;344:299–302.

45. Warhurst DC. Drug-resistance in *Plasmodium falciparum*. Infection 1999;27 Suppl 2:S55–S58.

46. Achari A, Somers DO, Champness JN, et al. Crystal structure of the anti-bacterial sulfonamide drug target dihydropteroate synthase. Nat Struct Biol 1997;4:490–497.

47. Warhurst DC. Antimalarial drug discovery: development of inhibitors of dihydrofolate reductase active in drug resistance. Drug Discov Today 1998;3:538–546.

48. Bolin JT, Filman DJ, Matthews DA, et al. Crystal structures of *Escherichia coli* and *Lactobacillus casei* dihydrofolate reductase refined at 1.7 A resolution. I. General features and binding of methotrexate. J Biol Chem 1982;257:13650–13662.

Chapter 6

THE VECTOR AND MEASURES
AGAINST MOSQUITO BITES

Matius P. Stürchler

ABSTRACT

It is not without reason that the main emphasis of the massive effort of the World Health Organization (WHO) to eradicate malaria in the 1950s and 1960s was the fight against malaria vectors—had WHO succeeded in eliminating the *Anopheles* mosquito, there would be no more malaria today. It did not, but we have available today powerful and easy-to-use measures to physically protect the traveler from malaria infection by mosquito bites. These range from repellents applied to the skin to permethrin-impregnated protective clothing to mosquito nets. Additional knowledge of the vector itself, its behavior, feeding habits, and distribution helps to define areas and times of high risk. *Anopheles* mosquitoes are not usually found above an altitude of 2,500 meters, and they are mainly active during the night. Preventive measures during nighttime and at dawn and dusk (but not during the day) may achieve increased compliance without a substantial increase in malaria transmission. As no malaria chemosuppression, even with the most modern of medications, can boast an efficacy of 100%, measures against mosquito bites constitute an important, simple, and effective way to significantly reduce the risk of malaria and other mosquito-borne diseases; such measures should be a mainstay preventive measure for every traveler to a malarious area. This chapter will briefly outline important aspects of the malaria vector (behavior, breeding, flight range, etc.) and then continue with a detailed and practical guide for personal protective measures for the traveler against mosquito bites.

Key words: *anopheles*; insecticide; malaria; mosquito; net; personal protection measures; repellent; transmission; vector.

THE VECTOR

The genus *Anopheles* comprises over 420 different species. Around 70 transmit malaria, and only about 50 are medically important vectors.[1,2] In general, adults in temperate (and possibly subarctic and arctic) regions live about 4 to 5 weeks on average. In hot tropical areas, life expectancy is shorter, probably 1 to 2 weeks on average. Normally, *Anopheles* do not fly more than 2 km, but in certain circumstances, they can regularly fly 3 to 5 and even up to 7 km.[1,3,4] There are, however, several accounts of long-distance migration, assisted in almost all instances by the wind. Distances of 100 km or more have been recorded. The distance mosquitoes fly is determined largely by the environment: if suitable hosts and breeding places are nearby, mosquitoes do not have to disperse far, but if one or both are more distant, greater dispersal will be necessary.[1]

Classification

The classification of the arthropods is a matter of considerable controversy, and several different schemes have been proposed (Table 6–1).[5–7]

Behavior and Breeding Sites

In search of a blood meal, the female mosquito is guided by several cues, the most important being heat, moisture, carbon dioxide (CO_2), and odor.

Sight also plays an important role. During daytime, movement and dark-colored clothing may initiate an orientation toward a person.[8,9] Carbon dioxide, released mainly from breath but also from skin, serves as a long-range airborne attractant and can be detected by mosquitoes at distances of up to 36 m. At close range, skin temperature and moisture serve as attractants.[9]

The periodicity of biting times is basically controlled by endogenous (circadian) rhythms, but environmental factors such as wind, temperature, and moonlight are capable of modifying biting activity. In some species (e.g., *Anopheles implexus*), biting patterns are known to be different in different microhabitats. Most mosquitoes are zoophagic, exophagic (i.e., they feed outdoors), and exophilic (they rest outdoors), but some enter houses to feed and are termed endophagic. Several important vector species are largely endophagic and endophilic (they rest inside after engorging). Some mosquitoes bite predominantly in forests or woods, others fly outside to feed, and some bite mainly in and around farms whereas many anthropophagic species bite in towns and villages. While most mosquitoes bite at ground level, feeding may be at different heights, depending on species and the main host.[1] With exophilic species, indoor spraying has less impact on vector control.[1,10] In sub-Saharan Africa, 80% to 90% of malaria transmission takes place during the second part of the night.[11] *Anopheles gambiae*, the principal vector of malaria in Africa, bites predominantly indoors and after midnight.[1] If there are numerous

Table 6–1. **Proposed Classification of the Genus *Anopheles***

Phylum	Class	Order	Family	Subfamily	Genus	Species
Arthropoda	Hexapoda (Insecta)	Diptera	Culicidae	Anophelinae	*Anopheles*	*Anopheles* spp

breeding sites throughout the year, the dry and rainy seasons may have less effect on anopheline populations, and feeding may be all through the night. Under certain conditions, *Anopheles* may develop a night-and-day feeding pattern.[10]

In summary, *Anopheles* mosquito biting activity varies considerably, depending on local factors and species, as can be seen in Table 6–2.[1,10,12–17] Depending on human behavior and geographic location (foresters, children, rural vs. urban population, etc.), the risk of getting bitten may be quite different. As it is not possible and practical to know when different local vectors have their peak activity for each malaria-endemic area, and as activity may be quite different depending on microclimate, it is best to advise the traveler that malaria is transmitted almost exclusively from dusk to (and including) dawn although dawn does not seem to be the main activity time for many *Anopheles* species.

Anopheles larvae can be found in different types of large and more-or-less permanent habitats (fresh- and saltwater marshes, mangrove swamps, grassy ditches, rice fields, edges of streams and rivers, ponds, and borrow pits) but can also be found in small and often temporary breeding places (e.g., puddles, hoofprints, wells, discarded tins, water storage pots, water-filled tree holes, and leaf axils of epiphytic plants). *Anopheles* prefer clean and unpolluted water.[7] There are some exceptions, though, like *Anopheles stephensi*, an important malaria vector especially in and around town, which is also able to breed in brackish[18] and even polluted

Table 6–2. **Approximate Biting Behavior of Some Malaria Vectors**

Vector	Dusk	Night (→ 24:00)	Night (24:00 →)	Dawn
		Time of Evening/Morning		
A. albimanus	++ outdoors			
A. arabiensis		+	++	
A. culicifacies		++		
A. darlingi*	+	+	+	+
A. dirius		++	+	
A. gambiae†			++ indoors	
A. maculatus	++	++		
A. minimus	+	+	+	+
A. nuneztrovari		++	++	
A. punctulatus		++		
A. sundaicus		++	++	
A. triannulatus	+	+		

++ = peak biting activity; *A.* = *Anopheles.*
*Principal vector in Amazonia.
† Principal vector in Africa.

waters.[19] Some mosquitoes of the *Anopheles gambiae* complex, such as *Anopheles melas* and *Anopheles merus,* can breed in salt water.[19] In short, given the right climatic conditions, minimal amounts of water will allow *Anopheles* to breed.

Transmission Potential

Although the salivary glands may contain as many as 60,000 to 70,000 sporozoites, only a few are injected into a person during a mosquito's blood meal.[1] It can be expected that at least half of the bites from an *Anopheles* that carries sporozoites of *Plasmodium falciparum* in its salivary glands will give a blood infection followed by a clinical attack in nonimmune subjects.[20] A mosquito, once infective, remains so throughout life.[1]

Below 15°C, sporogony in the extrinsic cycle (the development stage of *Plasmodium* in the mosquito) cannot be completed.[7] In other words, if the average temperature in a certain geographic region stays below 15°C, malaria transmission cannot take place. There are few data available on the maximum altitude at which malaria is still transmitted, and this is certainly dependent on the local climate and microclimate. To be sure that no transmission can occur, maximum isotherm during the whole year should not exceed 15°C. In general, malaria should not be transmitted above 2,500 m although transmissions at altitudes of 2,600 m (Kenya and Bolivia) and even more (2,773 meters by mosquitoes breeding in thermal springs) occurred in the early half of the 20th century.[21]

Risk of Transmission to Travelers

There are several indicators that estimate the transmission rate of malaria. Some are better suited than others to describe the malaria risk to nonimmune individuals. While the prevalence and incidence of malaria in the indigenous population are of importance to local health issues, they provide only an indirect and imprecise measure of the risk of malaria to travelers. In most cases, the situation of the traveler does not correspond to that of the indigenous population. The fraction of nonimmune people in the local population may vary drastically due to population movements and/or age distribution.[22] This can have a large effect on the incidence of malaria cases; transmission may be quite low with a high incidence recorded in the indigenous population or vice versa. Local mortality is not a suitable parameter, either. Data from Africa suggest that there is no marked variation in malaria mortality and prevalence when the entomological inoculation rate (EIR)—the number of infective bites per person per year in a defined area—is 1 or higher.[22,23] With decreasing EIR, there is a shift in the incidence of malaria attacks, from earlier to later in life.[22]

One of the best ways to describe the risk of transmission is by the EIR. It is a more direct measure of transmission intensity than traditional epidemiologic measures of malaria prevention or hospital-based measures of infection or disease incidence.[23] Annual EIR is defined as the number of infective bites per person per year in a defined area. The daily EIR is calculated as:

$$h' = mas$$

where h' is the daily number of infective mosquito bites received per person, m is the anopheline density in relation to humans, a is the average number of persons bitten by one mosquito in a day, and s is the proportion of mosquitoes with sporozoites in their salivary glands. The annual EIR may range from about 0.001 to several thousand infective bites per year and person.[22–24] The drawbacks of the EIR are that (1) the entomological methods are not standardized and that (2) to be representative of the year, the estimate of the biting rate and the sporozoite index must be repeated monthly or more frequently for at least a year or the complete transmission season.[22,24] Generally, the higher the EIR, the greater is the risk for the traveler of acquiring malaria even though the local malaria mortality and prevalence may stay the same over a wide range of different EIRs. For a comparison of EIRs in different areas of the world, see Chapter 2, "Global Epidemiology of Malaria."

The distribution of the malaria vector is discussed in more detail in Chapter 2, "Global Epidemiology of Malaria." Distribution is worldwide, not only in tropical regions but also in subtropical and some temperate regions.

PERSONAL PROTECTION MEASURES

Not traveling to endemic areas is the best way to avoid malaria. This is what should be advised to persons at higher risk than the average traveler for severe malaria, like pregnant women,[25–28] infants, and possibly those who have undergone a splenectomy.[29–31] Particularly among infants, the development of severe malaria can be very rapid, and death can occur within hours of the onset of illness.[29,32] Case-fatality rates among imported malaria cases in Europe average 1.1% and range from between 0% to 3.6% (German travelers).[33,34]

If travel to a malarious area cannot be avoided, several options, which should usually be combined for greater efficacy, are available. Chemoprophylaxis and standby emergency self-treatment (SBET) are dealt with in detail in other chapters of this book. Physical and chemical measures (personal protection measures) complement chemoprophylaxis and SBET. Travelers to malaria-endemic regions should become well acquainted with these personal protection measures (PPMs) because such measures, if used properly, can reduce the rate of mosquito bites substantially (in one study, from over 1,000 bites to 1 bite per hour).[35]

Schoepke and colleagues[36] reported that only 1.8% (1,594) of travelers questioned in a survey and visiting malaria-endemic areas in tropical Africa systematically and regularly adhered to all PPMs (air-conditioned room, bednet, adequate clothing, insecticides and/or coils) although only two-thirds of the travelers were apparently aware that such actions might be beneficial. The largest group of travelers (66,542 or 74.3%) reported regular use of some PPMs while 19% (17,061) reported irregular use, and 4.8% (4,319) used no PPMs at all. Compliance increased in periods when more mosquito bites were noticed and was higher among first-time travelers to tropical Africa and among persons staying in hotels on the beach than among those on safari or those on longer stay. When comparing zero PPMs to maximum PPMs, a significant but modest reduction of malaria to approximately 50% was noticed. Among the separate measures, only air-conditioned rooms and clothing covering arms and legs significantly reduced the malaria risk in this study. In a study of in-flight travelers to South African game parks, 89% (2,528) reported using PPMs, 21% of whom used only a single measure while 67% used several.[37] In Germany, only 7% of those infected with malaria reported using a mosquito net, 5% reported using a repellent, and 6% used a repellent plus a mosquito net.[38]

There is an obvious need not only to explain PPMs to travelers but also to convince travelers of their ease of use and to emphasis the regular use of not only one but a combination of several PPMs. In the case of long-term residency in malaria-endemic areas (where malaria prophylaxis is not a feasible option) and in the case of limited compliance with prophylaxis, PPMs may be the only possible preventive measures.

PPMs available to the traveler are the following:

1. Chemical measures
   - Repellents (skin application)
   - Insecticides
2. Physical measures
   - Clothing
   - Mosquito nets
   - Screens, air-conditioning, coils, vaporizers
3. Behavior

Chemical Measures

Many studies have shown that repellents and insecticides, when properly used, significantly reduce the biting rate of mosquitoes. In nonimmune travelers, this inevitably leads to a reduction in the risk of acquiring malaria even if not all bites can be avoided, because not all *Anopheles* mosquitoes (even in a holoendemic area) are infected. In Africa, sporozoite rates generally range from around 1% to 10%[22,39–44] but rarely may reach peaks of up to 25%.[45]

Repellents: DEET

The function of repellents should be to reduce the attractiveness of humans as a target for mosquitoes and other biting insects. Repellents interfere in a complex fashion with factors (such as heat, moisture, CO_2, and odor) that attract female mosquitoes to a human target.[8] There are many compounds on the market, but only a few offer adequate protective properties over an acceptable time span. Others have no effect at all and are a waste of money and a potential hazard because of the false feeling of security they engender.

N,N-diethyl-3-methylbenzamide (DEET) (previously N,N-diethyl-m-toluamide), the most widely used synthetic broad-spectrum insect repellent in the world, was developed in the 1960s by the U.S. Department of Agriculture (Figure 6–1).[46] Today, it is still one of the most effective repellents available, showing activity against mosquitoes, biting flies, chiggers, fleas, and ticks.[9,47,48] Although products with DEET concentrations from 2% to 100% are available on the market, ideal concentrations for travelers are from 10% to 35% because of increased toxicity and proportionally little gain of added protection at higher concentrations.[9,47,49–51] Mathematic models of the effectiveness and persistence of mosquito repellents show that the protection offered by a repellent is proportional to the logarithm of the concentration of the product. This curve tends to form a plateau at higher repellent concentrations, providing relatively less added protection for each incremental dose of DEET that exceeds a 50% concentration.[52–54]

Safety. Preparations containing less than 50% DEET are almost free of side effects when applied to the skin of adults.[47] Toxicity is remarkably low, with an oral lethal dose in 50% of test animals (LD_{50}) in rats of 2,000 mg/kg of body weight or more,[55] as compared, for instance, to caffeine, with an LD_{50} of 355mg/kg of body weight. It is generally regarded as safe for dermal use, as evidenced by over four decades of human experience, and experimental studies have confirmed that DEET-related toxicity is minimal after systemic absorption.[56] Transdermal absorption depends on site of application, formulation, and dose: up to a fourfold difference in transdermal bioavailability was observed in monkeys among different sites of the body surface.[57] Mean hourly absorption for the first 12 hours, when measured by carbon-14 (^{14}C) radioisotopic technique, was < 1% of the der-

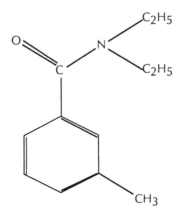

Figure 6–1. Molecular structure of N,N-diethyl-3-methylbenzamide (previously N,N-diethyl-m-toluamide)(DEET) ($C_{12} H_{17} NO$).

mal dose (4 μg/cm^2) after application on the ventral surface of the forearm. Once absorbed, DEET undergoes extensive metabolism before being excreted in urine. Elimination appears to be fast, and bioaccumulation is thus unlikely. DEET can enhance the skin penetration of some drugs like hydrocortisone or nifedipine. Dermatitis is the major local adverse effect associated with the dermal use of DEET-containing insect repellent formulations. Allergic reactions, cardiovascular (e.g., hypotension, bradycardia) and neurologic toxicities (e.g., convulsions and seizures, particularly among children and after ingestion) and even death have been reported.[48,58,59] Given only 14 to 32 cases of seizures in the United States since 1960 and 50 to 80 million people using DEET each year, the observed incidence of recognized seizures is about 1 per 100 million users.[55] Compared with the estimates of over 200 million people who use DEET products worldwide annually[49,60] and the annual use of DEET-containing insect repellents by about 30% of Americans and 25% of the population of the United Kingdom, the risk of serious medical effects appears to be low;[46,51] serious reactions are extremely rare, and even skin irritation and allergic responses are uncommon.[49,51] If properly used, DEET can be regarded as safe.

Use in Pregnancy. There are limited data on the use of DEET during pregnancy. Animal studies have yielded mixed results. While DEET skin application of up to 5,000 mg/kg/d for 30 days in rabbits during gestation did not yield significant differences between controls and treated mothers,[60] doses of 1,000 mg/kg/d in rats did result in a significant reduction in implantation and an increase in prenatal mortality.[61,62] Studies of the oral application of DEET to rats did show a slight increase in postimplantation loss and a statistically significant decrease in mean fetal body weight per litter in the high-dose group (750 mg/kg/d). At lower doses and in rabbits, no evidence of treatment-related developmental toxicity was reported.[55] On mutagenicity, the Environmental Protection Agency (EPA) Reregistration Eligibility Decision (RED) Facts Report concludes that the required battery for DEET has been met, that the results are all negative, and that DEET is not mutagenic under the conditions of the test assays.[55] These data seem to indicate that at least in animal testing, DEET had no effect on the fetus until very high doses of administration were reached. How far these results are applicable to humans is difficult to say, but they are an indicator that DEET is most probably no problem during pregnancy, when applied properly. To be on the safe side, the same precautions that are applied to children should be applied to pregnant women (see below). Malaria during pregnancy does almost certainly pose a much greater risk for the unborn infant and the mother. If travel to a malaria-endemic area cannot be avoided during pregnancy, a combination of different PPMs, including a repellent, should be used.

Formulations. DEET is available in different formulations and application forms such as pump spray, aerosol spray, lotion, stick, gel, soap, and impregnated towelettes.[46] Newer formulations using sustained-release technology and new polymers in which DEET is encapsulated in hydrogel emulsions, lipospheres, microcapsules, and microparticles offer longer protection times. Compared with alcohol-based formulations, absolute bioavailability with a liposphere solution was reduced from 45% to 16%, a threefold reduction in the amount of DEET absorbed.[63] While safer and more pleasant to use, these formulations achieve their extended protection by (1) regulating DEET evaporation by controlling the release of DEET and /or lowering the vapor pressure of DEET in the formulation; (2) preventing or reducing DEET transdermal absorption by retaining DEET in the superficial layers of the skin; and (3) being more resistant to loss from being wiped off and from sweating.[56,58]

Controlled-release formulations have been shown to be equally effective in the field at up to half the concentration of a standard ethanol-based formulation. Mean complete protection time (the time from application of the repellent to the time of the first confirmed bite) for the controlled-release preparation containing 35% DEET was 12 hours for the arms and 6.7 hours for the head.[64]

Duration of Protection. Repellents are lost from skin through mechanical removal,[65] evaporation, and absorption. Mechanical removal through friction with clothing and other objects is the single greatest source of loss. Repellents are easily washed off by water and lose their effect in seconds to minutes; they should therefore be re-applied after bathing. Sweating also washes off repellents and may be particularly profuse under hot conditions and exercise; in such circumstances, repellents have to be re-applied more often. There is a significant negative correlation between protection time and temperature. With every rise of 10°C, protection time is halved because hot weather increases volatility; wind can additionally and significantly reduce protection time.[8,49] The same repellent applied at the same dose per unit area under identical ambient conditions will give a different protection time on different individuals.[66] Depending on these factors, the duration of protection by a certain product may vary markedly under different conditions. As declarations of average protection time by the manufacturer usually represent laboratory data and not field conditions, it is prudent to divide the specified duration of protection by two or three and to adjust for temperature, kind of activity, exposure to wind, and mechanical removal.[67]

Practical Guidelines for Application. If the following rules (in part taken from the EPA) are applied, the use of DEET-containing repellents may generally be regarded as safe; the following guidelines should also be used when applying any other repellent:

- Combine repellent with other PPMs such as permethrin-impregnated (long) clothing to reduce exposed skin surface to a minimum.

- Use repellent only if exposed to mosquitoes (*Anopheles* mosquitoes are mainly active from dusk until dawn).[10]
- Do not apply repellent to mucous membranes; macerated, inflamed, or irritated skin; cuts; wounds; or eczema.
- Avoid contact of repellent with eyes and mouth. Do not apply repellent to children's hands, because they are likely to put them into their mouths.
- Use just enough repellent to lightly cover the skin. Do not saturate the skin. Two to four tablespoons should be sufficient to cover the arms, legs, and face of an average adult.[68]
- Repellents should be applied only to exposed skin, clothing, or both. Do not apply repellents underneath clothing.
- To apply a repellent to the face, dispense it onto the palms, rub the hands together, and apply a thin layer to the face.
- After applying, wipe or wash the repellent from the palms to prevent inadvertent contact with eyes, mouth, or genitals.
- Do not inhale aerosol formulations. Be careful to not let the spray drift into the eyes.
- Once indoors, wash treated areas with soap and water.
- Newer, extended-release preparations (which lead to a steadier release of repellent from the skin) should be preferred as protection times similar to those of higher-dosed standard formulations can be achieved with lower concentrations.
- Use products with a DEET concentration of 10% to 35%. If exposure is prolonged, these products can be applied several times.
- If using a sunscreen and a repellent at the same time, apply the repellent *after* the sunscreen.

Use in Children. In their study of 9,086 human exposures to DEET reported to the Poison Control Centers from 1985 to 1989, Veltri and colleagues found no relationship between age, gender, or concentration of DEET and the severity of the reaction by any of the various measures of severity available in the database.[46] Children less than 6 years of age were not more likely to develop adverse effects from DEET-containing products than older children or adults, and the effects that occurred in children were not more serious. The occurrence of adverse effects appeared to be related to the route of exposure rather than to the age or gender of the patient or to the concentration of DEET in the product formulation. Nonetheless, it seems prudent to

1. use repellents containing ≤ 10% DEET in children[9,69] because of a larger surface-to-volume ratio[49] compared to adults,
2. reduce the total amount of applied repellent by covering all possible areas with clothing, and
3. avoid applying a repellent to children's hands.

Other Precautions. DEET can damage plastics, synthetic fabrics, leather, and painted or varnished materials, so care must be taken not to apply it to surfaces such as eyeglass frames, watch crystals, walls, or furniture. DEET does not damage natural fibers, such as cotton or wool, and has no effect on nylon.

Other Repellents

Synthetics. Of the synthetic compounds, only the new product KBR 3023 (1-piperidinecarboxylic acid [2-2-hydroxy-ethyl]-ester 1-methyl-propyl-ester) was as effective as DEET in one study[70] and seems to have less potential for side effects than DEET[71] although it has been less extensively tested than DEET.

IR35/35 (ethyl-butylacetylaminoproprionate [EPAAP]) seems to have less potential for side effects than DEET. Particularly in laboratory settings, it has been shown to be less effective than DEET or KBR 3023.[71] At a concentration of 20%, it showed good protection times of around 8 hours for *Aedes aegypti* and *Anopheles stephensi*.[11]

Dimethyl phthalate (DMP) reportedly offers only 1.5 hours of protection at a concentration of 40%,[11] markedly shorter than protection with DEET. There is not much experience concerning its potential for adverse events and its efficacy against different vectors.[71]

Ethylhexanediol (Rutgers 612) is less effective than DEET, with protection times varying between 1.5 to 6 hours and between different vectors.[11,71]

The same precautions applied for DEET should be applied when any of the above repellents are used.

Natural Oils and Derivatives. Limited experience with natural oils used as insect repellents means their true safety profile, unlike that of DEET, has yet to be determined. One death after the ingestion of citronella oil by a 21-month-old child and by two deaths after the ingestion of eucalyptus oil have been reported.[51] None of the plant-derived chemicals tested to date demonstrate the broad effectiveness and duration of DEET.[9] Plants whose essential oils have been reported to have repellent activity include citronella (*Cymbopogon nardus*), cedar, verbena, pennyroyal, rosemary, basil, thyme, allspice, garlic, peppermint, eucalyptus (*Eucalyptus maculata citriodon*), *Lantana*, and neem (*Azadirachta indica*).[9,11] Combinations of plant derivatives have also been used, with varying success. Unlike synthetic insect repellents, plant-derived repellents have been relatively poorly studied. When tested, most of these essential oils tended to give short-lasting protection, usually less than 2 hours,[9] and, as has been jestingly remarked, some have such an unpleasant odor that one might well "repel" other persons in one's vicinity who would perhaps be more attractive targets for mosquitoes. Others are simply useless and may even attract mosquitoes.[67] The oil of the neem tree seems to be one of the few promising exceptions and has shown promising results in studies in India.[11] In general, the use of DEET or another synthetic product is advised over natural oils and their derivatives. Besides being generally less effective, they cannot be considered to be safer as there is only limited experience, and severe adverse reactions have been reported.

Insecticides: for Textile Impregnation and Knockdown Activity

Some of the most useful insecticides available today for use on clothing or nets or in the house originally derive from the pyrethrum plant *Chrysanthemum cinerariaefolium*, which contains pyrethrins toxic to insects (Figure 6–2). They are called pyrethroids and are produced synthetically, with the advantage of knowing the exact concentration and composition of a certain compound. A summary of available pyrethroids and their properties is provided in Table 6–3.[72–76]

A good insecticide to use on clothing should fulfill as many of the following points as possible:[77]

- Rapid acting (i.e., rapid knockdown after contact)
- Long lasting
- Safe
- Little or no color and odor
- Resistant to weathering, washing, and light-induced chemical breakdown

Insecticides can be used as stand-alone measures, but it is advisable to combine them with a repellent applied to exposed skin. Although insecticides themselves do show some repellent properties, it is not enough to wear impregnated clothing. Mosquitos are known to selectively pick patches of untreated skin in persons who have applied a repellent to the skin.

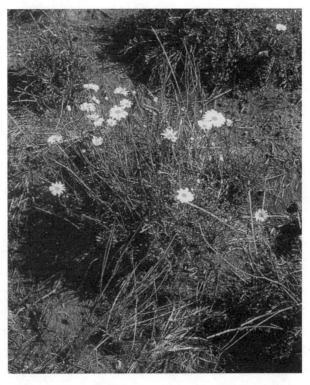

Figure 6–2. *Chrysanthemum cinerariaefolium.* (Courtesy of D. Stürchler). (See Color Plates)

Table 6–3. **Available Pyrethroids and Their Properties**

Compound	Properties/Comments
Permethrin ($C_{21}H_{20}Cl_2O_3$)	The most commonly recommended insecticide for impregnation of bednets and clothing. There are no reports of adverse side effects. An odorless, colorless crystalline solid or viscous liquid that is pale brown and stable in air and light. Half-life of < 5 days when in water.
	Formulations: Dusts, emulsifiable concentrates, smoke, and UVL and wettable powder formulations.
	Toxicity: Moderately to practically nontoxic via oral route, with a reported LD_{50} for technical permethrin in rats of 430 to 4,000 mg/kg. Slightly toxic via dermal route, with a reported dermal LD_{50} in rats of over 4,000 mg/kg and in rabbits of > 2,000 mg/kg. Reproductive effects are not likely to be seen in humans under normal circumstances. Reported to show no teratogenic and mutagenic activity.
	Metabolism and elimination in humans and animals: Efficiently metabolized by mammalian livers. Its metabolites are quickly excreted and do not persist significantly in body tissues. When permethrin is administered orally to rats, it is rapidly metabolized and almost completely eliminated from the body in a few days. Only 3% to 6% of the original dose was excreted unchanged in feces of experimental animals. May persist in fatty tissues, with half-life of 4 to 5 days in brain and body fat. Does not block or inhibit cholinesterase enzymes.
	Environment: Toxic to aquatic organisms, so should not be disposed into water. Degrades fairly quickly in soil, with half-life of between 30 and 38 days.
Deltamethrin ($C_{22}H_{19}Br_2NO_3$)	30 times as powerful as permethrin; recommended dosage is much lower than that of permethrin. Toxicity to humans is higher than that of permethrin, and there have been complaints about irritant effect during the impregnation process although people sleeping under dry nets usually experience no side effects. Appearance: colorless crystalline powder; white or slightly beige powder.
	Formulations include emulsifiable concentrates, wettable powders, ULV and flowable formulations and granules.
	Toxicity: LD_{50} is from 2–2.6 mg/kg (IV) to 10,000 mg/kg (percutaneous), depending on animal, study, and route of administration. Studies have shown many cases of dermal poisoning after agricultural use with inadequate handling precautions and many cases of accidental or suicidal poisoning by the oral route at doses estimated at 2–250 mg/kg. Oral ingestion caused epigastric pain, nausea, vomiting, and coarse muscular fasciculations. Doses of 100–250 mg/kg caused coma within 15–20 min. Suspected chronic exposure effects in humans include choreoathetosis, hypotension, prenatal damage, and shock. (Workers exposed for over 7–8 years to deltamethrin during its manufacture experienced transient cutaneous and mucous membrane irritation, which could have been prevented by use of gloves and face masks. No other ill effects were seen.) No teratogenic activity.
	Metabolism and elimination in humans: Physical signs of poisoning can include dermatitis after skin contact; exposure to sunlight can make it worse. Severe swelling of the face, including lips and eyelids, can occur. Symptoms and consequences of poisoning include sweating, fever, anxiety, and rapid heartbeat. If swallowed, symptoms may include feeling sick, vomiting, diarrhea, twitching of arms and legs, and convulsions if poisoning is severe. (People working with permethrin reported burning sensation and tightness and numbness on the face, sniffing and sneezing, other abnormal sensations in the face, dizziness, tiredness, red skin rashes, cold burning and numbness of the skin, eye watering, headache, heartburn, and skin spots. If proper precautions such as wearing gloves and an apron were used, few to no adverse events were reported.)
	Environment: Toxic to aquatic organisms (not fish), so should not be disposed into water. Degrades within 1–2 weeks in soil. Rapidly adsorbed in surface water, mostly by sediment, in addition to uptake by plants and evaporation into air.

Continued on next page

Compound	Properties/Comments
Lambda Cyhalothrin ($C_{23}H_{19}ClF_3NO_3$)	Newly developed insecticide, similar to deltamethrin. Causes nasal irritation to some people sleeping under freshly treated nets, even when nets are dry. A colorless solid at room temperature, but may appear yellowish in solution.
	Formulations: Emulsifiable concentrate, wettable powder or ULV liquid; commonly mixed with buprofezin, pirimicarb, dimethoate, or tetramethrin.
	Toxicity: Moderately toxic in the technical form, but may be highly toxic via some routes in formulation (e.g., inhalation). Available data indicate moderate toxicity via oral route in test animals. Tingling, burning or numbness sensations (particularly at point of skin contact), tremors, incoordination of movement, paralysis or other disrupted motor functions, and confusion or loss of consciousness may be observed. (Since most pyrethroids are generally absorbed poorly through the skin, the latter two systemic effects are unlikely unless the compound has been ingested.) Effects are generally reversible due to rapid breakdown of the compound in the body. Observed toxicity may vary not only according to the concentration of the active ingredient, but also according to the solvent vehicle. The principal toxic effects noted in chronic studies in animals were decreased body weight gain and food consumption. Unlikely to cause chronic and reproductive effects in humans under normal conditions. Available evidence suggests that it is nonmutagenic and nongenotoxic.
	Environment: Highly toxic to many fish and aquatic invertebrate species, so should not be disposed into water. Reported field half-life in soil is 4–12 weeks. Has extremely low water solubility and is tightly bound to soil, therefore is not expected to be prevalent in surface waters.
Cyfluthrin ($C_{22}H_{18}Cl_2FNO_3$)	More toxic to insects than permethrin but less toxic than lambda cyhalothrin and deltamethrin. No side effects reported, but testing has been very limited. Appearance: pasty yellow mass.
	Formulation: Emulsifiable concentrates, wettable powder, aerosol, granules, liquid, oil-in-water emulsion, and ULV oil spray.
	Toxicity: Considered moderately toxic to mammals; a skin and eye irritant in humans. (Pyrethroid poisonings are rare. The main reason for their low toxicity in humans is that they are rapidly broken down in the human body by liver proteins and eliminated fairly quickly. Also, pyrethroids are not well absorbed into the blood stream, contributing to their moderate acute toxicity in mammals.) May cause itching, burning, or stinging if it comes in contact with human skin; these sensations can progress to a numbing effect that may last up to 24 hours. Skin irritation is usually delayed for 1–2 hours following exposure but may occur immediately. Dermal irritation may be worsened by sweating, exposure to sun or heat, and application of water. (The only long-term effects of exposure to cyfluthrin were the retardation of weight gain and changes in some organ weights associated with body weight effects in the high-dose groups [rats, dogs]. No developmental abnormalities were observed at the highest dose tested.)
	Metabolism and elimination in humans and animals: Cyfluthrin metabolism in mammals occurs in two phases (biphasic)—an initial fast phase and a slower second phase. Laboratory tests show that about 60% of an IV dose is eliminated in the urine in the 1st 24 hours, with only an additional 6% eliminated in the next 24 hours. Similarly, 20% of the administered dose was eliminated in the feces in the 1st day, followed by 3%–4% the next day. Another test with a single oral dose showed that 98% was eliminated by 48 hours.
	Environment: Highly toxic to marine and freshwater organisms and should not be disposed into water. Sensitive to breakdown by sunlight. Half-life is 48 hours (surface) to 63 days. Broken down quickly in surface water. Because it is relatively nonsoluble and less dense than water, it will float on the surface film of natural waters.
Other pyrethroids	The toxicities of cypermethrin, flumethrin, and alphacypermethrin range between those of permethrin and deltamethrin. However, these insecticides have not yet been fully tested for efficacy and safety in the treatment of mosquito nets or clothing.

IV = intravenously; LD_{50} = lethal dose in 50% of test animals; ULV = ultra low-volume.
Data from Rozendaal et al.[72] and Extension Toxicology Network.[73–76]

Permethrin. Permethrin (Figure 6–3) is a quick-acting synthetic pyrethroid insecticide with additional repellent properties.[78] People who are sleeping in a room in which there is a treated mosquito net but who are sleeping outside of the net may also get some protection from permethrin (1) because of its repellent properties (fewer mosquitoes in the room) and (2) because mosquitoes alighting on the net die, which further reduces mosquito density. The spray form is non-staining, nearly odorless, and resistant to degradation by heat or sun. It maintains its potency for at least 2 weeks, even through several launderings.[77,79] *It should not be applied to the skin.*

The following formulations of permethrin are available:[72]

1. Solutions (emulsifiable concentrates) that can be mixed with water to produce a milky liquid.
2. Oil-in-water emulsion formulations made especially for the treatment of fabrics; they adhere well and do not produce an unpleasant odor during treatment.
3. Wettable powders or suspension concentrates (flowable concentrates) are less suitable for treating fabrics since they are more easily dislodged. The period of effectiveness is reduced, and dislodged particles may cause skin irritation.
4. Prepared sprays. These may be a good option for the traveler, who does not have time, facilities, or patience to soak clothing or other fabrics in a solution.

Application with sprays is mentioned here first because this may be the most practical way for the traveler to impregnate fabrics. Compliance is an important factor, not to be forgotten. Calculating impregnation doses on the basis of surface area may already be too demanding for the average traveler.

The following are advantages of sprays:[72]

- Both application and drying are quick.
- For thicker fabrics, application on only the outer surface may reduce losses of insecticide by inward penetration.

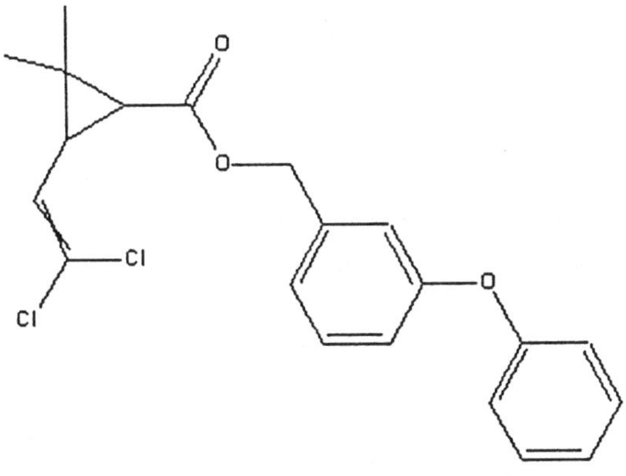

Figure 6–3. Molecular structure of permethrin ($C_{21}H_{20}Cl_2O_3$).

• Less insecticide can be used if it is applied only to the parts where contact with insects is likely to occur.

Two of the disadvantages are (1) uneven distribution of the insecticide and (2) loss of considerable quantities of insecticide into the atmosphere.

To apply permethrin spray to clothing, spray each side of the exposed area of the fabric for 30 to 45 seconds, just enough to moisten it, and then allow it to dry for 2 to 4 hours before wearing.[9] This is best done in the open. Spraying of the walls, curtains, and other objects where mosquitoes might rest, particularly in the sleeping room, can further reduce mosquito density by killing insects and by the additional repellent effect. Tents and other fabrics where insects might make contact can also be treated. Together with the physical measures discussed below, the mosquito burden can be significantly reduced.

Soaking of fabrics leads to an even distribution and concentration of the active agent. It is questionable, however, if this procedure is practical for most travelers because of its complexity.[72] With the advent of preimpregnated nets and the anticipated difficulties of soaking clothing and nets, sprays seem to be more practical for travelers. (A more detailed description for dedicated, compliant travelers can be found in the WHO publication by Rozendaal and colleagues.)[72]

If possible, the soaking of fabrics should be done outdoors or in well-ventilated areas. Gloves should be worn. The insecticide mixture should not come in contact with the skin, particularly the lips, mouth, eyes, and any open wounds. Fumes should not be inhaled. Care should be taken with the disposal of used chemicals to prevent possible environmental contamination.

To treat mosquito nets and other fabrics, the following steps should be taken:[72,80]

1. Be sure the fabric to be treated is clean and dry.
2. Calculate the surface area (in square meters) of the fabric to be treated.
3. Determine the amount of water needed to completely soak the fabric.
4. Partially fill a bowl or bucket with a known quantity of water (note this in milliliters).
5. Soak the fabric in the water.
6. Wring it gently and/or allow it to finish dripping, collecting the runoff in the container.
7. Measure the difference between the initial amount and the remaining amount of water. The difference in grams is equal to the number of milliliters of water absorbed by the fabric. Divide the volume of water the fabric takes up by the area of the fabric, to obtain the volume per square meter of fabric.
8. Prepare the solution for treatment. Of course, the fabric should be dry before being soaked a second time.

The amounts of permethrin needed to impregnate different fabrics are shown in Table 6–4.[72,81] Mosquito nets and other fabrics can also be impregnated inside a plastic bag. This avoids contact with toxic vapors. The plastic bag should be filled with the needed amount of mixture. Once the fabric has been put into the bag and the opening is tightly sealed, the bag is shaken and vigorously kneaded to distribute the insecticide evenly.[11,72] A further possibility that has been reported to the author is to seal the muzzle of a spray can tightly with the opening of a plastic bag to produce a vapor inside the bag, and then to again vigorously knead the content for even distribution.

After treatment, the fabric should be allowed to dry completely, first on the ground (for even distribution) and then by hanging. Exposure to bright sunlight may partially destroy pyrethroid insecticides, so it is preferable to keep wet fabrics away from sunshine.

Gas chromatography tests of clothing (100% cotton twill and 50% cotton/50% polyester olive drab) treated with 0.125 mg/cm^2 of permethrin and worn by test subjects showed that 24% to 48% of the chemical remained after 10 to 30 days of wearing whereas aging without being worn (patches packed in aluminum foil and stored at constant temperature) did not appreciably reduce the amount of permethrin during the 30 days of the test. Knockdown time for *Aedes aegypti* and *Anopheles quadrimaculatus* was increased fivefold after 30 days. The amount remaining and unchanged after 2 weeks to 1 month (0.033 to 0.061 mg/cm^2) appeared sufficient to effectively protect against some arthropods that attack man; minimum effective doses to give a quick kill (on contact) for mosquitoes, flies, fleas, and ticks, depending on the length of contact and on the insect, lay between 0.008 and < 1.0 mg/cm^2.[77,79] Schreck and colleagues[77] concluded that permethrin at starting concentrations (i.e., concentrations in clothing at the beginning of a test) of 0.125 to 0.25 mg/cm^2 would be quick-acting, with only momentary contact, against most of the test species. With these concentrations, a 100% kill of *Aedes aegypti* was still achieved after 33 to 50 cold rinses whereas washing with hot water and soap rapidly reduced permethrin concentrations and concomitant effectiveness.

In conclusion, properly impregnated clothing (0.125 to 0.25 mg/cm^2) can be expected to remain effective for at least 2 weeks to 1 month even after several launderings with soap in cold or lukewarm water or after exposure to weathering.[54,77,79]

Table 6–4. **Amounts of Permethrin Needed to Impregnate Different Types of Fabric**

Fabric	Dose (g/m^2)*
Wide-mesh netting (> 2 mm)	0.10–0.25[†]
Standard mosquito mesh (1.5 mm)	0.20–0.50[†]
Cotton cloth (sheeting, shirts)	0.70–1.20
Thick fabrics (jackets, trousers)	0.65–1.25

*1 g/m^2 = 0.1 mg/cm^2.
[†]It has been proposed to increase World Health Organization (WHO) standard recommendations for permethrin of 0.25% to 0.5–1.0% because of increased vector resistances to permethrin.

Although the treatment rate of 0.5% permethrin aerosols to clothing is only 10% of the 0.125 mg/cm^2 rate described above, the reduced application rate was effective because of only slight penetration of the cloth. Virtually all the permethrin is concentrated at the outer surface and is in contact with a landing insect.[82] Sprayed clothing should thus also offer protection for at least 2 weeks. Table 6–5 shows the approximate duration of the residual efficacy of permethrin applied to clothing and nets under various conditions.[11,54,77,79,83]

To prolong the duration of efficacy,

- avoid unnecessary handling of treated fabrics;
- treat fabric soon after washing, so that it will not need to be washed again for some time after treatment;
- store the fabric in a plastic bag or box (this avoids both deterioration of the insecticide and the accumulation of dust);
- use alternative methods of cleaning (e.g., shaking or brushing with a soft brush; if washing cannot be postponed, the fabric should be washed in cold water without using soap);
- use colored nets that do not show dirt or dust; and
- time treatment in accordance with the seasonal patterns of biting and disease transmission.

Permethrin degrades fairly quickly, once it has been mixed with water (it has a half-life of < 5 days when in water).[73] Sprays made of a concentrate mixed with water remain effective only for a limited amount of time, once mixed.

Resistance to pyrethroids has been detected in several species of mosquitoes, for instance, *Aedes aegypti* in Puerto Rico and Indonesia and *Anopheles gambiae* in West Africa. This development is most probably due to the agricultural and domestic use of pyrethroids. Resistances have never developed in some areas where impregnated bednets were used extensively.[81] Particularly worrisome is the appearance of target

Table 6–5. Approximate Duration of Residual Efficacy of Permethrin

Fabric Item	Time (mo)
Clothing worn daily and washed weekly	1–2
Clothing washed 8 times with soap in lukewarm water	2
Clothing exposed to weathering	≥ 1
Unused mosquito net	> 6 (1–2 yr in airtight bag)
Mosquito net used daily	4–8
Net used daily and washed after 1 month in cold water	2–3
Net used daily and washed weekly in cold water	1
Mosquito net, with permethrin integrated into the net during manufacture	≥ 12

Data from Carnevale P,[11] Guillet PF,[54] Schreck CE et al.,[77] Schreck CE et al.,[79] and Rozendaal JA.[83]

site resistance (knockdown resistance); cross-resistance patterns have also been documented.[81,84] It is questionable how big the impact of resistance on protective efficacy is going to be;[85] pyrethroids should continue to be used as a highly effective protective measure against mosquito bites. It is interesting to note that dichlorodiphenyltrichloroethane (DDT) continues to be effective in Africa, India, Brazil, and Mexico, despite the malaria vector's being physiologically resistant to DDT. This effect seems to stem from the additional repellent properties of DDT.[86] As pyrethroids also exhibit repellent properties, they can be expected to remain effective even against resistant vectors, particularly if used to spray rooms.

Deltamethrin. Deltamethrin has proven to be a powerful insecticide that is 30 times more powerful than permethrin. Thus, it should be used in much lower concentrations. It has proven to be highly effective in laboratory tests, in which it exhibited acaricidal effects of between 78% and 100%, even at concentrations several times lower (0.012 to 0.75 mg/m^2) than recommended.[78] Its toxicity to humans is higher than that of permethrin, and there have been complaints about an irritant effect during the impregnation process although people sleeping under dry nets do not usually experience any side effects.[72] Unlike permethrin, it is mainly used to impregnate bednets and as a general insecticide (e.g., in agriculture) although trials with impregnated scarves and wristbands have shown promising results.[87] Permethrin at higher doses seems to be equally effective[78] and less toxic than deltamethrin, and it is also more readily available to the consumer (e.g., in sprays). There also seem to be almost no data on deltamethrin used in clothing. These factors make permethrin much more suitable for the traveler. If available, deltamethrin can be used, with the appropriate precautions, to impregnate bednets and spray the surroundings, but it should not be used on clothing.

Lambda Cyhalothrin and Cyfluthrin. Lambda cyhalothrin and cyfluthrin have been used to impregnate bednets but should not be used for clothing. They are more toxic, and there is no experience in regard to impregnated clothing.

Other Pyrethroids. Other pyrethroids have not yet been fully tested for efficacy and safety in the treatment of mosquito nets and clothing[72] and should not be used for these purposes until more data are available.

Nonpyrethroid Insecticides with Superior Efficacy. Nonpyrethroid insecticides (such as pirimiphos-methyl [an organophosphate] and particularly, carbosulfan [$C_2OH_{32}N_2O_3S$]) have been shown to be very effective in areas of pyrethroid-resistant *Anopheles gambiae* for the treatment of bednets.[88] They may be an alternative in areas of pyrethroid resistance, but the safety of these insecticides will have to be carefully considered.[89] It is clear that these substances are not meant for the impregnation of clothing or for use by the traveler but rather for local mosquito control programs in developing countries.

Physical Measures

Physical measures such as clothing, bednets, screens, and air-conditioned mosquito-proof rooms, already briefly mentioned above, are important complementary PPMs. Air-conditioned rooms can be kept closed all the time. Screened and tightly fitting windows and doors prevent mosquito entry. Additional protection can be gained by spraying the room with an insecticide (see above) and burning a coil.

As with repellents and insecticides, the goal of physical PPMs is to reduce the average number of mosquito bites per time period to reduce the risk of malaria transmission. As no one PPM alone is 100% effective, it is advisable to combine different PPMs for greater efficacy.

Clothing

Probably, the most effective thing to do is to impregnate clothing with permethrin. Even without the additional use of a repellent, persons wearing permethrin-impregnated clothing in Alaska had a 93% rate of protection from mosquito bites[35] although this also depends on the propensity of certain mosquito species and other vectors to bite through clothing. When tested against the tsetse fly (*Glossina* sp) in one study, there was no significant difference in protection between DEET alone and DEET in combination with permethrin-impregnated clothing (76% to 87% vs. 91%), and wearing preimpregnated coveralls alone offered only 34% protection for untreated and exposed skin.[90] It is still best to use both permethrin-impregnated clothing and a repellent in combination although the increase in protection due to the impregnated clothing may vary.

Clothing should be light colored as dark-colored clothing may initiate mosquito orientation toward a person.[8,9,72] Fabrics of tighter weave or texture and greater thickness may increase protection from mosquito bites[72] although there are not much data available. A compromise between comfort and protection has to be found.

Long, loose-fitting clothing reduces the area of exposed skin and thus the amount of repellent that has to be applied. As some species of mosquitoes (e.g., *Culiseta impatiens*) are reluctant to bite through clothing,[35] nonimpregnated fabrics covering the skin already increase protection against mosquito bites.

Boots can protect the ankles from biting insects. Long trousers tucked into the socks offer some protection, as do collars and hats.[72] Face veils may be worn in areas of particularly high biting pressure.

Mosquito Nets

Mosquito nets, which have been used for the last 2,000 years,[80] are easy to install, can be readily removed, are reasonably priced, and will last for years when treated with care. In an unscreened room, a medium-mesh (mesh size of 1.2 to 1.5 mm [Figure 6–4A], which protects against anopheline mosquitoes)[72,80] insecticide-treated mosquito net offers protection and comfort during the night, and not only from mosquitoes—the author once had a rat crawl over his mosquito net while on the island of Flores, in Indonesia. Mesh sizes below 1.2 mm impede ventilation whereas mesh sizes above 1.5 mm should be used only when the net is impregnated.[80]

The three most common materials used for the construction of bednets are nylon, polyester, and cotton, alone or in combination. Less common is polyethylene. They decrease vector-human contact, lower malaria transmission, and decrease morbidity and mortality.[80] Their quality depends on the thickness and strength of the threads and on the production process. The threads can be woven or knitted. Woven nets have the disadvantage that the threads can slide over each other, thus creating enlarged holes. In woven nets made of stiff polyethylene fibers, this does not seem to be a problem.[72] Synthetic nets cost less and are less likely to rot than cotton nets.[72] Good-quality (thick, strong threads) nylon, polyester, and polyethylene are more durable than cotton. Permethrin-impregnated polyester and nylon have been shown to produce higher anopheline mortality than cotton treated with similar amounts of permethrin. Nets having a denier of 100 (indicating weight, which translates into strength) provide the best protection against tearing. Reinforced bottom borders help prevent tearing while the net is being tucked in.[80]

The superior efficacy of impregnated bednets, leading to a significant reduction in malaria cases, has been proven in many studies.[80,91,92] It has to be noted that the effect of insecticide-treated materials on the incidence of malaria cases varies depending on vector and personal behavior.[93] Some mosquitoes tend to bite more at night while others prefer to bite in the morning or evening hours. (On how to impregnate a net, see above.)

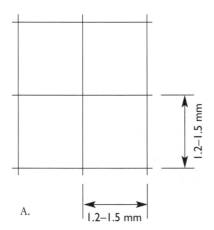

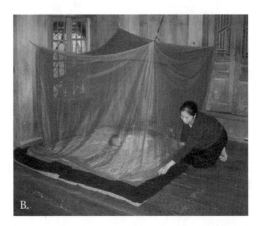

Figure 6–4. *A.* Optimum mesh size between 1.2–1.5mm. *B.* A rectangular mosquito net (PermaNet®) in which deltamethrin is integrated into the polyester during polymerization. Note the thick mattress (to protect against mosquito bites from below), the tightly fitting border, and the vertical sides that reduce chance contacts with the net's surface. (Courtesy of The Vestergaard Frandsen Group.)

Nets come in many different sizes and forms.[72] If possible, a rectangular (Figure 6–4B) net should be preferred because the chances of touching the net and getting bitten while sleeping are lower with this construction.[80] An overlapping entrance is possible. The traveler may find it difficult, though, to find the appropriate supports for this kind of net. This is the advantage of conical or circular nets, which can be hung from a single support. However, more care has to be taken to avoid contact with the net surface during sleep. Wedge-shaped nets are convenient for travelers because of their small volume. Because of their shape, they have less surface area.

Self-supporting nets look a bit like tents and are easy to set up indoors. They are usually small and are convenient for protecting babies and infants. There are even mosquito nets available for hammocks.

When buying a tent, one must take care to chose a model in which all openings can be tightly closed with a mosquito net, preferably with a zipper. Spraying the inner side of the tent (e.g., with permethrin) will further increase protection.[94]

The following should be observed when using a mosquito net:

- If a bednet is used, it should be tucked under the mattress to offer complete protection.
- Any holes should be mended as soon as possible.
- Avoid contact with the net surface.
- An impregnated net should be used; this also offers some protection against smaller insects that might crawl through the net openings.
- The mattress or floor should be "mosquitotight" and thick enough to prevent mosquitoes from biting through the fabric.
- The bednet should be of sufficient size to cover the entire bed or sleeping area.
- The net should be lowered before darkness to avoid having mosquitoes inside the net. Again, impregnated nets have an advantage here, as they kill off mosquitoes captured accidentally inside the sleeping space.

Preimpregnated nets are now available commercially. In particular, nets in which permethrin or deltametherin is integrated into the synthetic material during polymerization (Olyset Net®, PermaNet®) seem to offer protection times of 1 year or longer (Figure 6–4B).[11] According to data from the manufacturer, PermaNet® achieved a 100% knockdown rate after 21 washes in standardized washing tests at 30°C when mosquitoes were exposed for 3 minutes, which indicates that these nets probably stay effective over a long period of time without having to be reimpregnated. With permethrin, preimpregnated nets have proven to be just as effective as nets impregnated with such insecticides as cyfluthrin, deltamethrin, and lambda cyhalothrin.[95] When stored in their original packaging, preimpregnated nets keep their efficacy for several years.[11]

In summary, a good net for the traveler should (1) be from synthetic fabric (nylon, polyester, or polyethylene), (2) be preimpregnated, (3) have a denier of around 100, and (4) be easy to set up (rectangular vs. other shapes).

Screens, Air-Conditioning, Coils, Vaporizers

Keeping a room free of mosquitoes while still having enough ventilation to be comfortable can be achieved with the help of tightly fitting mosquito screens on windows, doors, and other openings. Air-conditioning helps achieve the same goal. It can therefore be of advantage for the traveler to ask his or her travel agent if the booked hotels offer screened or air-conditioned rooms or if a good mosquito net is available; if not, it is advisable for the traveler to take along a mosquito net. Houses should have screened doors that close automatically, and care should be taken that there are no openings through which mosquitoes can enter the building. The additional application of insecticides on walls, screens, curtains, and fissures further improves protection and kills mosquitoes that make it through the first line of defense.

If a room is already infested with mosquitoes, a coil containing natural pyrethrum or synthetic pyrethroids[96] may be burned a few hours before going to bed, to clear the room of mosquitoes, and the room can be sealed tightly thereafter. Possible airway irritation can be avoided in this way. Another possibility is to burn a coil during the night although a certain caution is advisable, especially concerning local products, because of possible toxicity.[11] Coils may differ markedly in their active ingredients; while some contain allethrin or another pyrethroid, others may contain DDT (less effective) or lindane. This leads to different toxicities and efficacies, depending on the product.[11] The efficacy of coils containing pyrethrum has been proven in several studies.[97,98] Coils burn down in 6 to 8 hours, and liberated pyrethrum or pyrethroids act mainly as repellents and partially as insecticides.[11] Inhalative toxicity is minimal. Very rarely, the smoke can produce an irritation of the airways when the coils are burned for long periods in rooms lacking even minimal ventilation.[97] One should not rely on coils alone for protection.[11] As always, it pays of to combine different PPMs.

Electrical devices that vaporize pyrethroids produce effects similar to those of coils. They are at least as effective as, if not superior to, mosquito coils although electricity may be a problem.[96,97] All products producing some kind of repellent and/or insecticidal vapor lose their efficacy if there is too much ventilation. On the other hand, a minimum amount of ventilation is desirable to avoid possible inhalational toxicity.

What Does Not Work

Contrary to public opinion, oral thiamine (vitamin B_1) does not protect against mosquito bites.[97,99,100] Acoustic devices that produce ultrasound waves have also been shown to be ineffective, as are light traps, which may electrocute flies and numerous useful insects but not mosquitoes.[97] Such devices can not reduce the frequency of blood meals taken by mosquitoes.[101] Eating garlic is of no avail, either.[67] In the end, the traveler should stick to well-tried and proven PPMs and avoid throwing money down the drain for more exotic, useless, and sometimes expensive methods and devices.

Behavior

Depending on regional mosquito activity and personal behavior, the risk of getting bitten by mosquitoes may differ markedly among travelers.[11] Is the traveler staying at a hotel with well-screened rooms, mosquito nets, or air-conditioning or is he or she sleeping under the sky? Is there a lot of evening, morning, or nighttime activity? Is the traveler staying mainly in large cities or in the countryside? It is important to make the traveler knowledgeable about the different risks of acquiring malaria that depend on the mode and route of travel. The itinerary can often be changed so as not to enter a malaria-endemic area. Most of South Africa, for instance, is malaria free, and if the big game parks in the north of the country are left in favor of the very nice Cape region with its vineries, the risk of malaria is virtually zero. Most big cities in Southeast Asia can be counted as malaria free, but that is not so for the countryside. Last but not least, there are many nontropical areas in the world that offer a unique holiday experience without the risk of malaria. Choose your road wisely, and you will circumvent many dangers, toils, and snares.

Summary

The traveler should know about the different PPMs available to him or her (Table 6–6) and where they are *easily* obtainable. The traveler should be made aware that it is paramount to combine as many of these measures as possible to optimize efficacy. On the other hand, a reasonable compromise should be found to optimize compliance; it is better to have the traveler use a repellent *regularly* during nighttime than to insist on use during the entire day, which might result in poor compliance. Travel of small children or pregnant women to malaria-endemic areas should be strongly discouraged. If a particular destination cannot be avoided (in favor of a malaria-free area), the traveler should take particular care to use PPMs in addition to chemoprophylaxis or standby emergency self-treatment (see Table 6–6). It is important to realize that behavioral changes are very difficult to achieve

Table 6–6. **Travelers' Malaria Survival Kit**

Consider not traveling to a malaria-endemic area.

Consider malaria chemoprophylaxis or standby emergency self-treatment (depending on destination).

Consider impregnating your clothes with permethrin.

Consider taking along an impregnated mosquito net (depending on accommodations).

Consider using a mosquito coil and an insecticide to reduce mosquito pressure.

Take along a repellent (preferably one containing DEET).

Take along light-colored long-sleeved shirts and long trousers and socks.

Take along proper shoes and a hat.

Choose a hotel that offers air-conditioning or well-screened rooms/mosquito nets.

in the traveler. Thorough written and oral information is necessary not only to inform but also to convince the traveler of the importance of PPMs.

REFERENCES

1. Service MW. Mosquitoes (Culicidae). In: Lane RP, Crosskey RW, editors. Medical insects and arachnids. London: Chapman & Hall, 1993.
2. World Health Organization. Division of Vector Biology and Control. Geographical distribution of arthropod-borne diseases and their principal vectors. Geneva, Switzerland: World Health Organization Vector Biology and Control Division, 1989.
3. Charlwood JD, Alecrim WA. Capture-recapture studies with the South American malaria vector Anopheles darlingi, Root. Ann Trop Med Parasitol 1989;83:569–576.
4. Faye O, Fontenille D, Herve JP, et al. [Malaria in the Saharan region of Senegal. 1. Entomological transmission findings]. Ann Soc Belg Med Trop 1993;73:21–30.
5. Lane RP. Introduction to the arthropods. In: Lane RP, Crosskey RW, editors. Medical insects and arachnids. London: Chapman & Hall, 1993.
6. Marquardt WC, Grieve RB, Demaree RS. Parasitology and vector biology. San Diego (CA) and London: Harcourt Academic, 2000.
7. Service MW. Medical entomology for students. Cambridge: Cambridge University Press, 2000.
8. Maibach HI, Akers WA, Johnson HL, et al. Insects. Topical insect repellents. Clin Pharmacol Ther 1974;16:970–973.
9. Fradin MS. Mosquitoes and mosquito repellents: a clinician's guide. Ann Intern Med 1998;128:931–940.
10. Tadei WP, Thatcher BD, Santos JM, et al. Ecologic observations on anopheline vectors of malaria in the Brazilian Amazon. Am J Trop Med Hyg 1998;59:325–335.
11. Carnevale P. [Protection of travellers against biting arthropod vectors]. Bull Soc Pathol Exot 1998;91:474–485.
12. Braack LE, Coetzee M, Hunt RH, et al. Biting pattern and host-seeking behavior of Anopheles arabiensis (Diptera: Culicidae) in northeastern South Africa. J Med Entomol 1994;31:333–339.
13. Singh S, Singh RP, Jauhari RK. Biting activity of the malaria vector, Anopheles culicifacies, on man and cattle in Doon valley, India. Appl Parasitol 1995;36:185–191.
14. Rattanarithikul R, Konishi E, Linthicum KJ. Observations on nocturnal biting activity and host preference of anophelines collected in southern Thailand. J Am Mosq Control Assoc 1996;12:52–57.
15. Rubio-Palis Y, Curtis CF. Biting and resting behaviour of anophelines in western Venezuela and implications for control of malaria transmission. Med Vet Entomol 1992;6:325–334.
16. Samarawickrema WA, Parkinson AD, Kere N, Galo O. Seasonal abundance and biting behaviour of Anopheles punctulatus and An. koliensis in Malaita Province, Solomon Islands, and a trial of permethrin impregnated bednets against malaria transmission. Med Vet Entomol 1992;6:371–378.
17. Kumari R, Sharma VP. Resting and biting habits of Anopheles sundaicus in Car Nicobar Island. Indian J Malariol 1994;31:103–114.
18. Roberts D. Mosquitoes (Diptera: Culicidae) breeding in brackish water: female ovipositional preferences or larval survival? J Med Entomol 1996;33:525–530.

19. Gilles HM, Warrell DA, Bruce-Chwatt LJ. Bruce-Chwatt's essential malariology. London: E. Arnold, 1993.
20. Rickman LS, Jones TR, Long GW, et al. *Plasmodium falciparum*-infected *Anopheles stephensi* inconsistently transmit malaria to humans. Am J Trop Med Hyg 1990;43:441–445.
21. Reiter P. Global-warming and vector-borne disease in temperate regions and at high altitude [letter]. Lancet 1998;351:839–840.
22. Trape J-F, Rogier C. Combating malaria morbidity and mortality by reducing trasmission. Parasitol Today 1996;12:236–240.
23. Beier JC, Killeen GF, Githure JI. Short report: entomologic inoculation rates and *Plasmodium falciparum* malaria prevalence in Africa. Am J Trop Med Hyg 1999;61:109–113.
24. Hay SI, Rogers DJ, Toomer JF, Snow RW. Annual *Plasmodium falciparum* entomological inoculation rates (EIR) across Africa: literature survey, internet access and review. Trans R Soc Trop Med Hyg 2000;94:113–127.
25. Nahlen BL. Rolling back malaria: in pregnancy. N Engl J Med 2000;343:651–652.
26. McGregor IA. Thoughts on malaria in pregnancy with consideration of some factors which influence remedial strategies. Parassitologia 1987;29:153–163.
27. Klufio CA. Malaria in pregnancy. P N G Med J 1992;35:249–257.
28. Canadian recommendations for the prevention and treatment of malaria among international travellers. Committee to Advise on Tropical Medicine and Travel (CATMAT). Can Commun Dis Rep 2000;26 Suppl 2:1–42.
29. Goujon C. Aspects pédiatriques de la prévention et du traitement du paludisme. Med Hyg 2000;58:1117–1120.
30. Boone KE, Watters DA. The incidence of malaria after splenectomy in Papua New Guinea. BMJ 1995;311:1273.
31. Snow RW, Craig M, Deichmann U, Marsh K. Estimating mortality, morbidity and disability due to malaria among Africa's non-pregnant population. Bull World Health Organ 1999;77:624–640.
32. Phillips RE, Solomon T. Cerebral malaria in children. Lancet 1990;336:1355–1360.
33. Muentener P, Schlagenhauf P, Steffen R. Imported malaria (1985–95): trends and perspectives. Bull World Health Organ 1999;77:560–566.
34. Schlagenhauf P, Muentener P, Steffen R. Importierte Malaria in Europa. Symposium Medical 2000;6.
35. Lillie TH, Schreck CE, Rahe AJ. Effectiveness of personal protection against mosquitoes in Alaska. J Med Entomol 1988;25:475–478.
36. Schoepke A, Steffen R, Gratz N. Effectiveness of personal protection measures against mosquito bites for malaria prophylaxis in travelers. J Travel Med 1998;5:188–192.
37. Waner S, Durrhiem D, Braack LE, Gammon S. Malaria protection measures used by in-flight travelers to South African game parks. J Travel Med 1999;6:254–257.
38. Importierte Infektionskrankheiten (in Deutschland): Malaria. Epidemiol Bull 2000: 231–233.
39. Trape JF, Zoulani A. Malaria and urbanization in central Africa: the example of Brazzaville. Part II: Results of entomological surveys and epidemiological analysis. Trans R Soc Trop Med Hyg 1987;81:10–18.
40. Coene J. Malaria in urban and rural Kinshasa: the entomological input. Med Vet Entomol 1993;7:127–137.

41. Anderson RA, Knols BG, Koella JC. *Plasmodium falciparum* sporozoites increase feeding-associated mortality of their mosquito hosts *Anopheles gambiae* s.l. Parasitology 2000;120:329–333.

42. Shililu JI, Maier WA, Seitz HM, Orago AS. Seasonal density, sporozoite rates and entomological inoculation rates of *Anopheles gambiae* and *Anopheles funestus* in a high-altitude sugarcane growing zone in western Kenya. Trop Med Int Health 1998;3:706–710.

43. Bockarie MJ, Service MW, Barnish G, et al. Malaria in a rural area of Sierra Leone. III. Vector ecology and disease transmission. Ann Trop Med Parasitol 1994;88:251–262.

44. Temu EA, Minjas JN, Coetzee M, et al. The role of four anopheline species (Diptera: Culicidae) in malaria transmission in coastal Tanzania. Trans R Soc Trop Med Hyg 1998;92:152–158.

45. Shiff CJ, Minjas JN, Hall T, et al. Malaria infection potential of anopheline mosquitoes sampled by light trapping indoors in coastal Tanzanian villages. Med Vet Entomol 1995;9:256–262.

46. Veltri JC, Osimitz TG, Bradford DC, Page BC. Retrospective analysis of calls to poison control centers resulting from exposure to the insect repellent N,N-diethyl-m-toluamide (DEET) from 1985–1989. J Toxicol Clin Toxicol 1994;32:1–16.

47. Are insect repellents safe? [editorial]. Lancet 1988;2:610–611.

48. Brown M, Hebert AA. Insect repellents: an overview. J Am Acad Dermatol 1997;36:243–249.

49. Mafong EA, Kaplan LA. Insect repellents. What really works? Postgrad Med 1997;102:63, 68–69, 74.

50. Buescher MD, Rutledge LC, Wirtz RA. The dose-persistence relationship of deet against *Aedes aegypti*. Mosq News 1983;43:364–366.

51. Goodyer L, Behrens RH. Short report: the safety and toxicity of insect repellents. Am J Trop Med Hyg 1998;59:323–324.

52. Buescher MD, Rutledge LC, Wirtz RA. Test of commercial repellents on human skin against *Aedes aegypti*. Mosq News 1982:428–433.

53. Rutledge LC, Wirtz RA, Buescher MD, Mehr ZA. Mathematical models of the effectiveness and persistence of mosquito repellents. J Am Mosq Control Assoc 1985;1:56–62.

54. Guillet PF. La protection personelle des voyageurs contre les piqûres de moustiques. Med Hyg 2000;58:1099–1104.

55. Environmental Protection Agency Reregistration Eligibility Decision (RED). DEET. Washington (DC): U.S. Environmental Protection Agency, 1998.

56. Salafsky B, He YX, Li J, et al. Short report: study on the efficacy of a new long-acting formulation of N, N-diethyl-m-toluamide (DEET) for the prevention of tick attachment. Am J Trop Med Hyg 2000;62:169–172.

57. Moody RP, Benoit FM, Riedel D, Ritter L. Dermal absorption of the insect repellent DEET (N,N-diethyl-m-toluamide) in rats and monkeys: effect of anatomical site and multiple exposure. J Toxicol Environ Health 1989;26:137–147.

58. Qui H, Jun HW, McCall JW. Pharmacokinetics, formulation, and safety of insect repellent N,N-diethyl-3-methylbenzamide (DEET): a review. J Am Mosq Control Assoc 1998;14:12–27.

59. Tenenbein M. Severe toxic reactions and death following the ingestion of diethyltoluamide-containing insect repellents. JAMA 1987;258:1509–1511.

60. N,N-diethyl-m-toluamide (Deet) Pesticide Registration Standard. Washington (DC): U.S. Environmental Protection Agency, 1980.

61. Gleiberman SE, Volkova AP, Nikolaev GM, Zhukova EV. [Study of the embrotoxic properties of the repellent diethyltoluamide]. Farmakol Toksikol 1975;38: 202–205.

62. Hayes WJ. Pesticides studied in man. Baltimore: Williams & Wilkins, 1982.

63. Domb AJ, Marlinsky A, Maniar M, Teomim L. Insect repellent formulations of N,N-diethyl-m-toluamide (deet) in a liposphere system: efficacy and skin uptake. J Am Mosq Control Assoc 1995;11:29–34.

64. Schreck CE, Kline DL. Personal protection afforded by controlled-release topical repellents and permethrin-treated clothing against natural populations of *Aedes taeniorhynchus*. J Am Mosq Control Assoc 1989;5:77–80.

65. Rueda LM, Rutledge LC, Gupta RK. Effect of skin abrasions on the efficacy of the repellent deet against *Aedes aegypti*. J Am Mosq Control Assoc 1998;14:178–182.

66. Maibach HI, Khan AA, Akers W. Use of insect repellents for maximum efficacy. Arch Dermatol 1974;109:32–35.

67. Rudin W. Repellentien. Fortbildungsveranstalltung der Fachgesellschaft für Tropenmedizin. 2000 Feb; Bern, Switzerland.

68. Bug off! How to repel biting insects. Consumer Reports 1993;58:451–454.

69. Garrettson L. Commentary—DEET: caution for children still needed. J Toxicol Clin Toxicol 1997;35:443–445.

70. Yap HH, Jahangir K, Chong AS, et al. Field efficacy of a new repellent, KBR 3023, against *Aedes albopictus* (SKUSE) and *Culex quinquefasciatus* (SAY) in a tropical environment. J Vector Ecol 1998;23:62–68.

71. Rudin W. Tropentauglicher Schutz vor Stechmücken. Ars Medici 2000:764–768.

72. Rozendaal JA, World Health Organization. Vector control: methods for use by individuals and communities. Geneva: World Health Organization, 1997.

73. EXTOXNET (Extension Toxicology Network) Pesticide Information Profiles: Permethrin. Vol. 2000. A pesticide information project of Cooperative Extension Offices of Cornell University, Oregon State University, University of Idaho, and University of California at Davis and the Institute for Environmental Toxicology, Michigan State University, 1996.

74. EXTOXNET (Extension Toxicology Network) Pesticide Information Profiles: Deltamethrin. Vol. 2000. A pesticide information project of Cooperative Extension Offices of Cornell University, Oregon State University, University of Idaho, and University of California at Davis and the Institute for Environmental Toxicology, Michigan State University, 1995.

75. EXTOXNET (Extension Toxicology Network) Pesticide Information Profiles: Lambda cyhalothrin. Vol. 2000. A pesticide information project of Cooperative Extension Offices of Cornell University, Oregon State University, University of Idaho, and University of California at Davis and the Institute for Environmental Toxicology, Michigan State University.

76. EXTOXNET (Extension Toxicology Network) Pesticide Information Profiles: Cyfluthrin. Vol. 2000. A pesticide information project of Cooperative Extension Offices of Cornell University, Oregon State University, University of Idaho, and University of California at Davis and the Institute for Environmental Toxicology, Michigan State University.

77. Schreck CE, Posey K, Smith D. Durability of permethrin as a potential clothing treatment to protect against blood-feeding arthropods. J Econ Entomol 1978;71:397–400.

78. Kocisova A, Para L. Possibilities of long-term protection against blood-sucking insects and ticks. Cent Eur J Public Health 1999;7:27–30.

79. Schreck CE, Carlson DA, Weidhass DE, et al. Wear and aging tests with permethrin-treated cotton-polyester fabric. J Econ Entomol 1980;73:451–453.

80. Sexton JD. Impregnated bed nets for malaria control: biological success and social responsibility. Am J Trop Med Hyg 1994;50:72–81.

81. Chandre F, Darrier F, Manga L, et al. Status of pyrethroid resistance in *Anopheles gambiae* sensu lato. Bull World Health Organ 1999;77:230–234.

82. Schreck CE, Snoddy EL, Spielman A. Pressurized sprays of permethrin or deet on military clothing for personal protection against *Ixodes dammini* (Acari: Ixodidae). J Med Entomol 1986;23:396–399.

83. Rozendaal JA. Impregnated mosquito nets and curtains for self-protection and vector control. Trop Dis Bull 1989;7:R1–R41.

84. Brogdon WG, McAllister JC. Insecticide resistance and vector control. Emerg Infect Dis 1998;4:605–613.

85. Lengeler C. Insecticide-treated materials for malaria control: many good news, few worries: new challenges in tropical medicine and parasitology. Oxford (GB): Oxford, 2000.

86. Roberts DR, Andre RG. Insecticide resistance issues in vector-borne disease control. Am J Trop Med Hyg 1994;50:21–34.

87. Lwin M, Lin H, Linn N, et al. The use of personal protective measures in control of malaria in a defined community. Southeast Asian J Trop Med Public Health 1997;28:254–258.

88. Kolaczinski JH, Fanello C, Herve JP, et al. Experimental and molecular genetic analysis of the impact of pyrethroid and non-pyrethroid insecticide impregnated bednets for mosquito control in an area of pyrethroid resistance. Bull Entomol Res 2000;90:125–132.

89. Fanello C, Kolaczinski JH, Conway DJ, et al. The kdr pyrethroid resistance gene in *Anopheles gambiae*: tests of non-pyrethroid insecticides and a new detection method for the gene. Parassitologia 1999;41:323–326.

90. Sholdt LL, Schreck CE, Mwangelwa MI, et al. Evaluations of permethrin-impregnated clothing and three topical repellent formulations of deet against tsetse flies in Zambia. Med Vet Entomol 1989;3:153–158.

91. Cheng H, Yang W, Kang W, Liu C. Large-scale spraying of bednets to control mosquito vectors and malaria in Sichuan, China. Bull World Health Organ 1995;73:321–328.

92. Lines JD, Zaim M. Insecticide products: treatment of mosquito nets at home. Parasitol Today 2000;16:91–92.

93. Kroeger A, González M, Ordóñez-Gonzáles J. Insecticide-treated materials for malaria control in Latin America: to use or not to use? Trans R Soc Trop Med Hyg 1999;93:565–570.

94. Bouma MJ, Parvez SD, Nesbit R, Winkler AM. Malaria control using permethrin applied to tents of nomadic Afghan refugees in northern Pakistan. Bull World Health Organ 1996;74:413–421.

95. Curtis CF, Myamba J, Wilkes TJ. Comparison of different insecticides and fabrics for anti-mosquito bednets and curtains. Med Vet Entomol 1996;10:1–11.

96. Curtis CF. Personal protection methods against vectors of disease. Rev Med Vet Entomol 1992;80:543–553.

97. Holzer RB. [Malaria prevention without drugs]. Schweiz Rundsch Med Prax 1993;82:139–143.

98. Charlwood JD, Jolley D. The coil works (against mosquitoes in Papua New Guinea). Trans R Soc Trop Med Hyg 1984;78:678.

99. Khan AA, Maibach HI, Strauss WG, Fenley WR. Vitamin B1 is not a systemic mosquito repellent in man. Trans St Johns Hosp Dermatol Soc 1969;55:99–102.

100. Kodkani N, Jenkins JM, Hatz CF. Travel advice given by pharmacists. J Travel Med 1999;6:87–93.

101. Nasci RS, Harris CW, Porter CK. Failure of an insect electrocuting device to reduce mosquito biting. Mosq News 1983;43:180–184.

USEFUL WEB SITES

http://ace.orst.edu/info/extoxnet/
   Detailed description of chemical and toxicologic properties of different insecticides and repellents.

http://konops.imbb.forth.gr/AnoDB/Species/malariaspecies.html
   List of malaria vectors throughout the world.

http://www.expediamaps.com/
   Locations of places (city, country, etc.).

Chapter 7

STRATEGIES OF MALARIA PREVENTION IN NONIMMUNE VISITORS TO ENDEMIC COUNTRIES

Robert Steffen

ABSTRACT

The primary principle in medicine is, *primum non nocere* (first, do not harm).[1] This is paramount in preventive medicine even more than in therapy; adverse events will impair previously healthy persons (who are more likely to complain), and there may be situations in treatment that force one to accept a greater risk. With this dogma in mind, we must analyze the pros and cons of each of the four strategic options available for malaria prophylaxis in nonimmune visitors to endemic countries: information, personal protection measures (PPMs) against mosquito bites, chemoprophylaxis (i.e., chemosuppression), and prompt assessment and treatment of symptoms suggestive of malaria, including emergency self-therapy in special circumstances (Figure 7–1).

All considerations must be based on recent epidemiologic and pharmacologic data (Table 7–1). Whenever possible, recommendations should be based on evidence. Analyzing the data, one becomes aware that there is great variability in the

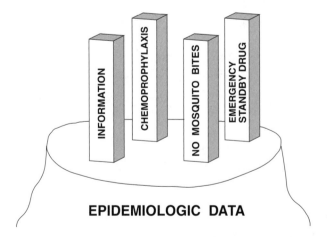

Figure 7–1. Strategy of malaria prophylaxis in nonimmune visitors to endemic countries.

risk of malaria transmission, depending mainly on the duration of stay and on the destination. The risk for nonimmune travelers varies enormously between countries and even within a country. Risk is highest in some Pacific islands, Papua New Guinea, and tropical Africa. For travelers with no chemoprophylaxis, the risk of symptomatic malaria infection is estimated to be 2.4% per month of stay in West Africa and 1.5% per month of stay in East Africa.[2] More recent seroepidemiologic surveys using *Plasmodium falciparum* circumsporozoite antibodies confirm a high rate of infection in travelers returning from sub-Saharan Africa. Antibodies were detected in the sera of more than 20% of travelers who had visited Kenya for 2 to 16 weeks, with individual travelers at a risk 8.7 times greater (48.8%) than the risk of those on package tours (5.6%).[3,4] There is intermediate risk on the Indian subcontinent. There is a low risk of transmission in frequently visited tourist destinations in Latin America and Southeast Asia (Figure 7–2), but some small areas of Brazil, India, and Thailand pose a considerable risk. Differing meteorologic conditions may cause annual and seasonal fluctuations in risk.

Key words: chemoprophylaxis; emergency self-treatment; personal protection measures; prevention; strategies; travelers' malaria.

Table 7–1. **Main Factors for Deciding Which Strategy for Which Traveler**

Travel characteristics
- Destination: with risk/limited risk/no risk
- Duration: short/"usual 1–4 weeks"/long term
- Travel style (e.g., outdoor camping/air-conditioned hotel)

Host factors
- Behavior (e.g., compliance)
- Pregnancy: particularly high risk
- Personal history (e.g., history of psychiatric disorders, seizures)

Entomological inoculation rate (EIR)
- Inoculation rate/morbidity
- Infectivity
- Season/meteorology

Parasite
- Resistance (both in *P. falciparum* and *P. vivax)*
- Species/mortality

Medical infrastructure
- At destination, including risk of overdiagnosis (mainly a problem in Africa)
- In residence country (e.g., case-fatality rate)

Medication
- Availability of malaria medication at origin and at destination for long-term residents
- Adverse events of chemoprophylaxis
- Costs vs. budget

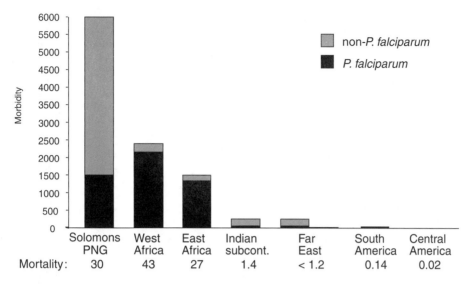

Figure 7–2. Morbidity and mortality in 100,000 nonimmune travelers exposed for 1 month without chemoprophylaxis (Australian, German, and Swiss malaria registers). Mortality rates assume a case-fatality rate of 2%. (*P.* = *Plasmodium*; PNG = Papua New Guinea; subcont. = subcontinent.)

INFORMATION

Travelers visiting countries where malaria is endemic should obtain essential information on the following:

- Location of endemic regions and areas free (or with negligible risk) of transmission (Figure 7–3). While some travelers arrive in endemic areas unaware that they should take protective measures, other travelers may take unnecessary measures against malaria where there is no transmission. This information can be found in the World Health Organization (WHO) source,[5] which is annually updated. Many national travel health advisory boards publish similar lists. Sloppy information may result in an unnecessary scare (e.g., a traveler to Rio de Janeiro is warned that there is malaria in Brazil, when there is no risk of transmission in Rio de Janeiro itself).
- Mode and period of transmission. Infected mosquitoes bite almost exclusively at night, particularly around midnight. Travelers without this information will not understand, for example, why they have to avoid mosquito bites during nighttime.
- Incubation period. This is a minimum of 6 days for *P. falciparum* and may be up to several months and occasionally even longer than 1 year for other *Plasmodium* species. Intelligent travelers should at least be able to appreciate why a prophylactic regimen should be continued for 4 weeks after they leave the transmission area. To obtain better compliance, it may be beneficial to explain in simple terms that the parasite needs to undergo reproduction while "hiding"

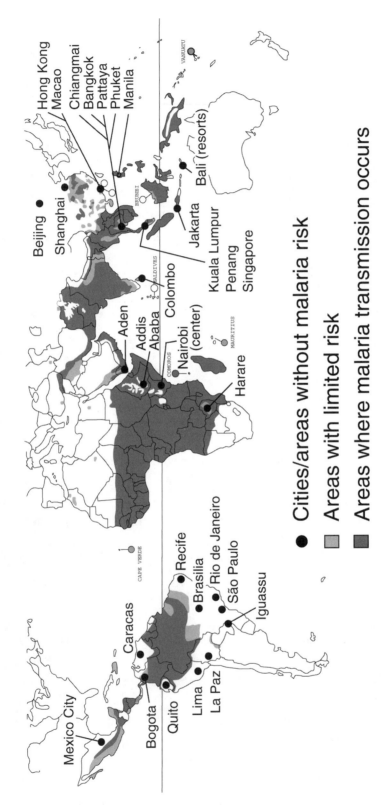

Figure 7–3. Worldwide malaria endemicity. (Adapted from World Health Organization data, 1997.) (See Color Plates)

● Cities/areas without malaria risk

▨ Areas with limited risk

■ Areas where malaria transmission occurs

in the liver, before it invades red blood cells, and that the antimalarials so far prescribed act only on this latter stage. (An exception is Malarone, which has recently been licensed for chemoprophylaxis in some countries [Figure 7–4]).

- Early symptoms. These are usually flulike, with fever, chills, headache, generalized aches and pains, and malaise. These symptoms may or may not occur with classic periodicity.
- Options for prevention. First, travelers should know that preventive measures against mosquito bites are the first line of defence. Second, chemoprophylaxis should be used when indicated, but travelers should be cautioned that (1) this strategy is not 100% effective, even when compliance is perfect, and that (2) the chemoprophylactic agent may cause adverse reactions.
- Necessity for medical consultation. Medical consultation is needed within 24 hours of the occurrence of symptoms suggestive of malaria as complications may develop very rapidly thereafter. The best advice is to "think and act malaria" when febrile symptoms occur.

It seems that no studies so far have ascertained the benefit of pretravel information relating to malaria, but such benefit is so plausible that it appears unethical to let travelers leave for endemic zones without such information. On the other

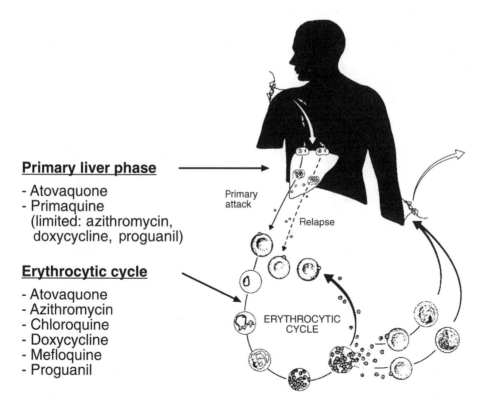

Primary liver phase

- Atovaquone
- Primaquine
  (limited: azithromycin,
  doxycycline, proguanil)

Erythrocytic cycle

- Atovaquone
- Azithromycin
- Chloroquine
- Doxycycline
- Mefloquine
- Proguanil

Figure 7–4. Site of action of antimalarials.

hand, one should also take care not to overload travelers with information; it is, for instance, irrelevant that only female *Anopheles* transmit malaria (at least, this author has never been able to determine the sex of a mosquito that was trying to bite him). It is probably best to inform travelers both verbally and in writing since they tend to confuse information that is given only verbally.[6,7]

MEASURES AGAINST MOSQUITO BITES

Mosquitoes use visual, thermal, and (most important) olfactory stimuli to locate the human host required for their blood meal and thus for their reproduction cycle. To prevent mosquito bites between dusk and dawn, one has a variety of options that are best combined, none being 100% effective.

Safe Areas

Staying in air-conditioned rooms or in rooms protected by wire mesh usually is safe, but few tourists will renounce outdoor activities just to avoid mosquito bites. Additionally, mosquitoes may enter rooms with air conditioners, particularly when tourists leave the windows open during the night, as many do to avoid being disturbed by a loud air conditioner. According to a large survey, air-conditioned rooms have been demonstrated to be the most effective protective tool.[8]

Sleeping under a mosquito net has been shown to be efficacious in many studies,[9] but mosquito nets are not available in the most frequently visited tourist resorts because the rooms are air-conditioned. Impregnation (soaking) of such a net with insecticide offers additional protection for 2 to 3 months, even when the net is slightly damaged.

Personal Protection: Clothing, Repellents, Insecticides

Perfumes and fragranced soaps or lotions should be avoided because their fragrances may attract mosquitoes.

Outdoors, one should use clothing to cover arms, legs, and ankles, in particular. This has been shown to be an effective tool for protection.[8]

Mosquito bites may penetrate thin clothes (i.e., clothes < 1 mm thick and with openings of > 0.02 mm). Obviously, thin clothes are preferred in a tropical climate; therefore, it is recommended to spray clothing with repellents or (even better) insecticides. Uncovered skin should be protected with a repellent. Dark colors attract *Anopheles* mosquitoes; light colors are thus to be preferred.

Repellents are chemicals that cause insects to turn away.[10] Unprotected skin only a few centimeters from a treated area may be attacked by hungry mosquitoes. Repellents are effective for only a limited time period and appear to protect females less.[11] Most repellents contain N,N,diethyl-methyl-toluamide (DEET), a very effective substance that has been used for more than 40 years. Some others contain ethyl-buthylacetylaminopropionate (EBAAP), picaridin (1-piperidincarboxyl-acid,2-[2-hydroxyethyl]-1-methyl-propylesther [Bayrepel]), dimethylphtalate (DMP), ethylexanediol, ind-alone, or a mixture of these. While older-generation DEET formulations are rapidly lost through sweating, newer ones containing polymers or other substances last longer but are frequently considered too sticky. In particular, seasoned travelers prefer lotions for the face and sprays for the rest of the body.

There is risk of DEET toxicity, which usually occurs when the product is mis-used.[12] This toxicity is due to the absorption of 9% to 56% of the chemical through the skin, with higher rates for alcohol-based solutions. Toxicity is especially a concern in infants, in whom three cases of lethal encephalopathy with high concentrations (up to 100%) have been observed.[10] The concentration is therefore limited to 35% in many countries. Any formulation with a higher concentration is not recommended (use no DEET or EBAAP of > 10% concentration in children). For these reasons, many consider repellents to be contraindicated in the following populations:

1. Infants below the age of 1 year; mosquito nets are preferred. (Also, one must avoid applying repellents on children's hands because the chemical is likely to be transferred from the hands into the eyes or mouth.)
2. Long-term residents, for fear of accumulated toxicity.
3. Pregnant women (although no teratogenicity has been demonstrated).

Natural repellents, such as citronella oil or other plant extracts, are rarely used anymore as their effectiveness is usually limited to less than an hour and as they are likely to cause an allergic reaction. Oral vitamin B is an ineffective repellent.[13]

Insecticides are poisons that target the nerves of insects and other cold-blood-ed animals and thus kill them. Synthetic pyrethroid insecticides such as permethrin and deltamethrin are more photostable and less volatile than the natural product pyrethrum (obtained from the flowers of *Chrysanthemum cinerariaefolium*). Pyrethrum acts as an insecticide as well as a repellent. Pyrethroid-containing sprays should be used to eliminate mosquitoes from living and sleeping areas during evening and nighttime hours. Most experts consider them to be nontoxic.[14] Mos-quito coils containing pyrethroids may be used although these coils last only a few hours. Many products are of questionable quality and may cause irritation of the mucous membranes.

Clothing sprayed with permethrin or deltamethrin provides residual protection for 2 to 4 weeks; the spraying causes no stains and minimal odor. This measure is considered nontoxic for adults whereas it is questionable for infants and children. Permethrin, however, should not be applied directly to the skin.

Ultrasonic devices and "bug zappers" that lure and electrocute insects are inef-fective measures against mosquito bites.

In summary, there is general agreement that for that visitors to endemic areas, PPMs against *Anopheles* mosquito bites are the first line of defense against malaria[5] although only a few PPMs have a proven efficacy in travelers.[8,15] PPMs, with all the above-mentioned options, seem nevertheless to be indicated for those who are at greatest risk of frequent mosquito bites. For those at low or intermediate risk, preference should be given to convenient measures with proven effectiveness, such as using air-conditioned rooms and wearing appropriate clothing.

CHEMOPROPHYLAXIS

The prevention of malaria symptoms after infection requires a disruption of the plasmodial life cycle. Several agents are available that act at one or more points in the parasite's cycle (see Figure 7–4). "Chemoprophylaxis" is essentially a misnomer as most currently marketed drugs actually do not prevent infection. Rather, these agents act by suppressing the proliferation and development of the malarial parasite, and they would better be termed chemosuppressive agents.

Decision To Use

All antimalarial agents have considerable potential for causing adverse events. The incidence of these reactions varies, depending on surveillance method and study design. Self-reports of side effects suggest that reactions to drugs are reported by 16% to 90% of users.[16] The highest rates of adverse events (of any degree) and discontinuation of chemoprophylaxis were usually observed in chloroquine/proguanil users,[2,15,17] but mefloquine more often resulted in neuropsychiatric adverse events.[16,17] Serious reactions to drugs are of more concern than the subjective reports mentioned above. Chloroquine (alone or with proguanil) and mefloquine, as used in prophylaxis, may cause severe neuropsychiatric events (including psychosis and seizures) in approximately 1 in 10,000 users, usually resulting in hospitalization.[2,18] Another agent currently recommended for chemoprophylaxis by WHO is doxycycline.[5] The limited available information suggests that the adverse drug reaction rates of doxycycline are similar to those of mefloquine, but data on hospitalizations in travelers are scarce. Fatalities have been associated with mefloquine[19,20] and with chloroquine (mostly suicidal).

There is a consensus that chemoprophylaxis must be recommended for travelers to endemic areas whenever the benefit of avoiding symptomatic infections exceeds the risk of serious adverse events (i.e., events that require hospitalization). This is the case for most stays (except very short ones) in areas with high or intermediate transmission, such as tropical Africa, some Pacific areas, certain provinces in Brazil, and parts of the Indian subcontinent. When the risk of acquiring an infection is low, such as in the most frequently visited destinations in Southeast Asia and Latin America, the frequency of adverse experience due to prophylactic medication is greater than any expected benefit (Figure 7–5). According to WHO and various European expert groups, instead of prescribing chemoprophylaxis, it is

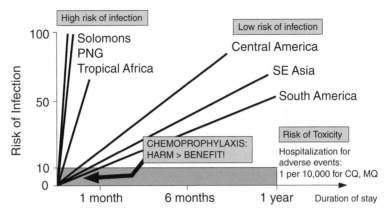

Figure 7–5. Risk of malaria infection without chemoprophylaxis vs. hospitalization for adverse events (per 100,000 travelers). (CQ = chloroquine; MQ = mefloquine; PNG = Papua New Guinea; SE = Southeast.)

more appropriate to insist on PPMs against mosquito bites and to recommend consulting a doctor within 24 hours of the onset of suggestive symptoms during short stays in areas of low malarial endemicity. If the traveler stays in an area where there is no competent medical infrastructure, then standby or presumptive treatment may be an alternative strategy.

Thus, with respect to chemoprophylaxis, the first decision in low-risk situations is whether or not to recommend it. This approach is, however, only exceptionally endorsed by the U.S. Centers for Disease Control and Prevention (CDC)[21] and by various other national expert groups, which (mainly for legal reasons) prescribe chemoprophylaxis for all travelers.

Choice of Agent

The selection of a prophylactic agent is often complex, and although there are generalized guidelines to minimize confusion, recommendations for travelers need to be tailored on an individual basis. Efficacy and tolerability are the most important factors to consider.

Travel health professionals implementing WHO recommendations or national guidelines should be aware of (1) destination factors (such as the degree of endemicity), (2) the predominant *Plasmodium* species, and (3) the extent of drug resistance (Figure 7–6), as this will define the efficacy of a particular agent.

The travelers' medical history and other characteristics (such as age and pregnancy) may also influence the choice of prophylaxis; most regimens have clearly defined contraindications and precautions that must be observed to ensure tolerability. The duration and mode of travel have also been shown to be important, as have medication factors such as compliance and acceptability (discussed in Chapter YY). It must be clearly stated that homeopathic drugs are no option for the prophy-

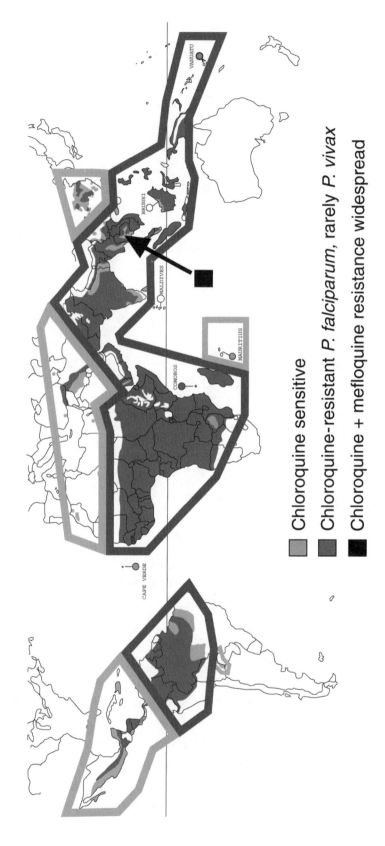

Figure 7–6. Drug resistance in plasmodia. (*P.* = *Plasmodium.*)

Chloroquine sensitive

Chloroquine-resistant *P. falciparum*, rarely *P. vivax*

Chloroquine + mefloquine resistance widespread

laxis of malaria as they have no effectiveness; consequently, many cases of life-threatening malaria treated with such a regimen have been anecdotally reported.

STANDBY EMERGENCY TREATMENT

When symptoms suggestive of malaria occur while abroad or after return, the traveler must obtain competent medical care within 24 hours of the onset of symptoms. Medical assessment must include blood sample screening, either by microscopic examination or with an appropriate rapid diagnostic test kit. Most travelers anywhere have access to competent medical attention within the specified time frame. Only a small minority may find themselves with symptoms suggestive of malaria in a location remote from established medical facilities. Travelers in such a situation may be advised to carry antimalarial medication for standby emergency treatment (SBET) and, possibly, a malaria test kit. These emergency supplies can be used for self-diagnosis and self-therapy or can be made available to the consulted physician.

For travelers using this approach, it is imperative to provide

- precise instructions on how to recognize malaria symptoms,
- the recommendation to seek local medical care if at all possible,
- an indication of the time frame within which medical attention must be procured,
- information on the precise use of the SBET medication,
- warning about the potential for adverse events, and
- advice on the necessity to also seek medical advice as soon as possible after initial SBET, to ensure that the therapy was successful or to obtain the proper treatment in case of erroneous self-diagnosis.

The SBET strategy is a logical one, and when first recommended to Swiss travelers visiting Thailand, no increase in the rate of imported malaria was reported. However, SBET in practice also entails great inconveniences and has disadvantages (resulting in both over- and underuse), such as the following:

1. Difficulty in explaining malaria symptoms to people who are not medical professionals.
2. Noncompliance with the advice to consult a medical professional within 24 hours in case of febrile illness during or after a visit to a malaria-endemic area.[22,23]
3. Overdiagnosis of malaria (partly for financial reasons) by physicians in endemic countries.[2]
4. Misuse of SBET (e.g., for travelers' diarrhea).
5. Frequent serious adverse events with agents used for SBET, such as quinine, chloroquine, and mefloquine.[18] Fatalities are associated with halofantrine, the cardiotoxic potential of which has been established. Sudden deaths associated with the therapeutic use of this drug have led WHO to state that "halofantrine is

no longer recommended for standby treatment, following reports that it can result in prolongation of the Q-Tc intervals and ventricular dysrhythmias in susceptible individuals. These changes can be accentuated if halofantrine is taken with other antimalarial drugs that can decrease myocardial conduction."[5,24] An electrocardiogram [ECG] with a normal Q-Tc interval prior to departure apparently does not preclude the risk of a fatal adverse event with this drug.[25]

6. Inability of travelers to perform self-diagnostic tests reliably, which essentially limits SBET to use by trained people.[26–28]
7. Recrudescence of malaria when artemisinin products bought in developing countries are used.
8. Increased cost of medication when newer agents are prescribed.

In summary, SBET is a logical approach, but it has numerous practical shortcomings that have not been solved satisfactorily. Newer agents, such as artemisinin benflumetol and atovaquone/proguanil, at least offer the option of SBET with unlikely recrudescence and with lower rates of adverse events.

CONCLUSION

There is no simple universal approach that is optimal for all nonimmune travelers visiting malaria-endemic areas. Information and a varying degree of PPMs are indicated for all travelers. With respect to chemoprophylaxis, this author feels that the dogma of "first, do not harm" has priority. Furthermore, travelers to low-risk destinations now often bluntly refuse to use prophylactic medication at those destinations. The alternate solution of SBET, as shown, is far from satisfactory. A reasonably priced prophylactic drug (ultimately, a vaccine, perhaps) taken only just before departure might solve the dilemma, but whether the future agent tafenoquine offers this option[29] remains to be demonstrated.

REFERENCES

1. Hippocrates. Corpus hippocraticum. First book on epidemics. Chapter 11.
2. Steffen R, Fuchs E, Schildknecht J, et al. Mefloquine compared with other malaria chemoprophylactic regimens in tourists visiting east Africa. Lancet 1993;22:299–303.
3. Jelinek T, Löscher T, Nothdurft HD. High prevalence of antibodies against circumsporozoite antigen of *Plasmodium falciparum* without development of symptomatic malaria in travelers returning from sub-Saharan Africa. J Infect Dis 1996;174:1376–1379.
4. Jelinek T, Bluml A, Loscher T, Nothdurft HD. Assessing the incidence of infection with *Plasmodium falciparum* among international travelers. Am J Trop Med Hyg 1998;59:35–37.
5. World Health Organization. International travel and health. Geneva, World Health Organization, 2001.

6. Behrens RH, Bradley DJ, Snow RW, Marsh K. Impact of UK malaria prophylaxis policy on imported malaria. Lancet 1996;9023:344–345.

7. Debrunner JF. Tropenreisende: was sie wissen, was sie meinen und was sie lernen [dissertation]. Zürich: Universität Zürich, 1999.

8. Schoepke A, Steffen R, Gratz N. Effectiveness of personal protection measures against mosquito bites for malaria prophylaxis in travelers. J Travel Med 1998;5:188–192.

9. Curtis CF, Myamba J, Wilkes TJ. Comparison of different insecticides and fabrics for anti-mosquito bednets and curtains. Med Vet Entomol 1996;10:1–11.

10. Fradin MS. Mosquitoes and mosquito repellents: a clinician's guide. Ann Intern Med 1998;128:931–940.

11. Golenda CF, Solberg VB, Burge R, et al. Gender-related efficacy difference to an extended duration formulation of topical N,N-diethyl-m-toluamide (DEET). Am J Trop Med Hyg 1999;60:654–657.

12. Goodyear L, Behrens RH. Short report: the safety and toxicity of insect repellents. Am J Trop Med Hyg 1998;59:323–324.

13. Khan AA, Maibach HI, Strauss WG, Fenley WR. Vitamin B1 is not a systemic mosquito repellent in man. Trans St Johns Hosp Dermatol Soc 1969;55:99–102.

14. Gratz NG, Steffen R, Cocksedge W. Why aircraft disinsection? Bull World Health Organ 2000;78:995–1004.

15. Croft A. Extracts from "Clinical Evidence." Malaria: prevention in travellers. BMJ 2000;321:154–160.

16. Schlagenhauf P. Mefloquine for malaria chemoprophylaxis 1992–1998: a review. J Travel Med 1999:122–133.

17. Barrett PJ, Emmins PD, Clarke PD, Bradley DJ. Comparison of adverse events associated with use of mefloquine and combination of chloroquine and proguanil as antimalarial prophylaxis: postal and telephone survey of travellers. BMJ 1996;313: 525–528.

18. Weinke T, Trautmann M, Held T, et al. Neuropsychiatric side effects after the use of mefloquine. Am J Trop Med Hyg 1991;45:86–91.

19. MacBride AR, Lawrence CM, Pape SA, Reid CA. Fatal toxic epidermal necrolysis assiociated with mefloquine prophylaxis. Lancet 1997;349:101.

20. Schlagenhauf P, Abo El Ela H, Niederberger W, et al. Drug safety database analysis of the events suicide, attempted suicide and suicidal ideation reported in association with the use of Lariam® chemoprophylaxis [abstract]. Proceedings of the ISTM Conference; 2001 May 27–31; Innsbruck.

21. Centers for Disease Control and Prevention. Health Information for the international traveler 2001–2002. Atlanta: U.S. Department of Health and Human Services, Public Health Service; 2001.

22. Schlagenhauf P, Steffen R, Tschopp A, et al. Behavioural aspects of travellers in their use of malaria presumptive treatment. Bull World Health Organization 1995;73:2:215–221.

23. Schlagenhauf P, Phillips-Howard PA. Malaria: emergency self-treatment by travelers. In: DuPont HL, Steffen R, editors. Textbook of travel medicine and health. 2nd ed. Hamilton (ON): B.C. Decker, 2001.

24. World Health Organization. Drug alert: halofantrine. Wkly Epidemiol Rec 1993;68:268–270.

25. Matson PA, Luby SP, Redd SC, et al. Cardiac effects of standard-dose halofantrine therapy. Am J Trop Med Hyg 1996;54:229–231.

26. Funk M, Schlagenhauf P, Tschopp A, Steffen R. MalaQuick versus ParaSight F as a diagnostic aid in travellers' malaria. Trans R Soc Trop Med Hyg 1999;93:268–272.
27. Trachsler M, Schlagenhauf P, Steffen R. Feasibility of a rapid dipstick antigen-capture assay for self-testing of travellers' malaria. Trop Med Int Health 1999;4:442–447.
28. Jelinek T, Amsler L, Grobusch MP, Nothdurft HD. Self-use of rapid tests for malaria diagnosis by tourists. Lancet 1999;354:1609.
29. Lell B, Faucher JF, Missinou MA, et al. Malaria chemoprophylaxis with tafenoquine: a randomised study. Lancet 2000;355:2041–2045.

Chapter 8

DRUGS USED IN MALARIA CHEMOPROPHYLAXIS

"...the simplicity, in theory, of prophylaxis against malaria is only equaled by its difficulty in practice...everything about malaria is so moulded and altered by local conditions that it becomes a thousand different diseases and epidemiological puzzles..."
—Hackett (1937)

8.1 Chloroquine and Combinations
Ashley M. Croft and Katie G. Geary

ABSTRACT

Chloroquine is a cheap, relatively well-tolerated, and exceptionally important antimalarial drug that has been in continuous use for over 50 years. Its usefulness is now limited by increasing *Plasmodium falciparum* resistance to the drug. The combination of chloroquine plus proguanil retains some effectiveness in areas of multidrug resistance although it should no longer be first-line chemoprophylaxis. Chloroquine alone is effective chemoprophylaxis in those malaria-endemic countries where there is no *Plasmodium falciparum* resistance. Chloroquine is safe in pregnancy. It should not be used by those suffering from epilepsy nor by people with generalized psoriasis. Chloroquine users with mild psoriasis or light-sensitive skin should use sunblocking preparations. Travelers who plan to use chloroquine chemoprophylaxis should be advised of the range and approximate frequencies of the nonserious adverse effects (mainly gastrointestinal and neuropsychologic) they may expect to encounter from this drug; around 2% of users may need to discontinue chloroquine and start alternative chemoprophylaxis because of such effects. Rare or serious adverse effects from chloroquine use may be cardiac, dermatologic, neuropsychiatric, or ophthalmologic. There is some evidence that the concurrent use of chloroquine and other quinoline derivatives (e.g., amodiaquine, mefloquine, primaquine, quinidine, quinine, and tafenoquine) can result in serious drug interactions. In addition to using chemoprophylaxis, all travelers to malaria-endemic areas should use bite avoidance measures of proven effectiveness.

Key words: adverse effects; amodiaquine; chloroquine; malaria; mefloquine; primaquine; prophylaxis; resistance; tafenoquine; travel.

BACKGROUND

Development of Chloroquine

Chloroquine is a 4-aminoquinoline drug, chemically related to other quinoline derivatives such as amodiaquine, mefloquine, primaquine, quinidine, quinine, and tafenoquine.[1] The chemical formula of chloroquine is 7-chloro-4-(4'-diethyl-amino-1'-methylbutylamino) quinoline.[2] Chloroquine's chemical structure is shown in Figure 8.1–1.

Chloroquine was one of a large series of 4-aminoquinolines investigated through the collaborative antimalaria drug discovery program that took place among the Allied powers during World War II. After the war, it was found that the chemical had already been synthesized and studied by the Germans as early as 1934, under the name resochin. Although chloroquine was developed primarily as an antimalaria drug, it was subsequently found to be effective also in the treatment of hepatic amebiasis, some collagen-vascular and granulomatous diseases (notably rheumatoid arthritis and discoid lupus erythematosus), and various dermatologic disorders.[3,4]

Chloroquine is an off-patent drug and is available today under a great variety of trade names. Travel medicine specialists should be aware of these alternative names as they can otherwise cause confusion when the physician takes a travel history. The principal trade names of chloroquine are listed in Table 8.1–1.

Antimalaria Effects

Chloroquine is a blood schizonticide, acting mainly on the large ring-form and mature trophozoite stages of the parasite. It is ineffective against the exoerythrocytic-tissue stages of plasmodia. Chloroquine is thus not a causal prophylactic

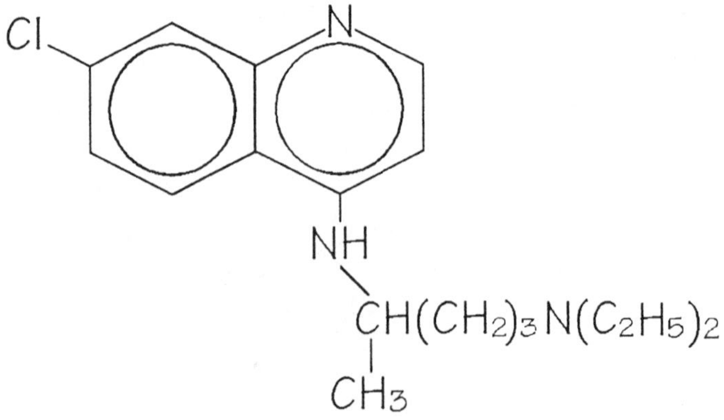

Figure 8.1–1. Chemical structure of chloroquine.

Table 8.1–1. **Synonyms and Trade Names of Chloroquine (a 4-Aminoquinoline)**

Aralen	Malaquin
Arechin	Malarex
Avloclor	Malarivon
Bemaphate	Matalets
Chinamine	Nivaquine
Chlorocon	Nivaquine B
Chlorquim	Resochin
Chlorquin	Resochine
Cidanchin	Resoquine
Delagil	Roquine
Gontochin	Sanoquin
Imagon	Siragan
Iroquine	Tanakan
Klorokin	Tresochin
Luprochin	Trochin

Adapted from Warrell DA. Treatment and prevention of malaria. In: Gilles HM, Warrell DA, editors. Bruce-Chwatt's essential malariology. 3rd ed. London: Edward Arnold, 1993. p. 164–195.

agent and does not prevent the initial establishment of infection. However, chloroquine is highly effective against sensitive strains of *Plasmodium falciparum*, and in addition, it is gametocidal against *Plasmodium vivax*, *Plasmodium malariae*, and *Plasmodium ovale.*[2]

In acute clinical malaria, chloroquine at therapeutic doses rapidly controls symptoms and parasitemia; thick smears of peripheral blood are generally negative for parasites by 48 to 72 hours. Chloroquine, like quinine, does not prevent relapses in vivax malaria, but it substantially lengthens the interval between relapses.

Mechanism of Action against Plasmodia

All the blood schizonticides are weak bases, and it is believed that this property causes them to concentrate in and raise the pH of acidic vesicles within sensitive malaria parasites.[5] Chloroquine's primary mechanism of action is thought to be the inhibition of the proteolysis of hemoglobin in the parasite's food vacuole.[6] Because hemin (i.e., free heme) obtained from the proteolysis of hemoglobin is toxic and lyses membranes, it is necessary for the parasite to polymerize toxic hemin into nontoxic hemozoin ("malaria pigment"). Chloroquine is believed to inhibit this polymerization process.[7]

A second mechanism through which chloroquine may act against plasmodia is through the drug's ability to alkalinize the plasmodial food vacuole (the secondary lysosome) at concentrations 1,000-fold less than those that alkalinize vesicles in mammalian cells, thereby preferentially inhibiting parasite growth.[8]

Pharmacokinetics

Chloroquine is rapidly and almost completely absorbed from the gastrointestinal tract, after which it is localized in the tissues, mainly concentrated in cell lysosomes.[9,10] The drug is sequestered in the liver, spleen, kidney, lungs, melanocytes, and neural tissue.[11] Because of extensive tissue binding, a loading dose of chloroquine is necessary when it is desirable to achieve swift therapeutic concentrations in plasma.[12]

Chloroquine is metabolized by alkylation in the liver and is excreted slowly by the kidneys, with a half-life of from 3 to 6 or 7 days in a normal healthy adult, depending on the amount and frequency of drug intake.[13] Chloroquine's principal metabolites are desethyl- and bisdesethyl-chloroquine; of these, the former has approximately equivalent antimalaria activity.[14] Following daily administration of chloroquine, about 10% appears in the feces and about 60% in the urine, of which approximately two-thirds is the parent compound.[13]

Parasite Resistance to Chloroquine

The resistance gradient of plasmodia to antimalaria drugs is conventionally characterized as S (sensitive), R1 resistance (low-level resistance), R2 resistance (intermediate-level resistance), and R3 resistance (high-level resistance).[15] Resistance results from a number of factors, including the remarkable adaptability of *Plasmodium*, the widespread use of antimalaria drugs for prophylaxis, and the use of suboptimal treatment regimens for clinical illness.[16]

Parasite resistance to chloroquine was first observed in Thailand in 1957 and on the Colombian-Venezuelan border in 1959. The first cases of chloroquine resistance in Africa were reported from Kenya and Tanzania in 1978.[17] From this initial focus in East Africa, resistance spread to the Comoros Islands, Madagascar, Uganda, and Zambia. By the late 1980s, chloroquine resistance had spread widely through Southeast Asia, South America, and Africa and had been detected also in the western Pacific, India, and southern China.[18]

From the mid-1980s onward, *Plasmodium vivax* resistance to chloroquine was reported in New Guinea and then elsewhere in Oceania.[19,20]

Plasmodium falciparum resistance to chloroquine is now established in almost all malaria-endemic areas of the world although there are countries (principally those where *Plasmodium vivax* is the predominant species) where there has been no reported resistance as yet.[21] These countries are listed in Table 8.1–2. In the rural areas of these countries, chloroquine alone remains effective as malaria chemoprophylaxis.

Chloroquine-resistant strains of *Plasmodium falciparum* are at a biologic advantage over chloroquine-sensitive strains, having a more robust metabolism and preferential tropism for uptake by mosquitoes.[2] It seems likely, therefore, that *P. falciparum* resistance to chloroquine will eventually spread to all areas of the world endemic for falciparum malaria.[22]

Table 8.1–2. **Malaria-Endemic Regions with No Reported Chloroquine Resistance***

Northern Central America/ Caribbean Region	*Near East*
Belize	Armenia
Costa Rica	Azerbaijan
Dominican Republic	Georgia
Haiti	Iraq
Honduras	Turkey
Mexico	

* Wholly resistance-free countries.
Reprinted with permission from World Health Organization. International travel and health—vaccination requirements and health advice. Geneva: World Health Organization, 2000.

Travel medicine specialists can obtain regularly updated country-by-country information on chloroquine resistance patterns from the World Health Organization (WHO) Web site at www.who.int/ith/english/country.htm.

CHLOROQUINE IN MALARIA PROPHYLAXIS

Because of its relatively favorable adverse effect profile, its safety in pregnancy, and its low cost, chloroquine has been extensively used in malaria prophylaxis both by indigenous residents of malaria-endemic areas and by nonimmune travelers to those areas. In most industrialized countries, the currently recommended dose of chloroquine for adult travelers is 300 mg of the base (or 500 mg of chloroquine phosphate), taken orally once a week with food. The pediatric dose is 5 mg of the base per kilogram (or 8.3 mg of the salt per kilogram), once weekly.[21] Because of the bitter taste of the drug, chloroquine syrup is preferred for children.[23]

Chloroquine prophylaxis should be started 2 weeks before travel, to allow time for the traveler to change to a different antimalaria drug if unacceptable adverse effects are encountered. Chemoprophylaxis must be maintained throughout the period of travel and should continue for 4 weeks after departure from the malaria-endemic area. The reasons for this latter requirement are (1) to protect against infection acquired at or shortly before the time of departure and (2) to ensure that schizonticidal concentrations of chloroquine are still present in the blood when merozoites emerge from the liver after a maximum pre-patent period.[2]

As explained above, chloroquine cannot be relied on to prevent hypnozoites of *Plasmodium vivax* and *Plasmodium ovale* from developing in the liver. It is recommended, therefore, that any chloroquine-using traveler who has experienced prolonged exposure to these infections (e.g., for 6 months or more) should undergo terminal prophylaxis with primaquine after leaving the malaria-endemic area. Before primaquine terminal prophylaxis is started, the returning traveler's glucose-6-phosphate dehydrogenase (G6PD) status should be determined.[13]

Chloroquine Alone

At the time of writing (December 2000), there are just two malaria-endemic regions where *Plasmodium falciparum* chloroquine resistance has not yet been reported: (1) parts of northern Central America and the northern Caribbean regions and (2) parts of the Near East.[21] Table 8.1–2 lists those countries (in these particular regions) that have not as yet submitted to WHO any reports of parasite resistance to chloroquine.

Nonimmune travelers to rural areas in regions of continuing chloroquine sensitivity should be prescribed weekly chloroquine and should take proven measures to avoid mosquito bites.[24] Travelers who remain in the towns do not need to take malaria chemoprophylaxis.[25]

In some cases, apparent chemoprophylaxis failures of chloroquine are due to the fact that adult travelers, who may vary in weight from 40 kg to over 100 kg, are prescribed a fixed dose of the drug rather than a dose titrated against their weight.[26] It is thus good clinical practice to adjust the dosage of chloroquine to the traveler's weight. For instance, travelers weighing more than 75 kg might be better protected by taking chloroquine 300 mg every 5 or 6 days rather than once weekly.[13]

Chloroquine plus Proguanil

The fixed combination of chloroquine 300 mg weekly plus proguanil 200 mg daily has been widely recommended since the 1980s for travelers to malaria-endemic areas with *P. falciparum* resistance to chloroquine. The efficacy and tolerability of this regimen is further considered below.

Other Chloroquine Combinations

During the Vietnam War, a combined chloroquine/primaquine tablet was taken weekly by U.S. troops, in an early attempt to overcome *P. falciparum* resistance to chloroquine. This combination of two quinoline derivatives was poorly tolerated, however, and commonly gave rise to severe nausea, diarrhea, abdominal cramps, and headache.[27] Typically, the symptoms occurred within 24 hours of taking the drugs and lasted approximately 24 to 36 hours. In some cases, so-called drug fever (comprising a shaking chill and a low-grade fever in the absence of any infective cause) was also associated with the weekly ingestion of this fixed chloroquine combination.[28]

From the late 1970s onward, as chloroquine-resistant strains of *P. falciparum* became even more widespread in the Far East, Australian troops experimented with a fixed combination of chloroquine plus dapsone and pyrimethamine (Maloprim).[29] Gastrointestinal disturbances were experienced by approximately 31% of users of chloroquine plus Maloprim. By the late 1980s, this triple drug combination was no longer considered to be effective prophylaxis against malaria since true drug failures were being documented, as shown by adequate plasma concentrations of chloroquine, dapsone, and pyrimethamine, despite the presence of confirmed clinical illness.[29]

Table 8.1–3. **Contraindications to the Use of Chloroquine**

1. Family history of epilepsy.

2. History of generalized psoriasis.

3. Concurrent use of any other quinoline derivative (e.g., amodiaquine, mefloquine, primaquine, quinidine, quinine, and tafenoquine), whether for additional malaria prophylaxis or for treatment. (Chloroquine users should avoid these drugs.)

4. Severe pruritus resulting from chloroquine treatment. (An alternative drug should be used for prophylaxis.)

Adapted from World Health Organization. International travel and health—vaccination requirements and health advice. Geneva: World Health Organization, 2001.

Contraindications to the Use of Chloroquine

WHO has published a list of the contraindications to the use of chloroquine by travelers.[21] This list is summarized in Table 8.1–3.

There are no reports of teratogenic effects in humans when chloroquine has been used as an antimalaria drug; it may therefore be administered during pregnancy.[13] However, any prospective travelers who are pregnant or who are contemplating pregnancy should be advised that pregnant women are twice as attractive as nonpregnant women to anopheline mosquitoes and that because of the relative immunosuppression that accompanies pregnancy, pregnant women are particularly prone to develop severe disease.[30,31]

EVIDENCE OF EFFICACY IN TRAVELERS

Chloroquine Alone

There is no systematic review of the use of chloroquine or any chloroquine combination as prophylaxis in nonimmune travelers. One published randomized controlled trial (RCT) compared chloroquine with sulfadoxine plus pyrimethamine (Fansidar) in 173 Austrian industrial workers based in Nigeria.[32] This study found no evidence of a difference in the incidence of malaria.

Chloroquine plus Proguanil

There are two published RCTs of the use of chloroquine plus proguanil in nonimmune general travelers. One RCT in Scandinavian travelers to East Africa found 4 cases of *P. falciparum* malaria in 384 travelers randomized to chloroquine plus proguanil and 3 cases in 383 participants randomized to a combination of chloroquine with sulfadoxine plus pyrimethamine (Fansidar); the difference was not statistically significant.[33] An RCT in Dutch travelers to Africa found 7 cases of falciparum malaria in 1,640 travelers randomized to chloroquine plus proguanil and 5 cases in 830 travelers randomized to proguanil alone; the difference was not statistically significant.[34]

A controlled clinical trial carried out in French troops in central Africa during 1996 compared 270 soldiers taking a combined daily tablet consisting of chloroquine (136 mg) plus proguanil (200 mg) with an equivalent group of 171 soldiers taking doxycycline hyclate (100 mg daily).[35] Although adverse effects resulting in drug discontinuation were significantly higher in the doxycycline group (11 of 171 vs. 0 of 270, $p < .001$), only 0.6% of the doxycycline users developed *P. falciparum* malaria during the 4-month deployment, compared to 4.8% of the users of chloroquine plus proguanil ($p < .02$).

A recently concluded multicenter RCT in 1,083 nonimmune travelers to *P. falciparum*–endemic areas found that 3 of 511 travelers randomized to chloroquine plus proguanil developed *P. falciparum* malaria and that just 1 of 511 travelers randomized to atovaquone plus proguanil developed *P. ovale* malaria.[36]

EVIDENCE OF HARM IN TRAVELERS

Common Adverse Effects

Chloroquine Alone

Travelers who use chloroquine prophylaxis commonly experience a wide range of adverse effects, typically of a gastrointestinal, neuropsychologic, or dermatologic nature. Table 8.1–4 summarizes the relative frequencies of these common adverse effects. The data are derived from four retrospective questionnaire surveys carried out in nonimmune tourists and business travelers.[37–40]

Travel medicine specialists who advise travelers should warn them of the range and approximate frequencies of the nonserious adverse effects they may encounter from their malaria chemoprophylaxis. Travelers should be advised that most common adverse effects from antimalaria drugs are mild and self-limiting and should not be an occasion to stop chemoprophylaxis. Where the adverse effects are severe or prolonged, however, medical advice should be sought, and alternative chemoprophylaxis should be started.

Table 8.1-4. Common Adverse Effects of Chloroquine Prophylaxis in Nonimmune Travelers

Frequency (Incidence)*	Adverse Effects
Low (1–5%)	Abdominal pain, anxiety, depression, headache, muscle cramps, pruritus, rash, sleep disturbance, tingling, tiredness, visual difficulties, vivid dreams
Medium (6–10%)	Anorexia, diarrhea, dizziness, nausea, vomiting
High (> 10%)	None

*As the percentage of nonimmune travelers in whom the adverse effects occur.
Data from Huzly et al,[37] Corominas et al,[38] Durrheim et al,[39] and Petersen et al.[40]

Table 8.1–5. **Common Adverse Effects of Chloroquine plus Proguanil Prophylaxis in Nonimmune Travelers**

Frequency (Incidence)*	Adverse Effects
Low (1–5%)	Depression, dizziness, headache, mouth ulcers, pruritus, sleep disturbance, tingling, tiredness, visual difficulties, vivid dreams, vomiting
Medium (6–10%)	Abdominal pain, diarrhea, nausea
High (> 10%)	Anorexia

* As the percentage of nonimmune travelers in whom the adverse effects occur.
Data from Huzly et al,[37] Corominas et al,[38] Durrheim et al,[39] Petersen et al,[40] and Carme et al.[41]

Chloroquine plus Proguanil

Table 8.1–5 summarizes the relative frequencies of the common adverse effects associated with chloroquine-plus-proguanil chemoprophylaxis. These data are derived from five retrospective questionnaire surveys carried out in nonimmune tourists and business travelers.[37–41]

Other Chloroquine Combinations

Durrheim and colleagues analyzed the common adverse effects reported by a cohort of 29 travelers who took chloroquine-plus-mefloquine chemoprophylaxis. This group experienced an exceptionally high frequency of nonserious adverse effects, with only 48% reporting "no adverse effects."[39]

Rare or Serious Adverse Effects

General Observations

Adverse effects associated with the prophylaxis and treatment of malaria with chloroquine are generally less severe and less frequent than those associated with the use of chloroquine to treat collagen-vascular, granulomatous, and dermatologic disorders.

In an overdose, chloroquine is acutely cardiotoxic, causing hypotension, arrhythmias, and eventual cardiovascular collapse, convulsions, and death. Untreated chloroquine overdoses are rapidly fatal, in part due to the rapid and almost complete absorption of the drug.

Rare dermatologic adverse reactions to chloroquine include toxic epidermal necrolysis, vitiligo, and the bleaching of hair. Reported neuropsychiatric harms in travelers using chloroquine have included serious adverse effects such as psychotic episodes, personality changes, and convulsions; these effects, however, are relatively rare. Keratopathy and retinopathy, in some cases irreversible, have been reported in chloroquine users; these ophthalmologic disorders, however, appear to be more common with the higher chloroquine dosages used for treating the noninfective disorders.

The following narrative illustrates some of the rare or serious adverse effects of chloroquine, with reference to published case reports of these harms.

Cardiovascular Harms

Adverse cardiac effects have been reported following the parenteral administration of chloroquine. These effects appear to be related to the early and transient high plasma concentrations of the drug and result also from chloroquine overdosage or abuse and from long-term oral treatment for rheumatologic conditions.[42] Cardiovascular harms from chloroquine have not been seen at the standard doses recommended for malaria prophylaxis.

There is one case in the literature of a Liberian businessman who presented after four Stokes-Adams attacks in 12 hours.[43] On admission to hospital, he was found to be in complete heart block, and a temporary pacemaker was inserted. Electrocardiography performed at this time showed right bundle-branch block (RBBB). He had no previous cardiac history, no symptoms of other systemic disease, and no family history of heart disease. On questioning, he was found to be self-medicating with chloroquine phosphate (chloroquine base, 155 mg; Avloclor) whenever he felt he had the symptoms of cerebral malaria, namely, a headache. This amounted to a weekly dose of six to eight chloroquine tablets over a period of 3 years. Permanent pacing was instituted in this patient due to his life-threatening dysrhythmias. This patient also demonstrated ocular changes due to chronic chloroquine ingestion; these changes are documented below.

Ogola and colleagues reported a second case of complete heart block, in a 27-year-old African woman.[44] She had presented with ophthalmic symptoms as well as increasing fatigability, dyspnea, and dizziness progressing to frank syncopal attacks over a 2-year period. She admitted to taking two chloroquine tablets (300 mg base) daily over that 2-year period, for supposed "chronic malaria." Cardiac assessment revealed bibasal crepitations and a tender hepatomegaly. Her electrocardiogram (ECG) showed complete heart block and RBBB. She showed borderline cardiomegaly on chest radiography. A permanent artificial pacemaker was fitted. The same authors reported that RBBB and complete heart block were the common manifestations of chronic chloroquine toxicity, and they cited two additional cases in the literature from Nigeria and one additional case from Kenya.[45]

The presumed mechanism of action for heart block and RBBB derives from the quinidine-like effects of chloroquine, these being negatively inotropic and chronotropic and thus causing decreased conduction in excitable cardiac tissue.

The other presentations of serious cardiovascular harms from chloroquine include restrictive and dilated cardiomyopathy.[46]

The immediate discontinuation of chloroquine in cases of chronic toxicity has been shown to improve the heart failure but not the conduction abnormalities, which seem permanent once acquired. It would therefore seem that immediate discontinuation of chloroquine after the initial assessment might reverse some of the symptoms associated with chronic use of the drug. Hughes and colleagues reported two cases in which similar doses of chronic chloroquine intake resulted in clinical and histologic changes to the heart muscle. The first case was that of a young man who was found dead from a presumed Stokes-Adams attack, and the second was that of a 48-year-old man who was seen early enough for a pacemaker to be fitted and who subsequently improved.[47]

Guedira and colleagues reported a 43-year-old woman who developed juvenile chronic arthritis at the age of 10 years.[48] She was treated with chloroquine sulfate (200 mg daily). Over the next decade, she developed myalgia and skin pigmentation and continued to take daily chloroquine despite warnings. Thirteen years later, having continued intermittent self-therapy with chloroquine, she developed a third-degree heart block that required a pacemaker.

There is additional evidence for the cardiotoxic effects of chloroquine in reports of cases of deliberate self-harm, in which chloroquine was used in much higher doses than is common in either standard prophylactic or therapeutic use. Meeran and Jacobs described three cases of this kind, all illustrating the negative inotropic effect of chloroquine.[49] The first case was that of a 45-year-old Asian woman who had ingested a total dose of 4.5 g of chloroquine base. She collapsed at home. On arrival at hospital, she was asystolic and unresponsive to all resuscitative attempts. The second case was that of a young Madagascan woman who presented to casualty 3 hours after ingesting a similar amount of chloroquine and who was found to have an unrecordable blood pressure, a normal pulse rate of 70 bpm, and a questionably abnormal ECG. She responded well to gastric lavage with activated charcoal, adrenaline, and diazepam infusions, making a full recovery after 12 hours. The patient in the third case ingested a much lower dose of chloroquine (amounting to a total dose of 1.95 g) together with an unknown amount of alcohol. He was assessed within 45 minutes of ingestion. He was cardiovascularly stable, with a blood pressure of 130/80 mm Hg and a normal ECG. He had a gastric lavage with activated charcoal, but despite this, his blood pressure dropped. He recovered spontaneously without further complications. This patient's cardiovascular response to chloroquine seems to show that the absorption rate was quite high despite the rapid use of activated charcoal.[49]

These case reports give some insight into the manifestations of chloroquine toxicity and chloroquine's potential for being acutely toxic even at relatively low doses.

Dermatologic Harms

Toxic epidermal necrolysis secondary to chloroquine use has occasionally been described in the literature. Phillips-Howard and Buckler reported a 59-year-old man who took chloroquine (300 mg) (Nivaquine) and pyrimethamine (12.5 mg) plus dapsone (100 mg) (Maloprim) weekly, starting 5 days before his departure to the Republic of South Africa.[50] He was also taking aspirin and propranolol, a combination he had used for the previous decade with no ill effect. Furthermore, he had traveled extensively and had previously taken pyrimethamine plus dapsone without ill effect; this journey was the first on which he took chloroquine as well. Within 1 day of arrival overseas, he noticed bullous erythema on exposed areas of his skin; this resolved over 2 to 3 days, to return within 4 hours of his next weekly ingestion of malaria chemoprophylaxis, affecting his soft palate, uvula, and epiglottis. This acute attack settled over a period of 10 days, aided by a single 5-mg dose of dexamethasone. The resolving skin lesions, however, left scars on his legs. The authors commented that they had found one other reported case in the literature of toxic epidermal necrolysis during treatment with chloroquine.[50]

Binding of chloroquine to skin melanin may be responsible for some of chloroquine's cutaneous adverse effects, such as the relatively high frequency (8% to 20%) of reversible pruritus that commonly occurs in black Africans within a few hours of starting treatment.[51] This pruritus may be severe enough to warrant withdrawal of chloroquine treatment.

Reversible depigmentation as a result of chloroquine use has occasionally been reported, invariably in black Africans. Selvaag reported the case of a 6-year-old girl of Ethiopian origin, resident in Norway, who presented with vitiligo following a visit to her grandparents in Eritrea.[52] She had been prescribed chloroquine (250 mg weekly) as prophylaxis against malaria. She used no other systemic medication nor any topical agent. She had a past medical history of eczema, but there was no personal or familial history of autoimmune disease. She had taken a total of ten doses of chloroquine before her return to Norway. Her depigmentation was first noticed after 3 weeks of therapy, but it was not accompanied by subjective complaints of ill health nor by any evidence of visual impairment, and she continued to play as normal. On stopping chloroquine use, she underwent a rapid and complete repigmentation of the affected areas over 3 months.[52]

Hyperpigmentation secondary to chloroquine use may occasionally be seen in white skin. Reversible bleaching of the hair has also been reported, following long-term chloroquine treatment.[53]

Chloroquine may aggravate psoriasis, especially in patients with light-sensitive disease.[54] Although most of the published cases involve patients using high-dose chloroquine for collagen-vascular disorders, there has been one reported case of aggravated psoriasis in a traveler taking chloroquine (500 mg weekly).[55] WHO advises that chloroquine should not be prescribed at all for people with generalized psoriasis.[21] When recommending chloroquine prophylaxis to travelers with mild psoriasis or with light-sensitive skin, it is good clinical practice to advise that they use sunblock preparations as well.[56]

Neuropsychiatric Harms

Barrett and colleagues reported a British traveler who was taking chloroquine (300 mg base weekly) plus proguanil (200 mg daily) and who had two seizures while asleep; she underwent hospital investigation after her return to Britain, but the outcome was not given.[57] Petersen and colleagues reported one Danish traveler who experienced severe depression secondary to chloroquine prophylaxis.[40]

In a narrative review of the published literature, Phillips-Howard and ter Kuile quoted an incidence for all neuropsychiatric adverse effects secondary to chloroquine prophylaxis of 1 in 13,600 users and an incidence for extrapyramidal symptoms of 1 in 5,000 users.[58] The authors concluded that chloroquine has a small therapeutic window, being toxic in high doses. They found that the central nervous system (CNS) symptoms of chloroquine overdose typically start with dizziness, vomiting, and headache and progress rapidly to CNS depression and visual disturbance.[58]

At least seven cases of tonic-clonic seizures have been described in users of prophylactic chloroquine.[59–61] Most of the patients described were female, and most had never previously had a seizure although two had evidence of a low seizure threshold. The seizures occurred between day 1 and day 33 following the initial dose of chloroquine. In three of the patients, a drug-drug interaction was thought to have precipitated the seizure: one patient had been taking sulfadoxine plus pyrimethamine (Fansidar) for 1 month prior to and concurrently with chloroquine, and two patients had been taking concurrent dapsone (100 mg) plus pyrimethamine (12.5 mg) (Maloprim).

Lysack and Lysack reported psychiatric symptoms in a previously healthy 23-year-old traveler who took mefloquine and chloroquine as malaria prophylaxis.[62] He was embarking on a journey to India and had started with mefloquine (250 mg salt [Lariam] weekly). He took the first dose of mefloquine on arrival in India, then started to experience anxiety, depression, and sleep disturbance. He took both of the next two doses, and his symptoms progressed to severe suicidal ideation, paranoia, and both visual and auditory hallucinations. He discontinued mefloquine; a week later, he started chloroquine (300 mg base weekly) for malaria prophylaxis. A severe "anxiety attack" followed, 3 hours after ingestion of the first chloroquine dose; 7 hours later, he experienced neurologic symptoms including paresthesias and paresis. These symptoms were initially localized to both his hands and feet, but they became generalized within 15 minutes. He also experienced alternating bouts of racing heartbeat and rapid breathing followed by a slow heart rate and slow breathing. The paresthesias took the form of sharp "electric shocks." These acute symptoms gradually resolved over the next 6 hours. However, the patient was still troubled by persisting episodic fatigue, vertigo, tinnitus, depression, and suicidal ideation 9 months later, without further chloroquine exposure. All but the fatigue, tinnitus, and vertigo had spontaneously resolved by 12 months after the onset of the acute neuropsychiatric symptoms.[62]

Lovestone reported a case of chloroquine-induced mania in a previously fit 33-year-old entertainer with no past history of family or personal psychiatric illness.[63] This patient had been started on chloroquine (300 mg weekly) plus proguanil (200 mg daily), as antimalaria prophylaxis. After each dose of chloroquine, he had noticed a brief period of arousal. On return from holiday, he took a double dose of chloroquine in error, following which he became irritable and overactive. He continued to take his medication for a week, with increasing psychiatric disturbance. He was admitted to a psychiatric hospital, experiencing flight of ideas and expressing delusions of grandeur and reference. He was diagnosed as hypomanic and was prescribed a single 5-mg dose of haloperidol. His mental state returned to normal within 3 days. At this point, he was given a further 300-mg dose of chloroquine, after which his hypomanic symptoms returned. He made a full recovery and was discharged from hospital after a further 3 days. He had a brief recurrence of symptoms 3 weeks later without further chloroquine provocation. This episode resolved spontaneously, and he remained well in the year of follow-up. His physicians surmised that chloroquine may have exerted its toxic effects through the dopaminergic pathway.[63]

Four patients taking a higher-dose treatment regimen of chloroquine experienced convulsions after taking between 500 and 1,000 mg of chloroquine per day for 14 days for treatment of amebiasis. The initial complaints were of headache, nausea, blurring of vision, and dizziness, followed by seizures on days 3, 5, 6, and 12 following the commencement of chloroquine therapy.[64]

In a small series of patients, Umez-Eronini and Eronini reported that normal therapeutic levels of chloroquine (25 mg/kg) induced involuntary movements.[65] This series included patients of both genders, and the preponderance of young patients was striking, the age range being from 12 to 26 years. Reactions to chloroquine included protrusion of the tongue, involuntary pulling of the neck to one side, fasciculation of facial muscles including those of the tongue, excessive salivation, and (in one case) paresthesia of the right side of the face and neck. After cessation of chloroquine, the symptoms abated. This occurred spontaneously in one patient, but medication was used in the others to control the symptoms. In one patient, a further dose of chloroquine was administered 3 months later for an attack of malaria, and the neurologic symptoms returned. In another patient, who had used chloroquine without ill effect prior to this reaction, a further similar reaction was witnessed 8 months later, following treatment with two chloroquine sulfate tablets for an acute attack of malaria.[65]

In a letter to the *Lancet*, Ragan and colleagues reported the occurrence of psychotic symptoms in four aid workers who had self-administered treatment doses of chloroquine (either orally or by injection) in response to fever of presumed malaria origin.[66] Three of these patients developed symptoms after an interval of 48 hours, and the fourth patient developed symptoms within 2 weeks. The clinical picture was not compatible with that of cerebral malaria. Two of the aid workers suffered a recurrence of the symptoms several months after their return home without further exposure to chloroquine. The authors surveyed 69 other aid workers and discovered a further four patients with cases of lesser severity, two of whom had taken chloroquine prophylactically. The authors speculated that other factors besides chloroquine (such as stress and marijuana or other psychoactive agents) might have been implicated in the development of the psychotic symptoms.[66]

Three other cases of serious neuropsychiatric adverse effects were reported by Steffen and colleagues in a cohort of 40,726 travelers using chloroquine at the standard prophylactic dose of 300 mg base per week.[61]

Ophthalmologic Harms

The main ophthalmologic adverse effects of chloroquine are keratopathy and retinopathy.

Keratopathy may occur within a few weeks of starting chloroquine and is characterized by corneal deposits. Typically, these deposits are initially asymptomatic, but they progress to symptoms such as photophobia, the seeing of halos around lights, and blurring of vision. Chloroquine-induced keratopathy is entirely reversible on stopping administration of the drug.

Chloroquine-induce retinopathy is potentially more serious, is not reversible, is generally progressive, and can continue to progress even after cessation of chloroquine therapy; this may be due to the long half-life of the drug and to its accumulation in tissues.[67] It appears that retinopathy is rarely if ever associated with the weekly use of chloroquine in malaria prophylaxis.[68]

In patients taking treatment doses of chloroquine, cases of both keratopathy and retinopathy have been reported, particularly when chloroquine has been misused for prophylaxis or for self-medication. Waddell reviewed 22 cases of maculopathy presenting in clinics in Uganda over a 5-year period.[69] The visual loss was insidious, and the early lesions were detectable only through careful ophthalmoscopy. It was difficult to establish the true dosages of chloroquine taken by the patients in this series as oral chloroquine was freely available without prescription; in addition, some patients had had chloroquine injections at their health centers, and in some cases, full courses of chloroquine were taken once or twice a month, sometimes continuing for decades. It was therefore difficult to determine accurately a toxic threshold for the total dose of chloroquine although a safe daily threshold of 5.1 mg/kg/day for the phosphate (i.e., one 300-mg tablet daily for a 62-kg user) was suggested.[69]

There are two further published reports of visual loss secondary to chronic and toxic chloroquine ingestion for presumed malaria; both patients presented with initial heart block and progressed to permanent visual loss.[43,44] In the first case, repeated chloroquine use resulted in bilateral scotomata and loss of central vision; in the second case, the continuous daily ingestion of chloroquine (600 mg base) over 3 years for "chronic malaria" resulted in chloroquine retinopathy and permanent blindness.

A retrospective survey of 558 career missionaries, carried out to assess the association between total body burden of chloroquine and the development of retinopathy, detected only one case of retinopathy; the patient had taken chloroquine in high doses as an anti-inflammatory agent for a connective-tissue disorder for at least 6 years prior to the survey.[70] The authors speculated that while the daily dose of chloroquine is a risk factor in the development of ophthalmologic disturbances, the total cumulative dose of the drug may also be important.

Bernstein found that the accumulation of 100 mg of chloroquine daily for 1 year may cause retinopathy and that the risk increases if the daily dose exceeds 300 mg.[71] Experience in rheumatology also suggests that the incidence of retinal toxicity is related to the size of the daily chloroquine dose.[72]

Miscellaneous Harms

A case of chloroquine-induced endocrine disturbance was described by Munera and colleagues.[73] A woman with hypothyroidism, well stabilized on thyroxine sodium (125 μg daily), took chloroquine plus proguanil daily for 2 months as malaria prophylaxis for a holiday in Africa. At 4 weeks, her thyroid-stimulating hormone (TSH) concentration was found to be very high (44.8 mU/L [normal range, 0.35 to 6.0 mU/L]), but it returned to normal within a week of stopping administration of chloroquine plus proguanil. Rechallenge with chloroquine plus proguanil a year later again resulted in raised levels of TSH, a lowered concentration of free triiodothyronine (T_3), and a normal free thyroxine (T_4) concentration. This patient's liver function was not tested, but the authors speculated: "Chloroquine... seems to have enhanced the induction of liver enzymes. Chloroquine probably increased the catabolism of thyroid hormones by enzymatic induction."[73]

Other serious adverse effects of chloroquine use have also been noted but have not been widely published in the literature. These include hypoglycemia following chloroquine therapy for the treatment of collagen-vascular diseases. Myalgia and proximal muscle weakness have also been reported, both on clinical and histologic grounds, often associated with skin manifestations and/or cardiac or ophthalmologic symptomatology.[48]

CONCLUSION

No other antimalaria drug has matched the speed of action, safety, and breadth of activity exhibited by chloroquine when it was first introduced in the 1940s. Despite the extensive spread of chloroquine-resistant strains of *Plasmodium falciparum* from the late 1950s onward and the more recent emergence of chloroquine-resistant *Plasmodium vivax* in Oceania, chloroquine is still by far the most widely used antimalaria drug in the world.[2]

Chloroquine alone is a cheap and effective chemoprophylactic drug for travelers to the rural areas of those malaria-endemic countries (currently fewer than 12) where there is no reported *Plasmodium falciparum* resistance to chloroquine.[21] Travelers weighing more than 75 kg should take a single 300-mg dose of chloroquine every 5 or 6 days rather than 300 mg once weekly.[13] All travelers to malaria-endemic areas should also use proven methods for avoiding mosquito bites.[24]

Chloroquine is safe in pregnancy.[13]

People who are epileptic and people with generalized psoriasis should not use chloroquine.[21] Travelers who have mild psoriasis or light-sensitive skin and who use chloroquine should be advised to use sunblock preparations in addition.[56]

There is some evidence that the concurrent use of chloroquine and other quinoline derivatives can result in serious drug-drug interactions.[27,39,62] Chloroquine users should therefore avoid the concurrent use of any other quinoline derivative (e.g., amodiaquine, mefloquine, primaquine, quinidine, quinine, and tafenoquine), whether for additional malaria prophylaxis or for treatment.

As a matter of good clinical practice, prospective users of chloroquine chemoprophylaxis should be advised of the range and approximate frequencies of the common and nonserious adverse effects they may expect to encounter from this drug.

The combination of chloroquine plus proguanil, although still widely recommended for areas where there is *P. falciparum* resistance to chloroquine, and although relatively well tolerated by general travelers, is of declining efficacy in preventing *P. falciparum* malaria[35,36] and should no longer be used as first-line chemoprophylaxis.

REFERENCES

1. Webster LT. Drugs used in the chemotherapy of protozoal infections. In: Gilman AG, Rall TW, Nies AS, Taylor P, editors. Goodman and Gilman's the pharmacological basis of therapeutics. 8th ed. New York: McGraw-Hill, 1992. p. 978–998.
2. Warrell DA. Treatment and prevention of malaria. In: Gilles HM, Warrell DA, editors. Bruce-Chwatt's essential malariology. 3rd ed. London: Edward Arnold, 1993. p. 164–195.
3. Dubois EL. Antimalarials in the management of discoid and systemic lupus erythematosus. Semin Arthritis Rheum 1978;8:33–51.
4. Isaacson D, Elgart M, Turner ML. Antimalarials in dermatology. Int J Dermatol 1982;21:379–395.
5. Krogstad DJ, Schlesinger PH. A perspective on antimalarial action: effects of weak bases on *Plasmodium falciparum*. Biochem Pharmacol 1986;35:547–552.
6. Goldberg DE, Slater AF, Beavis R, et al. Hemoglobin degradation in the human malaria pathogen *Plasmodium falciparum*—a catabolic pathway initiated by a specific aspartate protease. J Exp Med 1991;173:961–969.
7. Slater AF, Cerami A. Inhibition by chloroquine of a novel haem polymerase enzyme activity in malaria trophozoites. Nature 1992;355:167–169.
8. Schlesinger PH, Krogstad DJ, Herwaldt BL. Antimalarial agents—mechanisms of action. Antimicrob Agents Chemother 1988;32:793–798.
9. Walker O, Daurodu AH, Adeyokunnu AA, et al. Plasma chloroquine and desethylchloroquine concentrations in children during and after chloroquine treatment for malaria. Br J Clin Pharmacol 1983;16:701–705.
10. Frisk-Holmberg M, Bergqvist Y, Termond E, et al. The single dose kinetics of chloroquine and its major metabolite desethylchloroquine in healthy subjects. Eur J Clin Pharmacol 1984;26:521–530.

11. White NJ, Miller KD, Churchill FC, et al. Chloroquine treatment of severe malaria in children. Pharmacokinetics, toxicity and new dosage recommendations. N Engl J Med 1988;319:1493–1500.
12. Gustafsson LL, Walker O, Alvan G, et al. Disposition of chloroquine in man after single intravenous and oral doses. Br J Clin Pharmacol 1983;15:471–479.
13. Strickland GT. Malaria. In: Strickland GT, editor. Hunter's tropical medicine. 7th ed. Philadelphia: W.B. Saunders, 1991.
14. White NJ. Malaria. In: Cook GC, editor. Manson's tropical diseases. 20th ed. London: W.B. Saunders, 1996.
15. Krogstad DJ. *Plasmodium* species (malaria). In: Mandell GL, Bennett JE, Dolin R, editors. Principles and practice of infectious diseases. 4th ed. New York: Churchill Livingstone, 1995. p. 2415–2427.
16. Knell AJ. Malaria. Oxford: Oxford University Press, 1991.
17. Centers for Disease Control. Chloroquine-resistant malaria acquired in Kenya and Tanzania—Denmark, Georgia, New York. MMWR Morb Mortal Wkly Rep 1978;27:463–464.
18. White NJ. Antimalarial drug resistance: the pace quickens. J Antimicrob Chemother 1992;30:571–585.
19. Rieckmann KH, Davis DR, Hutton DC. *Plasmodium vivax* resistance to chloroquine. Lancet 1989;2:1183–1184.
20. Nosten F, ter Kuile F, Chongsuphajaisiddhi T, et al. Mefloquine-resistant falciparum malaria on the Thai-Burmese border. Lancet 1991;337:1140–1143.
21. World Health Organization. International travel and health—vaccination requirements and health advice. Geneva: World Health Organization, 2000.
22. Le Bras J, Longuet C, Charmot G. Transmission humaine et résistance des plasmodies. Rev Prat 1998;48:258–263.
23. Lobel HO, Kozarsky PE. Update on prevention of malaria for travelers. JAMA 1997;278:1767–1771.
24. Croft A. Malaria: prevention in travellers. BMJ 2000;321:154–160.
25. Bradley DJ, Warhurst DC. Guidelines for the prevention of malaria in travellers from the United Kingdom. Commun Dis Rep CDR Rev 1997;7:R137–R152.
26. Hansford CH. Malaria prophylaxis dosage. Lancet 1995;345:1049.
27. Pettyjohn FS. United States Army aviation medicine in the Republic of Vietnam. Mil Med 1968;133:478–483.
28. Colwell EJ, Boone SC, Brown JD, et al. Investigations on acute febrile illness in American servicemen in the Mekong delta of Vietnam. Mil Med 1968;134:1409–1414.
29. Rieckmann KH, Yeo AET, Davis DR, et al. Recent military experience with malaria chemoprophylaxis. Med J Aust 1993;158:446–449.
30. Lindsay S, Ansell J, Selman C, et al. Effect of pregnancy on exposure to malaria mosquitoes. Lancet 2000;355:1972.
31. Starr M. Malaria affects children and pregnant women most. BMJ 2000;321:1288.
32. Stemberger H, Leimer R, Widermann G. Tolerability of long-term prophylaxis with Fansidar: a randomized double-blind study in Nigeria. Acta Trop 1984;41:391–399.
33. Fogh S, Schapira A, Bygbjerg IC, et al. Malaria chemoprophylaxis in travellers to east Africa: a comparative prospective study of chloroquine plus proguanil with chloroquine plus sulfadoxine-pyrimethamine. BMJ 1988;296:820–822.

34. Wetsteyn JCFM, de Geus A. Comparison of three regimens for malaria prophylaxis in travellers to east, central, and southern Africa. BMJ 1993;307:1041–1043.

35. Baudon D, Martet G, Pascal B, et al. Efficacy of daily antimalarial chemoprophylaxis in tropical Africa using either doxycycline or chloroquine-proguanil; a study conducted in 1996 in the French Army. Trans R Soc Trop Med Hyg 1999;93:302–303.

36. Hogh B, Clarke PD, Camus D, et al. Atoquone-proguanil versus chloroquine-proguanil for malaria prophylaxis in non-immune travellers: a randomised, double-blind study. Malarone International Study Team. Lancet 2000;356(9245):1888–1894.

37. Huzly D, Schönfeld C, Beurle W, Bienzle U. Malaria chemoprophylaxis in German tourists: a prospective study on compliance and adverse reactions. J Travel Med 1996;3:148–155.

38. Corominas N, Gascón J, Mejías T, et al. Reacciones adversas asociadas a la quimio-profilaxis antipalúdica. Med Clin (Barc) 1997;108:772–775.

39. Durrheim DN, Gammon S, Waner S, et al. Antimalarial prophylaxis—use and adverse events in visitors to the Kruger National Park. S Afr Med J 1999;89:170–175.

40. Petersen E, Rønne T, Rønn A, et al. Reported side effects to chloroquine, chloroquine plus proguanil, and mefloquine as chemoprophylaxis against malaria in Danish travelers. J Travel Med 2000;7:79–84.

41. Carme B, Péguet C, Nevez G. Chimioprophylaxie du paludisme: tolerance et observance de la mefloquine et de l'association proguanil/chloroquine chez des touristes français. Bull Soc Pathol Exot 1997;90:273–276.

42. Piette JC, Guillevin L, Chapelon C, et al. Chloroquine cardiotoxicity. N Engl J Med 1987;317:710–711.

43. Edwards AC, Meredith TJ, Sowton E. Complete heart block due to chronic chloroquine toxicity managed with a permanent pacemaker. BMJ 1978;1:1109–1110.

44. Ogola ESN, Muita AK, Adala H. Chloroquine related complete heart block with blindness: case report. East Afr Med J 1992;69:50–52.

45. Oli JM, Ihenacho HNC, Talwar RS. Chronic chloroquine toxicity and heart block, a report of two cases. East Afr Med J 1980;57:505–507.

46. Nicolas X, Touze JE. La toxicité cardiaque des antipaludiques. Med Trop (Mars) 1994;54:361–365.

47. Hughes JT, Esiri M, Oxbury JM, et al. Chloroquine myopathy. QJM 1971;40:85–93.

48. Guedira N, Hajjaj-Hassouni N, Srairi JE, et al. Third degree heart block in a patient under chloroquine therapy. Rev Rhum Engl Ed 1998;65:58–62.

49. Meeran K, Jacobs MG. Chloroquine poisoning—rapidly fatal without treatment. BMJ 1993;307:49–50.

50. Phillips-Howard PA, Buckler WJ. Idiosyncratic reaction resembling toxic epidermal necrolysis caused by chloroquine and Maloprim. BMJ 1988;296:1605.

51. Sowunmi A, Walker O, Salako LA. Pruritus and antimalarial drugs in Africans. Lancet 1989;ii:213.

52. Selvaag E. Vitiligo caused by chloroquine phototoxicity. J R Army Med Corps 1998;144:163–165.

53. Tanenbaum L, Tuffanelli DL. Antimalarial agents: chloroquine, hydroxychloroquine and quinacrine. Arch Dermatol 1980;116:587–591.

54. Baker H. The influence of chloroquine and related drugs on psoriasis and keratoderma blenorrhagica. Br J Dermatol 1966;78:161–166.

55. Olsen TG. Chloroquine and psoriasis. Ann Intern Med 1981;94:546–547.

56. Luzzi GA, Peto TEA. Adverse effects of antimalarials—an update. Drug Saf 1993;
    8:295–311.
57. Barrett PJ, Emmins PD, Clarke PD, et al. Comparison of adverse events associated
    with use of mefloquine and combinations of chloroquine and proguanil as anti-
    malarial prophylaxis: postal and telephone survey of travellers. BMJ 1996;313:
    525–528.
58. Phillips-Howard PA, ter Kuile FO. CNS adverse events associated with antimalarial
    agents—fact or fiction? Drug Saf 1995;12:370–383.
59. Fish DR, Espir MLE. Convulsions associated with prophylactic antimalarial drugs:
    implications for people with epilepsy. BMJ 1988;297:526–527.
60. Fish DR, Espir MLE. Malaria prophylaxis and epilepsy. BMJ 1988;297:1267.
61. Steffen R, Fuchs E, Schildknecht J, et al. Mefloquine compared with other malaria
    chemoprophylactic regimes in tourists visiting east Africa. Lancet 1993;341:
    1299–1303.
62. Lysack JT, Lysack CL. A severe adverse reaction to mefloquine and chloroquine pro-
    phylaxis. Aust Fam Physician 1998;21:1119–1120.
63. Lovestone S. Chloroquine-induced mania. Br J Psychiatry 1991;159:164–165.
64. Torrey EF. Chloroquine seizures. JAMA 1968;204:867–870.
65. Umez-Eronini EM, Eronini EA. Chloroquine induced involuntary movements. BMJ
    1977;1:945–946.
66. Ragan E, Wilson R, Li F, et al. Psychotic symptoms in volunteers serving overseas.
    Lancet 1985;2:37.
67. Parfitt K, editor. Martindale— the complete drug reference. 32nd ed. London: Pharma-
    ceutical Press, 1999.
68. Winstanley PA. Chemotherapy for falciparum malaria: the armoury, the problems
    and the prospects. Parasitol Today 2000;16:146–153.
69. Waddell KM. Eye damage from chloroquine as an antimalarial: misuse makes safe
    medicines unsafe. Trop Doct 1997;27:10–12.
70. Robert-Lange W, Frankenfield DL, Moriarty-Sheehan M, et al. No evidence for
    chloroquine-associated retinopathy among missionaries on long-term malaria
    chemoprophylaxis. Am J Trop Med Hyg 1994;51:389–392.
71. Bernstein HN. Ophthalmologic considerations and testing in patients receiving long-
    term antimalarial therapy. Am J Med 1983:75(1A Suppl):25–34.
72. Mackenzie AH. Dose refinements in long-term therapy of rheumatoid arthritis with
    antimalarials. Am J Med 1983;75(1A Suppl):40–45.
73. Munera Y, Hugues FC, Le Jeunne C, Pays JF. Interaction of thyroxine sodium with
    antimalarial drugs. BMJ 1997;314:1593.

8.2 Azithromycin
Jeanine Bygott and Graham Fry

ABSTRACT

Azithromycin is a macrolide antibiotic, structurally related to erythromycin although having very different pharmacokinetics. Azithromycin is a semisynthetic compound, which is considered the prototype of new macrolide structures identified as azalides. It is known under the trade name of Zithromax (Pfizer). Azithromycin is normally indicated for respiratory tract infections, otitis media, skin and soft-tissue infections, disseminated mycobacterial infections, and genital chlamydial infection. Azithromycin has been shown to have antimalarial activity in vitro and in animal and (more recently) human studies. Azithromycin has been developed as a single agent for malaria prophylaxis against multidrug-resistant *Plasmodium falciparum* although it may be more effective in combination with other agents.

Key words: azithromycin; chemoprophylaxis; malaria.

PHARMACOLOGY AND MODE OF ACTION

Absorption, Distribution, and Metabolism

Azithromycin is rapidly absorbed and has good oral bioavailability at 37%. Absorption is reduced if the drug is taken with food, which significantly delays the onset and extent of absorption by 40% to 50%.

Azithromycin is lipid soluble and distributes extensively in body fluids and tissues. It shows excellent tissue penetration and attains high intracellular concentrations. Tissue concentrations of azithromycin may be as high as 10 to 100 times its blood concentrations. Such high tissue concentrations confer theoretic benefits in the treatment of infections due to intracellular pathogens, such as malaria. The high tissue concentration results in a half-life of 68 hours and excretion over several days.

Azithromycin is metabolized by the liver by demethylation. It is eliminated primarily via biliary excretion and in the feces.

Mode of Action

Azithromycin attains high intracellular concentrations, and its antimalarial effect may rest on its ability to accumulate in lysosomes and on its high tissue concentrations.

In malaria, azithromycin mainly works as a suppressive chemoprophylactic agent. It has only partial causal prophylactic activity in the human challenge model. Initial studies in the rodent model showed that azithromycin had a causal prophylactic efficacy superior to that of doxycycline.[1] However, a subsequent study

by Anderson and colleagues in 10 human volunteers showed that the causal prophylactic regimen of azithromycin, used for 7 days after challenge, was successful in
only 40% of cases.[2]

TOLERABILITY

Collectively, macrolides are considered to be one of the safest anti-infective agents
in clinical use. No studies have been done to compare their tolerability with that of
other chemoprophylactic agents. The overall incidence of adverse reactions with
azithromycin is 12%, with less than 1% of patients discontinuing treatment
because of adverse reactions. The most frequent adverse reactions are those that
affect the gastrointestinal system, such as nausea and diarrhea. The poor gastrointestinal tolerance of macrolides is related to their stimulant effect on gut motility.
The overall incidence of gastrointestinal reactions with azithromycin is 9.6%. Photosensitivity, dizziness, and headache may occur. Rare adverse events include tinnitus, taste disturbance, angioedema, and cholestatic jaundice.

CONTRAINDICATIONS, PRECAUTIONS, AND DRUG INTERACTIONS

The use of azithromycin is contraindicated in those with a known sensitivity to
macrolide antibiotics and in cases of hepatic impairment.

Azithromycin is not known to be harmful in pregnancy and is classified in pregnancy as class B (no evidence of teratogenicity in laboratory animals but no well-
controlled clinical studies). Only small amounts are excreted in breast milk.

Macrolide antibiotics may interact with many commonly used drugs. However,
fewer interactions occur with azithromycin than with other macrolides because
azithromycin does not affect hepatic metabolism. Pharmacokinetic drug interactions may occur from its antibiotic effect on microorganisms of the enteric flora and
through enhanced gastric emptying due to a motilin-like effect. Azithromycin may
thus theoretically interfere with the oral contraceptive pill. Azithromycin has not
been reported to have any effect on prothrombin time in patients receiving warfarin.

ADMINISTRATION

Azithromycin is available in 250-mg capsules and as an oral suspension (100 mg/
5 mL and 200 mg/5 mL). The adult dose is 250 mg daily; the pediatric dose for children (> 6 months of age) is 5 mg/kg/d.

Used as a malaria prophylactic, azithromycin requires daily dosing, starting the
day before exposure, continued during exposure, and continued for 4 weeks after
departure from the malarial region.

EFFICACY

Studies on the efficacy of azithromycin as a chemoprophylactic agent are limited (Table 8.2–1).[2–5]

Initial field trials suggested a moderate prophylactic efficacy of 83% against *Plasmodium falciparum* in malaria-immune Kenyans, with a 250-mg single daily dose.[3]

Efficacy in semi-immune Indonesians in Irian Jaya showed the protective efficacy of azithromycin compared with placebo to be 71.6% against *Plasmodium falciparum* malaria and 98.9% against *Plasmodium vivax* malaria.[4] Corresponding figures for doxycycline in the same study were 96.3% against *Plasmodium falciparum* and 98% against *Plasmodium vivax* malaria. The conclusions from this study involving 300 subjects were that azithromycin offered excellent protection against *Plasmodium vivax* malaria but only modest protection against *Plasmodium falciparum* malaria. Azithromycin was well tolerated but is clearly less efficacious than doxycycline, mainly because of the poor efficacy against *P. falciparum*, especially in the malaria-naive population.

These results were confirmed in a later study done in 1999 in western Thailand in a partially immune population.[5] This study of 276 adults showed azithromycin's efficacy to be 69% for *Plasmodium falciparum* malaria and 98% for *Plasmodium vivax* malaria.

A trial in Gambia with weekly azithromycin (20 mg/kg) among 226 partially immune children showed a beneficial effect on the clearing of current parasitemia

Table 8.2–1. **Summary of Studies of Azithromycin as Malaria Chemoprophylaxis**

Reference	Site of Study	Subjects	No. of Subjects	Outcome
2	Water Reed Institute (Washington, D.C.)	Nonimmune adults challenged with *P. falciparum*–infected mosquitoes	20	Azithromycin continued for 7 days after challenge: 60% efficacy; azithromycin continued for 28 days after challenge: 100% efficacy
3	Western Kenya	Partially immune adults	213	Daily azithromycin (250 mg daily): 82.7% efficacy; weekly azithromycin (1,000 mg weekly): 64.2% efficacy. daily doxycycline (100 mg daily): 92.6% efficacy
4	Irian Jaya, Indonesia	Partially immune adults	300	Daily azithromycin: 71.6% protective efficacy against *P. falciparum* malaria; 98.9% efficacy against *P. vivax* malaria (doxycycline: 93% and 96%, respectively)
5	Western Thailand	Partially immune adults	276	Azithromycin: 69% protective efficacy against *P. falciparum* malaria; 98% efficacy against *P. vivax* malaria

P. = *Plasmodium.*

rather than any significant effect as a prophylactic agent.[6] Based on these results, further development of azithromycin as a single agent against *Plasmodium falciparum* malaria has been discontinued.

Studies to examine the efficacy of combining azithromycin with other chemoprophylactic agents are under way. In vitro studies to assess the use of combinations of drugs including azithromycin for drug-resistant *P. falciparum* malaria have been done.[7] The results suggest that a chloroquine/azithromycin combination should be evaluated as a malaria prophylaxis regimen and that quinine/azithromycin should be evaluated as a treatment regimen in areas of drug resistance.

INDICATIONS

Studies performed to date are small and suggest that azithromycin is less effective than either mefloquine or doxycycline for prophylaxis of *P. falciparum* malaria. Azithromycin should be considered for chemoprophylaxis only in highly selected groups. It is considered to be safe for children and for women in pregnancy and is available in suspension. However, in view of the serious possible consequences of malaria in pregnancy, this suboptimal antimalarial would not routinely be recommended.

SUMMARY

There is insufficient evidence to recommend azithromycin as an alternative stand-alone antimalarial prophylactic agent for *Plasmodium falciparum* malaria except in circumstances in which other and more effective antimalarials are not available or are contraindicated. Azithromycin may be useful for chemoprophylaxis of *Plasmodium vivax* malaria in appropriate geographic areas. Azithromycin as a combined malaria prophylactic agent is being assessed, but such research is not sufficiently advanced to suggest that this will be a viable option.

REFERENCES

1. Anderson SL, Ager AL, McGreevy P, et al. Efficacy of azithromycin as a causal prophylactic agent against murine malaria. Antimicrob Agents Chemother 1994;38:1862–1863.
2. Anderson SL , Berman J, Kuscher R, et al. Prophylaxis of *Plasmodium falciparum* malaria with azithromycin administered to volunteers. Ann Intern Med 1995;123:771–773.
3. Andersen SL, Oloo AJ, Gordon DM, et al. Successful double-blinded, randomized, placebo-controlled field trial of azithromycin and doxycycline as prophylaxis of malaria in western Kenya. Clin Infect Dis 1998;26:146–150.
4. Taylor WR, Richie TL, Fryauff DJ, et al. Malaria prophylaxis using azithromycin; a double-blind, placebo-controlled trial in Irian Jaya, Indonesia. Clin Infect Dis 1999;28:74–81.

5. Heppner D, Wongsrichanalai C, Walsh DS, et al. Azithromycin for the prophylaxis of malaria in Thailand. Proceedings of the 48th Annual Meeting of the American Society of Tropical Medicine and Hygiene; 1999 Nov 28–Dec 2.
6. Sadiq ST, Glasgow KW, Drakley CJ, et al. Effects of azithromycin on malariometric indices in The Gambia. Lancet 1995;346:881–882.
7. Ohrt C, Willingmyre G, Lee P, et al. In vitro assessment of azithromycin drug combinations for drug-resistant falciparum malaria. Proceedings of the 48th Annual Meeting of the American Society of Tropical Medicine and Hygiene; 1999 Nov 28–Dec 2.

8.3 Mefloquine
Patricia Schlagenhauf

ABSTRACT

Mefloquine is an orally administered blood schizonticide for the chemoprophylaxis of malaria, and it has been used for this indication by approximately 20 million travelers. Steady-state pharmacokinetics of weekly prophylaxis in long-term travelers have shown that toxic accumulation does not occur and that weekly dosing is associated with protective levels of the drug. Food increases the bioavailability of mefloquine. The pharmacokinetics of mefloquine is highly stereospecific, and all pharmacokinetic parameters except t_{max} are significantly different for the (+) and (−) enantiomers.

Cumulative evidence suggests a high protective efficacy of mefloquine (> 91%) in nonimmune travelers to areas of chloroquine-resistant *Plasmodium falciparum* (CRPF), except for clearly defined regions of multidrug resistance. Mefloquine resistance is associated with halofantrine and quinine resistance but not with chloroquine resistance. Penfluridol has been shown to reverse *P. falciparum* mefloquine resistance in vitro.

There is some controversy regarding the tolerability of mefloquine for malaria chemoprophylaxis, mainly due to the profile of mefloquine-associated adverse events (AEs), which are characterized by a predominance of neuropsychiatric AEs. A review of studies shows that in the reporting of any AE, the incidence lies in the range of 12% to 90% and that where there is a comparator, the incidence is equivalent to the incidence reported for almost all alternative regimens. When some measure of subjective severity is applied to the rating of AEs, it appears that 11% to 17% of travelers are incapacitated by AEs to some extent. A Cochrane systematic review of mefloquine studies in adult travelers found no significant difference in tolerability in mefloquine users compared to that of users of comparator regimens. Major studies and worldwide monitoring have shown that serious events are rare. No performance deficit or functional impairment was observed in five clinical toxicity studies of mefloquine prophylaxis, including a study of driving performance.

There is limited data regarding use of mefloquine in pregnancy. Early animal studies documented teratogenic and embryotoxic effects associated with the use of high-dose mefloquine. Two studies showed a relatively high incidence of spontaneous abortions in mefloquine users. Cumulative evidence, however, is reassuring and has led the World Health Organization (WHO) and the Centers for Disease Control and Prevention (CDC) to sanction the use of mefloquine in pregnant women during the second and third trimesters. Mefloquine prophylaxis is recommended for travelers to high-risk areas of CRPF. The risk of malarial infection and the proven efficacy of mefloquine to prevent malaria should be weighed against the risk of drug-associated AEs.

Key words: adverse events; mefloquine; pharmacokinetics; protective efficacy; resistance; use in pregnancy.

DESCRIPTION, PHARMACOLOGY, AND MODE OF ACTION

Because of its potent antimalarial activity in animal models, mefloquine (Figure 8.3–1) was selected from nearly 300 quinoline methanol compounds for further investigation in the 1960s by the Walter Reed Army Institute of Research.[1] Today, mefloquine is used clinically as a 50:50 racemic mixture of the erythroisomers, and all clinical studies with the drug have used this mixture. The commercial form is available as tablets containing 250 mg of mefloquine base. The mefloquine formulation available in the United States contains 250 mg of mefloquine hydrochloride (equivalent to 228 mg of mefloquine base). Mefloquine has been available for malaria chemoprophylaxis in Europe since 1985. Since 1990, it has been available in the United States, and it has been used by approximately 20 million nonimmune travelers. Comprehensive reviews of mefloquine have been published.[2,3]

Mefloquine is a potent long-acting blood schizonticide and is effective against all malarial species, including *P. falciparum* resistant to chloroquine and

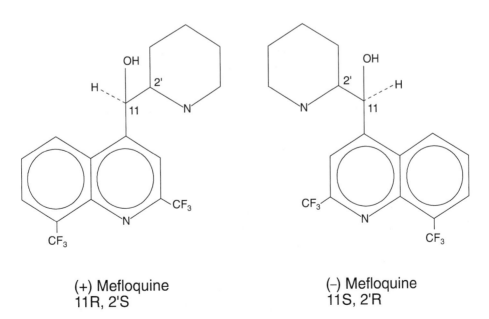

(+) Mefloquine
11R, 2'S

(–) Mefloquine
11S, 2'R

Figure 8.3–1. Mefloquine is a antimalarial agent available as the racemic mixture of (+) and (–) erythroisomers.

pyrimethamine/sulfonamide combinations. The exact mechanism of activity is unclear, but mefloquine is thought to compete with the complexing protein for heme binding, and the resulting drug complex is toxic to the parasite.[4]

PHARMACOKINETICS

The major pharmacokinetic properties of the orally administered blood schizonticide mefloquine in healthy volunteers have been previously reviewed.[2] Mefloquine is characterized as having a mean absorption half-life of 2.1 hours, peak blood concentrations within a mean of 17.6 hours, a large mean volume of distribution of 22.1 L/kg, a slow mean systemic clearance of 0.042 L/h/kg, and a long terminal elimination half-life ranging from 14 to 28 (mean, 18.1) days. Mefloquine is metabolized in the liver, and the main metabolite is the corresponding carboxylic acid, which is devoid of antimalarial activity. There is marked interindividual and ethnic variation in pharmacokinetic parameters.

Food increases the bioavailability of mefloquine. In an open two-way crossover study, the pharmacokinetic parameters C_{max} and area under the concentration-time curve (AUC) of both mefloquine and its metabolite were significantly higher when 750 mg of mefloquine was administered after food than when it was administered under fasting conditions.[5] It is thus recommended that travelers using mefloquine take the drug after a meal to maximize bioavailability and optimize prophylactic efficacy although it can be conjectured that the increased availability may lead to an increased incidence of AEs.

Dosage

On the basis of its long half-life of approximately 18 days, it was originally recommended that mefloquine (250 mg) be taken in alternate weeks for long-term malaria chemoprophylaxis. An unacceptably high failure rate with this regimen in Peace Corps volunteers suggested that trough plasma levels of mefloquine were inadequate to prevent clinical malaria. In 1993, Pennie and colleagues reported on the steady-state pharmacokinetics of weekly mefloquine (250 mg) in long-term travelers.[6] The results of this study support mefloquine weekly dosing for long-term prophylaxis because toxic accumulation did not occur and because weekly dosing was associated with significantly higher trough levels (mean, 1,144 µg/L) and thus gave better protection than the alternate-week regimen.

Stereochemistry

Mefloquine (MQ) is a chiral antimalarial agent, commercially available as the racemic mixture of (+) and (–) enantiomers. The pharmacokinetics of MQ enantiomers were studied at steady state in healthy volunteers and were found to be highly stereospecific.[7]

Plasma concentrations of the (–) enantiomer were significantly higher than those observed for the (+) enantiomer, and all main pharmacokinetic parameters (except t_{max}) were significantly different between the two enantiomers. The mean terminal half-life at steady state for the (–) enantiomer is 430 hours, compared to 172 hours for the (+) enantiomer. MQ appears to cross the blood-brain barrier stereoselectively, with a much higher brain penetration of the (+) enantiomer.[8]

Hemodialysis

MQ and its metabolite are not appreciably removed by hemodialysis.[9] No special dosage adjustments are indicated for dialysis patients to achieve concentrations in plasma similar to those in healthy volunteers.

Lack of Bioequivalence of a Generic Product

An open-label randomized two-way crossover study with a 750-mg dose was performed to assess the bioequivalence between a generic form of MQ (Mephaquin) versus the original preparation (Lariam).[10] The pharmacokinetic parameters of both formulations were significantly different, with Lariam having a higher mean maximum plasma concentration (1,018 ng/mL vs. 656 ng/mL), a more rapid rise to maximum concentration (13 hours vs. 46 hours), and a larger area under the plasma concentration-time curve (AUC 432 versus 338 ug/h/mL). The relative bioavailability of the generic product was 0.78 (range, 0.38 to 1.37).

Loading Dose

To reach steady-state levels of MQ in a reduced time frame (4 days rather than 7 to 9 weeks with the regular 250-mg/week regimen), some studies[11-14] have used a loading-dose strategy of 250 mg of MQ daily for 3 days, followed thereafter by weekly MQ dosage. This strategy has also been suggested for last-minute travelers to high-risk areas with CRPF. The advantage is the rapid attainment of MQ protective levels (620 ng/mL) within 4 days, but this is offset to some extent by a higher proportion of individuals with AEs using the loading-dose strategy.[11,12]

EFFICACY IN NONIMMUNE TRAVELERS

MQ is currently recognized as a highly effective malaria chemoprophylaxis for nonimmune travelers to high-risk areas with CRPF. Rapid emergence of drug-resistant parasites is a serious threat to all travelers to malaria-endemic areas. There is a paucity of information about the drug susceptibility of parasites in many regions. This section considers the situation, taking into account published efficacy studies, reports of prophylactic failures, reports of MQ failure from the literature, and reports of in vitro resistance. The main emphasis is on chemoprophylactic efficacy.

Efficacy Studies

Studies conducted in 1993 showed a high efficacy of MQ in travelers. The protective effectiveness of MQ in a large cohort of travelers to East Africa was 91%, which was significantly higher than that of other regimens used at that time, namely, chloroquine/proguanil (72%) and chloroquine monoprophylaxis at various doses (10% to 42%).[15] Long-term prophylaxis with MQ proved highly effective in Peace Corps volunteers stationed in sub-Saharan Africa, with an incidence of 0.2 infections per month in 100 volunteers. Weekly MQ was considered 94% more effective than prophylaxis with chloroquine and 86% more effective than prophylaxis with the chloroquine/proguanil regimen.[16] MQ was shown to be highly efficacious (100%) in the prevention of malaria in Indonesian soldiers in Irian Jaya.[17] Rieckmann and colleagues[18] found MQ to be 100% effective against *P. falciparum* in Australian soldiers deployed in Papua New Guinea. Pergallo and colleagues[19] reported on the effective use of MQ by Italian troops in Mozambique from 1992 to 1994. When chloroquine/proguanil was the recommended regimen, an attack rate of 17 cases per 1,000 soldiers per month was noted. The rate dropped significantly to 1.8 cases per 1,000 per month when chloroquine/proguanil was replaced by MQ.

The effectiveness of long-term MQ in United Nations peacekeeping forces in Cambodia in 1993 was 91.4%.[20] Conversely, MQ was found to be not completely effective in the prevention of malaria in Dutch marines in western Cambodia during the period of 1992 to 1993. The attack rate in marines varied significantly, according to the geographic location of the battalions. Of 260 persons assigned to the Sok San area, 43 developed malaria (16%, 6.4 per 1,000 person-weeks), compared to 21 of 2,029 persons stationed elsewhere (1%, 0.5 per 1,000 person-weeks). MQ-resistant parasites were isolated from Dutch and Khmer patients.[21]

MQ showed high prophylactic efficacy in American troops using it during Operation Restore Hope in Somalia in 1992 and 1993. Sanchez and colleagues[22] reported prophylactic efficacy in an uncontrolled cross-sectional survey of troops at one location (Bale Dogle). MQ users had a malaria rate of 1.15 cases per 10,000 person-weeks, compared to 5.49 cases per 10,000 person-weeks for doxycycline users. From this and other reports,[23] MQ was shown to be more effective than doxycycline in U.S. troops deployed in Somalia. The lower efficacy of doxycycline was attributed to poorer compliance.

Mefloquine was shown to provide a high degree of protection in Dutch military personnel (n = 125) deployed as part of a disaster relief operation in Goma, Zaire (1994). Despite evidence of exposure to *P. falciparum* (as shown by the presence of *P. falciparum* circumsporozite [CS] antibodies in 11.2% of the group), no one developed overt malaria, a fact that was attributed to the MQ prophylaxis.[24]

In a German population-based case-control study, MQ was considered to be 94.5% effective in preventing malaria in tourists traveling to Kenya.[25]

Prophylactic Failures

In many geographic regions, the mapping of prophylactic failures, mainly in non-immune individuals, has been used to detect early resistance development (although it should be emphasized that prophylactic failures do not prove resistance). MQ blood concentrations of 620 ng/mL are considered necessary to achieve 95% prophylactic efficacy. A prophylactic failure is defined as confirmed *P. falciparum* infection in persons with MQ blood levels in excess of the 95% protective level of 620 ng/mL as defined by Lobel and colleagues[16,26] in their studies of Peace Corps volunteers in Africa. Using this definition, a recent analysis of 44 confirmed *P. falciparum* cases acquired in sub-Saharan Africa[26] showed 5 volunteers with MQ-resistant *P. falciparum*. Other confirmed cases were attributed to poor compliance, and the authors concluded that the prevalence of MQ-resistant *P. falciparum* in sub-Saharan Africa is still low.

Failure of MQ for prophylaxis, despite protective serum levels of MQ, was documented in two U.S. soldiers deployed in Somalia[27] and was later documented in other compliant soldiers.[28] Two reports of *Plasmodium falciparum* resistant to both MQ and halofantrine have been documented, one from Sierra Leone[29] and one from Ivory Coast.[30] A further report cited MQ failure in an Italian soldier returning from duty in Mozambique (serum MQ = 920 ng/mL),[31] and a recent report describes MQ prophylaxis failure in a native resident of Kenya.[32]

In the assessment of prophylactic failures, attention should be paid to the samples available for analysis. The concentration of MQ in serum is significantly greater than that in whole blood, with an overall mean ratio of 1.28.[33]

MQ has been shown to delay the onset of falciparum malaria in returned travelers. Malaria in individuals using MQ chemoprophylaxis tends to present much later (mean interval from return to diagnosis is 43.8 days) compared to malaria in those using chloroquine/proguanil (for which the mean interval from return to diagnosis is 14.03 days).[34]

Literature Reports of Mefloquine Resistance

The first report of MQ resistance came from Thailand in 1982. This region remains a focus of resistance, particularly the Thailand-Cambodia border, where prophylaxis breakdown has been observed. Reports of treatment or prophylactic failure with MQ alone or as part of a triple combination (Fansimef) have come from several parts of Asia (Burma, China, Vietnam, Irian Jaya, Cambodia, India, Malaysia, Philippines, southern Yemen, and southern Iran) and (to a lesser extent) from Africa and from the Amazon basin in South America, as geographically represented by Mockenhaupt in a review of MQ resistance.[35] In addition, there has been a report of MQ-resistant *Plasmodium vivax* malaria in Papua New Guinea. The breakthrough occurred during prophylaxis with MQ (250 mg/week).[36] MQ-resistant malaria acquired in the Amazon basin was reported in 1992 by Chia and colleagues.[37]

Reports of In Vitro Resistance

Recently, Le Bras and colleagues[38] reported on the in vitro resistance of *Plasmodium falciparum* from imported African isolates to MQ (5.2%), chloroquine (46%), and cycloguanil (42%). MQ resistance was low, but the proportion had increased from 3.8% in the period of 1991 to 1994 to 8.5% in 1995 to 1997. Northern Cameroon appears to be a focus of MQ resistance.[39]

Data on Imported Malaria

The trends in imported malaria cases point toward the superior efficacy of MQ versus other regimens (including chloroquine/proguanil) in the protection of nonimmune travelers. An interesting analysis assessed the impact of the United Kingdom's malaria policy on imported malaria cases when British guidelines (May 1993) recommended MQ as an alternative to chloroquine/proguanil for tourists to Kenya and other areas with CRPF. A threefold reduction in imported malaria against stable malaria transmission on the Kenyan coast was attributed to the increased use of MQ by travelers.[40] A similar pattern of data on imported malaria (tourists returning from Kenya) was also observed for other countries after the adaptation of the more effective MQ regimen.[41]

RESISTANCE

Resistance has been concisely defined by Peters[42] as "the ability of a parasite to survive in the presence of concentrations of a drug that normally destroy parasites of the same species or prevent their multiplication." MQ resistance is considered to be a result of drug pressure, cross-resistance, and (to a lesser extent) innate resistance.[35] Of these factors, drug pressure appears to be the major determinant of resistance development.

Cross-resistance is now seen to be the second major factor in the development of resistance.[43] There is recent evidence that exposure of parasite populations to antimalarial drug pressure may select for resistance not only to the drug providing the pressure but also to other novel drugs. This was clearly illustrated in the northern part of Cameroon, West Africa, in the detection of a high level of MQ resistance attributed to cross-resistance with quinine,[39] a drug that had been widely deployed for therapy in the area (MQ was not used). Resistance to MQ appears to be distinct from chloroquine resistance, as shown by the activity of MQ against CRPF and by the inability of verapamil to reverse MQ resistance (although verapamil does modulate chloroquine resistance). Moreover, in vitro studies have documented an inverse relationship between chloroquine and MQ resistance. However, MQ resistance is associated with halofantrine resistance[44,45] and quinine resistance.[39,45]

Innate resistance means the existence of small subpopulations of intrinsically resistant malarial parasites within any infecting parasite biomass. The actual existence of natural resistance to MQ is still controversial and may partly be explained by cross-resistance to other drugs.[35]

The basis of resistance to antimalarials (including MQ) may be the amplification of certain genes that enable the parasites to pump the antimalarial drug out of the cell. Two multidrug-resistant (MDR) genes have been identified for *P. falciparum*, namely, pfmdr1 and pfmdr2. A recent report supports the hypothesis that the pfmdr1 gene confers a true multidrug-resistance phenotype that is lost by mutation. Assessments of pfmdr1 sequence polymorphisms showed that the tyrosine-86 allele of pfmdr1 is associated with increased sensitivity to MQ and increased resistance to chloroquine and quinine.[46] Penfluridol, a psychotropic drug, has been reported to reverse the resistance to MQ in *P. falciparum* in vitro.[47]

TOLERABILITY IN NONIMMUNE TRAVELERS

There is some controversy among international experts regarding the tolerability of MQ prophylaxis versus that of alternative regimens such as doxycycline, chloroquine/proguanil, and (more recently) atovaquone/proguanil. It is generally accepted that all antimalarial drugs are associated with AEs, and this factor is intrinsic in the risk-benefit analysis deciding whether or not to take an antimalarial and determining which agent will provide the best protection with minimal toxicity.

All Adverse Effects

An overview of the studies and databases comparing malaria chemoprophylactic agents used in travelers (Tables 8.3–1 and 8.3–2) shows largely disparate results due to differing designs, definitions, methodologies, and study populations. The incidence of any AE during the use of MQ lies in the range of 12% to 90% and (when there is a comparator) is usually equivalent to the incidence reported for almost all chemoprophylactic regimens. Peace Corps volunteers using long-term prophylaxis reported similar rates of mild AEs in both chloroquine- and MQ-using groups,[16] similar to the findings of Steffen and colleagues in a survey of returning European travelers.[15] A more recent retrospective survey of British travelers showed equal rates for any side effects (41%) and for stopping or changing medication in MQ users and in users of chloroquine/proguanil.[48] The highest incidence of AEs was reported in British soldiers in a retrospective analysis,[49] with a rate of 90% in the MQ group versus 89% in the chloroquine/proguanil (C+P) group. In Australian travelers, 38% of MQ users reported some AE, compared to 21% of doxycycline users.[50] Conversely, in the deployment of U.S. troops in Somalia, Sanchez and colleagues[22] reported superior compliance and tolerability in MQ users versus doxycycline users, particularly with regard to photosensitivity (5.2% in MQ users vs. 21.2% in doxycycline users) and gastrointestinal symptoms (12.8% in MQ users vs. 34.6% in doxycycline users). In a recent study comparing MQ

Table 8.3–1. **Incidence of Adverse Events in Mefloquine and Comparator Groups during Chemoprophylaxis (1992 to 2000)**

Study	Population	Methodology	Incidence of All Adverse Events (%)				Incidence of Moderate* Adverse Events (%)			
					C				C	
			MQ	C+P	A+P	DX	MQ	C+P	A+P	DX
Croft, 1995	U.K. soldiers	I/Q	90	89	—	—	—	—	—	—
Phillips, 1996	Australian travelers	Q	38	—	—	21	11.2	—	—	6.5
Barrett, 1996	U.K. travelers	TI/Q	41	41	—	—	17	16	—	—
Hopperus Buma, 1996	Dutch marines	Q	30	—	—	—	—	—	—	—
Schlagenhauf, 1996	Swiss travelers	I/Q/O	—	—	—	—	11.2	—	—	—
Steffen, 1993	European travelers	Q	24	35	—	—	13	16	—	—
Lobel, 1993[†]	Peace Corps volunteers	I/Q	41	46	—	—	—	—	—	—
Boudreau, 1993[†]	U.S. marines	I/Q/O	43	46	—	—	—	—	—	—
Overbosch, 2000	International travelers	I/D	68	—	71	—	29[‡]	—	14[‡]	—

MQ = mefloquine; C = chloroquine; C+P = chloroquine/proguanil; DX = doxycycline; A+P = atovaquone/proguanil; Q = questionnaire; D = diary; I = interview; TI = telephone interview; O = other.
* Interferes with daily activities.
[†] Central nervous system symptoms only.
[‡] Treatment-related neuropsychiatric adverse events.

Table 8.3–2. **Incidence of Serious* Adverse Events during Malaria Chemoprophylaxis (1992 to 2000)**

Report	Population	Methodology	Incidence	
			C	
			MQ	C+P
CANADA Safety Monitoring, 1992	Canadian travelers	S	1/20,000	—
Steffen et al., 1993	European travelers	Q	1/10,595	1/5,100
Croft et al., 1996	U.K. soldiers	I/Q	1/6,000[†]	—
Barrett et al., 1996	U.K. travelers	Q	1/607[‡]	1/1,181[‡]
Roche Drug Safety, 1997	Prophylaxis users worldwide[§]	S	1/20,000[ǁ]	—

C+P = chloroquine/proguanil; I = interview; MQ = mefloquine; Q = questionnaire; S = spontaneous reporting.
* CIOMS definition.
[†] Used for > 3 months.
[‡] Sample size small for detection of serious adverse events.
[§] Source: Roche Drug Safety Report for 1997.
[ǁ] Lowest reporting ratio: 2/100,000 (Netherlands). Highest reporting ratio: 17/100,000 (U.K.).

with atovaquone/proguanil, the overall frequency of AEs was not significantly different between the two regimens (68% vs. 71%).[51]

Prompting increases the reported incidence of AEs,[52] as demonstrated in a study of MQ tolerability in Dutch marines, in which the incidence of self-reported MQ-related AEs was low but increased with specific questioning. In any analysis of AEs, the underlying background incidence of symptoms such as fatigue, sleep disturbance, and dizziness should be kept in mind.

Moderate and Severe Adverse Events

When some measure of severity is applied to the reporting of AEs and when the reports are normally subjective ratings by the travelers, it appears that between 11% and 17%[15,48,50,53] of travelers using MQ are incapacitated by AEs to some extent. The extent of this incapacitation is often difficult to quantify, and a good measure of the impact of AEs is the extent of the curtailment of chemoprophylaxis. In a study of 5,120 Italian soldiers who were deployed in Somalia and Mozambique from 1992 to 1994 and who used either C+P or MQ, the rate of prophylaxis discontinuation in the C+P users was 1.5%, compared to a significantly lower rate (0.9%) of discontinuation in MQ users.[54] This contrasts with a recent study comparing MQ and atovaquone/proguanil (A+P), in which subjects receiving the A+P regimen had a significantly lower rate of drug-related AEs that caused the discontinuation of prophylaxis (5% in MQ users vs. 1% in A+P users).[51]

Serious Adverse Events

Serious AEs are those that (1) constitute an apparent threat to life, (2) require or prolong hospitalization, or (3) result in severe disability.[55] For MQ users, the incidence is estimated at between 1 in 6,000 and 1 in 10,600 (Table 8.3–2), compared to a rate in chloroquine users of 1 in 13,600. In a retrospective cohort analysis, serious neuropsychiatric AEs involving hospitalization were noted for 1 in 607 MQ users versus 1 in 1,181 C+P users.[48] A recent database analysis of suicide cases reported in association with MQ prophylaxis showed 8 reports of suicide (all men) reported for approximately 20 million MQ (Lariam) users, which must be viewed against a high background incidence of suicide in male groups worldwide.[56]

Neuropsychiatric Adverse Effects

Neuropsychiatric disorders include two broad categories of symptoms: (1) central and peripheral nervous system disorders (including headache, dizziness, vertigo, and seizures) and (2) psychiatric disorders (including major psychiatric disorders, affective disorders, and anxiety and sleep disturbances). In Peace Corps volunteers using long-term MQ prophylaxis, Lobel and colleagues found incidences of strange dreams (25%), insomnia (9%), and dizziness (8.4%) similar to those reported by users of chloroquine (respective incidences of 26%, 6.5%, and 10%). No severe neuropsychiatric reactions were causally associated with MQ use in this study.[16] Steffen and colleagues reported similar findings in an analysis of tourists (n = 139,164) returning from East Africa. Headache was observed in 6.2% of MQ users versus 7.6% of C+P users, and dizziness, depression, and insomnia were experienced by 7.6%, 1.8%, and 4.2%, respectively, of mefloquine users versus 5.5%, 1.7%, and 6.3%, respectively, of the C+P group.[15] In this same large cohort study, serious neuropsychiatric AEs were observed at a rate of 1 in 10,600 cases. A total of 5 probably associated hospitalizations were reported: 2 cases of seizures, 2 psychotic episodes, and 1 case of vertigo. The rate of such events in MQ users was 1 in 13,600 cases, with 3 associated hospitalizations for neuropsychiatric events (1 seizure and 2 psychotic episodes). Croft and World[57] reported on the experience of the British army with MQ, which indicated that the incidence of severe neuropsychiatric reactions arising during a period of prophylaxis lasting 3 months is not higher than 1 in 6,000. In a randomized double-blind placebo-controlled ongoing monitoring of AEs in Canadian travelers using MQ (n = 251) or placebo (n = 238), there was no significant difference in the number or severity of AEs reported by either group. One clinically significant neuropsychiatric AE, a moderate to severe anxiety attack, occurred in 1 of the 251 MQ users.[14] In a U. K. retrospective survey with telephone interviews,[48] significantly more neuropsychiatric AEs were reported by MQ users than by travelers taking C+P. Neuropsychiatric events classified as disabling were reported by 0.7% of MQ users and by 0.09% of C+P users (p = .021). Two travelers taking MQ (1 in 607) versus one traveler using C+P (1 in 1,181) were hospitalized for such events. Recently, a study comparing MQ and A+P showed a significantly higher incidence of any neuropsychiatric event in MQ users.[51] A retrospective survey of returned travelers suggested a causal relationship between neuropsychiatric events during travel and the use of MQ prophylaxis.[58] The precise role of antimalarial drugs in neuropsychiatric AEs is difficult to define, and the role of travel as a catalyst for such events should be considered, together with other confounding factors such as gender predisposition and the use of recreational drugs and alcohol.[59]

Meta-analysis

A meta-analysis evaluating the efficacy and tolerability of MQ prophylaxis included 10 trials in which 2,750 nonimmune adult participants were randomized to MQ, a placebo, or an alternative chemoprophylaxis.[60] Rates of withdrawal and overall incidence of AEs with MQ were not significantly higher than those observed with comparator regimens, and the authors concluded that no difference in tolerability between MQ and comparator regimens was detected. Withdrawals in MQ arms were (not surprisingly) higher than in placebo arms.

Risk Factors

Quinoline-type antimalarials have been associated with neuropsychiatric AEs of varying severity. In a review of severe psychiatric reactions and convulsions, Bem and colleagues identified individuals with a history of seizures or manic-depressive illness as being particularly at risk,[61] and WHO recommends that MQ be contraindicated for individuals with a personal or family history of such disorders. In terms of all AEs, studies have shown that women are significantly more likely to experience AEs.[48,50,53,61] This might be due to dose-related toxicity although studies have shown no association between body weight and AEs in malaria prophylaxis.[50,53] It might also be due to reporting bias, to greater compliance with prescriptions,[62] or to gender-related differences in drug absorption, metabolism,[50] or central nervous system (CNS) distribution.[50,63]

One tolerability study aimed to correlate nonserious AEs occurring during routine chemoprophylaxis with concentrations of racemic MQ, its enantiomers, or the carboxylic acid metabolite.[53] The disposition of MQ was found to be highly selective, but concentrations of enantiomers, total MQ, and metabolite were not found to be significantly related to the occurrence of nonserious AEs.[53] A role has been suggested for the concomitant use of MQ and recreational drugs[50, 58] or for an interaction between MQ and large quantities of alcohol[63] although the concomitant use of small quantities of alcohol does not appear to adversely affect tolerability.[13] Children tolerate MQ well, as do elderly travelers, who report significantly fewer AEs than their younger counterparts.[64] One report suggests that subjects experiencing AEs eliminate MQ more slowly than the population in general.[65] Careful screening of travelers, with particular attention to contraindications such as personal or family history of epilepsy, seizures, or psychiatric disorders, should minimize the occurrence of serious AEs.

Literature Case Reports

Numerous case reports in the literature address the issue of MQ tolerability. There is a predominance of neuropsychiatric or neuropsychologic AEs, including severe psychiatric reactions,[66–68] hallucinations and depression,[69] acute psychosis,[70–73] amnesia,[74] psychotic episodes,[75,76] acute depressive symptoms,[77] associated seizures,[78–81] and parasthesia.[82] A case of anxiety disorder in a 10-year-old boy has been documented.[67]

The dermatologic AEs associated with MQ have been reviewed;[83] cases reviewed include a case of fatal toxic epidermal necrolysis.[84] Cardiac toxicity has been reported,[85] including aberrant atrioventricular conduction triggered by MQ[86] and atrial flutter with 1:1 (AV) conduction.[87]

MEFLOQUINE AND PERFORMANCE IN USERS

That dizziness is frequently associated with the use of MQ has led to a concern that MQ prophylaxis may impair a user's performance and precision while driving, operating machinery, or using weapons. This factor became particularly important during the deployments of personnel (including military personnel) in Cambodia in 1992, in Mozambique in 1993, in Somalia in 1993, and in Angola in 1995. For the civilian population, the impact of MQ on driving performance, in particular, required clarification in view of the numbers of travelers who drive while using MQ prophylaxis.

No functional impairment was observed in 203 MQ-exposed U.S. marines taking a loading-dose regimen followed by weekly chemoprophylaxis (n = 46) or taking routine weekly chemoprophylaxis (n = 157),[11] and MQ (including the loading-dose regimen) was recommended as an option for deployed troops. Sleep disturbance, increased dream activity, and depressive feelings were, however, more frequent in MQ users than in chloroquine users. In a double-blind placebo-controlled crossover tolerability study with trainee pilots (n = 23) to quantitatively assess the performance impact of MQ at steady-state concentrations, no significant performance deficit was documented with MQ under laboratory conditions. Participants in this trial were assessed with questionnaires, computerized sleep monitors (actigraphs), a simplified sway meter, computerized psychomotor tests, and an instrument coordination analyzer.[12] Sleep disturbance and some loss of concentration (nonsignificant) were noted, however. The authors recommended further analysis with complex flight simulators and cautioned that their study was not a basis for recommending MQ prophylaxis for pilots.

The neurologic effects of MQ were examined in 95 healthy Australian volunteers in a double-blind placebo-controlled trial. MQ did not produce debilitating neurologic symptoms nor did it alter the results of sensitive tests of cerebral function, compared to placebo.[88] Balance and hearing were unaffected by MQ prophylaxis in Swedish volunteers, whom the investigators tested intensively for MQ toxicity, using subspecialized techniques such as posturography, nystagmus recording, and Békésy audiometry.[89] A study examining the impact of AEs on function found no significant deficit in computerized psychomotor tests in those experiencing moderate AEs.[53] In a controlled study examining the effects of MQ used alone and with alcohol on psychomotor and driving performance, no significant impairment was found in any test, relative to placebo.[13]

In summary, these studies (Table 8.3–3) suggest that if MQ is tolerated by an individual, it does not appear to undermine his or her performance.

SAFETY IN PREGNANCY

Malaria is a grave hazard for nonimmune female travelers, and pregnant women should be advised not to travel to malaria-endemic areas where there is a risk of exposure to CRPF. The use of antimalarial drugs prior to and during pregnancy is a major issue, and important data on MQ use in pregnancy are summarized in Table 8.3–4. Although the scope of this article is limited to MQ use in nonimmune travelers, major studies of MQ use in semi-immune pregnant women have been included in this section.

Table 8.3–3. **Studies of Mefloquine and Performance in Users, 1992 to 2000**

Study	Type of Analysis	Main Conclusions
Boudreau (1993)	DB trial with U.S. Marines, MQ (n = 46,* 157) vs. CQ (n = 156). Assessment: Q, I, A	No compromise in function due to dizziness or incoordination in the MQ users
Hessen-Soderman (1995)	Swedish volunteers, MQ (n = 10). Assessment: posturography, nystagmus recording, Békésy audiometry	Balance and hearing were not adversely affected by MQ prophylaxis.
Davis (1996)	DB, PC trial with Australian volunteers, MQ (n = 46) vs. P (n = 49). Assessment: PSY, electrocardiography, audiometry, biochemical variables	MQ did not impair neurologic or cardiovascular function apart from mild and transient Q-Tc prolongation. MQ-associated hypoglycemia was noted.
Vuurman (1996)	DB trial with Dutch volunteers, MQ (n = 20) vs. P (n = 20). Assessment: PSY, driving test, body sway, alcohol challenge	MQ caused no significant impairment in any test at any time, relative to placebo.
Schlagenhauf (1997)	DB, PC trial with Swiss trainee pilots, MQ* (n = 23) vs. P (n = 23). Assessment: Q, A, I, PSY, body sway, ICA	No significant performance deficit was observed for any test. Some sleep disturbance and decreased concentration was noted in the MQ group.

MQ = mefloquine; CQ = chloroquine; P = placebo; Q = questionnaire; I = interview; A = actigraphy; PSY = psychometric tests; ICA= Instrument Coordination Analyzer; DB = double-blind; PC = placebo-controlled.
* Denotes use of loading-dose regimen.

Early animal studies documented the teratogenic and embryotoxic effects associated with the use of high-dose MQ. However, recent experience is more reassuring although data are limited. A double-blind placebo-controlled study of MQ prophylaxis in 339 pregnant (at > 20 weeks of gestation) Karen women living on the Thailand-Myanmar border[90] showed that MQ prophylaxis was well tolerated. Apart from transient dizziness associated with the 10-mg/kg loading dose, no other significant adverse impact on mother, course of pregnancy, or infant survival or development (up to the age of 2 years) was observed. A higher overall rate of still-births was noted for MQ users (11 in 159 MQ users vs. 4 in 152 placebo recipients). The authors concluded that MQ is safe and effective for antimalarial prophylaxis in the second half of pregnancy.

A study of pregnant women in the Mangochi district of Malawi[91] showed no significant differences in the frequency of abortions or stillbirths between women receiving chloroquine prophylaxis and those receiving MQ prophylaxis during the second and third trimesters. A small proportion of women in this investigation also received antimalarial drugs in the first trimester. Fourteen women were treated with MQ and 53 with chloroquine. Where first-trimester drug exposure occurred, no adverse outcomes were identified in the MQ group; one baby was delivered breech, and all known birth weights were normal (mean, 3,009 g). One stillbirth

Table 8.3–4. **Major Reports Concerning Use of Mefloquine Prophylaxis in Pregnancy, 1992 to 2000**

Lead Author (Year)	Reference	Type of Analysis	Main Conclusions
Vanhauwere (1998)	93	Analysis of Roche International Spontaneous Reporting System to evaluate the teratogenic potential of MQ	26 congenital malformations in 646 deliveries, or a 4% birth prevalence (i.e., similar to incidence in general population). No specific pattern of malformations was observed.
Smoak (1997)	96	Analysis of pregnancies and outcomes in U.S. Army servicewomen exposed to MQ	72 soldiers used MQ during pregnancy, with 23 live births. High rate of spontaneous abortions (12/36). Authors concluded that MQ did not appear to cause gross congenital malformations.
Phillips-Howard (1996)	94	Literature review	No evidence to suggest that MQ is teratogenic
Steketee (1996)	92	Mangochi Malaria Research Project. Prospective monitoring of pregnant Malawi women using MQ (n = 1,032) or CQ (n = 3,077) during the period 1987–90. First trimester exposure to MQ (n = 14)	MQ was significantly more protective against LBW than CQ. MQ users had rates of abortions and stillbirths similar to those of CQ users. No congenital anomalies after first trimester exposure.
Nosten (1994)	90	Double-blind placebo-controlled trial of MQ prophylaxis in 339 Karen women (pregnancy > 20 weeks of gestation)	Overall rate of stillbirths higher in MQ users (1/159 vs. 4/152 in placebo users). Authors concluded that MQ is safe and effective for malaria prophylaxis in the second half of pregnancy.
Balocco (1992)	95	Case series of 10 women exposed to MQ in the first trimester	No malformations or perinatal pathologic symptoms

CQ = chloroquine; LBW = low birth weight; MQ = mefloquine.

occurred in the chloroquine-treated group. No congenital anomalies were noted in either group. Another analysis of this project[92] found that MQ was protective against low birth weight (LBW) and attributed this to its effect on reducing placental and umbilical-cord blood malaria infection. The proportion of low–birth weight babies born to women using MQ was 12.5%, significantly lower than the proportion born to women using chloroquine (15.5%).

Spontaneous reports received by Roche of women exposed to MQ (Lariam) before or during pregnancy were evaluated in regard to pregnancy, fetal outcome, and fetal congenital malformations.[93] In this study, 646 deliveries resulted in 26 congenital malformations, 33 other pregnancy-related and perinatal problems, and 587 normal infants. The prevalence of congenital malformations in infants born to women exposed to MQ was estimated at 4%, similar to the prevalence observed in the general population. Furthermore, the congenital malformations observed with MQ use did not show any specific pattern, and the authors of this analysis concluded that the teratogenicity observed at high doses in animal studies is not seen in humans.

No congenital defects were reported in a group of 99 European travelers to sub-Saharan Africa who were inadvertently exposed to MQ prior to or during their first trimester of pregnancy.[94] Some 10 Italian women, exposed to MQ prior to or during their first trimester of pregnancy, delivered without any malformations or perinatal pathologic symptoms.[95]

Additional information on the use of MQ in nonimmune pregnant women came from data on 72 U.S. servicewomen who inadvertently used MQ prior to becoming aware of their pregnancy. Of these 72 soldiers, 17 had elective abortions, 12 had spontaneous abortions, 1 had a molar pregnancy, and 23 gave live births; the pregnancy outcomes of 19 soldiers were unknown. All infants were healthy at birth, and there were no major congenital malformations. One infant died of viral pneumonitis at 4 months. Thirteen infants were reported healthy at 1 year of age, with normal cognitive and motor development. Regarding the high rate (33%) of spontaneous abortions observed in this cohort, the authors offered various explanations and cautioned that postmarketing surveillance of spontaneous abortion rates should be closely monitored to determine whether MQ exposure is a causal factor. The authors concluded that MQ does not appear to cause gross congenital malformations.[96]

A literature review of the use of antimalarials in pregnancy concluded that there was no evidence for MQ-associated teratogenicity.[94]

In summary, data are limited, but the increasing body of evidence on MQ use in pregnancy is reassuring. The use of the drug in the second and third trimesters for women at high risk has been sanctioned by WHO and CDC. Due to mefloquine's long half-life, pregnancy should be avoided for 3 months after prophylaxis is completed although inadvertent pregnancy while using MQ is not considered grounds for pregnancy termination.

MQ is secreted into breast milk in small quantities. Its effect, if any, on breast-fed infants is unknown.

DRUG INTERACTIONS

A retrospective analysis of a database of antimalarial tolerability data showed that co-medications commonly used by travelers have had no significant clinical impact on the safety of prophylaxis with MQ.[97] The information insert packaged with Lariam suggests that MQ users who are diabetics or who use anticoagulants should be checked before departure by a physician in case of drug interaction. Interactions can occur with other antimalarial drugs such as quinine, quinidine, chloroquine, and halofantrine. The coadministration of MQ with cardioactive drugs might contribute to the prolongation of Q-Tc intervals although in the light of currently available information, coadministration of MQ with such drugs is not contraindicated. Vaccination with oral live typhoid or cholera vaccines should be completed at least 3 days before the first dose of MQ.

COMMENTARY

Any malaria chemoprophylaxis involves a risk-benefit analysis to weigh possible drug-induced toxicity against the risk of acquiring malaria (particularly malaria caused by *Plasmodium falciparum*). Mefloquine has been used by over 20 million travelers, and while there is controversy regarding tolerability, several studies and a meta-analysis have shown that the reported incidence of minor and moderate AEs with MQ does not appear to be significantly higher than that found with other chemoprophylactic regimens. The profile of MQ-associated AEs is characterized by a predominance of neuropsychologic AEs, and careful prescribing could reduce the incidence of such events. There is consensus regarding efficacy, and studies of non-immune travelers have shown that MQ is effective in the prevention of CRPF malaria, except in clearly defined regions of multidrug resistance.

REFERENCES

1. Schmidt LH, Crosby R, Rasco J, Vaughan D. Antimalarial activities of various 4-quinolinemethanols with special attention to WR-142,490 (mefloquine). Antimicrob Agents Chemother 1978;13:1011–1030.
2. Palmer KJ, Holliday SM, Brogden RN. Mefloquine, a review of its antimalarial activity, pharmacokinetic properties and therapeutic efficacy. Drugs 1993;45:430–475.
3. Schlagenhauf P. Mefloquine for malaria chemoprophylaxis 1992–1998: a review. J Travel Med 1999;6:122–133.
4. Warhurst DC. Antimalarial interaction with ferriprotoporphyrin IX monomer and its relationship to the activity of the blood schizontocides. Ann Trop Med Parasitol 1987;81:65–67.
5. Crevoisier C, Handschin J, Barré J, et al. Food increases the bioavailability of mefloquine. Eur J Clin Pharmacol 1997;53:135–139.
6. Pennie RA, Koren G, Crevoisier C. Steady state pharmacokinetics of mefloquine in long-term travellers. Trans R Soc Trop Med Hyg 1993;87:459–462.
7. Gimenez F, Pennie RA, Koren G, et al. Stereoselective pharmacokinetics of mefloquine in healthy Caucasians after multiple doses. J Pharm Sci 1994;83:824–827.
8. Pham YT, Nosten F, Farinotti R, et al. Cerebral uptake of mefloquine enantiomers in fatal cerebral malaria. Int J Clin Pharmacol Ther 1999;37:58–61.
9. Crevoisier C, Joseph I, Fischer M, Graf H. Influence of hemodialysis on plasma concentration-time profiles of mefloquine in two patients with end-stage renal disease: a prophylactic drug monitoring study. Antimicrob Agents Chemother 1995;39:1892–1895.
10. Weidekamm E, Rüsing G, Caplain H, et al. Lack of bioequivalence of a generic mefloquine tablet with the standard product. Eur J Clin Pharmacol 1998;54:615–619.
11. Boudreau E, Schuster B, Sanchez J, et al. Tolerability of prophylactic Lariam regimens. Trop Med Parasitol 1993;44:257–265.
12. Schlagenhauf P, Lobel HO, Steffen R, et al. Tolerability of mefloquine in Swissair trainee pilots. Am J Trop Med Hyg 1997;56:235–240.

13. Vuurman EFPM, Muntjewerff ND, Uiterwijk MMC, et al. Effects of mefloquine alone and with alcohol on psychomotor and driving performance. Eur J Clin Pharmacol 1996;50:475–482.

14. MacPherson D, Gamble K, Tessier D, et al. Mefloquine tolerance randomised, double-blinded, placebo-controlled study using a loading dose of mefloquine in pre-exposed travellers [abstract 220]. Program and Abstracts of the Fifth International Conference on Travel Medicine; 1997 March 24–27; Geneva, Switzerland.

15. Steffen R, Fuchs E, Schildknecht J, et al. Mefloquine compared with other malaria chemo-prophylactic regimens in tourists visiting East Africa. Lancet 1993;341:1299–1303.

16. Lobel HO, Miani M, Eng T, et al. Long term malaria prophylaxis with weekly meflo-quine. Lancet 1993;341:848–851.

17. Ohrt C, Richie TL, Widjaja H, et al. A double-blind, placebo-controlled trial of meflo-quine versus doxycycline for the prophylaxis of malaria in Indonesian soldiers. Ann Intern Med 1997;126:963–972.

18. Rieckmann KH, Yeo AE, Davis DR, et al. Recent military experience with malaria chemoprophylaxis. Med J Aust 1993;158:446–449.

19. Pergallo MS, Sabatinelli G, Majori G, et al. Prevention and morbidity in non-immune subjects; a case-control study among Italian troops in Somalia and Mozambique, 1992–1994. Trans R Soc Trop Med Hyg 1997;91:343–346.

20. Axmann A, Félegyhazi CS, Huszar A, Juhasz P. Long term malaria prophylaxis with Lariam in Cambodia, 1993. Travel Med Int 1994;12:1:13–18.

21. Hopperus Buma AP, van Thiel PP, Lobel HO, et al. Long term malaria chemoprophylax-is with mefloquine in Dutch marines in Cambodia. J Infect Dis 1996;173:1506–1509.

22. Sanchez JL, DeFraites RF, Sharp TW, Hanson RK. Mefloquine or doxycycline prophy-laxis in US troops in Somalia. Lancet 1993;341:1021–1022.

23. Wallace MR, Sharp TW, Smoak B, et al. Malaria among United States troops in Soma-lia. Am J Med 1996;100:49–55.

24. Bwire R, Slootman EJH, Verhave JP, et al. Malaria anticircumsporozoite antibodies in Dutch soldiers returning from sub-Saharan Africa. Trop Med Int Health 1998;3:66–69.

25. Muehlberger N, Jelinek T, Schlipkoeter U, et al. Effectiveness of chemoprophylaxis and other determinants of malaria in travellers to Kenya. Trop Med Int Health 1998;3:357–363.

26. Lobel HO, Varma JK, Miani N, et al. Monitoring for mefloquine-resistant *Plasmodium falciparum* in Africa: implications for travelers' health. Am J Trop Med Hyg 1998;59:129–132.

27. Magill AJ, Smoak BL. Failure of mefloquine chemoprophylaxis for malaria in Somalia [letter]. N Engl J Med 1993;329:1206.

28. Wallace MR, Sharp TW, Romajzl PJ, Magill HO. Malaria among US troops in Somalia [abstract 107]. Clin Infect Dis 1994;(3)580.

29. Nozais JP. Un nouveau cas probable de resistance croisee de *Plasmodium falciparum* viv-a-vis de la mefloquine et de l'halofantrine, en provenance de Sierre Leone. Med Mal Infect 1992;22:421–423.

30. Delmont J, Faugere B, Doury JC, Bourgeade A. Paludisme a *Plasmodium falciparum* consectif a un echec de prophylaxie par mefloquine lors d'un sejour en Cote d'Ivoire. Med Mal Infect 1992;22:418–420.

31. Matteelli A, Chiodera A, Castelli F, et al. Failure of mefloquine chemoprophylaxis for malaria in Mozambique. J Travel Med 1995;2:260–261.

32. Kurtis JD, Koros JK, Duffy PE, Green MD. Malaria prevention for travelers [letter]. JAMA 1998;278:1767–1771.

33. Todd GD, Hopperus Buma AP, Green MD, et al. Comparison of whole blood and serum levels of mefloquine and its carboxylic acid metabolite. Am J Trop Med Hyg 1997;57:399–402.

34. Day JH, Behrens RH. Delay in onset of malaria with mefloquine prophylaxis. Lancet 1995;345:398.

35. Mockenhaupt FP. Mefloquine resistance in *Plasmodium falciparum*. Parasitol Today 1995;11:248–253.

36. Amor D, Richards M. Mefloquine resistant *P. vivax* malaria in PNG. Med J Aust 1992;156:883.

37. Chia JK, Nakata MM, Co S. Smear-negative cerebral malaria due to mefloquine-resistant *Plasmodium falciparum* acquired in the Amazon. J Infect Dis 1992;165:599–600.

38. Le Bras J, Durand R, Di Piazza JP, et al. *Plasmodium falciparum* resistance to mefloquine, chloroquine and cycloguanil and prevention of malaria in travelers from France to Africa. Presse Med 1998;27:1419–1423.

39. Brasseur P, Kouamouo J, Moyou-Somo R, Druilhe P. Multi-drug resistant falciparum malaria in Cameroon in 1987–1988. II. Mefloquine resistance confirmed in vivo and in vitro and its correlation with quinine resistance. Am J Trop Med Hyg 1992;46:8–14.

40. Behrens RH, Bradley DJ, Snow RW, Marsh K. Impact of UK malaria prophylaxis policy on imported malaria. Lancet 1996;9023:344–345.

41. Muentener P, Schlagenhauf P, Steffen R. Imported malaria in industrialized countries. Trends and perspectives. Bull World Health Organ 1999;77(7):560–566.

42. Peters W. Drug resistance in malaria parasites of animals and man. Adv Parasitol 1998;41:1–58.

43. White NJ. Why is it that antimalarial drug treatments do not always work? Ann Trop Med Parasitol 1998;92:449–458.

44. Peel SA, Bright P, Yount B, et al. A strong assocation between mefloquine and halofantrine resistance and amplification, overexpression and mutation in the P-glycoprotein gene homolog (pfmdr) of *Plasmodium falciparum* in vitro. Am J Trop Med Hyg 1994;51:648–658.

45. Cowman AF, Galatis D, Thompson JK. Selection for mefloquine resistance in *Plasmodium falciparum* is linked to amplification of the pfmdr1 gene and cross resistance to halofantrine and quinine. Proc Natl Acad Sci U S A 1994;91:1143–1147.

46. Duraisingh MT, Jones P, Sambou I, et al. The tyrosine-86 allele of the pfmdr 1 gene of *Plasmodium falciparum* is associated with increased sensitivity to the anti-malarials mefloquine and artemisinin. Mol Biochem Parasitol 2000;108:13–23.

47. Oduola AMJ, Omitowoju GO, Gerena L, et al. Reversal of mefloquine resistance with penfluridol in isolates of *Plasmodium falciparum* from south-west Nigeria. Trans R Soc Trop Med Hyg 1993;87:81–83.

48. Barrett PJ, Emmins PD, Clarke PD, Bradley DJ. Comparison of adverse events associated with the use of mefloquine and combination of chloroquine and proguanil as antimalarial prophylaxis: postal and telephone survey of travellers. BMJ 1996;313:525–528.

49. Croft A. Malaria prophylaxis. Toxicity of mefloquine is similar to that of other chemoprophylaxis. BMJ 1995;311:191.

50. Phillips MA, Kass RB. User acceptability patterns for mefloquine and doxycycline malaria chemoprophylaxis. J Travel Med 1996;3:40–45.
51. Overbosch, Schilthuis H, Bienzle U, et al. Malarone compared with mefloquine for malaria prophylaxis in non-immune travelers [abstract no. 271]. Proceedings of "New challenges in tropical medical parasitology," 18–22 September, 2000, Oxford.
52. Jaspers CA, Hopperus Buma AP, van Thiel PP, et al. Tolerance of mefloquine prophylaxis in Dutch military personnel. Am J Trop Med Hyg 1996;55:230–234.
53. Schlagenhauf P, Steffen R, Lobel H, et al. Mefloquine tolerability during chemoprophylaxis: focus on adverse event assessments, stereochemistry and compliance. Trop Med Int Health 1996;1:485–494.
54. Peragallo MS, Sabatinelli G, Sarnicola G. Compliance and tolerability of mefloquine and chloroquine plus proguanil for long-term malaria chemoprophylaxis in groups at particular risk (the military). Trans R Soc Trop Med Hyg 1999;93:73–77.
55. CIOM International reporting of adverse drug reactions. CIOMS Working Group Report. Geneva: World Health Organization, 1987.
56. Schlagenhauf P, Abo El Ela H, Neiderberger W, et al. Drug safety database analysis of the serious adverse events (SAE). Depression or suicide reported in association with the use of mefloquine. Proceedings of the 7th conference of the International Society of Travel Medicine; 2001 May 27-31; Innsbruck.
57. Croft AM, World MJ. Neuropsychiatric reactions with mefloquine chemoprophylaxis. Lancet 1996;347:326.
58. Potasman I, Beny A, Seligmann H. Neuropsychiatric problems in 2,500 long-term travelers to the tropics. J Travel Med 1999;6:122–133.
59. Schlagenhauf P, Steffen R. Neuropsychiatric events and travel: do antimalarials play a role? J Travlel Med 2000;7(5): 225-226.
60. Croft A, Garner P. Mefloquine for preventing malaria in non-immune adult travelers. In: Cochrane Collaboration. Cochrane database of systematic reviews. Issue 1. 2001.
61. Bem JL, Kerr L, Stürchler D. Mefloquine prophylaxis: an overview of spontaneous reports of severe psychiatric reactions and convulsions. J Trop Med Hyg 1992;95:167–179.
62. Phillips-Howard PA, ter Kuile FO. CNS adverse events associated with antimalarial agents. Fact or fiction? Drug Saf 1995;12:370–383.
63. Wittes RC, Sagmur R. Adverse reactions to mefloquine associated with ethanol ingestion. Can Med Assoc J 1995;152:515–517.
64. Mittelholzer ML, Wall M, Steffen R, Stürchler D. Malaria prophylaxis in different age groups. J Travel Med 1996;4:219–223.
65. Jerling M, Rombo L, Hellgren U, et al. Evaluation of mefloquine adverse effects in relation to the plasma concentration [abstract no. 95]. Proceedings of the Fourth International Conference on Travel Medicine; 1995 April 23–27; Acapulco, Mexico.
66. Hennequin C, Bouree P, Bazin N, et al. Severe psychiatric side effects observed during prophylaxis and treatment with mefloquine. Arch Intern Med 1994;20:2360–2362.
67. Clattenburg RN, Donnelly CL. Case study: neuropsychiatric symptoms associated with the antimalarial agent mefloquine. J Am Acad Child Adolesc Psychiatry 1997;36:1606–1608.
68. Lench P. Psychological problems after mefloquine and chloroquine. BMJ 1995;311:192.
69. Carme B, Nevez G, Peguet C, Bouko I. Intolerance neuropsychique au sours de la chimiprophylaxis antipalustre par la mefloquine. A propos de 5 observations. Bull Epi Herbdomadaire 1994;34:155.

70. Meszaros K. Acute psychosis caused by mefloquine prophylaxis? Can J Psychiatry 1996;41:196.

71. Hollweg M, Soyka M, Greil W. Mefloquininduzierte Psychosen—Probleme der Kausalzuordnung anhand zweier kasuistischer Berichte. Psychiatr Prax 1995;22:33–36.

72. Piening RB, Young SA. Mefloquine induced psychosis. Ann Emerg Med 1996;27: 792–793.

73. Grupp D, Rauber A, Froescher W. Neuropsychiatrische Stoerungen nach Malariaprophylaxe mit Mefloquin. Aktuelle Neurol 1994;21:134–136.

74. Marsepoil T, Petithory J, Faucher JM, et al. Encephalopathie et troubles amnesiques au cours des traitments par la mefloquine. Rev Med Interne 1993;14:788–791.

75. Recasens C, Zittoun C, Feline A. Un episode psychotique au retour d'un voyage en Afrique: implication possible de la mefloquine. Ann Psychiatr ;8:100–103.

76. Folkerts H, Kuhs H. Psychotische Episode infolge Malariaprophylaxe mit Mefloquine. Eine kasuistische Mitteilung. Nervenarzt 1992:63:300–302.

77. Caillon E, Schmitt L, Moron P. Acute depressive symptoms after mefloquine treatment. Am J Psychiatry 1992;149:712.

78. Ruff TA, Sherwen SJ, Donnan GA. Seizure associated with mefloquine for malaria prophylaxis. Med J Aust 1994;161:453.

79. Pous E, Gascon J, Obach J, Corachan M. Mefloquine-induced grand mal seizure during malaria chemoprophylaxis in a non-epileptic subject. Trans R Soc Trop Med Hyg 1995;89:434.

80. Adamolekun B. Epileptogenic potential of antimalarial drugs. West Afr J Med 1993;12:231–232.

81. Ries S. Zerebrale Krampfanfälle während einer Malariaprophylaxe mit Mefloquin. Dtsch Med Wochenschr 1993;118:1911–1912.

82. Olsen PE, Kennedy CA, Morte PD. Paresthesias and mefloquine prophylaxis. Ann Intern Med 1992;117:1058–1059.

83. Smith HR, Croft AM, Black MM. Dermatological adverse effects with the antimalarial drug mefloquine; a review of 74 published case reports. Clin Exp Dermatol 1999;24:249–254.

84. McBride SR, Lawrence CM, Pape SA, Reid CA. Fatal toxic epidermal necrolysis associated with mefloquine prophylaxis. Lancet 1997;349:101.

85. Nicolas X, Touze JE. La toxicite cardiaque des antipaludiques. Med Trop (Mars) 1994;54:361–365.

86. Richter J, Burbach G, Hellgren U, et al. Aberrant atrioventricular conduction triggered by antimalarial prophylaxis with mefloquine. Lancet 1997;349:101–102.

87. Fonteyne W, Bauwens A, Jordaens L. Atrial flutter with 1:1 conduction after administration of the antmalarial drug mefloquine. Clin Cardiol 1996;19:967–968.

88. Davis TME, Dembo LG, Kaye-Eddie SA, et al. Neurological, cardiovascular and metabolic effects of mefloquine in healthy volunteers: a double-blind, placebo controlled trial. Br J Clin Pharmacol 1996;42:415–421.

89. Hessen-Soederman AC, Bergenius J, Berggren I, et al. Mefloquine prophylaxis, and hearing, postural control and vestibular functions. J Travel Med 1995;2:66–69.

90. Nosten F, ter Kuile F, Maelankiri L, et al. Mefloquine prophylaxis prevents malaria during pregnancy: a double blind, placebo controlled study. J Infect Dis 1994;169:595–603.

91. Steketee RW, Wirima JJ, Slutsker L, et al. Malaria treatment and prevention in pregnancy: indications for use and adverse events associated with use of chloroquine or mefloquine. Am J Trop Med Hyg 1996;55:50–56.

92. Steketee RW, Wirima JJ, Hightower AW, et al. The effect of malaria and malaria prevention on offspring birthweight, prematurity and intrauterine growth retardation in rural Malawi. Am J Trop Med Hyg 1996;55 (1 Suppl):33–41.

93. Vanhauwere B, Maradit H, Kerr L. Post-marketing surveillance of prophylactic mefloquine (Lariam) use in pregnancy. Am J Trop Med Hyg 1998;58:17–21.

94. Phillips-Howard PA, Wood D. The safety of antimalarial drugs in pregnancy. Drug Saf 1996;14:131–145.

95. Balocco R, Bonati M. Mefloquine prophylaxis against malaria for female travellers of childbearing age. Lancet 1992;340:309–310.

96. Smoak BL, Writer JV, Keep LW, et al. The effects of inadvertent exposure of mefloquine chemoprophylaxis on pregnancy outcomes and infants of US Army service women. J Infect Dis 1997;176:831–833.

97. Handschin JC, Wall M, Steffen R, Starchier D. Tolerability and effectiveness of malaria chemoprophylaxis with mefloquine or chloroquine with or without co-medication. J Travel Med 1997;4:121–127.

8.4 Doxycycline

Carrie Beallor and Kevin C. Kain

ABSTRACT

Doxycycline is an inexpensive broad-spectrum antimicrobial agent effective for both the treatment and prevention of malaria. It is the chemoprophylactic drug of choice for those at risk of mefloquine-resistant *Plasmodium falciparum* malaria and is a useful alternative for the prevention of chloroquine-resistant and chloroquine-sensitive malaria. Doxycycline is contraindicated during pregnancy and in children less than 8 years of age. Doxycycline is highly efficacious against multidrug-resistant malaria but must be taken daily to be effective. Failure to adhere to the daily dosing regimen is the main reason for prophylactic failures. Overall, doxycycline is well tolerated, and serious adverse effects are rare. Taking doxycycline with food and fluids can reduce adverse effects such as gastrointestinal upset, and using appropriate sunscreens can decrease photosensitivity. Doxycycline prophylaxis has the added advantage of preventing travel-associated leptospirosis and rickettsial infections.

Key words: esophageal ulceration; malaria prevention; malaria treatment; photosensitivity; tetracycline.

DESCRIPTION

The tetracyclines form a class of antimicrobial agents with a broad spectrum of activity that includes action against gram-positive and gram-negative aerobic and anaerobic bacteria, mycoplasma, rickettsia, chlamydiae, and protozoa, including those that cause malaria. The first tetracycline, chlortetracycline (Aureomycin), was identified by Benjamin M. Duggar in 1944. Doxycycline and minocycline were derived semisynthetically in 1967 and 1972, respectively.[1,2] Tetracyclines can be divided into three groups on the basis of pharmacokinetics; two groups have been used for almost three decades in the treatment or prevention of malaria.[3–6] Tetracycline, a member of the short-acting group, is used in the therapy of falciparum malaria, and doxycycline (Figure 8.4–1), a long-acting compound, is used for both chemoprophylaxis and treatment of human malaria.

PHARMACOLOGY AND MODE OF ACTION

Tetracyclines, including doxycycline, are relatively slow-acting schizonticidal agents and are therefore not used alone for therapy. However, numerous studies

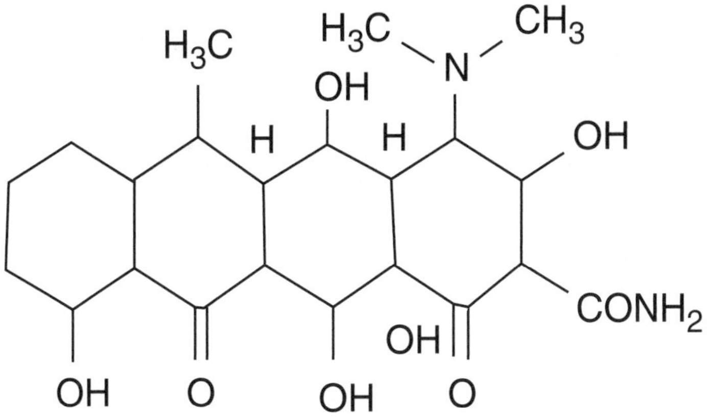

Figure 8.4–1. Structure of doxycycline.

have established the efficacy of doxycycline as a solo chemoprophylactic agent against *Plasmodium vivax* and *Plasmodium falciparum* malaria. In addition to its activity against the erythrocytic stage of the parasite, doxycycline is thought to possess pre-erythrocytic activity. However, studies examining its efficacy as a causal agent had unacceptable high failure rates, and doxycycline needs to be taken as a chemosuppressive for 4 weeks after leaving a malaria-endemic area to be optimally effective.[7–10]

The mechanism of action of tetracyclines in bacteria has been examined in detail. The mode of action is presumed to be similar in protozoa. Tetracyclines accumulate in bacteria by active transport; they reversibly bind primarily to the 30S ribosomal subunit at a position that blocks binding of the aminoacyl transfer ribonucleic acid (aminoacyl-tRNA) to the accepter site on the messenger ribonucleic acid (mRNA). This inhibits protein synthesis by preventing the incorporation of new amino acids into the growing peptide chain. Protein synthesis is also inhibited in mammalian cells, but since there is no active transport in these cells, selective activity against microorganisms is achieved.[1]

Doxycycline has several advantages over first-generation tetracyclines, including improved absorption, a broader spectrum, a longer half-life, and an improved safety profile. Doxycycline is well absorbed from the proximal small bowel (90% to 100% oral absorption), and in contrast to other tetracyclines, its uptake does not change significantly with food intake. Doxycycline may be taken with food or milk, and this approach decreases the gastrointestinal (GI) irritation occasionally associated with this drug. Doxycycline is highly protein-bound (93%), has a small volume of distribution (0.7 L/kg), and is lipid soluble. These features may explain its high blood levels and prolonged half-life, permitting a once-daily dosing regimen. The time to peak concentration (~ 2.5 µg/mL after a 200-mg dose) following oral ingestion is 2 to 3 hours. Doxycycline has a half-life of approximately 15 to 22 hours that is unaffected by renal impairment. Doxycycline is eliminated unchanged in the urine by glomerular filtration and largely unchanged in the feces by biliary and GI secretion. About 40% of the dose is eliminated in the urine in individuals with normal kidney function whereas those with renal dysfunction are able to eliminate it via the liver-biliary-GI route. Therefore, unlike other tetracyclines, doxycycline may be used in renal failure, and the dose does not need to be adjusted in cases of renal impairment. The drug is not effectively removed by peritoneal dialysis or hemodialysis.[1,2]

EFFICACY

Although doxycycline has a number of listed indications, there are relatively few studies evaluating its efficacy. A review of the literature from the past 15 years revealed eight randomized trials examining the efficacy of doxycycline as a chemoprophylactic against *Plasmodium* sp.[11–18] Four of these studies were recent, double blind, and placebo controlled. The results of these randomized trials are summarized in Table 8.4–1. Two of these trials evaluated semi-immune children or adults in Kenya, and two trials examined nonimmune populations in West Papua (Irian Jaya, Indonesia). In three of these studies, the currently recommended adult dose of doxycycline (100 mg base per day) was used.[9,10] The reported protective efficacy in these three trials was excellent, ranging from 92% to 100% against *Plasmodium falciparum* and *Plasmodium vivax* malaria. In comparative trials in areas with chloroquine-resistant falciparum malaria, doxycycline has been shown to be equivalent to mefloquine and atovaquone/proguanil and superior to azithromycin and chloroquine/proguanil.[14–19]

Table 8.4–1. **Recent Randomized, Double-Blind, Placebo-Controlled Trials of Doxycycline Efficacy**

Lead Author (Reference)	Year*	Population	Dose	Efficacy[†] (95% CI)
Weiss (15)	1995	Semi-immune Kenyan children aged 9–14 years	50 mg/d	Pf: 84% (66–92%) against developing parasitemia; 91% (61–98%) against developing clinical malaria
Ohrt (16)	1997	"Nonimmune" Indonesian adults newly arrived to Irian Jaya	100 mg/d	Pf: 98% (88–100%); Pv: 100% (90–100%)
Anderson (17)	1998	Semi-immune Kenyan adults	100 mg/d	Pf: 92.6% (79.9–97.5%)
Taylor (18)	1999	"Nonimmune" Indonesian adults recently (6–15 mo) arrived in Irian Jaya	100 mg/d	Pf: 96.3% (85.4–99.6%); Pv: 98% (88.0–99.9%)

Pf = *P. falciparum;* Pv = *P. vivax.*
* Year of study publication.
[†] Calculated as the percentage reduction in incidence density (cases of malaria/total person-years of follow-up).

Parasite resistance to doxycycline has not been reported to be an operational problem in any malaria-endemic area thus far. A distinct advantage of doxycycline over other chemoprophylatic agents such as mefloquine is that it can effectively prevent leptospirosis and rickettsial infections. However, recent reports from northern Thailand indicate that the agent of scrub typhus (Orientia tsutsugamushi) displays decreased susceptibility to doxycycline.[20] When doxycycline was first used as a chemoprophylactic agent against malaria, it was speculated that it might also provide protection against travelers' diarrhea. However, doxycycline used as a malaria chemoprophylactic has not been shown to decrease travelers' diarrhea. This is likely due to the presence of widespread tetracycline-resistant enteric pathogens, such as enterotoxigenic Escherichia coli.[21]

TOLERABILITY

The most commonly reported adverse events related to doxycycline use are GI effects, including nausea, vomiting, abdominal pain, and diarrhea. These adverse effects occur less frequently with doxycycline than with other tetracyclines, presumably because doxycycline is better absorbed and has less effect on intestinal flora. However, esophageal ulceration is a rare but well-described problem associated with doxycycline use. It generally presents with retrosternal burning and odynophagia 1 to 7 days after therapy is initiated.[22,23] In a study of ~10,000 U.S. troops deployed in Somalia, esophageal ulceration due to doxycycline was the most frequent cause of hospitalization attributed to the use of malaria chemoprophylaxis.[23] Gastrointestinal adverse effects can be reduced by taking doxycycline in an upright position, with food and a full glass of water.

Dermatologic reactions (especially an increased reaction to sunlight [photosensitivity]) are also a frequent adverse event associated with doxycycline use. These reactions range from mild paresthesias or exaggerated sunburn in exposed skin to photo-onycholysis (sun-induced separation of nails), severe erythema, bulla formation, and (rarely) Stevens-Johnson syndrome.[1] The reported rate of photosensitivity varies from ~4% to 16% or more of users, and the reaction is mild in the majority of cases.[19,24] The risk of photosensitivity may be reduced by the use of appropriate sunscreens (> SPF 15 and protective against both ultraviolet A [UVA] and ultraviolet B [UVB] radiation).[19,24]

Although doxycycline has a lesser effect on normal bacterial flora than other tetracyclines have, it still increases the risk of oral and vaginal candidiasis in predisposed individuals. Travelers with a past history of these problems who are prescribed doxycycline should be advised to carry an appropriate treatment course of antifungal therapy.

Other uncommon adverse events occasionally attributed to doxycycline include dizziness, lightheadedness, darkening or discoloration of the tongue, and (very rarely) hepatotoxicity, pancreatitis, or benign intracranial hypertension. Long-term (>12 years) and abnormally high-dose (1 g per day) doxycycline ingestion has been reported to induce hepatocellular necrosis, nephrotoxicity, leukopenia, anemia, hyperpigmentation, cardiac arrhythmia, and heart block, all of which were reversible (surprisingly) with drug discontinuation.[25]

Overall, a number of comparative studies have shown that doxycycline used as a chemoprophylactic agent is generally well tolerated and has relatively few reported side effects.[11,12,15–19,21,23] Pang and colleagues performed two controlled field trials examining the efficacy and tolerability of doxycycline in semi-immune children residing in an area of multidrug resistance in Thailand.[11,12] In the placebo-controlled trial, doxycycline provided a protective efficacy of 89% (95% CI: 51% to 96%) against *Plasmodium falciparum* and 96% (95% CI: 85% to 98%) against *Plasmodium vivax.*[12] In both trials, doxycycline was tolerated as well as or better than chloroquine[11] or placebo,[12] with no serious adverse events or photosensitivity reported. A randomized double-blind trial comparing the tolerability of mefloquine and doxycycline in soldiers deployed in Thailand found no significant differences between these agents.[21] Weiss and colleagues examined the efficacy and tolerability of primaquine, doxycycline, proguanil/chloroquine, and mefloquine compared to placebo in semi-immune children in Kenya. There were no significant differences in reported adverse events between placebo and any of the compared drugs.[15] Ohrt and colleagues compared mefloquine and doxycycline in a randomized placebo-controlled field trial in non-immune soldiers in West Papua (Irian Jaya). In this trial, both drugs were well tolerated, but doxycycline was better tolerated than mefloquine or placebo, with respect to the frequency of reported symptoms.[16] Significantly lower rates of GI symptoms, anorexia, neurologic symptoms, dizziness, headache, and fever were reported in individuals randomized to doxycycline versus mefloquine. The authors attributed this to the potential of doxycycline to prevent other infectious processes. Anderson and colleagues compared doxycycline and azithromycin in a field trial in semi-immune adults in western Kenya.[17] Both drugs were well tolerated compared to placebo, but there was one case of doxycycline withdrawal due to recurrent vaginitis. There were no significant differences observed in adverse event profiles between the treatment arms, except that azithromycin was protective against dysentery. Photosensitivity reactions were not reported as significant complaints in any of the above studies.

Most recently, a randomized comparative trial of doxycycline versus atovaquone/proguanil was performed in Australian military personnel deployed in Oceania. There were no malaria breakthough infections in either arm of this trial. Both drugs were well tolerated; however, atovaquone/proguanil was significantly better tolerated, with less reported GI (29% vs. 53%) and dermatologic (8% vs. 16%) adverse events.[19]

Adherence with doxycycline, despite its daily dosing schedule, has been reported to be relatively good in studies examining short-term use.[12,13,16,17] Estimating adherence rates in travelers is difficult because such studies require close daily monitoring. Ohrt and colleagues extended their initial comparative study of doxycycline and mefloquine but did not enforce adherence as they did in the first phase of the study.[16] This resulted in a drop in the protective efficacy of doxycycline from 99% (95% CI: 94% to 100%) to 89% (95% CI: 78% to 96%) against all malaria, suggesting a decrease in drug adherence if close monitoring is not done. Similar experience of declining effectiveness over time due to adherence issues has been reported by the U.S. military deployed in Somalia and in Dutch troops deployed in Cambodia.[23,26] U.S. troops in Somalia using doxycycline had fivefold higher attack rates by *Plasmodium falciparum* than did mefloquine users. These differences were attributed to poor adherence with daily doxycycline rather than to doxycycline resistance.[23] Collectively, these studies suggest that maintaining adherence with daily doxycycline may be challenging, especially for long-term travelers.

CONTRAINDICATIONS, PRECAUTIONS, AND DRUG INTERACTIONS

Doxycycline administration is not recommended in the following patients or conditions:[1,2,9,10]

1. Allergy or hypersensitivity to doxycycline or any member of the tetracycline class.
2. Infants and children under 8 years of age. Tetracyclines bind calcium and may cause permanent yellow-brown discoloration of teeth, damage to tooth enamel, and impairment of skeletal bone growth in this population. Doxycycline binds calcium less than other tetracyclines, and short courses of doxycycline (such as in the treatment of Rocky Mountain spotted fever) have not been reported to cause clinically significant staining of teeth.[27]
3. Pregnancy. Doxycycline crosses the placenta and therefore may cause permanent discoloration of teeth, damage to tooth enamel, and impairment of skeletal growth in the fetus.
4. Breastfeeding. Doxycycline is excreted in breast milk and therefore may cause permanent discoloration of teeth, damage to tooth enamel, impairment of skeletal growth, photosensitivity reactions, and thrush or vaginal candidiasis in breastfed infants.

Precautions should be taken when using doxycycline in individuals who are susceptible to photosensitivity reactions or who have vaginal yeast infections or thrush. In addition, certain susceptible individuals with asthma may experience an allergic-type reaction to sulfite, which is formed with the oxidation of doxycycline calcium oral suspension. Doxycycline is partially metabolized by the liver; in individuals with significant hepatic dysfunction, there may be a prolonged half-life, and a dose adjustment may be required.[1,2]

The safety of long-term use of doxycycline (> 3 months) has not been adequately studied.[24] Because lower doses of doxycycline and minocycline (a related tetracycline) are frequently used for extended periods to treat acne, it has been presumed that long-term use of doxycycline at an adult dose of 100 mg per day is safe. However, serious adverse events, including autoimmune hepatitis, fulminant hepatic failure, a serum-sickness-like illness, and drug-induced lupus erythematosus, have recently been reported with the use of minocycline for acne.[28] It is not known whether doxycycline causes similar adverse events.

A number of potentially important drug interactions have been associated with doxycycline use,[1,2] including those involving the following drugs and substances:

1. Antacids containing divalent or trivalent cations (calcium, aluminium, and magnesium). Doxycycline binds cations, and concomitant administration of antacids will decrease serum levels of doxycycline.
2. Oral iron, bismuth salts, calcium, cholestyramine or colestipol, and laxatives that contain magnesium. Concomitant ingestion of these compounds may decrease doxycycline absorption. The above agents should not be taken within 1 to 3 hours of doxycycline ingestion.
3. Barbiturates, phenytoin, and carbamazepine. These drugs induce hepatic microsomal enzyme activity and, if used concurrently with doxycycline, may decrease doxycycline serum levels and half-life and may necessitate a dosage adjustment.
4. Oral contraceptives. Concurrent use of doxycycline with estrogen-containing birth control pills may result in decreased contraceptive efficacy; generally, an additional method of birth control is advised. However, there are few examples of oral contraceptive failure attributable to doxycycline use, and serum hormone levels in patients taking oral contraceptives were reported to be unaffected by coadministration of doxycycline.[29]
5. Warfarin. By an unknown mechanism, the anticoagulant activity of warfarin compounds may be enhanced with concurrent use of doxycycline. Close monitoring of prothrombin time is advised if these drugs are used together.
6. Vitamin A. The use of tetracyclines with vitamin A has been reported to be associated with benign intracranial hypertension.[2]

INDICATIONS AND ADMINISTRATION

Doxycycline is currently recommended by the World Health Organization and the Centers for Disease Control and Prevention for the following uses:[9,10]

1. As the prophylactic agent of choice for those at risk for mefloquine-resistant *P. falciparum* malaria (evening or overnight exposure in rural border areas of Thailand with Myanmar [Burma] or Cambodia).

2. As an alternative to mefloquine or atovaquone/proguanil for the prevention of chloroquine-resistant *P. falciparum* malaria.
3. As an alternative to chloroquine for the prevention of chloroquine-sensitive *P. falciparum* malaria.

Doxycycline has a long half-life that permits once-daily dosing. The dosage of doxycycline recommended for chemoprophylaxis against drug-sensitive and drug-resistant malaria is 2 mg base/kg of body weight, up to 100 mg base daily.[9,10] Studies have examined lower-dose regimens, but such regimens have provided inadequate protective efficacy.[12,13] Doxycycline should be taken once daily, beginning 1 to 2 days before entering a malarious area, and should be continued while there. Because of its poor causal effect, it must be continued for 4 weeks after leaving the risk area. To decrease the occurrence of GI adverse events, it should be taken in an upright position with food and at least 100 mL of fluid. Doxycycline should not be taken within 1 to 3 hours of administering an oral antacid or iron.

REFERENCES

1. Joshi N, Miller DQ. Doxycycline revisited. Arch Intern Med 1997;157:1421–1426.
2. USP DI 2001. Drug information for the health professional. 1st ed. Vol. 1. Englewood, (CO): Micromedex, Inc., 2001. p. 2801–2812.
3. Colwell EJ, Hickman RL, Intraspert R, Tirabutana C. Minocycline and tetracycline treatment of acute falciparum in Thailand. Am J Trop Med Hyg 1972;21:144–149.
4. Colwell EJ, Hickman RL, Kosakal S. Tetracycline treatment of chloroquine-resistant falciparum malaria in Thailand. JAMA 1972;220:684–686.
5. Colwell EJ, Hickman RL. Quinine-tetracycline and quinine-bactrim treatment of acute falciparum malaria in Thailand. Ann Trop Med Parasitol 1973;67:125–132.
6. Clyde DE, Miller RM, DuPont HL, Hornick RB. Antimalarial effects of tetracycline in man. Am J Trop Med Hyg 1971;74:238–242.
7. Shmuklarsky MJ, Boudreau EF, Pang LW, et al. Failure of doxycycline as a causal prophylactic against *Plasmodium falciparum* malaria in healthy nonimmune volunteers. Ann Intern Med 1994;120:294–299.
8. Shanks DG, Barnett A, Edstein MD, Rieckmann KH. Effectiveness of doxycycline combined with primaquine for malaria prophylaxis. Med J Aust 1995;162:306–310.
9. Centers for Disease Control and Prevention. Health information for international travel—1999–2000. Atlanta (GA): Department of Health and Human Services, 1999.
10. World Health Organisation (WHO). International travel and health. Vaccination requirements and health advice 2000. Geneva, Switzerland: WHO, 2000.
11. Pang LW, Limsomwong N, Boudreau EF, Singharaj P. Doxycycline prophylaxis for falciparum malaria. Lancet 1987;1:1161–1164.
12. Pang LW, Limsomwong N, Singharaj P. Prophylactic treatment of vivax and falciparum malaria with low-dose doxycycline. J Infect Dis 1988;158:1124–1127.
13. Watanasook C, Singharaj P, Suriyamongkol V, et al. Malaria prophylaxis with doxycycline in soldiers deployed to the Thai-Kampuchean border. Southeast Asian J Trop Med Public Health 1989;20:61–64.

14. Baudon D, Martet G, Pascal B, et al. Efficacy of daily antimalarial chemoprophylaxis in tropical Africa using either doxycycline or chloroquine-proguanil; a study conducted in 1996 in the French Army. Trans R Soc Trop Med Hyg 1999;93:302–303.

15. Weiss WR, Oloo AJ, Johnson A, et al. Daily primaquine is effective for prophylaxis against falciparum malaria in Kenya: comparison with mefloquine, doxycycline, and chloroquine/proguanil. J Infect Dis 1995;171:1569–1575.

16. Ohrt C, Ritchie Tl, Widjaja H, et al. Mefloquine compared with doxycycline for the prophylaxis of malaria in Indonesian soldiers. Ann Intern Med 1997;126:963–972.

17. Anderson SL, Oloo AJ, Gordon DM, et al. Successful double-blinded, randomized, placebo-controlled field trial of azithromycin and doxycycline as prophylaxis for malaria in western Kenya. Clin Infect Dis 1998;26:146–150.

18. Taylor WRJ, Richie TL, Fryauff DJ, et al. Malaria prophylaxis using azithromycin: a double-blind, placebo controlled trial in Irian Jaya, Indonesia. Clin Infect Dis 1999;28:74–81.

19. Nasveld PE, Edstein MD, Kitchener SJ, Rieckmann KH. Comparison of the effectiveness of atovaquone/proguanil combination and doxycycline in the chemoprophylaxis of malaria in Australian Defense Force personnel. In: Program and abstracts of the 49th Annual Meeting of the American Society of Tropical Medicine and Hygiene; Houston, TX, 2000;62(3):139.

20. Watt G, Kantipong P, Jongsakul K, et al. Doxycycline and rifampicin for mild scrub-typhus infections in northern Thailand; a randomized trial. Lancet 2000; 356:1057–1061.

21. Arthur JD, Echeverria P, Shanks GD, et al. A comparative study of gastrointestinal infections in United States soldiers receiving doxycycline or mefloquine for malaria prophylaxis. Am J Trop Med Hyg 1990;43:606–618.

22. Adverse Drug Reactions Advisory Committee. Doxycycline-induced esophageal ulceration. Med J Aust 1994;161:490.

23. Wallace MR, Sharp TW, Smoak B, et al. Malaria among United States troops in Somalia. Am J Med 1996;100:49–55.

24. Schuhwerk M, Behrens RH. Doxycycline as first line malarial prophylaxis: how safe is it? J Travel Med 1998;5:102.

25. Westermann GW, Bohm M, Bonsmann G, et al. Chronic intoxication by doxycycline use for more than 12 years. J Intern Med 1999;246:591–592.

26. Hopperus Buma AP, van Thiel PP, Lobel HO, et al. Long-term prophylaxis with mefloquine in Dutch marines in Cambodia. J Infect Dis 1996;173:1506–1509.

27. Lochary ME, Lockhart PB, Williams WT. Doxycycline and staining of permanent teeth. Pediatr Infect Dis J 1998;17:429–431.

28. Gottlieb A. Safety of minocycline for acne. Lancet 1997;349:374.

29. Neeley JL, Abate M, Swinker M, D'Angio R. The effect of doxycycline on serum levels of ethinyl estradiol, norethindrone, and endogenous progesterone. Obstet Gynecol 1991;77:416–420.

8.5 Primaquine
Eli Schwartz

ABSTRACT

The arsenal of malaria chemoprophylaxis for travelers is very limited and has had serious disadvantages such as resistant malaria strains, adverse effects, and resultant reduced compliance. In the search for new solutions for malaria prophylaxis, primaquine was rediscovered.

Introduced in the early 1950s primaquine was found to be active against the early liver stages of both *Plasmodium falciparum* and *Plasmodium vivax* malaria. Although it is suitable as a causal prophylaxis for these strains, its use was abandoned. Since 1995, it has been reassessed in several studies conducted with both immune and nonimmune populations residing in endemic areas and was found to be highly effective for both *Plasmodium falciparum* and *Plasmodium vivax* malaria. It was also assessed among travelers to highly endemic areas, with similar results. Since it is active against the liver stage of malaria infection, there is no need to continue dosage for 4 weeks after exposure, which enhances compliance.

In all studies, primaquine was found to be very well tolerated. It is contraindicated for people with glucose-6-phosphate dehydrogenase (G6PD) deficiency and for pregnant women.

In conclusion, primaquine has been found to be a highly efficacious prophylactic drug for all types of malaria. Among the limited number of people who have used it, it seems to be very well tolerated in a dosage of up to 30 mg per day.

Key words: causal prophylaxis; *Plasmodium falciparum*; *Plasmodium vivax*; primaquine; prophylaxis.

INTRODUCTION

The current arsenal of drugs for malaria prophylaxis is limited. Moreover, the available drugs have serious disadvantages, such as inefficacy with drug-resistant malaria strains, intolerable adverse effects, contraindication during pregnancy, or prohibition for pediatric use. There is an urgent need to discover and develop more effective drugs to combat this widespread disease. But alongside new developments, there is value in re-examining an existing drug: primaquine, developed in the 1940s and since abandoned, is now making a comeback.

HISTORIC BACKGROUND

Primaquine is an 8-aminoquinoline. The first such compound to be synthesized was pamaquine, followed by primaquine, which was first synthesized during World War II. Primaquine was widely used as a curative agent for vivax malaria during the Korean War[1,2] and is still used for the radical cure of the malaria caused by species that have a liver hypnozoite stage, namely, *Plasmodium vivax* and *Plasmodium ovale.*

Early studies showed that primaquine is effective against infections of both *Plasmodium vivax* and *Plasmodium falciparum* in their early liver stage. In a study conducted in 1954, healthy "volunteers" (inmates of Illinois State Penitentiary) were inoculated with malaria. The study demonstrated that primaquine at a daily dose of 30 mg had a very powerful effect on the liver stage during the incubation period of vivax malaria and prevented blood-stage infection whereas primaquine given on the same day as sporozoite inoculation or after 5 days of liver-stage development was not effective.[3] Similar results were found with *P. falciparum* infections.[4] In vitro and animal studies supported the observation that primaquine was active against malaria parasites in the liver before they matured to invade the blood and cause disease.[5–7]

Primaquine has been found to be active also against the asexual blood forms but only at dangerously high doses, which does not allow its use for the treatment of acute malaria.[4]

Despite primaquine's effectiveness against the early liver stages of the parasite, it never gained widespread use as chemoprophylaxis. This was probably due to two principal reasons. The first was the reporting of severe adverse effects, including methemoglobinemia[8,9] and severe hemolytic reactions occurring only in glucose-6-phosphate dehydrogenase (G6PD)-deficient patients.[10,11] The second reason was probably the introduction of a new drug, chloroquine, which was relatively safe and highly potent. However, chloroquine-resistant strains of *Plasmodium falciparum* evolved in the early 1960s and spread rapidly to all endemic regions. Recently, chloroquine-resistant *Plasmodium vivax* strains have also made an appearance.[12]

As it was the only drug that acted against the liver hypnozoites, primaquine was not totally abandoned, and it continued to serve as the drug for radical cure of relapsing vivax and ovale malarias.[13]

CHEMISTRY AND PHARMACOKINETICS

Primaquine's structure is 6-methoxy-8-(4'-amino-1'-methylbutylamino) quinoline (Figure 8.5–1). Its action is to inhibit the mitochondrial respiration of the parasite in the primary and secondary (hypnozoite) liver stages, as well as in the gametocytes.[14]

A study done with Thai volunteers showed that after a single oral dose of 15 mg of primaquine, the peak level (mean = 65 ng/L) was reached after 2 hours (± 1 hour) and that the elimination half-life was 4.4 hours (± 1.4 hours). After chronic dosing with primaquine (15 mg daily for 14 days), no appreciable change in these parameters was seen.[15] These results are similar in kinetics to those that had been obtained in a study of Caucasian men.[16]

In a number of limited pharmacokinetic studies, primaquine was found to be rapidly absorbed from the gastrointestinal tract and rapidly excreted. Primaquine metabolizes into a carboxylic acid derivative that achieves high plasma concentrations after a single dose (mean = 730 [± 230] ng/mL; peak after 8 hours) and that accumulates with chronic administration (mean = 1,240 [± 560] ng/mL after 14 days). The elimination half-life of this metabolite is 24 to 30 hours.[15]

RE-INTRODUCTION AS A PROPHYLACTIC DRUG

In recent years, mefloquine has been the recommended antimalarial agent in areas with chloroquine-resistant strains. However, due to its adverse effects (mainly on the central nervous system), there is a hesitancy in using it as prophylaxis, and compliance to the drug appears to be low.[16–18] In addition, mefloquine-resistant strains of malaria are spreading alarmingly.[19] All of these factors are causing a search for alternatives.

The first study of primaquine as prophylaxis was conducted in Kenya, a hyperendemic area known to have a 90% incidence of new cases of falciparum malaria and with an estimate of nearly one infective mosquito bite per person per night.[20] Researchers entered 169 children (9 to 14 years of age) into a randomized study, with daily administration of either primaquine (15 mg daily [n = 32]), mefloquine, doxycycline, or chloroquine/proguanil. The participants were first treated with quinine and doxycycline daily for 7 days to clear their parasitemia. They were then given one of the prophylactic agents at the recommended doses for 11 weeks. A control group received vitamins daily. The efficacy at the end of a 3-week follow-up was 85% for primaquine, 84% for doxycycline, 77% for mefloquine, and 54% for chloroquine/proguanil. A major drawback to applying the results of this study to travelers is the fact that the study population was immune whereas travelers usually come from nonimmune populations.

Another study, published in the same year, was conducted in Irian Jaya (northeast Indonesia), an area endemic for both *Plasmodium falciparum* and *Plasmodium vivax* malaria, with a population of transmigrants who had relocated from a different part of Indonesia and who were most likely nonimmune. The study was completed by 121 Javanese males over 15 years of age, who were given doxycycline daily for 10 days, quinine daily for 4 days, and 0.5 mg/kg of primaquine base once a day for 14 days prior to the study treatment. After the radical-cure regimen, they were randomly assigned to either 0.5 mg/kg of primaquine (n = 43), placebo once a day, or 300 mg of chloroquine base once a week (the standard care for this area).

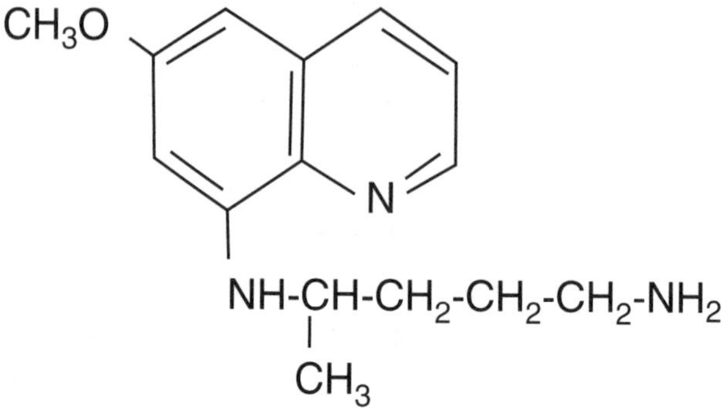

CH$_3$O

NH-CH-CH$_2$-CH$_2$-CH$_2$-NH$_2$

CH$_3$

Figure 8.5–1. Structure of primaquine.

After 52 weeks, efficacy against *Plasmodium falciparum* relative to placebo was 94.5% for primaquine and 33.0% for chloroquine, and efficacy against *Plasmodium vivax* was 90.4% for primaquine and 16.5% for chloroquine.[21]

A similar study was conducted in 1997 with Colombian soldiers (176 soldiers) who were on a mission in an area endemic to malaria.[22] They were given 15 mg of primaquine base twice a day (n = 122) or placebo for 15 weeks in the endemic area and for 1 week afterward. During administration and three weeks of follow-up, all cases of parasitemia were recorded. In the primaquine group, the protective efficacy was 88% against all types of malaria, 94% against *Plasmodium falciparum*, and 85% against *Plasmodium vivax* (Table 8.5–1). In a further study, in which chloroquine was added to primaquine, the results were not significantly different.[23]

Another recent study, again with transmigrants to Irian Jaya, showed similar results. Participants received 20 weeks of primaquine (n = 97) or placebo. Primaquine showed an overall protective efficacy of 93%, with 94% protective efficacy against *Plasmodium vivax* and 88% against *Plasmodium falciparum*.[24]

PROPHYLAXIS IN TRAVELERS

To date, there has been only one site testing primaquine in nonimmune travelers. The study population consisted of groups of Israeli rafters who traveled for a short period of time to the region of the Omo River, a highly endemic area in southern Ethiopia. The first groups experienced a 50% infection rate of vivax malaria despite mefloquine taken as prophylaxis; the onset was almost exactly 3 months after the group's return from the endemic area.[25] When deliberating what course to recommend to travelers on subsequent trips, the study's authors considered two options. The first was a full course of mefloquine followed by 2 weeks of primaquine (terminal prophylaxis); however, such a regimen would not be accepted by the travelers, and compliance would be low. The second possibility, which was recommended

Table 8.5–1. Summary of Studies of Primaquine for Malaria Prophylaxis

Lead Author	Site; Population	Subjects taking Primaquine	Efficacy (%)		Withdrawls from Study	Reference
			P. falciparum	P. vivax		
Weiss	Kenya; children	32	85	NA	0	20
Fryauff	Indonesia; transmigrants	43	95	90	0	21
Soto	Colombia; soldiers	122	94	85	3	22
Baird	Indonesia; transmigrants	97	88	94	0	24
Schwartz	Israel; travelers	106	NA	NA	1	26
Schwartz	Israel; travelers	110	NA	NA	0	27

NA = not assessed; *P. = Plasmodium.*

at the authors' travel clinic, was to use primaquine alone, on the basis that it had been proven to be effective against the early liver stages of both *Plasmodium falciparum* and *Plasmodium vivax*. The advantage of primaquine was that it could be used as causal prophylaxis due to its action against the liver stage of the parasites and that there would be no need for travelers to continue taking the drug for 1 month after leaving the malarious area.

An observational study followed those travelers, each of whom took antimalarial prophylaxis according to the recommendation of the medical center to which he or she went for pretravel consultation. This author's center was the only center that recommended primaquine as prophylaxis, at a dose of 15 mg of base daily for persons up to 70 kg in weight and 30 mg of base daily for persons over 70 kg in weight. Altogether, 158 travelers were studied, participating in 11 rafting trips. Among primaquine users, there was a 5.7% incidence of infection versus a 52% incidence of infection in travelers using other antimalarial prophylactic drugs (mefloquine, doxycycline, and chloroquine).[26]

Since then, more travelers have preferred to use primaquine when traveling to this area. To November 1999, the author has data on 216 travelers who used primaquine: 14 (6.5%) contracted malaria, 8 cases of which were from *Plasmodium falciparum*, 5 from *Plasmodium vivax*, and 1 from mixed infection. Follow-up of over 1 year revealed no cases of relapse or late infection. Only 1 (0.04%) traveler stopped taking primaquine (due to gastrointestinal upset).[27]

According to this study, primaquine gives the best results in areas where *Plasmodium falciparum* and *Plasmodium vivax* cocirculate.

The results of these studies[26,27] are somewhat different from those of studies done elsewhere, in that there were more cases of failure with *Plasmodium falciparum* whereas in other studies, primaquine was more efficacious against *Plasmodium falciparum* than against *Plasmodium vivax* (see Table 8.5–1). This may have been due to a reluctance to use higher doses of primaquine; an average dose of 0.25 mg/kg body weight was used as compared to 0.5 mg/kg body weight in most other studies. The author's center has recently started recommending a higher dose.

One advantage of our studies is that the travelers can be followed-up for a long period of time; thus, late infections (that would not be detected in studies that follow the cohort for only several weeks after the end of the study) can also be detected. For example, had the rafters been followed for only 1 month after their return from Ethiopia, a 100% protection rate for mefloquine prophylaxis would have been found; however, after 1 year, a failure of 50% occurred.[26]

TOLERABILITY

The most common adverse effects of primaquine are gastrointestinal effects that are dose dependent. In studies done during the early 1950s, it was found that doses of up to 30 mg/day were associated with minimal gastrointestinal upset; only doses of 45 mg/day or higher are associated with a significant rate of adverse effects.[1,4]

Recent studies also have shown minimal adverse effects. In the Colombian study,[22] two subjects (2%) who were taking an active drug withdrew from the study because of gastrointestinal complaints. In the Indonesian study,[24] primaquine was taken daily for 1 year with no withdrawals from significant adverse events. Complaints were similar in the placebo and drug groups.

In the author's study,[26] primaquine was well tolerated. There was only one case of withdrawal, which was due to nausea and vomiting (a rate of 1 per approximately 200 cases) (see Table 8.5–1).

TOXICITY

Primaquine can produce methemoglobinemia in normal individuals, but the effect is marked in people with congenital deficiency of the reduced form of nicotinamide adenine dinucleotide (NADH) methemoglobin reductase.[9]

Marked hemolysis occurs when the drug is administered daily to individuals with G6PD deficiency; therefore, testing for G6PD before treatment is recommended.

DOSAGE AND RECOMMENDATION

Since primaquine is a drug that acts on the liver stage of the malaria parasite, there is no need to continue taking it for 1 month after departure from the malarious area (as with most of the other antimalarial drugs that act on the erythrocyte stage of the malaria parasite). Therefore, the policy of the author's center is to have the traveler start taking it 1 day prior to entering the malarious area and to continue taking it for only 1 week after departure. Due to the short half-life of primaquine, it must be taken daily, preferably with food to avoid gastrointestinal upset. The doses used by the author's center are 15 mg (1 tablet) per day for people < 60 kg in weight and 30 mg (2 tablets) per day for people ≥ 60 kg in weight. Primaquine was recently listed in Canada as an option for malaria prophylaxis; the dose recommended there is 30 mg/day, to be taken up to 1 week after departure from the malarious area.[28]

The pediatric dose is 0.5 mg/kg/day. Due mainly to the fear of G6PD deficiency in the fetus, primaquine is not recommended for use by pregnant women.

Recently, a new compound—tafenoquine—that is similar to primaquine was synthesized. Its mode of action and toxicity, including its G6PD sensitivity, are similar to those of primaquine. Due to its very long half-life, however, it may be taken once a month, a fact that may increase compliance (it can be taken once before a trip of less than 1 month). More details about tafenoquine can be found in Chapter 8.7.

CONCLUSION

Primaquine is an effective drug against the liver stages of *Plasmodium falciparum* and *Plasmodium vivax* and is thus highly suitable for malaria prophylaxis. Its advantage is its ability to prevent early and late infection. Due to its mode of action, there is no need to continue taking it for 1 month after exposure, a fact that increases compliance. It seems to be very well tolerated although not enough trials have been conducted. It is contraindicated for G6PD-deficient people and during pregnancy.

Primaquine should be the prototype drug for the future development of malaria chemoprophylaxis.

REFERENCES

1. Alving AS, Arnold J, Robinson DH. Status of primaquine. JAMA 1952;149:1558–1562.
2. Garrison PL, Coker WG, Jastremsili B, et al. Status of primaquine: cure of Korean vivax malaria with pamaquine and primaquine: report to Council on Pharmacy and Chemistry. JAMA 1952;148:1562.
3. Arnold J, Alving AS, Hockwald RS, et al. The effect of continuous and intermittent primaquine therapy on the relapse rate of chesson strain vivax malaria. J Lab Clin Med 1954;44:429–438.
4. Arnold J, Alving AS, Hockwald RS, et al. The antimalarial action of primaquine against the blood and tissue stages of falciparum malaria (Panama, P-F-6 strain). J Lab Clin Med 1955;46:391–397.
5. Hollingdale MR. In vitro testing of antimalarial tissue schizonticides. In: Wernsdorfer WH, Trigg PI, editors. Primaquine. New York: John Wiley & Sons, 1984.
6. Puri SK, Dutta GP. Differential sensitivity of the pre-erythrocytic stages of *Plasmodium cynomolgi B* to the prophylactic action of primaquine. Trop Med Parasitol 1992;43:70–71.
7. Shoa B, Ye X. Tissue schizonticidal effect of trifluoroacetyl primaquine in *Plasmodium yoelli* infected mice and *Plasmodium cynomolgi* infected monkeys. Southeast Asian J Trop Med Public Health 1991;22:81–83.

8. Clayman CB, Arnold J, Hockwald RS, et al. Toxicity of primaquine in caucasians. JAMA 1952;149;1563–1568.

9. Cohen RJ, Sachs JR, Wicker DJ, Conrad ME. Methemoglobinemia provoked by malarial chemoprophylaxis in Vietnam. N Engl J Med 1968;279:1127–1131.

10. Georg JN, Sears DA, McCurdy PR, et al. Primaquine sensitivity in caucasians: hemolytic reactions induced by primaquine in G-6-PD deficient subjects. J Lab Clin Med 1967;70:80–93.

11. Clyde DF. Clinical problems associated with the use of primaquine as a tissue schizonticidal and gametocytocidal drug. Bull World Health Organ 1981;59:391–395.

12. Murphy GS, Basri H, Purnomo, et al. Vivax malaria resistant to treatment and prophylaxis with choloroquine. Lancet 1993;341:96–100.

13. Wyler DJ. Malaria chemoprophylaxis for the traveler. N Engl J Med 1993;329:31–37.

14. Bruce-Chwatt LJ. Essential malariology. London: William Heinemann, Ltd., 1980.

15. Ward SA, Mihaly GW, Edwards G, et al. Pharmacokinetics of primaquine in man. II. Comparison of acute vs. chronic dosage in Thai subjects. Br J Clin Pharmacol 1985;19:751–755.

16. Cook GC. Malaria prophylaxis: mefloquine toxicity should limit its use to teatment alone. BMJ 1995;311:190–191.

17. Van Tiemsdijk MM, Van der Klauw MM, Van Heest JAC, et al. Neuropsychiatric effects of antimalarials. Eur J Clin Pharmacol 1997;52:1–6.

18. Croft A, Garner P. Mefloquine to prevent malaria: a systematic review of trials. BMJ 1997;315:1412–1416.

19. Nosten F, ter Kuile F, Chongsuphajaisiddhi T, et al. Mefloquine-resistant falciparum malaria on the Thai-Burmese border. Lancet 1991;337:1140–1142.

20. Weiss WR, Oloo AJ, Johnson A, et al. Daily primaquine is effective for prophylaxis against falciparum malaria in Kenya: comparison with mefloquine, doxycycline, and chloroquine plus proguanil. J Infect Dis 1995;171:1569–1575.

21. Fryauff DJ, Baird JK, Basri H, et al. Randomised placebo-controlled trial of primaquine for prophylaxis of falciparum and vivax malaria. Lancet 1995;346:1190–1193.

22. Soto J, Toledo J, Rodriguez M, et al. Primaquine prophylaxis against malaria in nonimmune Colombian soldiers: efficacy and toxicity. Ann Intern Med 1998;129:241–244.

23. Soto J, Toledo J, Rodriguez M, et al. Primaquine prophylaxis against malaria in nonimmune Colombian soldiers. Clin Infect Dis 1999;29:199–201.

24. Baird JK, et al. Randomized pivotal trial of primaquine for prophylaxis against malaria in Javanese adults in Papua, Indonesia. Proceeding of the 49th Annual Meeting of the American Society of Tropical Medicine and Hygiene; 2000 Oct; Houston.

25. Schwartz E, Sidi Y. New aspects of malaria imported from Ethiopia. Clin Infect Dis 1998;26:1089–1091.

26. Schwartz E, Regev-Yochay G. Primaquine as prophylaxis for malaria for nonimmune travelers: a comparison with mefloquine and doxycycline. Clin Infect Dis 1999;29:1502–1506.

27. Schwartz E. New approach to malaria prophylaxis. The 48th Annual Meeting of the American Society of Tropical Medicine andHygiene; 1999 Nov; Washington, D.C.

28. Canadian recommendations for the prevention and treatment of malaria among international travelers. Can Commun Dis Rep 2000;26 Suppl 2:1–42.

8.6 Atovaquone/Proguanil
G. Dennis Shanks

ABSTRACT

The spread of drug-resistant malaria and the appreciation of side effects associated with existing antimalarial drugs emphasize the need for new drugs to prevent malaria. The combination of atovaquone and proguanil hydrochloride was previously shown to be safe and highly effective for the treatment of malaria, including multidrug-resistant *Plasmodium falciparum*. The prophylaxis regimen is 250 mg of atovaquone and 100 mg of proguanil hydrochloride (or an equivalent dose based on body weight in children), once daily. Field trials for malaria efficacy that used a fixed-dose combination of atovaquone and proguanil hydrochloride (Malarone) showed that in four placebo-controlled trials involving 417 subjects, the overall efficacy was 97%. Results of volunteer challenge studies indicate that both atovaquone and proguanil have causal prophylactic activity directed against the liver stages of *P. falciparum*, allowing the discontinuation of atovaquone/proguanil 1 week after leaving the malarious area. Atovaquone/proguanil is not effective against latent stages of relapsing malaria. Adverse events occurred with similar or lower frequencies in subjects treated with atovaquone/proguanil compared to placebo. Malarone was either superior to or as good as either weekly mefloquine or daily proguanil/chloroquine in safety and tolerance studies done in nonimmune Western travelers. One percent or less of patients discontinued participation in these safety studies because of a prophylaxis-related adverse event. Malarone is a promising new alternative for malaria prophylaxis in travelers to malaria-endemic areas.

Key words: atovaquone; malaria; Malarone; proguanil; prophylaxis; travel medicine.

Atovaquone/proguanil is a new antimalarial combination of atovaquone, which is also active against *Pneumocystis carinii*, and proguanil, which has been used as an antimalarial drug since the 1940s. Atovaquone is a hydroxynaphthoquinone with a novel mechanism of action (via inhibition of mitochondrial electron transport) and potent activity against *Plasmodium* spp.[1,2] Proguanil is metabolized to cycloguanil, which is a potent inhibitor of parasite dihydrofolate reductase.[3] Proguanil per se also has weak antimalarial activity.[4] Both proguanil and cycloguanil are synergistic with atovaquone against *Plasmodium falciparum* in vitro.[5] In more than 500 patients with acute falciparum malaria, the combination of atovaquone and proguanil hydrochloride was shown to be safe and highly effective for treatment of *P. falciparum* malaria, including multidrug-resistant strains.[6–14] Results in smaller numbers of patients indicate that atovaquone/proguanil is also effective for the treatment of *Plasmodium malariae* infections and erythrocytic stages of malaria caused by *Plasmodium vivax* or *Plasmodium ovale*.[15,16]

Atovaquone/proguanil is also safe and effective for malaria prophylaxis.[17] It is available as a fixed-dose combination (Malarone) containing 250 mg of atovaquone and 100 mg of proguanil hydrochloride per tablet. A pediatric-strength tablet containing 62.5 mg of atovaquone and 25 mg of proguanil hydrochloride is also available in some countries. The dose is based on body weight (Table 8.6–1).

PHARMACOLOGY AND MODE OF ACTION

The pharmacology and mode of action of atovaquone and proguanil have been reviewed previously[18,19] and are summarized below.

Pharmacokinetics of Atovaquone

Atovaquone is a highly lipophilic compound with low aqueous solubility and poor oral bioavailability that varies with dose and diet. In the fasted state, absorption of atovaquone increases in proportion to dose following single oral doses of between 25 and 450 mg but less than proportionally following a dose of 750 mg. Dietary fat taken concomitantly with atovaquone tablets increases the rate and extent of absorption of atovaquone. In the fed state, atovaquone shows linear pharmacokinetic behavior at doses of up to 750 mg but less-than-proportional behavior for doses greater than 750 mg. The mean absolute bioavailability of a 750-mg tablet dose taken with food is 23%.

Atovaquone is highly protein bound (> 99%), but there is no displacement of other highly protein-bound drugs in vitro, indicating that significant drug interactions arising from the displacement of drugs from plasma proteins are unlikely. There is negligible metabolism of atovaquone in man, as demonstrated by carbon-14 (^{14}C)–atovaquone administration and in vitro studies with human liver cells.

Table 8.6–1. **Recommended Dosing Regimen for Malaria Prophylaxis with Atovaquone/Proguanil**

Body Weight (kg)	Atovaquone/Proguanil Total Daily Dose*	Dosage Regimen
11–20	62.5 mg/25.0 mg	1 Malarone Pediatric tablet daily
21–30	125 mg/50 mg	2 Malarone Pediatric tablets as a single dose daily
31–40	187.5 mg/75.0 mg	3 Malarone Pediatric tablets as a single dose daily
> 40	250 mg/100 mg	1 Malarone tablet (adult strength) daily

* Prophylaxis should start 1 to 2 days before entering a malaria-endemic area and should continue daily until 7 days after leaving the area.

The main route of elimination of atovaquone in humans is hepatic. Only parent compound is recovered in the feces, with negligible amounts (< 1%) eliminated in the urine. The elimination half-life of atovaquone is not dependent on dose, frequency, dietary status, or proguanil hydrochloride coadministration. Overall, the elimination half-life is approximately 2 to 3 days in adults and 1 to 2 days in children.

Pharmacokinetics of Proguanil and Cycloguanil

Proguanil is rapidly absorbed, with peak plasma concentrations occurring between 2 to 4 hours after 200-mg single doses and 1 to 6 hours after a 400-mg dose. The absolute bioavailability is not known but is likely to be as high as 60%. Single-dose proportionality was demonstrated over the range of 50 to 500 mg. The extent of absorption is comparable when proguanil is administered with or without food. Proguanil is 75% protein bound, and the binding in vitro is unaffected by therapeutic concentrations of atovaquone.

Proguanil is metabolized to cycloguanil and 4-chlorophenyl biguanide. Metabolism to cycloguanil is mediated in the liver by cytochromes P-450 3A4 and 2C19. The latter enzyme exhibits genetic polymorphism leading to a bimodal frequency distribution of proguanil/cycloguanil concentrations. Poor metabolizers achieve markedly lower cycloguanil and moderately higher proguanil plasma concentrations. They are more common in East Asian and black populations (18% to 25%) than in Caucasians (3%).[20] In clinical trials of atovaquone/proguanil for treatment and prophylaxis of malaria, treatment success rates were similar in extensive and poor metabolizers.[21]

Less than 40% of proguanil is eliminated via the urine, and the rest is eliminated by hepatic transformation, with excretion of up to 20% of the metabolites in the urine. The half-life of proguanil and cycloguanil in adults and children is 12 to 15 hours. The renal clearance rates of both proguanil and cycloguanil are greater than the glomerular filtration rates, indicating active renal secretion.

Pharmacokinetics of Atovaquone and Proguanil in Combination

In a randomized three-period crossover study, there were no effects of atovaquone on any proguanil or cycloguanil pharmacokinetic parameters, nor were there any effects of proguanil/cycloguanil on any atovaquone pharmacokinetic parameters. Table 8.6–2 presents pharmacokinetic parameters after treatment with atovaquone/proguanil in healthy Caucasian adult volunteers and Thai children with malaria. Table 8.6–3 presents plasma concentration data for African adults and children receiving atovaquone/proguanil for malaria prophylaxis.

Recently completed pharmacokinetic studies indicate that no dosage adjustment is needed in elderly subjects, subjects with mild to moderate hepatic impairment, or subjects with mild to moderate renal impairment.[21] In patients with

Table 8.6–2. **Pharmacokinetic Parameters after Administration of Atovaquone/Proguanil**

Age Group and Parameter	Atovaquone*		Proguanil*		Cycloguanil*	
Adults[†]						
C_{max} (μg/mL)	11.8	(20)	0.52	(22)	0.09	(53)
AUC (h·μg/mL)	541	(35)	6.16	(23)	1.34	(44)
$t_{1/2}$ (h)	60	(23)	14.7	(17)	12.6	(43)
CL/F (L/h/kg)	0.003	(46)	68.8	(32)	—	
Vz/F (L/kg)	2.8	(37)	23.2	(30)	—	
Children[‡]						
C_{max} (μg/mL)	2.8	(51)	0.31	(35)	0.04	(40)
AUC (h·μg/mL)	162	(78)	4.65	(26)	0.79	(51)
$t_{1/2}$ (h)	31.8	(28)	14.9	(22)	14.6	(18)
CL/F (L/h/kg)	0.16	(56)	1.60	(44)	—	
Vz/F (L/kg)	8.1	(79)	32.7	(27)	—	

C_{max} = maximum concentration; AUC = area under the concentration-time curve; $t_{1/2}$ = elimination half-life; CL/F = apparent oral clearance; Vz/F = apparent volume of distribution.
*Values are given as mean (% CV).
[†] 18 healthy adults given 1,000 mg atovaquone and 400 mg proguanil HCl.
[‡] 9 children treated with ~20 mg/kg atovaquone and ~8 mg/kg proguanil HCl.
Data from Shanks GD, Kremsner PG, Sukwa TY, et al. Atovaquone and proguanil hydrochloride for prophylaxis of malaria. J Travel Med 1999;6 Suppl 1:S21–S27.

severe renal impairment (creatinine clearance < 30 mL/min), atovaquone maximum concentration (C_{max}) and area under the concentration-time curve (AUC) are reduced. As atovaquone is eliminated almost exclusively by biliary excretion, the decrease in atovaquone AUC in subjects with severe renal impairment is unexpected and unexplained. In addition, subjects with severe renal impairment had significantly higher elimination half-lives for proguanil and cycloguanil, with corresponding increases in AUC, resulting in the potential for drug accumulation with repeated dosing.[21] This could lead to plasma cycloguanil concentrations above those for which safety data are available, and pancytopenia has been reported in

Table 8.6–3. **Trough Plasma Drug Concentrations in 100 Adults and 121 Children Receiving the Recommended Prophylaxis Dose of Atovaquone/Proguanil**

Subject	Atovaquone (mean μg/mL ± SD)	Proguanil (mean ng/mL ± SD)	Cycloguanil (mean ng/mL ± SD)
Children 11–20 kg	2.5 ± 1.3	13.1 ± 8.2	7.9 ± 3.1
Children 21–30 kg	3.3 ± 1.9	16.2 ± 7.9	8.1 ± 2.2
Children 31–40 kg	4.0 ± 2.0	23.2 ± 12.0	10.3 ± 6.1
Children > 40 kg	2.8 ± 1.7	21.7 ± 10.4	8.8 ± 2.6
Adults > 40 kg	2.1 ± 1.2	26.8 ± 14.0	10.9 ± 5.6

SD = standard deviation.
Data from Shanks GD, Kremsner PG, Sukwa TY, et al. Atovaquone and proguanil hydrochloride for prophylaxis of malaria. J Travel Med 1999;6 Suppl 1:S21–S27.

patients with renal failure who used proguanil for malaria prophylaxis.[22,23] There-fore, atovaquone/proguanil should not be used for malaria prophylaxis in patients with severe renal impairment.

Pharmacokinetic and Pharmacodynamic Aspects

In clinical trials, atovaquone, proguanil, and cycloguanil plasma concentrations showed wide interindividual variability. Given the small numbers of patients who failed treatment or prophylaxis with the recommended dose of atovaquone and proguanil hydrochloride, it was not possible to define a concentration-response relationship.

In a study in Kenya, 5 of 81 patients treated with atovaquone/proguanil had recurrent parasitemia within 28 days.[12] These patients achieved higher plasma concentrations of atovaquone, proguanil, and cycloguanil than many adult and pediatric patients in this and other studies who were cured of malaria. Many of the adults and children who were successfully treated had 8-hour concentrations of cycloguanil below the limit of quantification. Low production of cycloguanil, therefore, does not predict treatment failure.

Plasma drug concentration data were obtained in two Zambian subjects who failed prophylaxis.[24] Their plasma atovaquone concentrations were higher than many subjects who did not develop malaria, but their plasma concentrations of proguanil were lower than most subjects who did not develop malaria. This suggests that synergy between atovaquone and proguanil/cycloguanil is important for effective malaria prophylaxis and that low plasma proguanil concentrations may have contributed to the lack of efficacy in the subjects who developed parasitemia.

Mode of Action

Atovaquone (Figure 8.6–1) is a hydroxynaphthoquinone with potent antimalarial activity. In vitro, the inhibitory concentration 50% (IC_{50}) against asexual erythro-

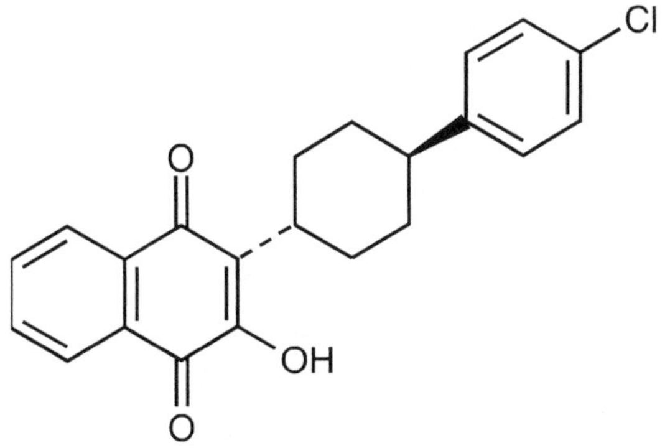

Figure 8.6–1. Chemical structure of atovaquone.

cytic stages of wild-type *Plasmodium falciparum* isolates ranges from 0.7 to 6.0 nM.[1,25,26] Atovaquone also has causal prophylactic activity against the pre-erythrocytic (hepatic) stages of *Plasmodium berghei*[27,28] and *Plasmodium falciparum*.[29]

The mechanism of action of atovaquone against *Plasmodium falciparum* is via the inhibition of mitochondrial electron transport.[2] Atovaquone has a novel mode of action, inhibiting the electron transport system at the level of the cytochrome b-c_1 complex. In malaria, there is an obligatory coupling of pyrimidine biosynthesis and electron transport, via ubiquinone/ubiquinol. Selectivity is achieved by virtue of the different sensitivities of the mammalian and *Plasmodium* electron transport systems to the hydroxynaphthoquinones (a 1,000-fold difference); thus, side effects are limited. Moreover, plasmodia are totally reliant on pyrimidine biosynthesis whereas mammalian cells are able to salvage pyrimidines. Atovaquone also causes collapse of the parasite mitochondrial membrane potential in *Plasmodium yoelii*[30] and *Plasmodium falciparum*.[31] Parasites highly resistant to atovaquone can be selected by exposure to sublethal concentrations of atovaquone in vitro[32,33] or by treatment of symptomatic *Plasmodium falciparum* infections with atovaquone alone.[7] Drug resistance is associated with point mutations in the cytochrome b gene.[33–35]

Proguanil is a biguanide that is metabolized to cycloguanil (Figure 8.6–2). Against asexual erythrocytic stages of *P. falciparum*, cycloguanil has potent activity (IC_{50}: 18 to 36 nM in standard culture medium[36] and 0.5 to 2.5 nM in a medium deficient in folic acid and *p*-aminobenzoic acid)[37] while proguanil (IC_{50}: 2.4 to 19.0 µM) has weak but measurable activity.[36] Proguanil is also active against the pre-erythrocytic (hepatic) stages of *Plasmodium berghei* in mice[38] and *Plasmodium falciparum* in man.[39] Cycloguanil is active against the hepatic stages of *Plasmodium yoelii* in vitro.[40]

The mechanism of action of proguanil, via its metabolite cycloguanil, is the inhibition of dihydrofolate reductase (DHFR). The affinity of malarial DHFR from

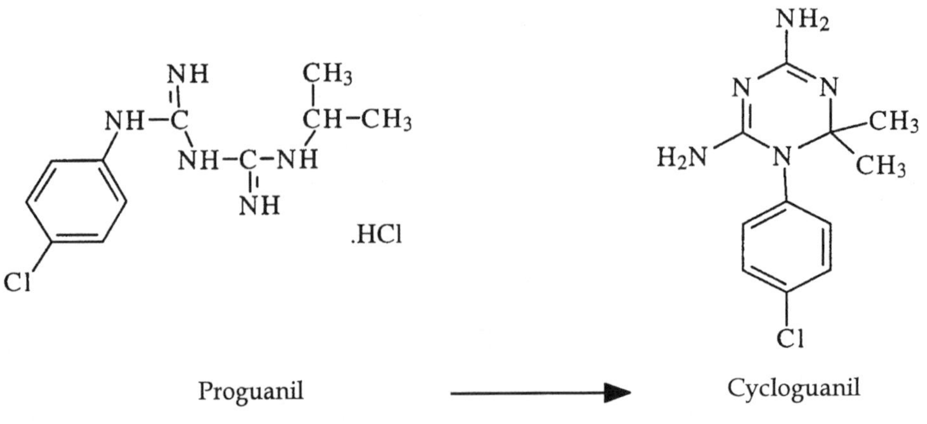

Proguanil ⟶ Cycloguanil

Figure 8.6–2. Chemical structure of proguanil and its metabolite, cycloguanil.

Plasmodium berghei is several hundred times stronger than erythrocyte DHFR, and plasmodia synthesize folate cofactors de novo and cannot use intact exogenous folates. Selective inhibition of parasite DHFR depletes tetrahydrofolate cofactors required for cellular metabolism, especially deoxyribonucleic acid (DNA) synthesis, and thus prevents growth.[41] Mutations in the DHFR gene are associated with resistance to proguanil/cycloguanil.[37]

Proguanil has antimalarial activity independent of its metabolism to cycloguanil. Cycloguanil-resistant parasites retain their sensitivity to high concentrations of proguanil.[36] *Plasmodium falciparum* transformed with a variant form of human DHFR selectable by methotrexate becomes resistant to cycloguanil with no change in the level of susceptibility to proguanil, thus providing direct evidence of intrinsic activity of proguanil against a target other than DHFR.[42] The additional mechanism of action of proguanil may involve mitochondrial toxicity, since proguanil (but not cycloguanil) is able to potentiate the ability of atovaquone to collapse mitochondrial membrane potential in *Plasmodium yoelii*.[31] The additional mechanism of action of proguanil probably explains the observation that both proguanil and cycloguanil are synergistic with atovaquone against the erythrocytic stages of *Plasmodium falciparum* in vitro.[5]

EFFICACY

The efficacy of atovaquone/proguanil has been demonstrated in three placebo-controlled studies in lifelong residents of endemic areas,[24,43,44] two placebo-controlled studies in nonimmune subjects,[45,46] and three active-controlled studies in nonimmune travelers or military personnel.[47–49] The causal prophylactic activity of atovaquone and proguanil separately have been demonstrated in volunteer challenge studies.[29,39] Efficacy studies have focused on malaria caused by *P. falciparum* because this is the commonest and most serious type of malaria and because drug resistance is the greatest problem, but recent data indicate that atovaquone/proguanil is also effective for the prophylaxis of malaria caused by *Plasmodium vivax*.[46]

Residents of Endemic Areas

Four randomized placebo-controlled clinical trials evaluated the prophylactic activity of the recommended dose of atovaquone/proguanil in subjects living in a malaria-endemic area.[24,43,44,46] Subjects were excluded from these studies if they would normally receive prophylaxis for malaria. All four studies enrolled adults who weighed > 40 kg, and one study also enrolled children who weighed 11 to 40 kg.[44]

Because unrecognized parasitemia may occur in subjects living in an endemic area, a curative course of atovaquone/proguanil was given before starting chemoprophylaxis. For the study in Irian Jaya, where both *P. vivax* and *Plasmodium falciparum* are common, subjects were also treated with a 2-week course of primaquine before starting chemoprophylaxis, to eradicate hypnozoites. Chemoprophylaxis was continued for 10 weeks,[24,43] 12 weeks,[44] or 20 weeks.[46] Giemsa-stained thick blood films were evaluated for the presence of parasitemia weekly or whenever symptoms suggestive of malaria occurred.

In these four studies, the efficacy of atovaquone/proguanil for the prevention of *P. falciparum* malaria ranged from 95% to 100%. Overall efficacy was 98% in life-long residents,[17] who were considered to be semi-immune, and 96% in recent transmigrants to Irian Jaya, who were considered to be nonimmune.[46] The overall efficacy in the four studies combined was 97% (Table 8.6–4).

Volunteer Challenge Studies

Drugs used for malaria prophylaxis can work in two ways: by killing parasites as they differentiate and develop in the liver (referred to as tissue schizonticidal or causal prophylactic drugs) or by killing parasites as they differentiate and develop within erythrocytes (referred to as blood schizonticidal or suppressive prophylactic drugs).[50] Volunteer challenge studies are essential for distinguishing between these two sites of prophylactic activity.

Volunteer challenge studies in the 1940s demonstrated that proguanil has causal prophylactic activity against *P. falciparum*. Proguanil was not consistently effective for causal prophylaxis if therapy was stopped within 1 or 2 days after challenge but was consistently effective when continued for 6 days after challenge.[39,51]

More recently, atovaquone has also been shown to have causal prophylactic activity against *P. falciparum* in human volunteers.[29] Parasitemia developed in 4 of 4 placebo recipients bitten by sporozoite-infected mosquitoes and in 0 of 6 subjects who received a single 250-mg dose of atovaquone 1 day before challenge. On days 6 and 7 after challenge, when parasites would first be expected to appear in peripheral blood, plasma levels of atovaquone were below the minimum inhibitory levels

Table 8.6–4. **Efficacy of Atovaquone/Proguanil for Malaria Prophylaxis***

| Study Location | Subjects with Parasitemia and at Risk | | | |
	Placebo[†]	Atovaquone/Proguanil[†]	Efficacy (%)[‡]	Reference
Kenya	28/54	0/54	100	43
Zambia	41/111	2/102	95	24
Gabon	25/134	0/113	100	44
Irian Jaya	23/147	1/148	96	46
Total	117/446	3/417	97	—

* In placebo-controlled trials of *Plasmodium falciparum* malaria prophylaxis in endemic areas.
[†] Number of subjects with parasitemia/number of subjects at risk.
[‡] % efficacy = 100 × [1 − (proportion with parasitemia in atovaquone/proguanil group ÷ proportion with parasitemia in placebo group)].

for blood-stage parasites, and subpatent parasitemia could not be found with sensitive detection methods (culture and polymerase chain reaction [PCR]).

The efficacy of a causal prophylactic regimen of atovaquone/proguanil has recently been confirmed in a human volunteer challenge trial. Sixteen nonimmune subjects were randomized to receive 1 tablet of Malarone (n = 12) or placebo (n = 4) daily for 8 days, starting 1 day before and continuing for 7 days after being bitten by *P. falciparum*–infected mosquitoes. During the 8-week follow-up period, parasitemia developed in 4 of 4 placebo recipients and 0 of 12 Malarone recipients (efficacy, 100%). Sensitive PCR assays of blood samples obtained 7 and 8 days after challenge identified subpatent parasitemia in placebo recipients but not in Malarone recipients.[45]

Plasmodium falciparum Malaria in Nonimmune Visitors to Endemic Areas

Three randomized active-controlled clinical trials evaluated the prophylactic activity of the recommended dose of atovaquone/proguanil in subjects from a non-endemic area who were traveling to a malaria-endemic area for up to 4 weeks[47,48] or 8 weeks.[49] Two studies enrolled more than 2,000 nonimmune subjects at travel clinics in Europe, Canada, and South Africa,[47,48] and one study enrolled 150 Australian Defence Force personnel.[49] The active control in these studies was chloroquine/proguanil,[47] mefloquine,[48] or doxycycline.[49] Based on the evidence of the causal prophylactic activity of atovaquone and proguanil,[29,39] prophylaxis with atovaquone/proguanil was stopped 7 days after the subjects left the malaria-endemic area.

In these three studies, a total of 3 cases of falciparum malaria occurred (all in subjects receiving chloroquine/proguanil). There were no cases of falciparum malaria in the 1,089 subjects who received atovaquone/proguanil.

In two of these studies,[47,48] serum was obtained before and after travel and was tested for antibodies to *P. falciparum* sporozoites. There were 25 subjects who developed antisporozoite antibodies, including 12 who had received atovaquone/proguanil, which provides a minimum estimate of the number of subjects who were actually bitten by an infected mosquito and thus would be expected to develop malaria had they not been receiving effective prophylaxis.

Malaria Caused by Other *Plasmodium* spp

In the placebo-controlled study in nonimmune transmigrants to Irian Jaya, *Plasmodium vivax* parasitemia developed in 16 of 147 subjects receiving placebo and in 3 of 148 subjects receiving atovaquone/proguanil. Protective efficacy was 81% (95% CI: 45% to 94%, $p = .003$).[46]

In the study by Høgh and colleagues, one subject developed malaria caused by *Plasmodium ovale* 28 days after completing the standard course of prophylaxis with atovaquone/proguanil.[47] Although atovaquone and proguanil have causal prophylactic activity directed against developing hepatic forms of *Plasmodium falciparum*,[29,39] neither drug is active against hypnozoites.[16,39] Thus, atovaquone/proguanil, like chloroquine and mefloquine, is a suppressive prophylactic drug for *Plasmodium vivax* and *Plasmodium ovale*, and relapse can occur after dosing is discontinued and drug elimination occurs. Travelers with intense exposure to *Plasmodium vivax* or *Plasmodium ovale*, and those who develop malaria caused by either of these parasites, will require additional treatment with primaquine.[16]

In the study by Lell and colleagues, *Plasmodium malariae* and *Plasmodium ovale* parasitemia developed in one subject each in the placebo group and in no subjects in the atovaquone/proguanil group.[44]

TOLERABILITY

Safety Evaluations in Residents of Endemic Areas

In three clinical trials in endemic areas,[24,43,44] there were 331 subjects (206 adults and 125 children) who received the recommended dose of atovaquone/proguanil for malaria prophylaxis, 67 who received twice the recommended dose, and 346 who received placebo. During the 10- or 12-week study period, adverse events attributed to the study drug occurred with similar or lower frequency in subjects receiving atovaquone/proguanil compared to placebo (Table 8.6–5). In the Kenyan study, the frequencies of common drug-related adverse events were not higher in patients receiving twice the recommended dose of atovaquone/proguanil compared to placebo.[43] No subjects in any of these studies discontinued treatment prematurely due to a treatment-related adverse event. No treatment-related effects

Table 8.6–5. **Common Drug-Related Adverse Events during Prophylaxis with Atovaquone/Proguanil or Placebo for 10 to 12 Weeks**

	Adults (%)		Children (%)	
Adverse Event	Placebo (n = 206)	Atovaquone/ Proguanil (n = 206)	Placebo (n = 140)	Atovaquone/ Proguanil (n = 125)
Headache	7	3	14	14
Abdominal pain	5	4	29	31
Diarrhea	3	< 1	1	0
Dyspepsia	4	2	0	0
Gastritis	2	3	0	0
Vomiting	< 1	< 1	6	7

Data from Shanks GD, Kremsner PG, Sukwa TY, et al. Atovaquone and proguanil hydrochloride for prophylaxis of malaria. J Travel Med 1999;6 Suppl 1:S21–S27.

were evident in either children or adults for any of the hematology or clinical chemistry parameters measured.

In the placebo-controlled study in nonimmune transmigrants to Irian Jaya, there were no drug-related serious adverse events, and only one subject discontinued prophylaxis with atovaquone/proguanil due to a drug-related adverse event (rash).[46]

Safety Evaluations in Nonimmune Visitors to Endemic Areas

Three recent studies evaluated the safety and tolerance of antimalarial prophylaxis in nonimmune travelers or military personnel and compared atovaquone/proguanil with mefloquine,[48] chloroquine/proguanil,[47] or doxycycline.[49] In these studies, there were 976, 1,022, and 150 subjects, respectively, who received the randomized study drug. Each study was conducted as a "double-blind, double-dummy" study (i.e., subjects randomized to arm A received active drug A and placebo for drug B, and subjects randomized to arm B received active drug B and placebo for drug A).

In the study that used mefloquine as the comparator, the overall frequency of adverse events, regardless of attributability to study drug, was not significantly different between the two groups, but drug-related adverse events occurred more frequently in subjects receiving mefloquine (Table 8.6–6). Subjects receiving atovaquone/ proguanil had a significantly lower rate of drug-related neuropsychiatric adverse

Table 8.6–6. **Common Drug-Related Adverse Events during Prophylaxis with Atovaquone/Proguanil or Mefloquine in Nonimmune Travelers**

	% of Subjects	
Adverse Event	Atovaquone/Proguanil (n = 493)	Mefloquine (n = 483)
Any event	30	42***
Any neuropsychiatric event	14	29***
Strange/vivid dreams	7	14***
Insomnia	3	13***
Dizziness	2	9***
Visual difficulties	2	3
Anxiety	< 1	4**
Depression	<1	4**
Any gastrointestinal event	16	19
Diarrhea	8	7
Nausea	3	8***
Abdominal pain	5	5
Mouth ulcers	6	4
Vomiting	1	2
Headache	4	7*

*p < .05; **p < .01; ***p < .001.
Data from Overbosch D, Schilthuis H, Bienzle U, et al. Malarone compared with mefloquine for malaria prophylaxis in non-immune travellers. Oxford 2000—new challenges in tropical medicine and parasitology; 2000 Sept 18–22; Oxford, U.K. p. 146.

events, nausea, and headache, and a significantly lower rate of drug-related adverse events that caused discontinuation of prophylaxis (1% vs. 5%, $p = .001$).[48]

In the study that used chloroquine/proguanil as the comparator, the overall frequency of adverse events, regardless of attributability to study drug, was not significantly different between the two groups, but drug-related adverse events occurred more frequently in subjects receiving chloroquine/proguanil (Table 8.6–7). Subjects receiving atovaquone/proguanil had a significantly lower rate of drug-related gastrointestinal adverse events and a significantly lower rate of drug-related adverse events that caused discontinuation of prophylaxis (0.2% vs. 2.0%, $p = .015$).[47]

In the study that used doxycycline as the comparator, the overall frequency of adverse events was lower in subjects receiving atovaquone/proguanil than in subjects receiving doxycycline (38% vs. 58%, $p < .05$) because of a lower rate of gastrointestinal events (29% vs. 53%), constitutional events (23% vs. 30%), and photosensitivity events (8% vs. 16%).[49]

In all three studies, no treatment-emergent effects were evident for any of the hematology or clinical chemistry parameters measured.

Postmarketing Surveillance Data

Malarone was first marketed in Switzerland in August 1997. It is approved in more than 35 countries for the treatment of *Plasmodium falciparum* malaria and has

Table 8.6–7. Common Drug-Related Adverse Events during Prophylaxis with Atovaquone/Proguanil or Chloroquine/Proguanil in Nonimmune Travelers

	% of Subjects	
Adverse Event	Atovaquone/Proguanil (n = 511)	Chloroquine/Proguanil (n = 511)
Any event	22	28*
Any gastrointestinal event	12	20***
Diarrhea	5	7
Nausea	3	7***
Abdominal pain	3	6*
Mouth ulcers	4	5
Vomiting	0	2**
Any neuropsychiatric event	10	10
Dizziness	3	4
Strange/vivid dreams	4	3
Insomnia	2	2
Visual difficulties	2	2
Headache	4	4

*$p < .05$; **$p < .01$; ***$p < .001$.
Data from Høgh B, Clark PD, Camus D, et al. Atovaquone/proguanil versus chloroquine/proguanil for malaria prophylaxis in non-immune travellers: results from a randomised, double-blind study. Lancet 2000;356:1888–1894.

been approved in Denmark and the United States for both prophylaxis and treatment of *P. falciparum* malaria since July 1998 and July 2000, respectively.

It is estimated from sales data that approximately 85,750 treatment packs of Malarone (12 tablets per pack) were sold worldwide between August 1997 and May 2000, and approximately 60% of the total sales were in Denmark. During the same period, there were 32 reports of adverse events submitted to the Glaxo Wellcome spontaneous-report databases; 88% were from Denmark. The indication for which Malarone was being used was specified in 22 cases: prophylaxis against malaria was the indication in 17 cases, and treatment of malaria was the indication in 5 cases.

Reported events most commonly involved the skin (11 reports) and the gastrointestinal tract (9 reports). These spontaneous reports did not identify unexpected events or events occurring at a frequency that warrants a change in prescribing information.[21]

CONTRAINDICATIONS AND INDICATIONS

Contraindications and Precautions

Atovaquone/proguanil is contraindicated for malaria prophylaxis in patients with severe renal impairment (creatinine clearance < 30 mL/min).

As with any drug, no one with a known hypersensitivity to either atovaquone or proguanil should be given the combination.

The safety and effectiveness of atovaquone/proguanil for the prophylaxis of malaria in children who weigh less than 11 kg has not been established.

Parasite relapse occurred commonly when *Plasmodium vivax* malaria was treated with atovaquone/proguanil alone. Travelers with intense exposure to *P. vivax* or *Plasmodium ovale*, and those who develop malaria caused by either of these parasites, will require additional treatment with a drug (such as primaquine) that is active against hypnozoites.

If malaria occurs after chemoprophylaxis with atovaquone/proguanil, patients should be treated with a different blood schizonticide.

The concomitant administration of atovaquone/proguanil and rifampicin or rifabutin is not recommended.

Drug Interactions

Concomitant administration of atovaquone/proguanil with rifampin or rifabutin reduces atovaquone levels by approximately 50% and 34%, respectively.[21] The mechanism for this interaction is unclear.

Administration of atovaquone/proguanil with the antiemetic metoclopramide reduces atovaquone levels by approximately 50%,[21] but this is not associated with a significant reduction in the efficacy of atovaquone/proguanil for treatment of malaria.[6]

Concomitant treatment with tetracycline has been associated with an approximately 40% reduction in plasma concentrations of atovaquone,[52] but tetracycline is synergistic with atovaquone in vitro[5] and enhances its efficacy in patients with acute malaria.[7]

Atovaquone is highly protein bound (> 99%) but does not displace other highly protein-bound drugs in vitro, which indicates that significant drug interactions arising from displacement are unlikely. Proguanil is metabolized primarily by CYP2C19. Potential pharmacokinetic interactions with other substrates or inhibitors of this pathway have not been studied.

Indications

Atovaquone/proguanil hydrochloride (Malarone) is approved in more than 35 countries for the treatment of acute uncomplicated malaria caused by *Plasmodium falciparum*, including malaria acquired in areas where multidrug-resistant strains of *P. falciparum* occur. The use of atovaquone/proguanil for this indication has been reviewed by Looareesuwan and colleagues.[6]

Malarone is also approved in at least two countries for the prophylaxis of malaria caused by *P. falciparum*, including in areas where chloroquine resistance has been reported. In the United States, it is approved for the prophylaxis of falciparum malaria in adults and in children who weigh at least 11 kg. There is currently no clinical information available regarding the use of atovaquone/proguanil in children who weigh < 11 kg.

Although atovaquone/proguanil is currently indicated only for the prophylaxis of malaria caused by *P. falciparum*, recent results indicate it is also effective for the prophylaxis of malaria caused by *Plasmodium vivax*.[46] Atovaquone/proguanil is also effective against the blood stages of *Plasmodium ovale* and *Plasmodium malariae*;[15] thus, there is no reason to prescribe an additional antimalarial drug for persons who travel to areas where they are exposed to multiple parasite species. Travelers with intense exposure to *Plasmodium vivax* or *Plasmodium ovale* should be given postexposure treatment with primaquine to reduce the risk of late (relapse) infections.

ADMINISTRATION

Atovaquone/proguanil is commercially available as fixed-dose tablets (Malarone, Glaxo Wellcome). Each Malarone tablet contains 250 mg of atovaquone and 100 mg of proguanil hydrochloride. Each Malarone Pediatric tablet contains 62.5 mg of atovaquone and 25 mg of proguanil hydrochloride. The dosage regimen for malaria prevention in adults and children who weigh at least 11 kg is shown in Table 8.6–1. Prophylaxis should start 1 day before entering a malaria-endemic area and should continue daily while the traveler is in the endemic area and for 7 days after the traveler leaves the area.

Atovaquone/proguanil should be taken with food or a milky drink (e.g., Ovaltine), which will increase the absorption of atovaquone and may minimize minor gastrointestinal upset from proguanil.

Although atovaquone suspension and proguanil tablets are available as separate drugs, atovaquone should never be used as monotherapy for malaria treatment or prophylaxis because of the potential for rapid emergence of parasite resistance.[7]

COMMENTARY

The early clinical trials program of atovaquone/proguanil has been much more extensive than for any previous drug developed for antimalarial prophylaxis. To date, more than 3,000 subjects have been enrolled in five placebo-controlled studies of atovaquone/proguanil; three active-controlled studies comparing atovaquone/proguanil to mefloquine, chloroquine/proguanil, or doxycycline; and one placebo-controlled study of atovaquone alone. In addition, the pharmacokinetics of atovaquone/proguanil have recently been evaluated in special population groups of elderly subjects and subjects with renal or hepatic impairment. Results from these studies provide a remarkably large body of information about a drug combination that was approved for malaria prophylaxis in only two countries by the end of 2000.

In both semi-immune and nonimmune populations, the efficacy of atovaquone/proguanil has been 95% to 100% for the prevention of *Plasmodium falciparum* malaria in all clinical studies in which protective efficacy could be calculated. The safety profile of atovaquone/proguanil has been uniformly favorable in all studies, with an adverse-event rate similar to that of placebo in placebo-controlled studies. In active-controlled studies, atovaquone/proguanil was better tolerated than mefloquine, chloroquine/proguanil, or doxycycline.

When considering options for chemoprophylaxis, it is important to evaluate each individual patient and his or her particular medical history and risk of malaria. A complete understanding of the appropriate uses for available drugs requires extensive practical postregistration experience in a variety of settings. Because atovaquone/proguanil is the newest member of the antimalarial prophylaxis armamentarium, it will undoubtedly be some time before its optimal role is established. However, there are some clear situations in which atovaquone/proguanil appears to be a good choice for malaria prophylaxis.

Because prophylaxis with atovaquone/proguanil can be discontinued 7 days after the traveler leaves a malaria-endemic area, it will find an important role for short-term travelers. The cost of prophylaxis also suggests that atovaquone/proguanil will be more acceptable to short-term travelers. Atovaquone is an expensive drug to manufacture, and the cost of atovaquone/proguanil is therefore relatively high. However, based on wholesale prices in the United States, the cost of atovaquone/proguanil is not much different from the cost of mefloquine until travel duration exceeds 3 weeks (Table 8.6–8). When considered against the thousands of dollars spent for the average business or vacation trip to a malaria-endemic area and the high costs associated with contracting malaria, the cost of highly effective and well-tolerated antimalarial prophylaxis should not be considered excessive by most travelers from the West.

Atovaquone/proguanil will also be preferred by travelers who are concerned about the side effects of prophylactic drugs. Because of widespread publicity about side effects associated with mefloquine,[53] many travelers are requesting alternatives or choosing not to use chemoprophylaxis, with potentially disastrous consequences.[54] The favorable side effect profile and high efficacy of atovaquone/proguanil provides a distinct advantage over other available drugs.

Atovaquone/proguanil will also play a role in areas where multidrug-resistant *P. falciparum* occurs. Resistance to chloroquine is widespread, pyrimethamine can no longer be used alone, and resistance to sulfadoxine/pyrimethamine is spreading. Resistance to mefloquine is not extensive at present, occurring with high frequency only in Southeast Asia;[55] it occurs less often in Africa.[56] Because there are currently no geographic differences in plasmodial sensitivity to it, atovaquone/proguanil is a good choice for chemoprophylaxis if the prescriber is uncertain about the resistance profile of the area to be visited. Atovaquone/ proguanil may become even more important in the future if the spread of multidrug resistance makes other options inadequate.

(This chapter was written by a U.S. Government employee and as such, cannot be copyrighted.)

Table 8.6–8. **Comparative Cost of Prophylaxis with Atovaquone/Proguanil (Malarone) or Mefloquine (Lariam) in the United States**

Duration of Travel	Number of Tablets*		Cost of Tablets (U.S.$)†	
	Malarone	Lariam	Malarone	Lariam
1 day	9	7	35	53
1 week	15	8	59	60
2 weeks	22	9	86	68
3 weeks	29	10	114	75

* Based on recommended dosing regimens of 1 tablet daily from 1 day before until 7 days after travel for Malarone and 1 tablet weekly from 3 weeks before until 4 weeks after travel for Lariam.
† Based on net wholesale price of U.S.$3.92 for Malarone and U.S.$7.55 for Lariam.
Data from World Health Organization. International travel and health. Geneva: World Health Organization, 2000; Shanks GD, Kremsner PG, Sukwa TY, et al. Atovaquone and proguanil hydrochloride for prophylaxis of malaria. J Travel Med 1996;6 Suppl 1:S21–S27; and First DataBank, Inc., San Bruno (CA), 94066; 2000 Oct 1.

ACKNOWLEGDMENTS

The author thanks Misba Beerahee, Jeffrey Chulay, and the Malarone International Study Team for assistance in preparing information for publication. Drs. Birthe Høgh, David Overbosch, Kevin Baird, Peter Nasveld, and Jonathan Berman are thanked for providing data in advance of publication.

REFERENCES

1. Hudson AT, Dickins M, Ginger CD, et al. 566C80: a potent broad spectrum anti-infective agent with activity against malaria and opportunistic infections in AIDS patients. Drugs Exp Clin Res 1991;17:427–435.

2. Fry M, Pudney M. Site of action of the antimalarial hydroxynaphthoquinone, 2-[trans-4-(4'-chlorophenyl) cyclohexyl]-3-hydroxy-1,4-naphthoquinone (566C80). Biochem Pharmacol 1992;43:1545–1553.

3. Ferone R. Dihydrofolate reductase from pyrimethamine-resistant *Plasmodium berghei*. J Biol Chem 1970;245:850–854.

4. Chulay JD, Watkins WM, Sixsmith DG. Synergistic antimalarial activity of pyrimethamine and sulfadoxine against *Plasmodium falciparum* in vitro. Am J Trop Med Hyg 1984;33:325–330.

5. Canfield CJ, Pudney M, Gutteridge WE. Interactions of atovaquone with other antimalarial drugs against *Plasmodium falciparum* in vitro. Exp Parasitol 1995;80:373–381.

6. Looareesuwan S, Chulay JD, Canfield CJ, Hutchinson DB. Malarone (atovaquone and proguanil hydrochloride): a review of its clinical development for treatment of malaria. Am J Trop Med Hyg 1999;60:533–541.

7. Looareesuwan S, Viravan C, Webster HK, et al. Clinical studies of atovaquone, alone or in combination with other antimalarial drugs, for treatment of acute uncomplicated malaria in Thailand. Am J Trop Med Hyg 1996;54:62–66.

8. Radloff PD, Philipps J, Nkeyi M, et al. Atovaquone and proguanil for *Plasmodium falciparum* malaria. Lancet 1996;347:1511–1514.

9. de Alencar FE, Cerutti C Jr, Durlacher RR, et al. Atovaquone and proguanil for the treatment of malaria in Brazil. J Infect Dis 1997;175:1544–1547.

10. Sabchareon A, Attanath P, Phanuaksook P, et al. Efficacy and pharmacokinetics of atovaquone and proguanil in children with multidrug-resistant *Plasmodium falciparum* malaria. Trans R Soc Trop Med Hyg 1998;92:201–206.

11. Bustos DG, Canfield CJ, Canete-Miguel E, Hutchinson DBA. Atovaquone/proguanil compared with chloroquine and chloroquine/sulfadoxine/pyrimethamine for treatment of acute *Plasmodium falciparum* malaria in the Philippines. J Infect Dis 1999;179:1587–1590.

12. Anabwani G, Canfield CJ, Hutchinson DBA. Combination atovaquone and proguanil hydrochloride versus halofantrine for treatment of acute *Plasmodium falciparum* malaria in children. Pediatr Infect Dis J 1999;18:456–461.

13. Mulenga M, Sukwa TY, Canfield CJ, Hutchinson DBA. Atovaquone and proguanil versus pyrimethamine/sulfadoxine for the treatment of acute falciparum malaria in Zambia. Clin Ther 1999;21:841–852.

14. Bouchoud O, Monlun E, Muanza K, et al. Atovaquone plus proguanil versus halo-fantrine for the treatment of imported acute uncomplicated *P. falciparum* malaria in non-immune adults: a randomised comparative trial. Am J Trop Med Hyg 2001. [In press]

15. Radloff PD, Philipps J, Hutchinson D, Kremsner PG. Atovaquone plus proguanil is an effective treatment for *Plasmodium ovale* and *P. malariae* malaria. Trans R Soc Trop Med Hyg 1996;90:682.

16. Looareesuwan S, Wilairatana P, Glanarongran R, et al. Atovaquone and proguanil hydrochloride followed by primaquine for treatment of *Plasmodium vivax* malaria in Thailand. Trans R Soc Trop Med Hyg 1999;93:637–640.

17. Shanks GD, Kremsner PG, Sukwa TY, et al. Atovaquone and proguanil hydrochloride for prophylaxis of malaria. J Travel Med 1999;6 Suppl 1:S21–S27.

18. Beerahee M. Clinical pharmacology of atovaquone and proguanil hydrochloride. J Travel Med 1999;6 Suppl 1:S13–S17.

19. Pudney M, Gutteridge W, Zeman A, et al. Atovaquone and proguanil hydrochloride: a review of nonclinical studies. J Travel Med 1999;6 Suppl 1:S8–S12.

20. Helsby NA, Edwards G, Breckenridge AM, Ward SA. The multiple dose pharmacokinetics of proguanil. Br J Clin Pharmacol 1993;35:653–656.

21. Glaxo Wellcome. [Data on file]. Research Triangle Park (NC); 2000.

22. Boots M, Phillips M, Curtis JR. Megaloblastic anemia and pancytopenia due to proguanil in patients with chronic renal failure. Clin Nephrol 1982;18:106–108.

23. Sirsat RA, Dasgupta A. Haematological complications of proguanil in a patient with chronic renal failure. Nephron 1997;75:108.

24. Sukwa TY, Mulenga M, Chisaka N, et al. A randomized, double-blind, placebo-controlled field trial to determine the efficacy and safety of Malarone (atovaquone/proguanil) for the prophylaxis of malaria in Zambia. Am J Trop Med Hyg 1999;60:521–525.

25. Basco LK, Ramiliarisoa O, Le Bras J. In vitro activity of atovaquone against the African isolates and clones of *Plasmodium falciparum*. Am J Trop Med Hyg 1995; 53:388–391.

26. Gay F, Bustos D, Traore B, et al. In vitro response of *Plasmodium falciparum* to atovaquone and correlation with other antimalarials: comparison between African and Asian strains. Am J Trop Med Hyg 1997;56:315–317.

27. Davies CS, Pudney M, Matthews PJ, Sinden RE. The causal prophylactic activity of the novel hydroxynaphthoquinone 566C80 against *Plasmodium berghei* infections in rats. Acta Leiden 1989;58:115–128.

28. Davies CS, Pudney M, Nicholas JC, Sinden RE. The novel hydroxynaphthoquinone 566C80 inhibits the development of liver stages of *Plasmodium berghei* cultured in vitro. Parasitology 1993;106:1–6.

29. Shapiro TA, Ranasinha CD, Kumar N, Barditch-Crovo P. Prophylactic activity of atovaquone against *Plasmodium falciparum* in humans. Am J Trop Med Hyg 1999; 60:831–836.

30. Srivastava IK, Rottenberg H, Vaidya AB. Atovaquone, a broad spectrum antiparasitic drug, collapses mitochondrial membrane potential in a malarial parasite. J Biol Chem 1997;272:3961–3966.

31. Srivastava IK, Vaidya AB. A mechanism for the synergistic antimalarial action of atovaquone and proguanil. Antimicrob Agents Chemother 1999;43:1334–1339.

32. Rathod PK, McErlean T, Lee PC. Variations in frequencies of drug resistance in *Plasmodium falciparum*. Proc Natl Acad Sci U S A 1997;94:9389–9393.

33. Korsinczky M, Chen N, Kotecka B, et al. Mutations in *Plasmodium falciparum* cytochrome *b* that are associated with atovaquone resistance are located at a putative drug-binding site. Antimicrob Agents Chemother 2000;44:2100–2108.

34. Srivastava IK, Morrisey JM, Darrouzet E, et al. Resistance mutations reveal the atovaquone-binding domain of cytochrome b in malaria parasites. Mol Microbiol 1999;33:704–711.

35. Syafruddin D, Siregar JE, Marzuki S. Mutations in the cytochrome b gene of *Plasmodium berghei* conferring resistance to atovaquone. Mol Biochem Parasitol 1999;104:185–194.

36. Watkins WM, Sixsmith DG, Chulay JD. The activity of proguanil and its metabolites, cycloguanil and *p*-chlorophenylbiguanide, against *Plasmodium falciparum* in vitro. Ann Trop Med Parasitol 1984;78:273–278.

37. Khan B, Omar S, Kanyara JN, et al. Antifolate drug resistance and point mutations in *Plasmodium falciparum* in Kenya. Trans R Soc Trop Med Hyg 1997;91:456–460.

38. Peters W, Davies EE, Robinson BL. The chemotherapy of rodent malaria, XXIII. Causal prophylaxis, part II: practical experience with *Plasmodium yoelii nigeriensis* in drug screening. Ann Trop Med Parasitol 1975;69:311–328.

39. Fairley NH. Researches on paludrine (M.4888) in malaria. An experimental investigation undertaken by the L.H.Q. Medical Research Unit (A.I.F.), Cairns, Australia. Trans R Soc Trop Med Hyg 1946;40:105–151.

40. Eriksson B, Courtier B, Bjorkman A, et al. Activity of dihydrofolate reductase inhibitors on the hepatic stages of *Plasmodium yoelii yoelii* in vitro. Trans R Soc Trop Med Hyg 1991;85:725–726.

41. Ferone R. Dihydrofolate reductase inhibitors. In: Peters W, Richards WHG, editors. Handbook of experimental pharmacology. Vol 68/II. Antimalarial drugs. New York: Springer-Verlag, 1984. p. 207–221.

42. Fidock DA, Wellems TE. Transformation with human dihydrofolate reductase renders malaria parasites insensitive to WR99210 but does not affect the intrinsic activity of proguanil. Proc Natl Acad Sci U S A 1997;94:10931–10936.

43. Shanks GD, Gordon DM, Klotz FW, et al. Efficacy and safety of atovaquone/proguanil for suppressive prophylaxis against *Plasmodium falciparum* malaria. Clin Infect Dis 1998;27:494–499.

44. Lell B, Luckner D, Ndjave M, et al. Randomised placebo-controlled study of atovaquone plus proguanil for malaria prophylaxis in children. Lancet 1998;351:709–713.

45. Berman JD, Chulay JD, Dowler M, et al. Causal prophylactic efficacy of Malarone (atovaquone/proguanil) in a human challenge model. Trans R Soc Trop Med Hyg 2001. [In press]

46. Baird K, Lacy M, Sismadi P, et al. Randomized, double-blind, placebo-controlled evaluation of Malarone for prophylaxis of *P. vivax* and *P. falciparum* malaria in non-immune transmigrants to Irian Jaya [abstract 17]. Proceedings of the 49th Annual Meeting of the American Society of Tropical Medicine and Hygiene; 2000 Oct 29–Nov 2; Houston (TX). Am J Trop Med Hyg Suppl 2000.

47. Høgh B, Clarke PD, Camus D, et al. Atovaquone/proguanil versus chloroquine/proguanil for malaria prophylaxis in non-immune travellers: results from a randomised, double-blind study. Lancet 2000;356:1888–1894.

48. Overbosch D, Schilthuis H, Bienzle U, et al. Malarone compared with mefloquine for malaria prophylaxis in non-immune travellers. Oxford 2000–new challenges in tropical medicine and parasitology; 2000 Sept 18–22; Oxford, U.K. p. 146.

49. Nasveld PE, Edstein MD, Kitchener SJ, Rieckmann KH. Comparison of the effectiveness of atovaquone/proguanil combination and doxycycline in the chemoprophylaxis of malaria in Australian Defence Force personnel [abstract 1391]. Proceedings of the 49th Annual Meeting of the American Society of Tropical Medicine and Hygiene; 2000; Oct 29–Nov 2; Houston (TX). Am J Trop Med Hyg Suppl 2000.

50. Chulay JD. Challenges in the development of antimalarial drugs with causal prophylactic activity. Trans R Soc Trop Med Hyg 1998;92:577–579.

51. Covell G, Nicol WD, Shute PG, Maryon M. Studies on a West African strain of *Plasmodium falciparum*. The efficacy of paludrine (proguanil) as a prophylactic agent. Trans R Soc Trop Med Hyg 1949;42:341–346.

52. Hussein Z, Eaves J, Hutchinson DB, Canfield CJ. Population pharmacokinetics of atovaquone in patients with acute malaria caused by *Plasmodium falciparum*. Clin Pharmacol Ther 1997;61:518–530.

53. Epstein K. The Lariam files. The Washington Post 2000 Oct 10. Available from: URL: http://washingtonpost.com/wp-dyn/articles/A38465-32000Oct38469.html.

54. Reid AJ, Whitty CJ, Ayles HM, et al. Malaria at Christmas: risks of prophylaxis versus risks of malaria. BMJ 1998;317:1506–1508.

55. Fontanet AL, Johnston DB, Walker AM, et al. High prevalence of mefloquine-resistant falciparum malaria in eastern Thailand. Bull World Health Organ 1993; 71:377–383.

56. Brasseur P, Kouamouo J, Moyou-Somo R, Druilhe P. Multi-drug resistant falciparum malaria in Cameroon in 1987–1988. II. Mefloquine resistance confirmed in vivo and in vitro and its correlation with quinine resistance. Am J Trop Med Hyg 1992;46:8–14.

8.7 Tafenoquine

Robert A. Gasser, Jr.

ABSTRACT

Tafenoquine is a new 8-aminoquinoline, an analogue of primaquine. Like primaquine, it inhibits liver-stage plasmodia schizonts, inhibits *Plasmodium vivax* hypnozoites (thereby preventing relapse), and possesses gametocidal activity, affording a transmission-blocking effect. In contrast to primaquine, tafenoquine has good schizonticidal effects against blood-stage plasmodia parasites. Tafenoquine also has a long serum half-life of about 2 weeks. The persistence of tafenoquine in blood, combined with its activity against liver-stage parasites, offers the prospect of effective single-drug prophylaxis for travelers, without the need for prolonged dosing regimens. Its ability to kill blood-stage parasites suggests that tafenoquine might have some limited role in treating malaria, not simply in preventing it. Based on a demonstrated risk of hemolysis, tafenoquine should not be administered to individuals with glucose-6-phosphate dehydrogenase (G6PD) deficiency.

Key words: 8-aminoquinoline; etaquine; G6PD deficiency; hemolysis; malaria; *Plasmodium*; primaquine; prophylaxis; relapse; tafenoquine; treatment.

BACKGROUND

The development of tafenoquine derives directly from the first attempts to develop synthetic antimalarial drugs. In 1891, Guttmann and Ehrlich reported their use of methylene blue to treat clinical malaria.[1] This initial report did not immediately lead to further progress, and quinine remained unchallenged as the only effective antimalarial drug for the next three decades. Following World War I, German scientists attempting to develop synthetic antimalarial drugs focused their efforts on agents chemically related to methylene blue. By 1925, this work, conducted by Schülemann and his colleagues, had identified the first clinically useful 8-aminoquinoline, pamaquine (also called plasmoquine, plasmochin, or plasmochine).[2] Although pamaquine was ineffective at eradicating the blood-stage parasites of human malaria and had substantial toxicity, it did afford protection against relapse. With combined quinine and pamaquine, both eradication of blood-stage parasites (clinical cure) and prevention of relapse (radical cure) could be reliably achieved.[2]

Two decades later (during the 1940s), wartime needs impelled a major American and British program to develop synthetic antimalarials.[3] Several important drugs emerged from this research, including primaquine, another 8-aminoquinoline. Like pamaquine, primaquine has only limited effectiveness in eradicating blood-stage parasites.[4–6] Nonetheless, compared to pamaquine, primaquine demonstrated both reduced toxicity and improved anti-relapse activity.[7] Its usefulness has been such that for almost 50 years, primaquine has remained virtually the only antimalarial used to prevent relapse of malaria caused by *P. vivax* or *Plasmodium ovale.*

Interest in potentially expanded roles for primaquine was encouraged by the global spread of resistance to other antimalarial drugs. By the 1980s, plasmodial resistance to chloroquine (the leading drug for prophylaxis and treatment of blood-stage infections) was common in Africa, South America, and Asia.[8] Resistance to alternative agents then in use, such as pyrimethamine/sulfadoxine and mefloquine, had already appeared.[8,9] During the mid-1990s, a number of studies suggested that primaquine might play some role in countering the clinical challenges posed by this widening resistance to other antimalarial agents. Used alone, primaquine may be useful as a prophylactic against *Plasmodium falciparum*[10–12] and *Plasmodium vivax,*[11,12] preventing blood-stage infection by killing the earlier, liver-stage parasites. When used in combination with chloroquine, primaquine may counteract chloroquine resistance in *P. vivax,* thus affording the drug a contributory role in the treatment of blood-stage infections.[13,14] However, despite its continuing clinical importance, primaquine's usefulness has remained limited by its short half-life, its adverse effects, and its limited ability to clear blood-stage parasites.

Worsening plasmodial resistance to available blood-stage schizonticidal drugs, the hope of achieving causal prophylaxis against *Plasmodium falciparum* (thereby ending the need to continue prophylaxis for weeks after leaving an endemic area), and the limitations of primaquine all combined to incite interest in the development of new 8-aminoquinolines.[15] During the 1980s, researchers at Walter Reed Army Institute of Research identified such a compound.[15,16] Initially identified as compound WR 238605, this drug was later called etaquine; it now possesses the generic name tafenoquine.[17]

CHEMISTRY AND MECHANISM OF ACTION

Tafenoquine is 2,6-dimethoxy-4-methyl-5-[(3-trifluoromethyl)-phenoxy]-8-[(4-amino-1-methylbutyl)amino] quinoline, formulated as the succinate salt (Figure 8.7–1).[16,18] Quantities of tafenoquine may be reported as the amounts of either the base or the salt. To interpret these quantities, 4 units of base contains the same amount of active drug as 5 units of salt (e.g., 100 mg base equals 125 mg salt).[19] Tafenoquine differs from primaquine by the addition of the 2-methoxy, 4-methyl, and 5-(3-trifluoromethyl)-phenoxy groups. The phenoxy group may retard tafenoquine's metabolism, prolonging an elimination half-life that is much longer than that of primaquine.[14,18] The 4-amino-1-methylbutyl side chain, common to both primaquine and tafenoquine, appears to be important for antiplasmodial activity.[7,20]

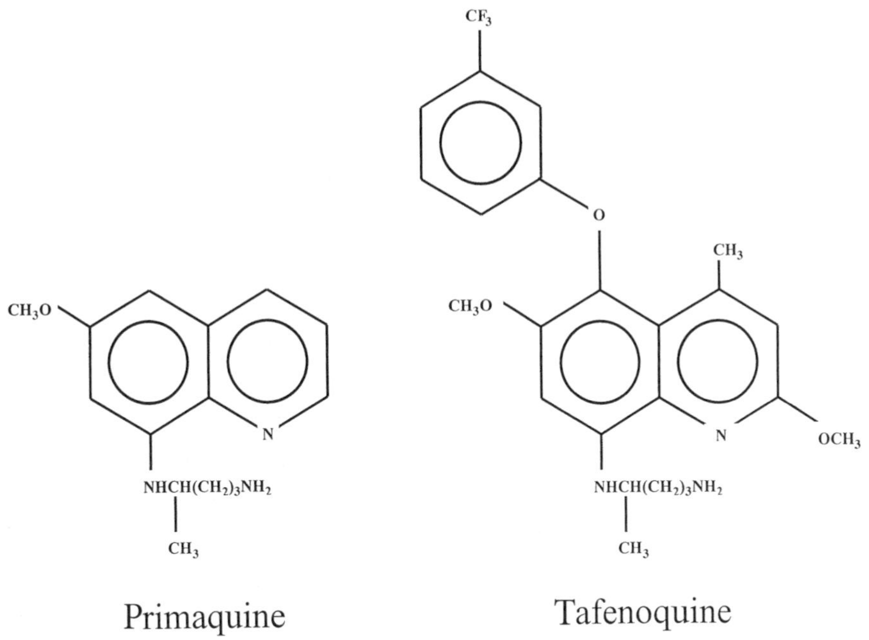

Figure 8.7–1. Structural formulas of primaquine and tafenoquine.

The precise mechanism of action of the 8-aminoquinolines, tafenoquine included, remains unknown. Several possible mechanisms for the antiplasmodial effects of these drugs have been proposed. The degree of pro-oxidant activity of 8-aminoquinolines is associated with their level of antiplasmodial activity. This correlation suggests that oxidant-mediated injury to the parasites accounts for the effects of these drugs.[21] Localization of primaquine within plasmodial mitochondria, followed by morphological changes in the parasite mitochondria, has been demonstrated.[22,23] These observations suggest drug-induced mitochondrial dysfunction. Additionally, primaquine has been shown to inhibit vesicle formation by the Golgi apparatus[24] and to inhibit membrane receptor recycling by endosomes.[25] These effects seem to be mediated by a mechanism that involves a direct effect of primaquine on the membrane components of these subcellular structures.[25] Like chloroquine[26,27] but unlike primaquine, tafenoquine inhibits polymerization of hematin within blood-stage parasites.[21] The ability to disrupt this essential parasite-specific metabolic process likely contributes to tafenoquine's activity against blood-stage plasmodia.

PHARMACOKINETICS

Tafenoquine was developed for oral administration. When the drug is taken with food, absorption is increased by approximately 50%,[28] and the severity of gastrointestinal adverse effects is diminished.[29] Absorption of tafenoquine is slow, and maximum plasma concentration is achieved approximately 12 to 13 hours after ingestion.[28,30] The drug demonstrates linear pharmacokinetics with increasing dose.[30] A dose of 600 mg (tafenoquine base) given to each of four fasting volunteers yielded peak concentrations in blood (C_{max}) ranging from 244 to 489 ng/mL, with the mean C_{max} being 401 ng/mL.[31] Tafenoquine blood levels are 1.8-times higher than simultaneous plasma levels, indicating that tafenoquine is concentrated within red blood cells at a level 2.8 times that of plasma.[30,32] This intraerythrocytic concentration of tafenoquine contrasts with the distribution of primaquine, which is not concentrated in red blood cells,[33] and may contribute to tafenoquine's greater schizonticidal effect against blood-stage plasmodia.

The bioavailability of tafenoquine has not been precisely determined, so its volume of distribution can only be estimated. Assuming a bioavailability of 100%, the volume of distribution could be as high as 2,550 L.[30] Dog studies suggested that at higher doses, bioavailability might be as low as 60%.[30,34] Using this lower estimate of bioavailability, tafenoquine's volume of distribution would be 1,530 L. This is still a very large volume of distribution and implies a high degree of drug binding in tissue.

The metabolic degradation of tafenoquine is complex, with C-hydroxylation of the 8-[(4-amino-1-methylbutyl)amino] side chain playing a prominent role.[18] Preclinical (animal model) studies suggested that the drug is eliminated via the gastrointestinal tract, possibly by biliary excretion, but not in the urine.[30] Data defining the route of excretion in humans have not yet been published. In contrast to primaquine, which has an elimination half-life of 5 to 6 hours,[33] the half-life of tafenoquine is prolonged, averaging about 14 days.[30,31]

CLINICAL USES

As with any antimalarial drug, there are at least four purposes for which the use of tafenoquine might be considered: (1) prophylaxis, (2) treatment of established blood-stage infections (clinical cure), (3) relapse prevention (radical cure), and (4) transmission blocking.

Prophylaxis

Prophylaxis against malaria may be achieved by one of two mechanisms. Causal prophylaxis is protection afforded by preventing the release of viable merozoites from the liver. This type of prophylaxis requires the killing or inhibition of sporozoites or liver-stage schizonts. Suppressive prophylaxis is protection provided by inhibiting or killing blood-stage parasites. When suppressive prophylaxis is used, parasites may successfully mature in the liver and invade red blood cells, but they are then prevented from achieving a mass in the blood sufficient to produce clinical illness. From a clinical viewpoint, the difference between the two mechanisms is significant. Causal prophylaxis may be discontinued once exposure to the bites of infective mosquitoes has ended and sufficient drug has been taken to assure that any liver-stage schizonts will not mature. At most, this would require continuing the prophylactic drug for several days after potential exposure has ended. In contrast, suppressive prophylaxis must be maintained past the period of the potential release of parasites from the liver into blood. Even for the nonrelapsing malarias, suppressive prophylaxis mandates continuing the drug for a few weeks after the end of exposure. This requirement holds even when the risk of exposure has been very brief (e.g., as little as a single overnight visit). Most drugs conventionally used for prophylaxis (chloroquine, doxycycline, and mefloquine) are employed as suppressive prophylactics. The need for weeks of continued drug use, despite the traveler's having departed the locale of risk, predisposes to noncompliance.[35] Causal prophylaxis, with its abbreviated requirement for postexposure dosing, may improve patients' compliance, reducing the risk of prophylactic failures.

Tafenoquine possesses causal prophylactic activity. Laboratory studies have shown that tafenoquine completely inhibits the development of liver-stage plasmodia schizonts in hepatocyte cell cultures, at doses that do not cause hepatocyte injury.[16] Used against the rodent malaria species *Plasmodium yoelii* in mice, tafenoquine completely suppressed liver-stage schizonts, at doses that were ineffective against blood-stage parasites.[14] In monkeys, tafenoquine was 14 times more potent as a causal prophylactic than was primaquine.[30]

Human studies have confirmed that tafenoquine is a very effective prophylactic agent against *Plasmodium falciparum* but are somewhat ambiguous on the issue of whether the basis of the observed protection is causal or suppressive. In the first reported study, tafenoquine protected 3 of 4 nonimmune volunteers experimentally challenged with chloroquine-sensitive *P. falciparum*.[31] The patient with the single case of tafenoquine failure developed parasitemia on day 31 after infectious challenge, 21 days later than two experimentally infected control subjects. Of note, the one prophylactic failure occurred in a patient whose peak tafenoquine blood level reached only 244 ng/mL whereas peak blood levels in the three protected subjects ranged from 417 to 489 ng/mL. This delay in parasitemia implied the suppression of parasitemia until tafenoquine blood levels dropped. These results do not permit discrimination of causal versus suppressive prophylaxis in the three protected subjects.

A second study evaluated the prophylactic effect of tafenoquine against *P. falciparum* in Gabon,[19] where most *P. falciparum* isolates are resistant to chloroquine.[36,37] Each of 410 subjects received three doses of the study drug, one dose on each of 3 consecutive days, and then no additional prophylactic drug. Tafenoquine, 25 mg base daily for 3 days, had no protective efficacy, but doses of 50, 100, or 200 mg base daily for 3 days all showed substantial protective efficacy through 10 weeks of follow-up. Tafenoquine, 200 mg daily for 3 days, provided 100% protection through 10 weeks. This study, too, could not distinguish a causal from a suppressive prophylactic effect. Nonetheless, the fact that a tafenoquine loading dose without subsequent maintenance doses provided such prolonged protection implies that tafenoquine might be used clinically as though it were a causal prophylactic, even if that is not its actual mechanism.

A third study, conducted among 513 semi-immune patients in Ghana, also examined tafenoquine's prophylactic activity against *P. falciparum*.[38] Subjects received a loading dose of study drug on each of 3 consecutive days, then a single weekly dose for 12 weeks. Doses of 200 mg of tafenoquine afforded a protective efficacy of approximately 86%, almost identical to that afforded by 250-mg doses of mefloquine. The protective efficacies of 50-mg and 100-mg doses of tafenoquine were similar.

In Kenya, a fourth study also evaluated tafenoquine for prophylaxis against *P. falciparum* in 249 semi-immune patients.[39] This study had four treatment arms: subjects received a loading dose of 400 mg of tafenoquine base daily for 3 days, followed by weekly placebo, or a loading dose of 200 mg of tafenoquine base daily for 3 days, followed by 200 mg of base weekly; or a loading dose of 400 mg of tafenoquine base daily for 3 days, followed by 400 mg of tafenoquine base weekly; or a loading dose of placebo daily for 3 days, followed by weekly placebo. Subjects were provided with weekly prophylactic doses of their study drug for 12 weeks and were then followed for an additional 4 weeks off prophylaxis. Malaria developed in 92% of the placebo controls. Given as loading and weekly maintenance doses at either 200 or 400 mg, tafenoquine provided a protective efficacy of about 90%. Subjects who received only the loading dose of tafenoquine, then placebo maintenance doses, showed equivalent protection lasting to 10 weeks.

The prophylactic efficacy of tafenoquine against *Plasmodium vivax* was demonstrated in a placebo-controlled trial in 205 nonimmune soldiers working along the northeastern border of Thailand. This region is notorious for the high incidence of chloroquine and mefloquine resistance in *Plasmodium falciparum*.[40] In this study, tafenoquine (400 mg base) was given as a daily dose for 3 consecutive days, followed by a single monthly dose of 400 mg. During 6 months, one *Plasmodium vivax* infection occurred in the tafenoquine group, and 20 *P. vivax* infections, 8 *Plasmodium falciparum* infections, and 1 mixed infection occurred in the placebo group.[41] These results equate to a 95% protective efficacy for tafenoquine against *Plasmodium vivax*. Such a high level of protection is particularly impressive in view of the well-documented presence of primaquine-refractory strains of *P. vivax* in Thailand.[5,42,43]

The preceding studies indicate that tafenoquine should be an excellent prophylactic agent against malaria caused by *Plasmodium falciparum*, including chloroquine-resistant and mefloquine-resistant strains, and against malaria due to *Plasmodium vivax*, even in areas where primaquine-refractory strains occur. Additionally, these studies suggest that a loading dose of tafenoquine taken just prior to exposure, without subsequent maintenance doses, could be protective for individuals whose period of exposure to infective mosquito bites will not exceed several weeks.

Clinical Cure

In contrast to the data available about tafenoquine's usefulness as a prophylactic agent, information about its effectiveness in curing disease is currently very limited. No reports of studies using tafenoquine to cure clinical cases of human malaria caused by any species have yet been published. Two studies that used tafenoquine to cure experimental *P. vivax* infections in monkeys have been reported. In the first study, six monkeys were infected by using the intravenous injection of chloroquine-resistant *P. vivax*–infected blood to directly establish blood-stage infections.[44] Therefore, no liver-stage infections occurred in these animals. Any antimalarial action of tafenoquine was restricted to blood-stage parasites. Once the establishment of patent parasitemia had been observed, the monkeys were treated with tafenoquine. In the low-dose group (0.8 mg/kg/d for 3 days), parasitemia was cleared in all three monkeys but recrudesced in one monkey 15 weeks later. In the high-dose group (3.2 mg/kg/d for 3 days), parasitemia was cleared in all three monkeys, without recrudescence. In both groups, clearance of parasitemia was slow, occurring 4 to 7 days after the start of treatment. The second study, which used similar tafenoquine doses against chloroquine-resistant *P. vivax* blood-stage infections, confirmed these results.[45] This study further demonstrated that the combination of chloroquine and tafenoquine gave additive effectiveness against blood-stage parasites, similar to that previously seen by combining chloroquine and primaquine.[13,14] These two studies suggest that tafenoquine might possess limited clinical usefulness as a blood-stage schizonticidal agent. If used in this role, however, its action may be so slow that it would require coadministration with a rapidly acting blood-stage schizonticide to achieve a clinically acceptable result. Such considerations remain speculative. Demonstration of tafenoquine's effectiveness in curing human malaria will be needed before it can be recommended for this purpose.

Radical Cure

For tafenoquine's third possible role—prevention of relapse, or radical cure—limited human data are available. A preliminary study in monkeys demonstrated that tafenoquine appeared to be 7 times more potent than primaquine in preventing relapse.[30] A subsequent human trial in Thailand compared three different tafenoquine regimens against placebo for this purpose.[29] First, blood-stage parasites were cleared, using chloroquine. Then, three tafenoquine regimens were evaluated: 300 mg base daily for 7 days; 500 mg daily for 3 days and repeated, beginning 1 week after the first dose; and 500 mg once. Lumped together, the subjects in the three tafenoquine regimens displayed a statistically significant 91% reduction in the annual incidence of *P. vivax* relapses, compared to those receiving placebo. The

number of subjects enrolled was too small to determine whether the observed outcome differences between the individual treatment arms were significant. A second
study, conducted during 1998 and 1999, compared the relapse-preventing efficacy
of primaquine with that of tafenoquine in nonimmune Australian soldiers who
had worked in Bougainville, North Solomons Province, Papua New Guinea.[46] Participants received one of several regimens consisting of either primaquine (a total
dose of 22.5 mg base daily for 14 days) or tafenoquine (a total dose of 400 mg daily
for 3 days). This open-label trial did not include a placebo arm. The rather high
dose of primaquine (22.5 mg instead of 15 mg) was warranted because primaquine-refractory strains of P. vivax are common in this area.[47,48] Failure rates
were calculated at 6 months postdeployment. Given the early and frequent relapse
patterns of the region's P. vivax strains,[49] this time period should have been sufficient to allow assessment of whether protection was being provided against relapse.
The failure rate was 1.9% for subjects under tafenoquine regimens and 3.3% for
those receiving primaquine. Viewed individually, each of these three studies has
limitations; taken together, they strongly suggest that tafenoquine will be very useful for preventing malaria relapses.

Transmission Blocking

The fourth potential role for tafenoquine—blocking transmission of malaria infection—is of minor importance in the clinical management of individual patients
but may be important if the drug becomes widely used within endemic areas or is
employed in public health efforts to suppress or eradicate the disease. Drugs may
achieve a transmission-blocking effect by one of two mechanisms. First, they may
suppress gametocyte formation or kill gametocytes within the patient. Alternatively, they may suppress sporogony within the mosquito after the insect ingests both
drug and gametocytes during an infected blood meal. Tafenoquine may exert both
effects. To date, the best data about these effects have come from experiments using
mice infected with the rodent malaria species, *Plasmodium berghei*.[50] Microgametocytes did not develop in mice that received tafenoquine on the same day
they were infected. When drug ingestion followed infection by 2 or 4 days, however, tafenoquine did not suppress the numbers of microgametocytes, delay their
appearance, or inhibit their ability to exflagellate. Tafenoquine had no discernible
effect on macrogametocyte development. Sporogony was evaluated by allowing
mosquitoes to feed on these mice. Even those mosquitoes that fed on mice that had
circulating gametocytes of both sexes never had sporozoite invasion of their salivary glands and could not transmit malaria to other mice. To further evaluate
tafenoquine's effect on sporogony, additional mosquitoes were fed first on mice
with untreated P. berghei infections, then, days later, fed again on tafenoquine-
treated mice.[50,51] These mosquitoes had fewer oocysts and slower oocyst development than mosquitoes fed on untreated mice. Sporozoite invasion of the salivary

glands of these mosquitoes was either diminished or absent, depending on the drug dose received by the mice on which the mosquitoes had fed. Although these data are promising, additional information derived from tafenoquine treatment of human infections will be needed before firm conclusions can be drawn about tafenoquine's usefulness in blocking malaria transmission.

TOXICITY AND ADVERSE EFFECTS

Tafenoquine is significantly less toxic than primaquine. In animal studies, substantially greater amounts of tafenoquine than primaquine were required to achieve similar levels of lethality.[30] In humans, the most notable adverse effects of tafenoquine are hemolytic reactions in G6PD-deficient individuals, gastrointestinal side effects, and methemoglobinemia. Minor and occasional adverse effects have included headaches[19,29,31] and mild transient elevations in serum levels of liver-associated enzymes.[38]

Primaquine has long been known to cause hemolysis in G6PD-deficient people, sometimes to a dangerous degree.[52–54] Given this precedent, tafenoquine's potential to induce similar hemolysis had been anticipated. That potential has now been realized unintentionally in two African subjects who received 400 mg of tafenoquine daily for 3 days.[39] In one of these subjects, tafenoquine-induced hemolysis was severe enough that hemoglobinuria ensued, and transfusion was required. In the second patient, an acute but asymptomatic decrease of 3 g/dL in blood hemoglobin level resulted. These events, confirming the precedent of primaquine, show that tafenoquine should not be administered to people with G6PD deficiency.

Gastrointestinal symptoms in people receiving tafenoquine are common but generally mild.[19,30,31,39] Specific symptoms have included abdominal pain, diarrhea, gas, and vomiting. These symptoms appear to be more frequent when larger doses of the drug are taken and much less frequent when the drug is taken with food.[29]

Tafenoquine almost invariably produces some degree of methemoglobinemia.[29,34,39] Peak methemoglobin levels are delayed after drug administration, occurring up to a week after peak drug levels occur. Higher doses of tafenoquine cause more severe methemoglobinemia. Tafenoquine doses of 200 mg daily for 3 days produced methemoglobin levels averaging 2.5%.[39] Doses of 300 mg daily for 7 days, or 500 mg daily for 3 days and repeated after a week, produced methemoglobin levels ranging from 3% to almost 15%.[29] The patients with these levels of methemoglobinemia were asymptomatic. This lack of symptoms is not surprising. Although cyanosis may occur with methemoglobin levels as low as 10%, symptoms resulting from impaired tissue oxygenation, such as fatigue, dyspnea, or headache, do not usually occur until methemoglobin levels exceed 20% to 25% or more.[55,56] Tafenoquine-induced methemoglobinemia is therefore not likely to pose a problem for most people. For members of selected groups that are more vulnerable to the effects of impaired oxygen delivery to tissue, this side effect may be an important consideration. Examples of such groups include aviators, mountaineers planning climbs to high altitudes, and patients with significant underlying cardiac or pulmonary disease.

INDICATIONS AND STRATEGIES FOR CLINICAL USE

At this time, tafenoquine is not commercially available, and regulatory authorities have not approved it for routine clinical use. Specific indications for tafenoquine's use and the dosing regimens to apply against those indications remain to be decided. However, the likely outlines of imminent recommendations are coming into focus. Any use of tafenoquine in G6PD-deficient individuals is contraindicated. Whether this precaution might eventually be softened to allow its use in the presence of partial G6PD activity will depend on information not yet obtained. Recommended indications for using tafenoquine for prophylaxis against *Plasmodium falciparum* and *Plasmodium vivax* and for relapse prevention (radical cure) of *P. vivax* malaria will likely come first. Except for long-term prophylaxis (longer than 1 to 2 months), regimens for these indications may be as brief as 3 days, using 200 to 400 mg of tafenoquine base daily. The ability to use a single drug, with so brief a regimen, for both prophylaxis and relapse prevention will be a significant advance.

Indications for using tafenoquine to cure clinical illness due to *Plasmodium falciparum* or *Plasmodium vivax* are likely to be slower in coming if they come at all. Given tafenoquine's slow schizonticidal action against blood-stage parasites, any regimens employing tafenoquine for clinical cure are likely to combine it with other (presumably faster-acting) antimalarials. Such combination therapy would offer the additional advantage of slowing the development of plasmodial resistance to tafenoquine. Despite their theoretic appeal, such combinations of tafenoquine with other antimalarials should be validated in clinical trials rather than introduced empirically. Drug combinations are not necessarily synergistic or even additive in effect. In vitro data have already suggested the possibility of an antagonistic interaction between tafenoquine and at least one other potential new antimalarial agent.[57]

Preventing the development of resistance to tafenoquine in plasmodia is not a major concern when the drug is used by travelers who depart endemic areas after brief visits. In contrast, if residents of malaria-endemic areas were to use tafenoquine, induction of resistance would become a much more serious issue. In these settings, tafenoquine's long half-life may foster resistance as blood drug levels wane and parasites receive prolonged exposure to subinhibitory drug levels.[17,58] Its prolonged elimination suggests that tafenoquine might be much more likely to induce resistance than its rapidly eliminated analogue, primaquine. If tafenoquine were to induce resistance by a mechanism that also counteracted primaquine, the subsequent ineffectiveness of both drugs could leave patients with no effective therapy for eradicating liver-stage plasmodia. These considerations should inhibit the use of tafenoquine in permanent residents of malaria-endemic regions.

At this time, a correlation between naturally existing primaquine refractoriness and tafenoquine refractoriness or resistance has not been shown. Tafenoquine failures have occurred in two patients with suspected primaquine-refractory *P. vivax*, but a firm correlation could not be established.[29] If some wild strains of *P. vivax* are already tafenoquine refractory, then concerns about the selective pressure exerted by prolonged subinhibitory tafenoquine blood levels assume even greater urgency.

(The views and assertions contained above are those of the author and do not claim to be the positions of the U.S. Air Force, the U.S. Department of Defense, or the U.S. Government.)

REFERENCES

1. Guttmann P, Ehrlich P. Über die Wirkung des Methylenblau bei Malaria. Berl Klin Wochenschr 1891 Sept 28;39:953–956.
2. Coggeshall LT, Craige B. Old and new plasmodicides. In: Boyd MF, editor. Malariology: a comprehensive survey of all aspects of this group of diseases from a global standpoint. Philadelphia: W.B. Saunders, 1949 p. 1071–1114.
3. Bruce-Chwatt LJ. History of malaria from prehistory to eradication. In: Wernsdorfer WH, McGregor I, editors. Malaria: principles and practice of malariology. New York: Churchill Livingstone, 1988. p. 1–59.
4. Arnold J, Alving AS, Hockwald RS, et al. The antimalarial action of primaquine against the blood and tissue stages of falciparum malaria (Panama, P-F-6 strain). J Lab Clin Med 1955;46:391–397.
5. Pukrittayakamee S, Vanijanonta S, Chantra A, et al. Blood stage antimalarial efficacy of primaquine in *Plasmodium vivax* malaria. J Infect Dis 1994;169:932–935.
6. Basco LK, Bickii J, Ringwald P. In-vitro activity of primaquine against the asexual blood stages of *Plasmodium falciparum*. Ann Trop Med Parasitol 1999;93:179–182.
7. Edgcomb JH, Arnold J, Yount EH Jr, et al. Primaquine, SN 13272, a new curative agent in vivax malaria: a preliminary report. J Natl Malaria Soc 1950;9:285–289.
8. World Health Organization. World malaria situation in 1990. World Health Stat Q 1992;45:257–266.
9. Hoffman SL, Rustama D, Dimpudus AJ, et al. RII and RIII type resistance of *Plasmodium falciparum* to combination of mefloquine and sulfadoxine/pyrimethamine in Indonesia. Lancet 1985;2:1039–1040.
10. Weiss WR, Oloo AJ, Johnson A, et al. Daily primaquine is effective for prophylaxis against falciparum malaria in Kenya: comparison with mefloquine, doxycycline, and chloroquine plus proguanil. J Infect Dis 1995;171:1569–1575.
11. Soto J, Toledo J, Rodriguez M, et al. Primaquine prophylaxis against malaria in non-immune Colombian soldiers: efficacy and toxicity. A randomized, double-blind, placebo-controlled trial. Ann Intern Med 1998;129:241–244.
12. Fryauff DJ, Baird JK, Basri H, et al. Randomised, placebo-controlled trial of primaquine for prophylaxis of falciparum and vivax malaria. Lancet 1995;346:1190–1193.
13. Baird JK, Basri H, Subianto B, et al. Treatment of chloroquine-resistant *Plasmodium vivax* with chloroquine and primaquine or halofantrine. J Infect Dis 1995:171:1678–1682.

14. Peters W, Robinson BL, Milhous WK. The chemotherapy of rodent malaria. LI. Studies on a new 8-aminoquinoline, WR 238,605. Ann Trop Med Parasitol 1993;87: 547–552.

15. Gutteridge WE. Antimalarial drugs currently in development. J R Soc Med 1989;82 Suppl 17:63–66.

16. Fisk TL, Millet P, Collins WE, Nguyen-Dinh P. In vitro activity of antimalarial compounds on the exoerythrocytic stages of *Plasmodium cynomolgi* and *P. knowlesi*. Am J Trop Med Hyg 1989;40:235–239.

17. Peters W. The evolution of tafenoquine—antimalarial for a new millennium? J R Soc Med 1999;92:345–352.

18. Idowu OR, Peggins JO, Brewer TG, Kelley C. Metabolism of a candidate 8-aminoquinoline antimalarial agent, WR 238605, by rat liver microsomes. Drug Metab Dispos 1995;23:1–17.

19. Lell B, Faucher JF, Missinou MA, et al. Malaria chemoprophylaxis with tafenoquine: a randomised study. Lancet 2000;355:2041–2045.

20. Bates MD, Meshnick SR, Sigler CI, et al. In vitro effects of primaquine and primaquine metabolites on exoerythrocytic stages of *Plasmodium berghei*. Am J Trop Med Hyg 1990;42:532–537.

21. Vennerstrom JL, Nuzum EO, Miller RE, et al. 8-Aminoquinolines active against blood stage *Plasmodium falciparum* in vitro inhibit hematin polymerization. Antimicrob Agents Chemother 1999;43:598–602.

22. Aikawa M, Beaudoin RL. *Plasmodium fallax*: high-resolution autoradiography of exoerythrocytic stages treated with primaquine in vitro. Exp Parasitol 1970;27:454–463.

23. Howells RE, Peters W, Fullard J. The chemotherapy of rodent malaria. XIII. Fine structural changes observed in the erythrocytic stages of *Plasmodium berghei berghei* following exposure to primaquine and menoctone. Ann Trop Med Parasitol 1970;64:203–207.

24. Hiebsch RR, Raub TJ, Wattenberg BW. Primaquine blocks transport by inhibiting the formation of functional transport vesicles: studies in a cell-free assay of protein transport through the Golgi apparatus. J Biol Chem 1991;266:20323–20328.

25. van Weert AW, Geuze HJ, Groothuis B, Stoorvogel W. Primaquine interferes with membrane recycling from endosomes to the plasma membrane through a direct interaction with endosomes which does not involve neutralisation of endosomal pH nor osmotic swelling of endosomes. Eur J Cell Biol 2000;79:394–399.

26. Slater AFG, Cerami A. Inhibition by chloroquine of a novel haem polymerase enzyme activity in malaria trophozoites. Nature 1992;355:167–169.

27. Ridley RG, Dorn A, Vippagunta SR, Vennerstrom JL. Haematin (haem) polymerization and its inhibition by quinoline antimalarials. Ann Trop Med Parasitol 1997;91:559–566.

28. Brueckner RP, Coster T, Kin-Ahn G, et al. Safety, pharmacokinetics, and antimalarial activity of WR 238605 in man [abstract]. Am J Trop Med Hyg 1997;57(3 Suppl):278–279.

29. Walsh DS, Looareesuwan S, Wilairatana P, et al. Randomized dose-ranging study of the safety and efficacy of WR 238605 (tafenoquine) in the prevention of relapse of *Plasmodium vivax* malaria in Thailand. J Infect Dis 1999;180:1282–1287.

30. Brueckner RP, Lasseter KC, Lin ET, Schuster BG. First-time-in-humans safety and pharmacokinetics of WR 238605, a new antimalarial. Am J Trop Med Hyg 1998;58:645–649.

31. Brueckner RP, Coster T, Wesche DL, et al. Prophylaxis of *Plasmodium falciparum* infection in a human challenge model with WR 238605, a new 8-aminoquinoline antimalarial. Antimicrob Agents Chemother 1998;42:1293–1294.

32. Kocisko DA, Walsh DS, Eamsila C, Edstein MD. Measurement of tafenoquine (WR 238605) in human plasma and venous and capillary blood by high-pressure liquid chromatography. Ther Drug Monit 2000;22:184–189.

33. Singhasivanon V, Sabcharoen A, Attanath P, et al. Pharmacokinetics of primaquine in healthy volunteers. Southeast Asian J Trop Med Public Health 1991;22:527–533.

34. Brueckner RP, Fleckenstein L. Simultaneous modeling of the pharmacokinetics and methemoglobin pharmacodynamics of an 8-aminoquinoline candidate antimalarial (WR 238605). Pharm Res 1991;8:1505–1510.

35. Kortepeter M, Brown JD. A review of 79 patients with malaria seen at a military hospital in Hawaii from 1979 to 1995. Mil Med 1998;163:84–89.

36. Brandts CH, Wernsdorfer WH, Kremsner PG. Decreasing chloroquine resistance in *Plasmodium falciparum* isolates from Gabon. Trans R Soc Trop Med Hyg 2000;94:554–556.

37. Pradines B, Mabika Mamfoumbi M, Parzy D, et al. In vitro susceptibility of African isolates of *Plasmodium falciparum* from Gabon to pyronaridine. Am J Trop Med Hyg 1999;60:105–108.

38. Hale BR, Owusu-Agyei S, Koram KA, et al. A randomized, double-blinded, placebo-controlled trial of tafenoquine for prophylaxis against *Plasmodium falciparum* in Ghana [abstract]. Am J Trop Med Hyg 2000;62(3 Suppl):139–140.

39. Shanks GD, Oloo AJ, Aleman GM, et al. A new primaquine analogue, tafenoquine (WR 238605), for prophylaxis against *Plasmodium falciparum* malaria. [Manuscript in preparation]

40. World Health Organization. World malaria situation in 1994. Wkly Epidemiol Rec 1997;72:269–274.

41. Walsh DS, Eamsila C, Sasiprapha T, et al. Randomized, double-blind, placebo controlled evaluation of monthly WR 238605 (tafenoquine) for prophylaxis of *Plasmodium falciparum* and *P. vivax* in Royal Thai Army soldiers [abstract]. Am J Trop Med Hyg 1999;61(3 Suppl):502.

42. Collins WE, Jeffrey GM. Primaquine resistance in *P. vivax*. Am J Trop Med Hyg 1996;55:243–249.

43. Looareesuwan S, Buchachart K, Wilairatana P. Primaquine-tolerant vivax malaria in Thailand. Ann Trop Med Parasitol 1997;91:939–943.

44. Cooper RD, Milhous WK, Rieckmann KH. The efficacy of WR238605 against the blood stages of a chloroquine resistant strain of *Plasmodium vivax*. Trans R Soc Trop Med Hyg 1994;88:691–692.

45. Obaldia N III, Rossan RN, Cooper RD, et al. WR 238605, chloroquine, and their combinations as blood schizonticides against a chloroquine-resistant strain of *Plasmodium vivax* in *Aotus* monkeys. Am J Trop Med Hyg 1997;56:508–510.

46. Nasveld PE, Edstein MD, Kitchener J, Rieckmann KH. Comparison of tafenoquine (WR238605) and primaquine in the terminal prophylaxis of vivax malaria in Australian Defence Force personnel serving in Bougainville, Papua New Guinea [abstract]. Am J Trop Med Hyg 2000;62(3 Suppl):315.

47. Rieckmann KH, Yeo AE, Davis DR, et al. Recent military experience with malaria chemoprophylaxis. Med J Aust 1993;158:446–449.

48. Schuurkamp GJ, Spicer PE, Kereu RK, et al. Chloroquine-resistant *Plasmodium vivax* in Papua New Guinea. Trans R Soc Trop Med Hyg 1992;86:121–122.

49. Coatney GR, Cooper WC, Young MD. Studies in human malaria: XXX. A summary of 204 sporozoite-induced infections with the Chesson strain of *Plasmodium vivax.* J Natl Malaria Soc 1950;9:381–396.

50. Coleman RE. Sporontocidal activity of the antimalarial WR-238605 against *Plasmodium berghei* ANKA in *Anopheles stephensi.* Am J Trop Med Hyg 1990;42:196–205.

51. Coleman RE, Clavin AM, Milhous WK. Gametocytocidal and sporontocidal activity of antimalarials against *Plasmodium berghei* ANKA in ICR Mice and *Anopheles stephensi* mosquitoes. Am J Trop Med Hyg 1992;46:169–182.

52. Clyde DF. Clinical problems associated with the use of primaquine as a tissue schizon-tocidal and gametocytocidal drug. Bull World Health Organ 1981;59:391–395.

53. Glader BE, Lukens JN. Glucose-6-phosphate dehydrogenase deficiency and related dis-orders of hexose monophosphate shunt and glutathione metabolism. In: Lee GR, Foerster J, Lukens J, et al., editors. Wintrobe's clinical hematology. 10th ed. Balti-more: Lippincott, Williams, & Wilkins, 1999. p. 1176–1190.

54. Hockwald RS, Arnold J, Clayman CB, Alving AS. Toxicity of primaquine in negroes. JAMA 1952;149:1568–1570.

55. Finch CA. Methemoglobinemia and sulfhemoglobinemia. N Engl J Med 1948;239:470–478.

56. Lukens JN. Methemoglobinemia and other disorders accompanied by cyanosis. In: Lee GR, Foerster J, Lukens J, et al., editors. Wintrobe's clinical hematology. 10th ed. Bal-timore: Lippincott, Williams & Wilkins, 1999. p. 1046–1055.

57. Fleck SL, Robinson BL, Peters W. The chemotherapy of rodent malaria. LIV. Combi-nations of 'Fenozan B07' (Fenozan-50F), a difluorinated 3,3'-spirocyclopentane 1,2,4-trioxane, with other drugs against drug-sensitive and drug-resistant para-sites. Ann Trop Med Parasitol 1997;91:33–39.

58. White NJ, Nosten F, Looareesuwan S, et al. Averting a malaria disaster. Lancet 1999;353:1965–1967.

Chapter 9

MALARIA PREVENTION FOR PARTICULAR TRAVELERS

9.1 Long-Term Travelers

Hans O. Lobel and A. Russell Gerber

ABSTRACT

There are few longitudinal studies of malaria prevention in long-term travelers. Peace Corps volunteers (PCVs) represent one category of long-term travelers on whom data about the effectiveness and safety of antimalarial drugs are available. Since 1985, a comprehensive and active epidemiologic surveillance system has allowed the monitoring of health and morbidity trends among PCVs. This system followed the epidemic spread of chloroquine-resistant *Plasmodium falciparum* malaria throughout Africa in the late 1980s. The introduction of mefloquine resulted in a return to pre-epidemic incidence levels of malaria within two years. In a study involving 6,230 person-months of observation, weekly mefloquine was 94% more effective than chloroquine and 86% more effective than proguanil/chloroquine in preventing confirmed *P. falciparum* malaria. Adherence to drug regimens was similar between the two groups: 5% of PCVs taking weekly mefloquine reported delayed or missed doses compared with 10% of those taking chloroquine. No serious adverse drug reactions were reported with any malaria chemoprophylactic regimen. The frequency of adverse events among PCVs taking mefloquine was 44% among persons using it for fewer than four months but 19% among those using it for more than one year ($p < .0001$). Yet fewer than 1% of PCVs discontinued mefloquine because of an adverse event. Doxycycline has been used for malaria prophylaxis in fewer than 10% of PCVs, and newer agents such as atovaquone/proguanil (Malarone) are just becoming available.

Key words: malaria; malaria chemoprophylaxis; mefloquine; Peace Corps volunteers; *Plasmodium falciparum*; travelers' health.

Little information is available about the use of malaria preventive measures by expatriates. U.S. Peace Corps volunteers are the only category of long-term trav-

elers (expatriates) on whom longitudinal data are available to assess the effectiveness and safety of antimalarial drugs. Review of the Peace Corps experience
with malaria control in sub-Saharan Africa provides a unique opportunity to
assess the implications of the development of chloroquine-resistant *Plasmodium
falciparum* (CRPF), the impact of changes of malaria chemoprophylactic regimens on malaria incidence, and other important lessons to be learned from the
Peace Corps experience.

Since 1985, the Peace Corps has implemented a comprehensive active surveillance system designed to monitor health and morbidity trends in Peace Corps volunteers (PCVs), a large group of development volunteers serving in developing
countries around the world. In the 1990s, the Peace Corps provided over 34,800
volunteers to over 100 countries in all regions: Africa, inter-America, Eastern
Europe, the Near East, Asia, and the Pacific. PCVs in sub-Saharan Africa, Papua
New Guinea, the Solomon Islands, and Vanuatu are especially at a high risk of
exposure to malaria. A full-time Peace Corps Medical Officer (PCMO) (often a
nurse practitioner, a physician's assistant, or a registered nurse) is assigned in each
country to provide for physical examinations, disease diagnosis and treatment, and
necessary health education for PCVs. Most serious illnesses are detected because
PCVs generally obtain health care either from the PCMO directly or with the
PCMO's authorization. In Africa, an Area Peace Corps Medical Officer (APCMO),
a physician, is assigned to supervise and coordinate the medical care provided to
PCVs within regions of countries.[1] Guidelines developed by the Peace Corps Office
of Medical Services (OMS) in Washington, D.C., provide detailed criteria and
instructions for the treatment and prophylaxis of malaria.

The data used for surveillance of health conditions among PCVs come from
several sources: (1) PCMOs worldwide who submit monthly epidemiologic surveillance data to OMS; (2) individual case reports concerning assaults, in-country
hospitalizations, and country-sponsored (regional) medical evacuations (mede-
vacs); (3) the OMS Deaths in Service database; and (4) selected Postal Service unit
data for returned PCVs. Data management and analysis are provided by the Surveillance and Epidemiology Unit of the OMS. The data are published annually in
Health and Safety of the Volunteer.

The monthly epidemiologic surveillance system was initiated in 1985. Each
month, each PCMO completes a form detailing the number of cases of 39 health
conditions (listed in Table 9.1–1), the number of hospitalizations and medical
evacuations, and the number of volunteers and trainees (the total at-risk population) in the country. These data are sent monthly to the OMS. Country-specific
data are tabulated, and monthly, quarterly, or annual incidence rates (cases per 100
PCVs per year) are computed (Figure 9.1–1). This information is used to guide
treatment and prevention measures for PCVs.

Table 9.1–1. **Health Conditions and Diseases Monitored by the Peace Corps Epidemiologic Surveillance System***

Assault injuries	Confirmed falciparum malaria
Alcohol problems	Confirmed nonfalciparum malaria
Cardiovascular problems	Presumed malaria
Dental problems	Medical evacuations
Dermatitis	Mental health counseling
Environmental concerns	Asthma
Febrile illnesses	Lower respiratory illnesses
Filariasis	Upper respiratory illnesses
Gastrointestinal problems	Reported pregnancy
Diarrhea	Non-STD gynecologic infections
Helminth infection	Genital ulcers
Hepatitis	Genital warts
Hospitalizations	Other STDs
Pedestrian injuries	Schistosomiasis
Bicycle injuries	Reported tuberculosis PPD conversions
Motorcycle injuries	Active tuberculosis
Motor vehicular injuries	PCV contacts with PCMO
Water injuries	Malaria chemoprophylaxis by agent
Other unintentional injuries	Vaccine and immunobiologic use by agent
	Typhoid vaccine

PCMO = Peace Corps medical officer; PCV = Peace Corps volunteer; PPD = purified protein derivative; STD = sexually transmitted disease.
* Data, (including number of PCVs in the country) collected monthly. Specified diseases require laboratory confirmation.

MALARIA AMONG PEACE CORPS VOLUNTEERS

PCVs typically live and work for 2- to 3-year terms in towns or rural areas. In countries with malaria transmission, PCVs may be exposed to malaria. The epidemiologic surveillance system distinguishes between laboratory-confirmed *Plasmodium falciparum* and nonfalciparum malaria and presumptive malaria. In addition, the number of PCVs using chemoprophylaxis is recorded in accordance with the drug(s) used, providing an estimate of the drug-specific denominators. PCVs in East Africa experienced a moderate increase of malaria in the early 1980s. In contrast, in West Africa, the incidence of *P. falciparum* among PCVs increased fourfold in 4 years, from 6 cases per 100 PCVs in 1986 to 42 cases per 100 PCVs in 1989. Malaria outbreaks occurred among volunteers in Benin and Togo in September and December 1986, followed by sharp incidence increases in 1988 in Ghana, Liberia, Mali, and Sierra Leone. Since chloroquine was used for prophylaxis before and at the time of the sudden increases in laboratory-confirmed malaria cases, these data strongly suggested that CRPF had become widespread. This hypothesis was supported by chloro-

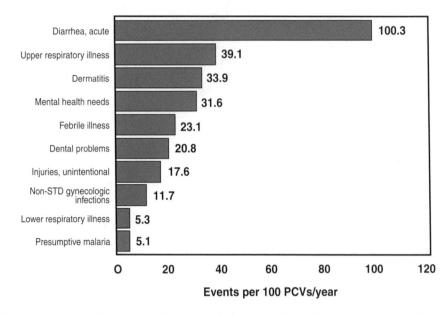

Figure 9.1–1. 1999 Africa region volunteer health profile; incidence of the 10 most commonly report-ed health-related events. STD = sexually transmitted disease. (Reproduced with permission from the Peace Corps Office of Medical Services. The 1999 annual report of volunteer health, 1999. p. 6.)

quine levels measured in PCVs with acute *P. falciparum* malaria; these levels were consistent with their reported histories of taking regular prophylaxis.[2]

Between 1986 and 1989, hundreds of confirmed *P. falciparum* infections occurred among PCVs in Africa taking weekly chloroquine phosphate prophylax-is, with or without concurrent use of daily proguanil (chloroguanide hydrochlo-ride.) The rapid increase of confirmed cases of *P. falciparum* infection led to an increase of patients in the small in-country Peace Corps hospitals, patients with severe organ involvement (renal failure, coma), and patients requiring medical evacuation. The limited ability to prevent malaria among PCVs led the Peace Corps in the late 1980s to consider the withdrawal of PCVs from Africa.

Because chloroquine prophylaxis, either alone or in combination with proguanil prophylaxis, seemed not to be effective any longer in reliably preventing *P. falci-parum* malaria, a more effective drug was needed. Of the newer antimalarials, mefloquine was recommended by the World Health Organization for prophylaxis for short-term travelers to West Africa and to areas with multidrug-resistant *P. falci-parum*.[3] In the United States, a New Drug Application for mefloquine was submit-ted to the Food and Drug Administration (FDA) in February 1986, and the drug was approved in 1989. This drug was made available to PCVs by the end of 1989, and routine surveillance of its efficacy and side effects was intensified because (1) meflo-quine had not been extensively used by U.S. citizens abroad, (2) FDA approval could not guarantee the safety and efficacy of the drug, and (3) no data were available on the use of mefloquine for long-term prophylaxis by nonimmune persons.

Because of concern that resistance to mefloquine might develop in Africa as it had in Southeast Asia, individual case reports (along with blood smears to confirm the diagnosis of malaria and blood samples to determine mefloquine concentration) on any PCVs in sub-Saharan Africa who were diagnosed with malaria were sent to the Centers for Disease Control (CDC).

Methods of Assessing Chemoprophylaxis

Estimates of the effectiveness of the malaria-prophylactic drugs used by PCVs—mefloquine, chloroquine, and chloroquine/proguanil—are based on observations, from October 1989 to May 1992, of PCVs in Benin, Ghana, Guinea, Liberia, Sierra Leone, and Togo (West Africa). Estimates of the tolerance of chemoprophylaxis are based on a study of 1,322 PCVs throughout sub-Saharan Africa.

Each episode of suspected malaria was documented as far as possible by blood slide examination, and the slides were sent to the CDC for reference examination. A detailed history of malaria prophylaxis was recorded, and if mefloquine had been used, a blood sample was collected to determine the blood concentration of mefloquine.[4] Each serious episode of adverse reaction was reported in detail by cable to the OMS in Washington, D.C. In addition, each PCV completed a questionnaire every 4 months, recording chemoprophylaxis use and any adverse health event perceived by the PCV to be associated with prophylaxis. A blood sample to determine the blood concentration of mefloquine was also obtained at that time from those using mefloquine prophylaxis. The incidence of malaria, the clinical tolerance of the prophylactic regimens, and the compliance with the drug regimens were compared between the regimens used (mefloquine, chloroquine, and chloroquine/proguanil).

In accordance with the manufacturer's recommendations listed in the FDA approval, the dosing regimen for adults was one tablet of mefloquine base every 2 weeks, after a loading dose regimen of one tablet weekly for the first 4 weeks. This regimen was used between October 1989 and November 1990. It was decided to change to weekly dosing with mefloquine at the end of November 1990 because biweekly mefloquine prophylaxis was found to be only 56% more effective than prophylaxis with chloroquine.

Results of Chemoprophylaxis

Effectiveness

An average of 421 PCVs were stationed in West Africa between October 1989 and May 1992, for a total of 13,487 person-months. Mefloquine every 2 weeks was used between October 1989 and November 1990, for a total of 3,328 person-months (Table 9.1–2).[5] Between December 1990 and May 1992, mefloquine was used weekly, for a total of 6,230 person-months. Between October 1989 and November 1990, 45 *P. falciparum* infections were diagnosed in PCVs using mefloquine every 2 weeks, indicating an incidence of 1.4 cases per 100 volunteers per month. The

Table 9.1–2. **Incidence of Infections Among Peace Corps Volunteers in West Africa**

Drug	Person-Months	Infections	Incidence*	Relative Risk (95% CI)
		Oct. 1989 to Nov.1990		
Chloroquine	844	26	3.1	1.00
Mefloquine every 2 weeks	3,328	45	1.4	0.44 (0.27–0.71)
Chloroquine and proguanil	1,828	39	2.1	0.70 (0.42–1.14)
		Dec. 1990 to May 1992		
Chloroquine	236	9	3.8	1.00
Mefloquine weekly	6,230	15	0.2	0.06 (0.03–0.14)
Chloroquine and proguanil	574	10	1.7	0.46 (0.19–1.12)

CI = confidence interval.

monthly incidence was 3.1 cases per 100 volunteers among users of chloroquine alone. Mefloquine used every 2 weeks was thus found to be only 56% more effective than chloroquine prophylaxis and 37% more effective than prophylaxis with chloroquine/proguanil.[6]

Prophylaxis with weekly mefloquine was 94% more effective than prophylaxis with chloroquine and 86% more effective than prophylaxis with chloroquine and proguanil. The addition of daily proguanil to weekly chloroquine did not siginificantly increase the effectiveness of chloroquine. Weekly mefloquine was 82% more effective than mefloquine used every 2 weeks. Blood samples were obtained within 5 days of diagnosis from 25 of the 60 volunteers who developed malaria while using mefloquine prophylaxis. The mean mefloquine blood concentration was 384 ng/mL (standard deviation [SD] 176 ng/mL). A probit analysis suggested that a prophylactic efficacy of 99% can be achieved at a mefloquine blood concentration of about 915 ng/mL, a 95% efficacy at a concentration of 620 ng/mL, and a 90% efficacy at a concentration of 462 ng/mL.[6]

Two years after the introduction of mefloquine, the incidence had declined to a pre-epidemic level (Figure 9.1–2).

Compliance

Compliance with taking chemoprophylaxis was not complete: 5% of PCVs who used weekly mefloquine, 6% of PCVs who used mefloquine every other week, and 10% of PCVs using chloroquine said that they had missed or delayed one or more doses.

Adverse Reactions

No serious adverse drug reactions or hospital admissions associated with any of the used chemoprophylactic regimens were reported. Except in the case of nausea, the

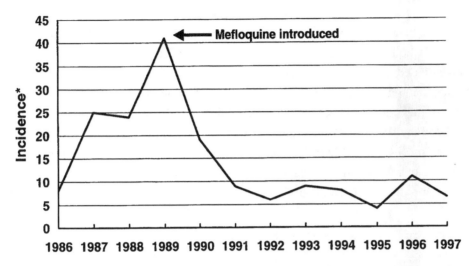

Figure 9.1–2. Incidence* of *Plasmodium falciparum* malaria among Peace Corps volunteers in West Africa, 1986 to 1997.

frequency and type of the mild adverse events reported were similar in mefloquine users and chloroquine users (Table 9.1–3). Importantly, only 6 (1.8%) of the mefloquine users reported that the adverse events interfered with their daily activities, compared with 11 (4.6%) of the chloroquine users ($p = .07$). Fifty-two (15.9%) mefloquine users sought medical advice for adverse events, as did 37 (15.5%) chloroquine users ($p = .994$). Few serious adverse health events could be attributed to any of the used drug regimens. Only 7 (0.9%) of 802 volunteers discontinued mefloquine prophylaxis because of adverse events.

A cohort of 152 PCVs who had used mefloquine for prophylaxis for more than 1 year was analyzed for changes in the rate of adverse reactions over time. The percentage of these PCVs who reported adverse events decreased with prolonged use of

Table 9.1–3. Side Effects of Mefloquine and Chloroquine

Side Effect	Mefloquine (N=802) (%)	Chloroquine* (N=520) (%)
Strange dreams	24.7	26.0
Nausea	8.7**	22.1**
Diarrhea	4.0	2.7
Dizziness	8.4	6.5
Insomnia	9.0	10.0
Weakness	5.2	2.5
Visual difficulties	6.5	7.5
Any event	40.6	45.8

* With or without proguanil.
** $p < .0001$.

mefloquine, from 44% of volunteers who had used mefloquine for less than 4 months to 40% of those who had used mefloquine between 4 and 7 months, 29% of those who had used the drug between 8 and 11 months, and 19% among those who had used mefloquine for more than 1 year (χ^2 for trend = 25.47, $p < .0001$), suggesting that the drug was well tolerated. A pharmacokinetic study showed that blood levels of mefloquine did not increase after steady state had been achieved.[7]

Between 1989 and 1999, 17,000 PCVs used mefloquine weekly, each for 2 to 3 years, for a total of 43,000 person-years of exposure to mefloquine. The long-term use of mefloquine for malaria prophylaxis has been well tolerated by users and has not been associated with an increase of adverse health events.

DISCUSSION AND CONCLUSION

Malaria presents a significant concern for PCVs in sub-Saharan Africa and in Oceania (Papua New Guinea, the Solomon Islands, and Vanuatu) because of the high levels of malaria transmission, the presence of CRPF, and the high risk of exposure to malaria in these regions. PCVs in these countries represent a unique group of nonimmune individuals who are highly exposed to malaria and other diseases. An intensive medical support mechanism is in place, and an epidemiologic surveillance system permits identification of significant health problems and assessment of the effect of control measures. The experience with malaria control measures is an excellent example. When the reduced effectiveness of chloroquine for malaria prophylaxis became apparent, first in East Africa and subsequently in West Africa, mefloquine was made available, and an intensified surveillance system that could measure the effectiveness and tolerance of mefloquine within a relatively short time was instituted. Since 1991, malaria has resumed its place as an important but not overwhelmingly threatening health problem. Continuation of the surveillance during the past 10 years has permitted the monitoring of the development of resistance to mefloquine in Africa, using well-defined criteria.[8] No evidence of resistance to mefloquine has been detected. This is important not only for PCVs but also for other expatriates exposed to malaria, for the military, and for short-term travelers in this setting.

The evidence that mefloquine was well tolerated by PCVs has been confirmed by data from 12 other prospective cohort studies (including 6 randomized double-blind placebo-controlled trials with 528 users of mefloquine and 7 comparative studies [N = 54,804]) that have failed to show important differences in adverse events among users of mefloquine, chloroquine, or placebo.[9]

It has not been possible to assess the effectiveness and tolerance of doxycycline in PCVs because few PCVs (< 10%) prefer to use this drug.

Significant resistance to mefloquine may develop in sub-Saharan Africa or Oceania, and new drugs are therefore needed. One such drug, atovaquone/

proguanil (Malarone), has recently been licensed by the FDA for treatment and prophylaxis. The need for daily dosing is a drawback for this drug, and only limited experience is currently available regarding its effectiveness and tolerance. Another drug, WR 238605 (tafenoquine), is being developed and is awaiting field trials among nonimmune persons.

The Peace Corps experience emphasizes the importance of epidemiologic information to treatment and to prophylaxis guidelines and practices. Organizationally, the Peace Corps medical care system is characterized by a well-defined at-risk population, centralized medical care, and excellent communication facilities—advantages that other temporary residents of developing countries may not have. However, such a system could be developed and adapted for use by private and other governmental volunteer organizations, international businesses, and international diplomatic communities. With the increasing availability of sophisticated telecommunications, computers, and digital cameras, such groups (individually alone or in combinations) could also provide medical care and monitor diseases and health conditions among their members, thus providing useful epidemiologic surveillance information needed for disease control and prevention efforts for both travelers and national populations in developing countries.[1]

REFERENCES

1. Bernard KW, Graitcer PL, van der Vlugt T, et al. Epidemiological surveillance in Peace Corps volunteers: a model for monitoring health in temporary residents of developing countries. Int J Epidemiol 1989;18:220–226.

2. Moran JS, Bernard KW. The spread of chloroquine-resistant malaria in Africa. JAMA 1989;262:245–248.

3. World Health Organization. Vaccination certificate requirements and health advice for international travel 1988. Geneva: World Health Organization, 1988. p. 46–52.

4. Bergquist Y, Hellgren U, Churchill F. High-performance liquid chromatographic assay for the simultaneous monitoring of mefloquine and its acid metabolite in biological samples using protein precipitation and ion-pair extraction. J Chromatogr 1988;432:253–263.

5. Lobel HO, Bernard KW, Williams SL, et al. Effectiveness and tolerance of long-term malaria prophylaxis with mefloquine. JAMA 1991;265:361–364.

6. Lobel HO, Miani M, Eng T, et al. Long-term malaria prophylaxis with weeky mefloquine. Lancet 1993;341:848–851.

7. Pennie RA, Koren G, Crevoisier C. Steady state pharmacokinetics of mefloquine in long-term travelers. Trans R Soc Trop Med Hyg 1993;87:459–462.

8. Lobel HO, Varma JK, Miani M, et al. Monitoring for mefloquine-resistant *Plasmodium falciparum* in Africa: implications for travelers' health. Am J Trop Med Hyg 1998;59:129–132.

9. Lobel HO, Kozarsky PE. Update on prevention of malaria for travelers. JAMA 1997;278:1767–1771.

9.2 Brief Exposure Malaria Prevention
J. Kevin Baird

ABSTRACT

This chapter discusses practical strategies for preventing malaria in travelers facing brief exposure. Personal protective measures may suffice where risk is relatively low, and new causal prophylactics provide practical protection against high-risk exposure. Estimating that risk represents the key element in deciding between personal protection measures and chemoprophylaxis. Primaquine and Malarone may be prescribed for prevention of malaria during brief exposure to risk. Malarone acts causally against *Plasmodium falciparum*, and primaquine acts causally against *P. falciparum* and *Plasmodium vivax*. Using these drugs precludes the necessity of 4 weeks of postexposure dosing common to the use of suppressive chemoprophylactics such as mefloquine or doxycycline.

Key words: brief exposure; causal prophylaxis; personal protection measures; risk.

INTRODUCTION

Travelers often face brief exposure to risk of malaria. This poses a special problem for health care providers who offer advice on preventing infection. Standard suppressive chemoprophylaxis requires a loading regimen and 4 weeks of postexposure dosing. A leisure ship carrying passengers out of Singapore bound for Hong Kong stops for 3 days at a port on the island of Borneo. Should chemoprophylaxis be prescribed? Do personal protective measures suffice? The answers require weighing specific risk factors and the practicality and availability of preventive measures. Two causal chemoprophylactics have recently emerged to create important options for travelers facing brief exposure to risk. This chapter brings these issues into focus.

What may be defined as brief exposure depends on the perspective of the traveler and the degree of inconvenience or risk imposed by indicated preventive measures. Compliance to recommended chemoprophylaxis using mefloquine requires a total of 5 weeks of dosing (1 week predeparture and 4 weeks postexposure), not including the period of travel. This represents the perspective for defining the term "brief exposure" in this discussion. While both risk of infection and safety of the drug play roles in this perspective, 1 week or less of exposure is considered brief.

SUPPRESSIVE VERSUS CAUSAL PROPHYLAXIS

Most practical references dealing with preventing malaria in travelers do not make the important distinction between suppressive and causal prophylactic drugs. This may be because no antimalarial licensed for prophylaxis exhibits causal activity. A recent and lone exception is Malarone (a fixed combination of atovaquone and proguanil), which exhibits causal activity against *Plasmodium falciparum* but perhaps not against *Plasmodium vivax*. Standard chemoprophylactics such as mefloquine, doxycycline, and chloroquine/proguanil exert suppressive activity. This means the drug kills plasmodia emerging from the liver and attempting development in the blood stream. This mechanism explains the necessity of continuing suppressive drugs for 4 weeks after exposure. In contrast, antimalarials having causal activity kill parasites in the liver, precluding the necessity of dosing long after exposure to biting mosquitoes.

In the context of brief risk of malaria, the distinction between causal and suppressive prophylactics is crucial. Figure 9.2–1 illustrates a hypothetical 7-day trip to a malarious area. The graph highlights the advantage of causal prophylaxis. Whereas this particular exposure would necessitate 42 doses of doxycycline, just 9 doses of a causal prophylactic drug such as primaquine would be indicated (commencing on the day of arrival and ending 2 days after return). Causal prophylactics are the prevention strategy of choice where chemoprophylaxis is indicated for brief moderate-to-high risk of malaria. Personal protective measures often suffice for brief exposure to low risk. The primary determinant in deciding between chemoprophylaxis and personal protective measures is the degree of risk.

GAUGING RISK WITH BRIEF EXPOSURE

Standard references on the prevention of malaria rarely deal explicitly with travelers facing brief risk. This may be the product of two biases: (1) chemoprophylaxis

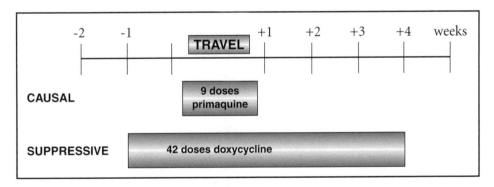

Figure 9.2–1. Comparison of causal versus suppressive chemoprophylactic regimens for a 1-week exposure to risk.

represents the most conservative recommendation for the prevention of malaria in people considered good candidates for such a measure, and (2) available chemoprophylactics have been suppressive rather than causal. Suppressive chemoprophylaxis for brief exposure constituted a heavy burden for the traveler. The point at which the risk, cost, and inconvenience of suppressive prophylaxis exceed the risk of infection is rarely clear. Travelers facing brief risk and the health care providers advising them typically weigh this formula in isolation. The availability of causal prophylactics now allows general recommendations for brief exposure to risk of infection. The crucial factor is the degree of risk; gauging it requires weighing the endemic risk at the destination (along with specific features of the itinerary such as location and style of accommodation) as well as the likelihood of contact with infectious anopheline mosquitoes during planned activities. Unlike longer trips, in which a broader range of activities and thus opportunities for exposure may be presumed, brief trips allow a reasonable assessment of risk by the evaluation of specific aspects of the itinerary. This assessment also provides a source of specific advice to the traveler for planning an itinerary that minimizes risk.

Table 9.2–1 lists five typical brief-exposure scenarios and the key factors in gauging risk of infection. The factors guide a reasonable estimation of risk and thus a decision to prescribe chemoprophylaxis, personal protective measures, or simply a modified itinerary. Whether the destination is urban or rural may be the most helpful factor. Most anopheline vectors shun urban habitats, favoring relatively pristine or pastoral environments instead. As a general rule, malaria transmission occurs in the countryside and not in the city. The risk of malaria tends to diminish as the size of the city increases. Cities on the Indian subcontinent represent important exceptions; the efficient vector *Anopheles stephensi* thrives in even the largest cities and actively transmits malaria. Another exception is Guyaquil, Equador, with an urban-adapted anopheline vector in residence. Travelers visiting large urban areas in Central and South America, Southeast and Southwest Asia, and Africa who refrain from excursions that put them in the countryside between dusk and dawn have little risk. However, just one overnight stay in the countryside carries a risk of exposure.

Table 9.2–1. **Gauging Risk of Infection after Brief Exposure**

Exposure	Typical Duration	Environment	Decisive Factors
Airport transit	1–24 hours	Rural	Local risk & season; night transit?
		Urban	Urban malaria? Leaving airport?
Seaport transit	1–3 days	Urban	Urban malaria? Leaving ship? Night excursion?
Business	1–7 days	Rural	Local risk & season; accommodation
		Urban	Urban malaria? accommodation; local itinerary
Holiday	1–7 days	Rural	Local risk & season; accommodation
		Urban	Urban malaria? accommodation; local itinerary
Local excursion	1–4 days	Rural	Local risk & season; accommodation

Assessing that risk requires considering the endemic risk (see Chapter 3), along with specific attributes of the itinerary, such as accommodations.

Accommodation where malaria transmission occurs is an important determinant of risk. Location and available amenities largely define that risk. Air-conditioned modern hotels at relatively cool elevations pose the lowest risk whereas more rustic accommodations (lacking air-conditioning and sealed doors and windows) at low elevations carry a relatively high risk. Campers in lowland endemic areas may be considered at highest risk.

Malaria transmission in some endemic areas may be limited to a particular season. However, areas where that season is strictly limited to a well-defined period are exceptional. Scheduling travel by low-risk season should be viewed as minimizing risk rather than as avoiding it. Although malaria risk often peaks during or immediately following rainy seasons, the dry season poses the highest risk in some areas. These patterns depend on the breeding habits of the local anopheline vectors. For example, *Anopheles maculatus* is an important vector of malaria on forested hillsides in Southeast Asia. It breeds in stagnant pools along rocky streams that appear only after heavy rainfall ceases. Health care providers who recommend travel out of season of risk should ascertain the seasonal pattern of malaria at the destination.

Travelers facing a relatively low risk of brief duration (as estimated by assessing the factors discussed above) may obtain adequate protection simply by diligently applying measures that minimize the likelihood of contact with biting anophelines (see below). While some travelers may find even the slightest risk of infection unacceptable and may demand chemoprophylaxis, others may need or wish to avoid exposure to drugs, even in the face of appreciable risk. The health care provider who interviews the individual traveler and who divines these personal preferences and attributes will recognize these as critical elements in the formulation of specific recommendations.

PERSONAL PROTECTIVE MEASURES

Personal protective measures are steps for avoiding contact with biting anopheline mosquitoes. These include avoidance and the use of nets, repellents, and certain types of clothing. The disciplined and appropriate application of these measures may greatly diminish risk but will almost never eliminate it completely. When exposure is relatively unlikely or brief, these measures alone may render the probability of infection acceptably low. (Chapter 6 details personal protective measures.)

CHEMOPROPHYLAXIS FOR BRIEF EXPOSURE

Appreciable risk of malaria from brief exposure should prompt a decision to prescribe causal prophylaxis in travelers considered good candidates for it. Two causal prophylactics are now available: primaquine and Malarone. These drugs are reviewed in depth elsewhere in this book (see Chapters 8.5 and 8.6). This discussion focuses on the decision to prescribe primaquine or Malarone for travelers facing brief exposure to risk.

Table 9.2–2 summarizes the key properties of primaquine and Malarone. The table lists differences between these drugs that may be weighed in deciding which is most appropriate for a given traveler. In general, primaquine may be considered superior when the risk of *Plasmodium vivax* infection occurs. Although Malarone exhibits good suppressive prophylactic activity against *P. vivax*, it has no apparent activity against latent hypnozoites of this parasite. Thus, the traveler facing brief risk of infection by *P. vivax* would have to take the drug for 7 days postexposure, and also consume the 14 days daily primaquine as terminal prophylaxis. Both drugs have shown good causal activity against *Plasmodium falciparum*. However, primaquine has little or no suppressive activity against *P. falciparum*. Although Malarone exhibits good suppressive activity against *P. falciparum*, a brief causal regimen may not apply that activity to breakthrough parasitemia (e.g., in the 3rd or 4th week after travel).

Table 9.2–2. **Key Properties and Dosing of Primaquine and Malarone as Casual Prophylaxis Against *Plasmodium falciparum* and *Plasmodium vivax* Infection**

	Primaquine		Malarone	
Property or Dose	P. falciparum	P. vivax	P. falciparum	P. vivax
Pre-exposure dosing	n/n	n/n	2 days	2 days
Exposure dose (adult dose)	0.5 mg/kg/d (two 15-mg tablets daily)	0.5 mg/kg/d (two 15-mg tablets daily)	ATQ 4.2 mg/kg/d + PGN 1.7 mg/kg/d (1 tablet [ATQ 250 mg + PGN 100 mg] daily)	ATQ 4.2 mg/kg/d + PGN 1.7 mg/kg/d (1 tablet [ATQ 250 mg + PGN 100 mg] daily)
Suppressive activity	No	Yes	Yes	Yes
Causal activity	Yes	Yes	Yes	No
Postexposure dose	2 days*	2 days*	7 days	7 days plus 14 days primaquine
Protective efficacy	>85%	>90%	>94%	81%[†]
Resistance	None known	None known	None known	None known
Pediatric use	Yes	Yes	Yes	Yes
Contraindications	G6PD deficiency; pregnancy	G6PD deficiency; pregnancy	Pregnancy	Pregnancy
Licensed in U.S.	No	No	Yes	No

ATQ = atovaquone; d = day; G6PD = glucose-6-phosphate dehydrogenase; n/n = not necessary; *P.* = *Plasmodium*; PGN = proguanil.
* Not firmly established in preventing relapse by *Plasmodium vivax* infection.
[†] Unpublished data from K. Baird.

It has been recommended that primaquine and Malarone be taken for 2 and 7 days after travel, respectively. These doses may represent a substantial proportion of the total dose administered to travelers who have brief exposure to risk. A traveler with a single day of risk takes only three daily doses of primaquine and eight doses of Malarone. Is this enough to prevent infection and (in the case of primaquine) relapse? None of the field trials of these drugs conducted in endemic areas address this issue. Those trials demonstrated good efficacy of 16- to 52-week dosing regimens, and none could evaluate postexposure parasitemia. Instead, the issue of prevention with a single dose must be addressed in the setting of an experimental challenge of volunteers in non-endemic areas. This work has been done with primaquine against *P. falciparum* and *P. vivax* and with Malarone against *P. falciparum.*

Arnold and colleagues[1] challenged 10 subjects with the Panama PF6 strain of *P. falciparum* on day 0 and then administered a single 30-mg dose of primaquine on day 1. No subject developed parasitemia. Arnold and colleagues[2] challenged 10 subjects with the primaquine-tolerant Chesson strain of *Plasmodium vivax* on day 0 and administered daily doses of 30 mg of primaquine on days –1 and 0 and on days 1 through 6. All of those subjects failed to develop parasitemia or relapse (after 12 months of follow-up). The single-dose experiment done with *Plasmodium falciparum* was not repeated with *Plasmodium vivax*. In summary, a single 30-mg daily dose of primaquine following exposure is apparently sufficient to prevent infection with *Plasmodium falciparum*, and it may suffice against relapse by *Plasmodium vivax*, but the data on this are incomplete. The recommendation for 2 days of postexposure dosing was intended to preclude *Plasmodium falciparum* infection and was estimated to prevent most *Plasmodium vivax* infection. A more conservative approach would be to recommend primaquine for the week following exposure to prevent relapse by *P. vivax* infection, where the available data show good protection. Shapiro and colleagues[3] administered single doses of 250 mg of atovaquone to six subjects the day before challenge, and none became patent.

Primaquine and Malarone both offer good options for practical protection from brief exposure to risk of malaria. The only clear preference for one over the other in most travelers is when there is risk of infection by *P. vivax* or *Plasmodium ovale*; in such cases, primaquine would effectively prevent relapse. Travelers with an inborn deficiency in glucose-6-phosphate dehydrogenase (G6PD) or those whose G6PD status is unknown should not receive primaquine. Malarone appears safe for such travelers. Commercially available qualitative tests for G6PD deficiency (e.g., the oxidized form of nicotinamide-adenine dinucleotide phosphate [NADP$^+$] spot test from Sigma Chemical Co., St. Louis, Missouri) require trained laboratory personnel but are relatively inexpensive (less than U.S. $1.00 per test), require no specialized equipment, use only a drop of blood, and can be completed in about 30 minutes.

The views expressed above are those of the author and do not purport to reflect or represent those of the U.S. Navy or the U.S. Department of Defense.

REFERENCES

1. Arnold J, Alving AS, Hockwald RS, et al. The antimalarial action of primaquine against the blood and tissue stages of falciparum malaria (Panama, P-F-6 strain). J Lab Clin Med 1955;46:391–397.
2. Arnold J, Alving AS, Hockwald RS, et al. The effect of continuous and intermittent primaquine therapy on the relapse rate of Chesson strain vivax malaria. J Lab Clin Med 1954;44:429–438.
3. Shapiro TA, Ranasinha CD, Kumar N, Barditch-Crovo P. Prophylactic activity of atovaquone against *Plasmodium falciparum* in humans. Am J Trop Med Hyg 1999;60:831–836.

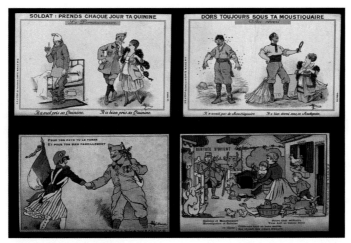

Figure 1–7 (see page 10)

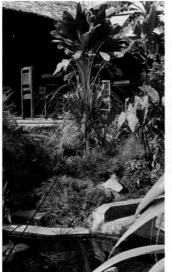

Figure 2–1 (see page 16)

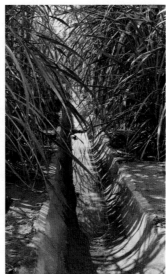

Figure 2–2 (see page 17)

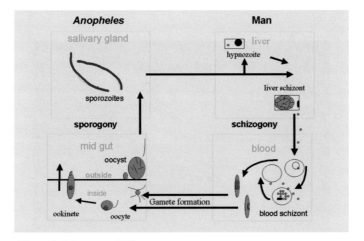

Figure 5–1 (see page 105)

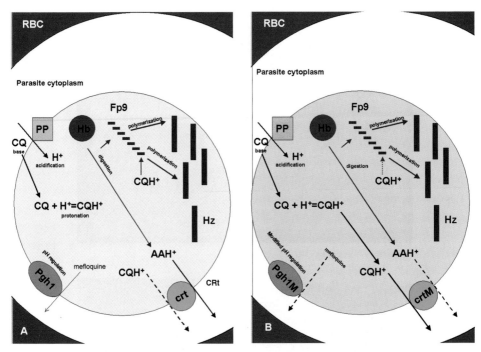

Figure 5–2 (see page 110)

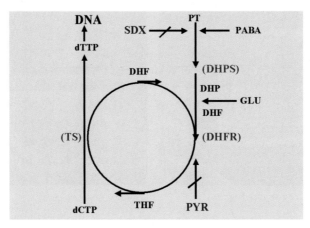

Figure 5–3 (see page 112)

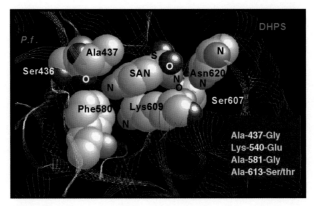

Figure 5–4 (see page 113)

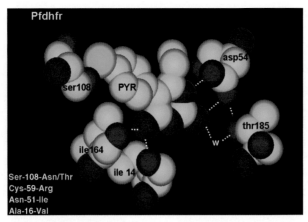

Figure 5–5 (see page 114)

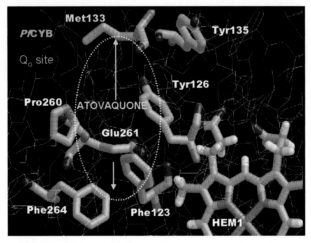

Figure 5–6 (see page 115)

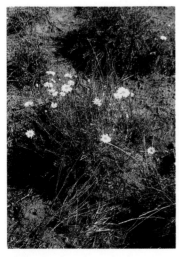

Figure 6–2 (see page 130)

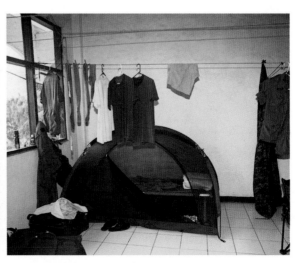

Figure 9.3–2 (see page 279)

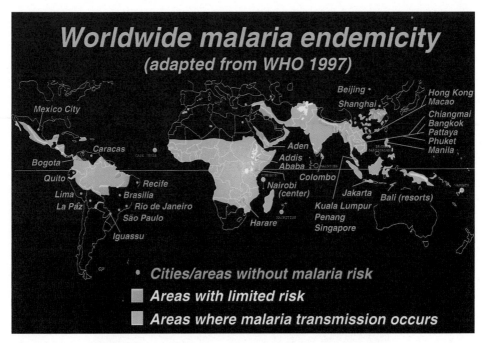

Figure 7–3 (see page 152)

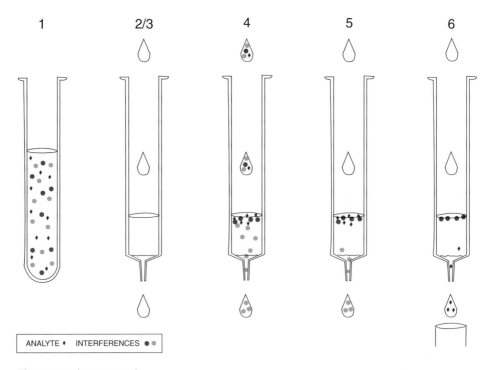

Figure 10–7 (see page 349)

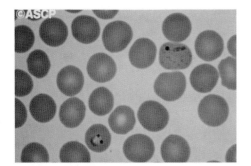

Figure 12–1 (see page 395)

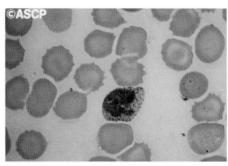

Figure 12–2 (see page 396)

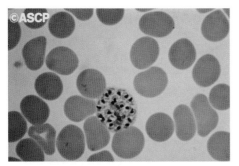

Figure 12–3 (see page 396)

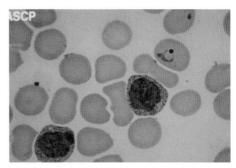

Figure 12–4 (see page 396)

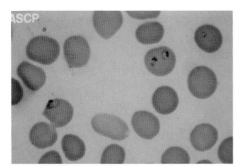

Figure 12–5 (see page 397)

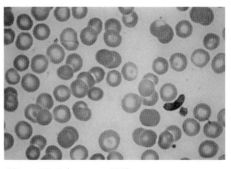

Figure 12–6 (see page 397)

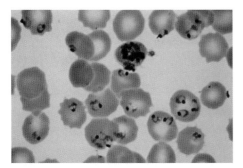

Figure 12–7 (see page 397)

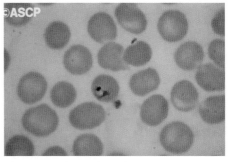

Figure 12–8 (see page 398)

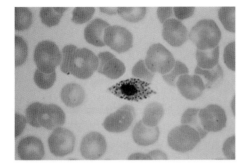

Figure 12–9 (see page 398)

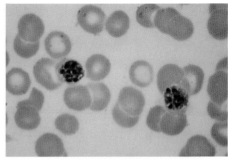

Figure 12–10 (see page 398)

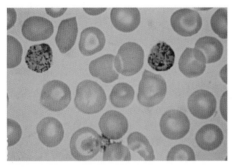

Figure 12–11 (see page 399)

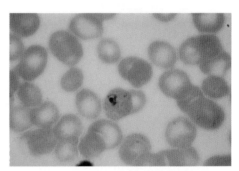

Figure 12–12 (see page 399)

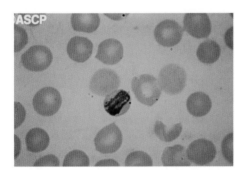

Figure 12–13 (see page 399)

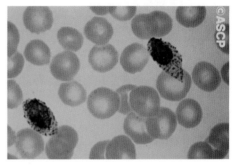

Figure 12–14 (see page 400)

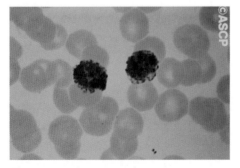

Figure 12–15 (see page 400)

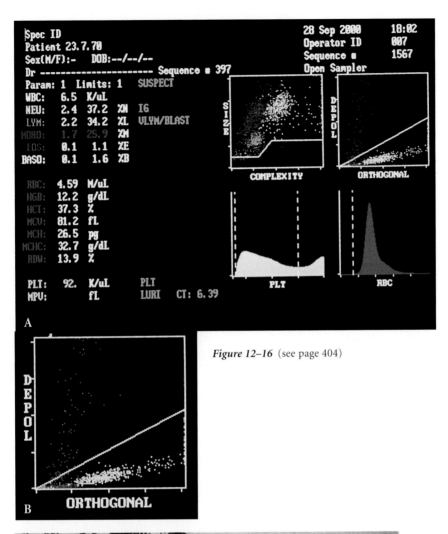

Figure 12–16 (see page 404)

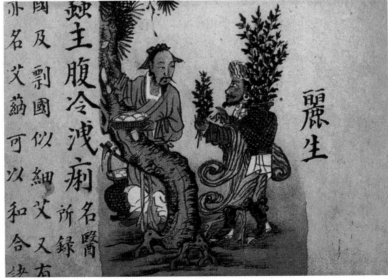

Figure 15–1 (see page 447)

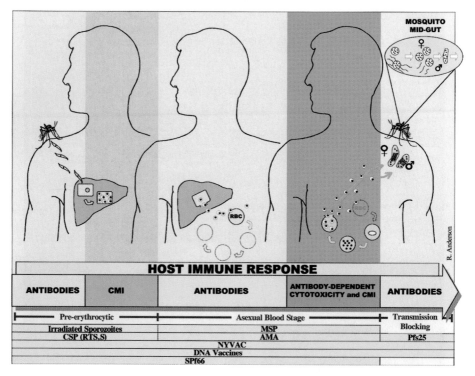

Figure 17–1 (see page 476)

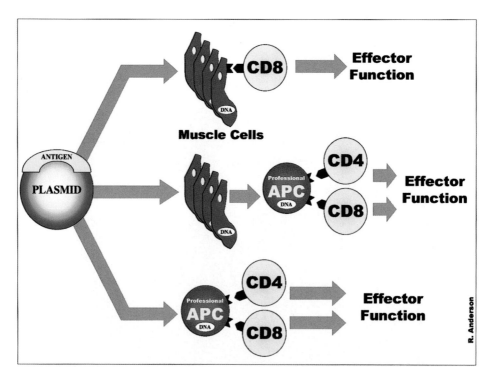

Figure 17–2 (see page 483)

9.3 *Military Perspective for Malaria Prevention*
Anne E. McCarthy

ABSTRACT

Malaria remains an important foe to military troops that deploy to tropical destinations. Preventive medicine personnel responsible for the health of these troops
are challenged with providing a mission-specific "universal" set of recommendations to minimize all health risks, including malaria. Successful preventive medicine programs incorporate the assessment of health risk, surveillance, and the
education of troops, commanders, and health care providers. Establishing the true
malaria risk for deploying troops may be hampered by differing exposure among
the troops, a paucity of information due to poor reporting, and unstable malaria
transmission within the country requiring military intervention. As with any
febrile illness, there is the need for early medical attention. As well, compliance with
malaria prevention measures, including personal protection measures and chemoprophylaxis, may be less than ideal.

Key words: malaria; military; preventive medicine.

ASSESSMENT OF MALARIA RISK

Throughout the history of armed conflicts, malaria has proven to be a serious
threat to military forces.[1-36] As modern military forces increasingly undertake missions to tropical locations throughout the world, there remains a significant risk of
many infectious diseases including malaria. Military medical personnel strive to
minimize the impact of all infectious diseases on troops deployed to foreign countries. They accomplish this through a comprehensive preventive medicine program
based on a detailed health threat assessment; a health surveillance program that
monitors health events during and following deployment; and an educational program to train soldiers, commanders, and health care providers about medical
threats and their prevention.

The assessment of health threat includes a thorough assessment of all potential
health risks that might diminish force effectiveness through troop morbidity or
mortality. Through the identification and evaluation of the health threats in areas
of planned deployment, medical personnel can prioritize these threats and implement specific preventive measures to reduce or eliminate them.

As with any travel medicine consultation, a risk assessment for the deploying
force as a whole is required. This entails detailed information about the group to be
protected, the specific activities of the group, the time and duration of the opera-

tion, and the precise geographic location. It is important to note that all groups of soldiers will not be at the same risk, a fact that presents a challenge to those providing preventive health advice.

The malaria threat to a military operation is complex. Troops are often deploying to areas where there has been a breakdown of the public health infrastructure due to ongoing strife, leading to inconsistent disease reporting and the failure to maintain routine preventive measures. Thus, the true malaria risk in many areas may not be known at a time when population migration and a breakdown in mosquito control measures may be re-introducing malaria to areas with previous successful mosquito eradication or control. To compound this problem, the itinerary of the deploying troops is seldom certain prior to departure. In fact, the geographic troop allocation in the destination country may not be finalized until after arrival. Also, individuals within a deploying force will not be facing the same malaria risk as they have varying job descriptions and accommodations. Some will be working in more urban environments, where there is potential for local mosquito control measures that decrease malaria risk, while others may be carrying out guard duty overnight in jungles or swamps, areas where compliance with personal protection measures against mosquitoes may be impossible. U.S. and Canadian experiences in Somalia revealed a much higher malaria attack rate in their special forces groups compared to that in the general military population in the country, illustrating the difficulties of protecting those at highest risk. The nature of special forces work often has these troops inhabiting areas of high malaria risk that require nighttime patrolling (often through swampy areas) where no local mosquito control measures are taken, due to security concerns. Because bednet use conflicts with the requirement for immediate mobility, these troops also have difficulties in minimizing mosquito contact while sleeping.

Despite the potential for different individual risks among deploying troops, the preventive medicine orders for each deployment strive to provide a mission-specific "universal" set of recommendations for minimizing health risk. The universal nature of these orders aids in the administration of immunization, preventative medicine briefings, and malaria prevention for the deploying military units. Mission-specific instructions also avoid multiple sets of nonuniform orders for the deploying troops that could result in confusion for the soldier on the ground, with the inherent risk of compromised compliance. In effect, these mission-specific orders require the provision of group health prevention methods that may not be applicable to each individual member of that group. They are based on a health risk assessment for the population as a whole rather than on an individual risk assessment for each deploying member.

Sources of information used for disease risk assessment include military and civilian disease-specific information, such as information from local government agencies, on-site evaluations by reconnaissance (RECCE/RECON) missions, reports from those working in the region, endemic disease reports, and reports of disease in travelers.

PREVENTIVE MEASURES AND MEDICAL SURVEILLANCE

Historically, it has been recognized that malaria can infect a large number of soldiers[22,32] and potentially cause significant morbidity and mortality, in effect compromising a unit's mission.[37] Effective chemoprophylaxis and personal protection measures (PPMs) against mosquitoes will decrease the likelihood of symptomatic malaria. PPMs include the use of long-sleeved shirts and long trousers from dusk to dawn, protected screened or air-conditioned quarters (Figure 9.3–1), the use of insect repellents containing diethyltoluamide (DEET), and the use of permethrin to impregnate bednets (Figure 9.3–2) and clothing. Troop insect control measures also include the choice of living accommodations, and local mosquito control measures are usually provided by the preventive medicine team deploying with the operation. It is also imperative that each of the deployed members recognizes the importance of seeking immediate medical attention in the event of a febrile illness, so that health care providers can make an early diagnosis and institute immediate treatment for this potentially life-threatening infection.

Despite a long history of infectious diseases compromising operation effectiveness, full compliance with preventive measures is seldom achieved.[38–41] Unfortunately, measures that require repeated actions to be effective deter compliance. Examples are the need for repeated application of insect repellents and repeated dosing of malaria chemoprophylaxis (which requires continuation even after departure from the malaria-endemic area).

During a deployment, medical surveillance is essential to monitor the health of military forces and to allow an immediate response to medical threats. Any increase in malaria cases during a deployment warrants an investigation. It is imperative to know which malaria chemoprophylaxis the troops are taking and whether or not the

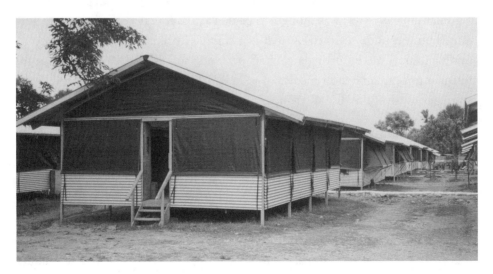

Figure 9.3–1. Canadian contingent living quarters, East Timor.

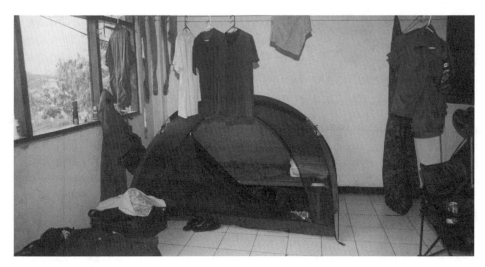

Figure 9.3–2. Military cot within bednet. (See Color Plates)

troops are compliant with the regimen. Malaria cases may also be due to a previously unrecognized change in malaria distribution, drug sensitivity, or predominant mosquito species within the country. As an example, during a U.S. military deployment in Somalia, one marine unit was noted to have an abrupt increase in malaria cases. An investigation of the outbreak revealed that the cases were due to a sudden change in malaria chemoprophylaxis from doxycycline (which has a very short half-life) to mefloquine (which has a very long half-life) in a highly malarious area and without the provision of a mefloquine loading dose or an overlap interval.[42]

Surveillance must also continue after deployment. It is important to document and investigate malaria cases that present after the return of troops from malaria-endemic areas since such cases may indicate a failure of malaria chemoprophylaxis or a failure of compliance. Malaria that occurred in U.S. soldiers following a deployment in Somalia in early 1992 was thought to be due to a failure in compliance with prescribed postexposure regimens as well as a failure of primaquine terminal prophylaxis.[43] Malaria cases occurring in military personnel following deployments have the potential to overcome local medical resources, whether because of the number of cases or because of the lack of diagnostic or treatment capability.[9,10,15,16,23,39,40,44–56]

Education About Malaria Risk and Preventative Measures

Medical education concerning the risk of malaria infection is essential for commanding officers, medical personnel, and individual soldiers. All must understand the appropriate means of avoiding symptomatic malaria infection and the requirement for early intervention in any febrile illness occurring during or following deployment. The commanding officer of a military unit must understand that he or she has the ultimate responsibility for the health of his or her troops; military medical personnel serve in an advisory capacity. The maintenance of the health of troops depends on the use of preventive measures specified by command instructions and enforced by command authority. This was well demonstrated in 1943 by Field Marshall William Slim, who commanded the British 14th Army during a time when malaria was decimating the ranks. He ordered daily mepacrine for chemoprophylaxis and then carried out surprise checks on entire units, in which every man was evaluated for compliance. If overall compliance was less than 95%, he fired the commanding officer. (He claimed to have fired only three.)[37]

IMPORTANCE OF EARLY DIAGNOSIS AND IMPROVED COMPLIANCE

The prevention of adverse outcomes with malaria in military members is essential. This requires early diagnosis and treatment for any febrile illness occurring after 1 week of troops' entering a malaria-endemic area and for at least 3 months after their departure from the area (up to 3 years if in areas of relapsing malaria). Getting military members to present to medical care urgently with their symptoms can be hampered if symptoms occur during much-needed time off; members often prefer to delay the medical examination until they officially return to work, a choice that obviously puts them at risk of severe and complicated malaria.

An ideal malaria chemoprophylactic drug for troops being deployed would allow one to "fire and forget"—that is, it would require infrequent dosing and would act as a causal agent, so that prolonged compliance would not be required following a deployment. Perhaps a long-acting causal agent such as tafenoquine will hold promise here. An effective malaria vaccine would be an asset for deploying troops but would not eliminate requirements for PPMs to minimize vector (and thus parasite) exposure. Other potential areas for improvement in compliance among military personnel include improved agents for prevention, such as permethrin impregnation of uniforms at the point of manufacture and improved insect repellents that leave no sticky residue. Another possible means of improving compliance with malaria prevention methods would be to use all the agents for malaria prevention at a time when there is no malaria risk. For example, when on exercise in a non–malaria-endemic country, troops should use DEET, permethrin, impregnated bednets, and even prophylaxis. Military members would have increased comfort with the appropriate use of these preventive tools and with the reassurance of their safety and tolerability. Such reassurance might go a long way to improve compliance with these measures when malaria is a risk.

SUMMARY

Military medical personnel play an integral role in deploying missions. They assess potential health threats before troops reach foreign soil, so that adequate preventive measures can be instituted. They use continuous surveillance and analysis of health outcomes during and following deployment, which is critical to the assessment of both the health of troops and the success of any preventive measures taken. Military medical personnel educate commanders and soldiers in how to protect themselves against medical threats, including malaria, emphasizing the requirement of ongoing compliance as well as early recognition and consultation with medical caregivers in the event of a febrile illness. Through their efforts to minimize the health risk for deployed troops, they assist commanders in the successful completion of the military mission.

REFERENCES

1. Hayes GJ. Medical aspects of the Vietnamese campaign. Clin Neurosurg 1966;14:380–385.
2. McCabe ME. Malaria—a military medical problem yet with us. Med Serv J Can 1966;22:313–332.
3. Bermudez R, Garcia Pont PH, Rivera JV. Malaria among Puerto Rican veterans of the Viet Nam conflict. Bol Asoc Med P R 1967;59:141–147.
4. Bourke AT, Joy RJ. Malaria as understood by soldiers. Mil Med 1967;132:366–370.
5. Gilbert DN, Greenberg JH. Vietnam: preventive medicine orientation. Mil Med 1967;132:769–790.
6. Moseley V. Falciparum malaria: a clinical note. A health hazard in veterans from Viet Nam. J S C Med Assoc 1967;63:353–356.
7. Sheehy TW. Malaria in servicemen from Vietnam. Ann Intern Med 1967;66:447.
8. Barrett O Jr. The problem of vivax malaria in Vietnam returnees. Mil Med 1968;133:211–214.
9. Gilbert DN, Moore WL Jr, Hedberg CL, Sanford JP. Potential medical problems in personnel returning from Vietnam. Ann Intern Med 1968;68:662–678.
10. Glatt W, Jarrold T. Malaria in Vietnam veterans. Postgrad Med 1968;44:80–83.
11. Goldstein E. A clinical study of falciparum and vivax malaria in Vietnam servicemen. Mil Med 1968;133:991–996.
12. Modell W. Malaria and victory in Vietnam. The first battle against drug-resistant malignant malaria is described. Science 1968;162:1346–1352.
13. Moore WL Jr, Hedberg CL, Sanford J. Medical problems from Vietnam. Ann Intern Med 1968;69:168–170.
14. Reback H. Medical problems from Vietnam. Ann Intern Med 1968;69:168.
15. Skrzypek G, Barrett O Jr. The problem of vivax malaria in Vietnam returnees. II. Malaria chemoprophylaxis survey. Mil Med 1968;133:449–452.
16. Barrett O Jr, Skrzypek G, Datel W, Goldstein JD. Malaria imported to the United States from Vietnam. Chemoprophylaxis evaluated in returning soldiers. Am J Trop Med Hyg 1969;18:495–499.
17. Blount RE. Malaria—a persistent threat. Ann Intern Med 1969;70:127–129.
18. Blount RE. Acute falciparum malaria. Field experience with quinine-pyrimethamine combined therapy. Ann Intern Med 1969;70:142–147.
19. Colwell EJ, Brown JD, Russell PK, et al. Investigations on acute febrile illness in American servicemen in the Mekong Delta of Vietnam. Mil Med 1969;134:1409–1414.

20. Glor BA. Falciparum malaria in Vietnam: clinical manifestations and nursing care requirements. Mil Med 1969;134:181–191.

21. Martelo OJ, Smoller M, Saladin TA. Malaria in American soldiers. Arch Intern Med 1969;123:383–387.

22. Skinner HG, Lewthwaite CJ. Malaria—a military problem. Trans R Soc Trop Med Hyg 1969;63:417–418.

23. Fisher GU, Gordon MP, Lobel HO, Runcik K. Malaria in soldiers returning from Vietnam. Epidemiologic, therapeutic, and clinical studies. Am J Trop Med Hyg 1970;19:27–39.

24. Bruce-Chwatt LJ. Malaria and its prevention in military campaigns. Z Tropenmed Parasitol 1971;22:370–390.

25. Byrne JP. Malaria, a new threat from an old foe. Ariz Med 1971;28:297–300.

26. McKelvey TP, Lundie AR, Vanreenen RM, et al. Chloroquine-resistant falciparum malaria among British service personnel in West Malaysia and Singapore. Trans R Soc Trop Med Hyg 1971;65:286–309.

27. Black RH. Malaria in the Australian army in South Vietnam: successful use of a proguanil-dapsone combination for chemoprophylaxis of chloroquine-resistant falciparum malaria. Med J Aust 1973;1:1265–1270.

28. Black RH. Letter: malaria in the Australian army in South Vietnam. Med J Aust 1973;2:564–565.

29. Fleming K. Experiences with malaria in the early phase of Australian army involvement in South Vietnam. Med J Aust 1974;2:834–837.

30. Bruce-Chwatt LJ. John Hull Grundy lecture. Mosquitoes, malaria and war; then and now. J R Army Med Corps 1985;131:85–99.

31. von Bonsdorff M. [Panorama of diseases in Finland's Army during the Second World War]. Nord Med 1991;106:134–136.

32. Beadle C, Hoffman SL. History of malaria in the United States Naval Forces at war: World War I through the Vietnam conflict. Clin Infect Dis 1993;16:320–329.

33. Sartin JS. Infectious diseases during the Civil War: the triumph of the "Third Army." Clin Infect Dis 1993;16:580–584.

34. Fenner F, Sweeney AW. Malaria in New Guinea during the Second World War: the Land Headquarters Medical Research Unit. Parassitologia 1998;40:65–68.

35. Kenyon G. Australian army infected troops and internees in second world war. BMJ 1999;318:1233.

36. Joy RJ. Malaria in American troops in the south and southwest Pacific in World War II. Med Hist 1999;43:192–207.

37. Crutcher JM, Sharp TW, Wallace MR, Hoffman SL. Malaria (part 1). Lessons from Somalia and General Slim. Navy Med 1994;85:16–19.

38. Croft AM, Clayton TC, World MJ. Side effects of mefloquine prophylaxis for malaria: an independent randomized controlled trial. Trans R Soc Trop Med Hyg 1997;91:199–203.

39. Talarmin F, Sicard JM, Mounem M, et al. [Imported malaria in Moselle: 75 cases in three years]. Rev Med Interne 2000;21:242–246.

40. Newton JA, Schnepf GA, Wallace MR, et al. Malaria in US Marines returning from Somalia. JAMA 1994;272:397–399.

41. Ledbetter E, Shallow S, Hanson KR. Malaria in Somalia: lessons in prevention [letter]. JAMA 1995;273:774–775.

42. Wallace MR, Sharp TW, Smoak B, et al. Malaria among United States troops in Somalia. Am J Med 1996;100:49–55.

43. Smoak BL, DeFraites RF, Magill AJ, et al. *Plasmodium vivax* infections in U.S. Army troops: failure of primaquine to prevent relapse in studies from Somalia. Am J Trop Med Hyg 1997;56:231–234.

44. Shomakov AO. [Imported malaria in the Kabardino-Balkarian republic]. Med Parazitol (Mosk) 1999;2:48–51.

45. Kortepeter M, Brown JD. A review of 79 patients with malaria seen at a military hospital in Hawaii from 1979 to 1995. Mil Med 1998;163:84–89.

46. Sighinolfi L, Libanore M, Ghinelli F. A double malarial infection in a soldier returning from Somalia [letter]. Eur J Epidemiol 1994;10:445–446.

47. Miller JH, Byers M, Whiteoak R, Warrell DA. Imported falciparum malaria in British troops returning from Kenya. J R Army Med Corps 1994;140:119–123.

48. Sergiev VP, Baranova AM, Orlov VS, et al. Importation of malaria into the U.S.S.R. from Afghanistan, 1981–89 [published erratum appears in Bull World Health Organ 1994;72(2):321]. Bull World Health Organ 1993;71:385–388.

49. Gunby P. Will civilian physicians see post-Somalia malaria? JAMA 1993;269:3091.

50. Malaria among U.S. military personnel returning from Somalia, 1993. MMWR Morb Mortal Wkly Rep 1993;42:524–526.

51. Cristau P, Desbaumes J, Giraud D. [Late manifestations of *Plasmodium falciparum* after leaving an endemic area {letter}]. Presse Med 1987;16:493.

52. Brittan JC, Preheim LC. Imported malaria: problems with diagnosis and prevention. J Fam Pract 1986;22:451–452.

53. Willerson D Jr. *Plasmodium malariae* imported from Vietnam. JAMA 1972;221:604.

54. Wenzel RP, Stotka VL. Imported malaria in Marine Corps personnel. N Engl J Med 1972;287:1153.

55. Greenberg JH. Public health problems relating to the Vietnam returnee. JAMA 1969;207:697–702.

56. Waterhouse BE, Riggenbach RD. Malaria. Potential importance to civilian physicians. JAMA 1967;202:683–685.

9.4 *Migrants*
Louis Loutan

ABSTRACT

It was estimated that at the end of the 20th century, some 150 million people were living outside the country of their birth, amounting to about 2.5% of the world's population, or 1 of every 40 people. Of these, 15 million (10%) are refugees. Population movements in and out of malarious areas precipitate, increase, or contribute to malaria transmission. International travel and migration are changing the epidemiology of imported malaria in Europe and North America. A growing proportion of imported cases are seen in arriving immigrants and refugees and in settled migrants returning to their countries of origin. Underestimating the risk of acquiring malaria, migrants visiting friends and relatives tend to take fewer protection measures such as chemoprophylaxis. They may take their children, who are unprotected and who have no immunity, putting them at high risk of developing severe malaria. New fields of travel medicine that need to be further developed are raising the awareness of the potential risks of diseases for travelers abroad and are promoting access to information (through effective channels of communication) for various communities of foreign-born residents or ethnic minorities. As medical providers and travel medicine doctors are caring for patients of diverse sociocultural backgrounds, it is essential that these health professionals acquire cultural competence.

Key words: chemoprophylaxis; cultural competence; immigrants; immunity; imported malaria; migrants; refugees; travelers.

INTRODUCTION

As we move into the 21st century, the effects of globalization on population movements become more apparent. Travelers by the hundreds of millions circulate around the globe, usually for short periods of time, then return home while migrants, primarily and usually traveling from poor to richer countries on one-way tickets, experience much longer journeys, often suffer hardships and restricted access to health care, and may never return to their country of origin. In their own way and with their own specific characteristics, they all participate in the growing mobility of populations, sharing some common factors related to travel and exposure to new environments and risks. As time passes, individuals and populations may move from one category of traveler or migrant to another (Table 9.4–1), thus creating the need for a comprehensive approach to mobility and its implications to health.

Table 9.4–1. **Various Categories of Travelers and Migrants**

Travelers	Migrants
Tourists	Foreigners
Expatriates	Refugees
Corporate travelers	Internally displaced persons
Military personnel	Immigrants
Diplomats	Asylum seekers
Students	Foreign workers
Pilgrims	Seasonal workers
Missionaries	Illegal migrants or aliens
Humanitarian workers	Returnees

THE GROWING COMPLEXITY OF POPULATION MOVEMENT

Population mobility is not a new phenomenon. Since the dawn of humanity, people have been moving in search of food, water, and more favorable environments or have been fleeing insecurity and war. Hunters and gatherers would move, following the migratory patterns of game, and nomads still have to constantly adjust to the fluctuations of available pasture and water sources. As humans have been able to control more of their environment and means of living, they have been able to settle and become more sedentary. Demographic pressure, economic disparities, and new means of transportation have lead to new migration patterns over the last centuries. Massive numbers of immigrants from Europe crossed the Atlantic to colonize the New World; other Europeans moved to Australia, New Zealand, or South Africa. With the end of the colonies, large numbers of former colonial citizens moved to European cities such as those of the United Kingdom and France. In the 1960s and 1970s, the industrialized nations' fast-growing economies and need for larger workforces led to the active recruitment of migrant workers from former colonies or surrounding countries (Indonesia, Morocco, Algeria, Turkey, Yugoslavia, etc.). In several industrialized countries, consequently, there are large communities of foreign-born residents who have various legal statuses and who represent several generations, at different levels of acculturation and integration in the country of residence. Often, they still have links with their country of origin and may return temporarily to visit relatives or friends.

Since the 1980s, with the buildup of the European Union (strengthening the links between the various members of the union, some of which had the labor force needed by others) and with the much slower pace of economic growth, immigration policies have become much more restrictive. As a result, seeking asylum or migrating illegally has become almost the only way to enter Europe for many people. In North America, immigrant and refugee quotas are still set every year for legal entry to Canada or the United States. This has not protected these two countries from the increasing number of asylum seekers and the growing influx of illegal migrants coming mainly from Latin American countries.

Population movements are by no means limited to south-north patterns. Practically any difference in economy and work opportunities between countries may trigger migratory movements. There are large movements between West African countries (e.g., from Ghana to Nigeria and from Sahelian countries to coastal states). Numerous migrants from Bangladesh move to the Persian Gulf States, Filipinos move to Southeast Asian countries, etc. Countries may establish administrative barriers to control or block these movements. When these barriers become too tight, illegal migration increases. Globalization of the economy, easy access to new means of communication, worldwide media networks that give basically everyone access to information, and rapid means of transportation all contribute to the increasing mobility of the world's people.

Today, a growing number of people seek to migrate to achieve a better life or to escape war, human rights violations, poverty, or environmental disasters. It was estimated that at the end of the 20th century, some 150 million people were living outside their country of birth, amounting to about 2.5% of the world's population, or 1 of every 40 people. Of these, 15 million (10%) are refugees, according to the United Nations High Commissioner for Refugees (UNHCR).[1] According to the United Nations Population Division, there were 120 million international migrants in 1990 (up from 75 million in 1965), with an annual growth rate of 1.9%.[2] In 1990, international migrants made up 18% of the total population in Australia and New Zealand, nearly 11% in West Asia, less than 9% in North America, over 6% in Western Europe, and less than 2.5% in Asia, Africa, and Latin America. Net international migration contributed to 45% of the population growth in the developed world from 1990 to 1995. In Europe, it contributed to almost 88% of the population growth during this period. The number of refugees has increased markedly, reaching a maximum of 18.2 million in 1993. Since then, the number of refugees has been decreasing (to 13.2 million in 1996), due to major repatriations.[3] By January 2000, the total number of people of concern to the UNHCR (including internally displaced people) was 22.3 million.[4] The number of people seeking asylum also increased drastically until 1992, then stabilized as the result of the more restrictive policies of the receiving countries. Between 1985 and 1995, over 5 million asylum applications were registered in the industrialized states. Due to the increasing instability and ensuing war in Kosovo, the number of refugees fleeing the Balkans and seeking asylum in other parts of Europe rose drastically in 1998 and 1999; there were 473,000 new applications in 1999, a 19.1% increase from 1998.[4] As security was restored in certain places, 2.5 million refugees were able to return to their country of origin in 1999. Table 9.4–2 gives statistics on people of concern to the UNHCR as of January 2000.

Table 9.4–2. **Persons of Concern to the United Nations High Commissioner for Refugees***

Region	Refugees	Asylum Seekers	Returned Refugees	IDPs and Others	Total From Region
Africa	3,523,250	61,110	933,890	1,732,290	6,250,540
Asia	4,781,750	24,750	617,620	1,884,740	7,308,860
Europe	2,608,380	473,060	952,060	3,252,300	7,285,800
Latin America and Caribbean	61,200	1,510	6,260	21,200	90,170
North America	636,300	605,630			1,241,930
Oceania	64,500	15,540			80,040
TOTAL	11,675,380	1,181,600	2,509,830	6,890,530	22,257,340

IDPs = internally displaced persons.
*As of January 1, 2000.

As the number of refugees and migrants going to industrialized countries increases, tighter border controls and administrative barriers are set to contain this influx of newcomers. This has lead to a significant increase in irregular migration and in the human trafficking of migrants. The United Nations estimates that 4 million people are victims of international trafficking each year.[5] Of these, 700,000 are women or children, of whom 175,000 are estimated to come from the former Soviet bloc; approximately 45,000 to 50,000 arrive in the United States. It is estimated that there are 5 million irregular migrants in the United States and 3 million in Western Europe.[6] Trafficking in migrants has become a very lucrative illegal market with worldwide ramifications. Having no legal status and living with the constant fear of being deported, illegal migrants represent a vulnerable population with very little access to health care.

These numbers of migrants illustrate the growing complexity of population movements worldwide, crossing back and forth over geobiologic boundaries and moving from one cultural environment to another, each individual experiencing a unique journey.

POPULATION MOVEMENT AND MALARIA

Population movement has long been recognized to facilitate the spread of diseases. In the 18th century, John Snow recognized the importance of travel and trade in the spread of cholera.[7] Over the centuries, epidemics of cholera and meningitis have traveled through the hajj pilgrimage. Large population displacements due to war, insecurity, and environmental or economic pressures have contributed to the spread of communicable diseases from one area to another, with massive outbreaks of dysentery, cholera, measles, and meningitis in refugee camps.[8] The arrival of displaced populations in a new environment with local transmission of vector-born diseases has also led to large outbreaks in these newly arrived nonimmune populations. Such outbreaks have been observed in southern Sudan (visceral leishmaniasis)[9] and in Nepal (Japanese encephalitis).[10]

Malaria is no exception. It has been spread or introduced by migratory movements of infected individuals or populations into areas where the vector was present, leading to local transmission. Newly arrived people may also change the local environment (e.g., by deforestation or irrigation), thus creating more favorable habitats for *Anopheles* mosquitoes. In Brazil, the development of mining activities and the settlement of workers led to a sharp increase in malaria transmission in the Amazonian region.[11] A similar situation has been observed in Thailand, in the eastern Trat province, where gem-mining activities are carried out. Malaria transmission has increased because of environmental changes related to open mining, which creates breeding sites for the mosquitoes. With migration, malaria is then exported elsewhere. Many of the workers come from the northwestern part of the country (in the Tak province), and their migratory movements have largely contributed to the spread of resistant strains of falciparum malaria into their home region; local transmission then further propagates the disease.[12] Population in transit through a malarious area may contribute to the introduction or spead of specific strains of malaria. In eastern Nepal (on the Terraï plain, where mainly vivax malaria is transmitted), an increase in falciparum malaria cases was observed with the arrival of refugees from Bhutan. In this case, it was during their travel through the neighboring Indian province of Assam, an area with *Plasmodium falciparum* transmission, that these refugees probably acquired the disease and brought it into Nepal (Shekar Koïrala, personal communication, November, 1999).

The movement of populations from endemic areas can also contribute to the re-introduction of malaria in areas where malaria has been eradicated. Failure to consider population mobility contributed to the failure of malaria eradication programs in the 1950s and 1960s.[13] R.M. Prothero looked extensively at the various population movement patterns in Africa in relation to malaria control and eradication.[14] He pointed to the existent extensive mobility of people in various parts of Africa (particularly of pastoralists or migrant workers across boundaries) and the seasonal or long-term patterns of movements from rural to urban areas, which could lead to the failure of the malaria eradication effort or to the re-introduction of malaria in malaria-free areas. A typology of population movement has been proposed; it is summarized in Table 9.4–3. In endemic areas of the world, urbanization has had a different impact on malaria transmission. In the majority of cases, water pollution has led to a decrease in vector population and transmission. Nevertheless, in some instances in Africa and Asia, some *Anopheles* species (e.g., *Anopheles stephensi*) have adapted to urban conditions, breeding in household water tanks or in periurban areas where people live in poor housing conditions.

Table 9.4–3. **A Typology of Population Movement**

		Circulation		
Daily	*Periodic*	*Seasonal*	*Long Term*	*Migratory*
Commuting	Trading	Fishing	Laboring	Urbanization
Trading	Pilgrimage	Pastoralism	Colonization	Colonization
Cultivation	Mining	Laboring	Seeking asylum	Seeking refuge
Woodcutting	Tourism		Trafficking	Seeking asylum
				Trafficking

Adapted from Martens P, Hall L. Malaria on the move: human population movement and malaria transmission. Emerg Infect Dis 2000;6:103–109.

Colonization of endemic unpopulated areas in the Amazon region by nonimmune or semi-immune settlers has resulted in the spread of malaria in Brazil. Agricultural developments in Swaziland and irrigation projects in Colombia have also led to increased transmission of the disease.[15]

Insecurity and war are presently major causes of mass population movements in various part of the world. Refugees and internally displaced persons within their own country resettled in malarious areas have paid a heavy toll to malaria. Malaria has been reported as a major cause of death in Cambodian refugee camps in Thailand and (to a lesser extent) among refugees from areas of low malaria endemicity who sought refuge in camps in highly endemic zones in western Ethiopia, Somalia, Sudan, Malawi, and Mozambique.[8] The forced migration of people from the Ethiopian highlands to resettlement in malaria-endemic areas in the lowlands has also led also to high mortality rates. Nomadic populations living often in arid or semiarid lands with a low level of seasonal transmission of malaria may be at high risk of malaria epidemics when they move into malarious areas because of droughts or insecurity.

Migration can also contribute to autochthonous transmission of malaria in more-temperate climates. Cases of vivax malaria contracted locally in the United States have been reported over the last years in the southern states of California and Georgia but also in the northern state of New York.[16] When local climatic conditions (temperature and humidity) are favorable, local *Anopheles* can transmit malaria parasites, particularly *Plasmodium vivax*, which can complete its cycle in the mosquito at a lower temperature than *Plasmodium falciparum*. It is probable that migrant workers coming from endemic areas in Latin America, infected with *Plasmodium vivax*, and working on local farms may be bitten by local mosquitoes, which can generate some local transmission in turn. One must also briefly mention airport malaria in Europe, due mainly to infected mosquitoes carried by intercontinental flights from endemic regions. Under certain climatic conditions, such mosquitoes can cause local transmission.

INTERNATIONAL TRAVEL AND MIGRATION: THE CHANGING EPIDEMIOLOGY OF IMPORTED MALARIA

Population mobility is not restricted only to neighboring regions or countries. The development of the travel industry has brought millions of nonimmune tourists to malarious areas. Returning home to industrialized countries, they may bring back malaria if adequate chemoprophylaxis is not taken regularly. Airplanes are also used by migrants leaving endemic countries for Europe or North America. Foreign-born residents in European countries may return to their country of origin, underestimating the risk of acquiring malaria. Thus, the profile of imported malaria in industrialized countries has changed during the last 20 years. (This topic is dealt with in detail in Chapter 18).

Imported Malaria in Europe and North America

Between the 1970s and the 1980s, many countries reported an increasing number of cases of imported malaria. Between 1977 and 1986, the incidence of malaria reported in Britain increased by 51% (from 1,529 to 2,309 cases), *Plasmodium falciparum*–related malaria increasing from one-fifth to one-third of all cases.[17] Attack rates were highest in immigrants who had settled in Britain and were visitors of friends or relatives (VFRs)—316 and 331 per 100,000 for such visitors to Africa and Asia, respectively, compared to 120 and 39 per 100,000 for tourists to those same regions. Between 1977 and 1986, the greatest rise in malaria cases has been in VFRs, with an increase of from 55% to 66% in all malaria cases in British residents. Of all cases reported in travelers with a known reason for travel, those of ethnic-minority travelers increased from 27.6% to 39.5% during this period. Of the 63 patients whose nationality was recorded, 54% were nonimmune whites, 9 were of Asian origin, and 4 were of African descent. Cases in new immigrants decreased twofold, while cases in foreign visitors increased fivefold. These visitors were mainly from Nigeria, Ghana, and India. Globally, malaria cases have increased, and while cases caused by *Plasmodium vivax* have decreased, those due to *Plasmodium falciparum* have increased, partly due to a decreased flow of new immigrants from areas endemic for vivax infection.[18,19] Many infections contracted in West Africa by settled immigrants in Britain were falciparum malaria. Between 1987 and 1992, 49% of 8,355 cases of malaria in the United Kingdom occurred in VFRs.[20] Immigrants and foreign visitors made up 11% and 19%, respectively, of the remaining cases. There was a marked difference in the percentage of tourists and VFRs using chemoprophylaxis (73% and 19%, respectively). In Britain, a significant proportion of imported malaria occurs in children less than 15 years of age.[21] In 1995, 14.9% of 2,055 cases reported were in this group, a higher proportion than the 9.3% of reported cases in the Netherlands between 1991 and 1994. The highest proportion of infection was acquired in Nigeria and Ghana, all due to *Plasmodium falciparum* and mostly in children of VFRs. The proportion of all cases of malaria in children from the Indian subcontinent was also high (34%) and was mostly due to *Plasmodium vivax.*

There are, on average, 300 cases of malaria reported every year in Switzerland.[22] Since 1988, when the reporting procedure was changed, there has been no significant increase in the overall number of cases reported. Nevertheless, the proportion of cases reported for foreigners has increased, rising from a third of all cases in 1982 to nearly 50% of cases in 1999; this is a much higher proportion than the 20% of the population of Switzerland that they represent. The destination from which infection had been acquired did not differ significantly, with the exception of the Americas.[23] In 1995 to 1996, in both Swiss and foreigners, 77% and 80% of cases, respectively, had been contracted in Africa; 12% and 19%, respectively, in Asia; and 3.6% and 0.4%, respectively, in the Americas. During this period, 12 patients died, 2 (17%) of whom were VFRs (one a 4-year-old girl who had visited her relatives in Zaire, the other a 36-year-old man returning from Ghana).

In the United States, there has been a regular increase of reported cases in U.S. civilians, from 89 cases in 1966 to 599 cases in 1995.[24] Cases in foreign civilians during this period increased from 32 to 461. A peak of 1,534 cases was recorded in 1980 due to the arrival of Southeast Asian refugees. Unfortunately, these figures do not reflect the proportion of all foreign-born residents who may have returned to their country of origin as VFRs. In an earlier report on *Plasmodium falciparum* malaria in American travelers to Africa (1981 to 1988), it was noted that patients who acquired malaria in East Africa were predominantly tourists (55%); of those who acquired malaria in West Africa, only 9% traveled for tourism, and 34% traveled to visit friends and relatives.[25]

For 2,117 reported cases in France in 1996 that could be analyzed, the patients' nationalities were known in 86.5% of cases. Patients from Europe, North America, and some other non-endemic countries represented 58% of cases, Africans represented 40%, Asians represented 1.8%, and Latin Americans made up 0.2%.[26]

Imported Malaria Seen in Hospitals

Hospital-based studies give a similar picture of change in the cases of imported malaria. In northern Italy, several reports illustrate the increasing proportion of imported cases seen in immigrants. In Verona, a sixfold increase was recorded between the periods of 1988 to 1989 and 1990 to 1991 (from 8% to 48%).[27] Of the 82 cumulative cases due to *Plasmodium falciparum*, immigrants had significantly less severe diseases as compared to short-term travelers. For 683 individuals admitted for malaria in 52 hospitals in the region of Lombardi during the period of 1991 to 1995, the proportion of immigrants increased from 34% in 1991 to 60% in 1995.[28] Overall, 52.4% were foreign born, and 6.3% had arrived in Italy for the first time. The proportion of severe falciparum malaria was 1.3% (4 of 312 cases) among immigrants, significantly less than in nonimmigrants (9.2%). Eight deaths were recorded, all in nonimmigrants. Immigrants cleared parasites faster than non-immigrants. The use of chemoprophylaxis was significantly lower in immigrants (7.4%) than in nonimmigrants (50.2%).

Of 286 patients with malaria in Amsterdam between 1991 and 1994, 114 (40%) were originally from malaria-endemic areas (92 immigrants and 22 asylum seekers).[29] There were also 11 children born in the Netherlands to immigrants. Whereas only 15% of patients with falciparum malaria were semi-immune immigrants in the period of 1979 to 1988, the percentage rose to 58% in 1988. Of the 18 patients with severe complicated malaria, 14 were Dutch adults and 4 were nonimmune children born to semi-immune parents. Two nonimmune women died. Overall, 8% of the settled immigrants took adequate chemoprophylaxis, compared to 38% of the Dutch citizens. Several other studies show the same trends in different clinical settings in Spain,[30] Norway,[31] France,[32–34] Switzerland,[35,36] the United Kingdom,[37] and Canada.[38]

This brief review of the literature illustrates the changing epidemiology of imported malaria in Europe and North America. Over the last decade, there has clearly been a significant increase of imported cases in migrants arriving from malaria-endemic countries either as new immigrants or asylum seekers or as settled migrants returning to their country of origin to visit friends and relatives. These reports also show that a higher proportion of migrants, as compared to tourists, do not take malaria prophylaxis and that they present with less severe or complicated disease.

MIGRANTS AS TRAVELERS

As there are currently no prospective studies looking at specific risk factors for acquiring malaria in migrants traveling to their country of origin, many of the explanations proposed here are (to some extent) hypotheses to be confirmed. Nevertheless, data from the above studies show that residents of foreign origin represent a growing proportion of imported cases, suggesting a higher risk of exposure or insufficient protection measures.

Are Migrants Visitng Friends or Relatives at High Risk?

In Britain, migrant VFRs have an incidence rate almost three times higher than that of tourists to Africa and eight times higher than that of tourists to Asia.[17,18] This may reflect longer visits made by VFRs. Migrant VFRs may also be more exposed as they visit their families in rural areas with higher transmission rates; the higher incidence may be also due to the time of visitation. Simple living conditions may put them at higher risk of exposure to mosquito bites at night when sleeping in non-air-conditioned closed rooms or when not using bednets. Many return home during summer holidays, a period corresponding to the rainy season in West Africa or to the monsoon season in India, when malaria transmission is at its peak. Asian immigrants who visit relatives in malarious areas are often unaware of the risk because they left the area at the height of the eradication programs in south Asia, when malaria transmission had almost entirely disappeared. Many also believe that they retain a lifetime immunity, and they return to endemic areas, unaware of the risk and having lost their immunity. This was illustrated by 53 Nigerians interviewed in the Nigerian Airways office in London. All had been residents in Britain for at least 2 years, and 45 had had malaria before coming to Britain. Asked about their most recent trip to Nigeria in the past 5 years, 36 (68%) answered that they had taken no antimalarial chemoprophylaxis;[39] 16 had taken tablets irregularly or had discontinued them on returning to Britain, and only 1 person had taken a full course of chemoprophylaxis. The usual reason given for not taking any tablets was that they preferred to treat the attacks when they occurred; this was linked to the belief that they had immunity from previous infection. Since they had not taken regular antimalaria prophylaxis before coming to Britain, they would not expect to do so when they returned to visit their relatives. Table 9.4–4 gives some possible risk factors for acquiring malaria for VFRs.

Stress has also been proposed as a possible cause for the relatively high percentage (19%) of malaria cases in the United Kingdom reported in visitors from endemic countries.[20] Why should semi-immune adults develop malaria soon after arrival in Britain? Stress associated with travel may alter the parasite-host equilibrium, allowing the parasite to escape immunologic control and to replicate and produce clinical malaria. Of 300 patients studied, 80% developed symptoms within 2 weeks of arrival.

Do Immigrants Maintain Some Protection Against Malaria?

Although immunity does wane when constant re-exposure stops, some immunity may be retained. Thus, the malaria contracted when visiting home may not be as dangerous as the malaria that infects nonimmune tourists. This may explain why several studies suggest that malaria in foreign-born immigrants in Europe is less

Table 9.4–4. **Potential Risk Factors for Acquiring Malaria in Migrants Visiting Friends and Relatives in Endemic Areas**

Lack of awareness regarding the waning of immunity

Lack of awareness regarding the need for chemoprophylaxis

Preference for treating attacks of malaria

Unawareness of the absence of immunity of their children

Living conditions with little protection from mosquitoes

Prolonged periods of exposure in areas with high level of malaria transmission

Visitation during rainy season and period of high malaria transmission in destination area

Visitation of areas where there is limited access to medical services severe than in nonimmune European travelers, with lower rates of complicated malaria and mortality and lower levels of parasitemia.[27,28,32] A comparable situation was reported in Madagascar recently.[40] In the central highlands (a region of malaria hyperendemicity before 1950), malaria had been eradicated only to reappear 30 years later. Residents more than 40 years of age who had been exposed during their childhood were less likely to have fever and had a lower spleen rate than younger individuals. Villagers more than 40 years of age were more likely to be protected against falciparum malaria than were younger members of the community. This suggests that prior exposure to malarial infection (three decades earlier, in this instance), may still confer some immunologic memory, which when recalled by a new malarial infection, provides some protection and reduces the severity of the disease. Studies have shown that CS protein and Pf155/RESA may persist in migrants from West Africa after the migrants have spent up to 13 years in France without returning to their native area.[41] Another possible reason for the lower case-fatality rate in migrants may be related to their knowledge of the disease. Having previously experienced malaria, they know the symptoms and may present earlier to see a doctor for treatment.

Hemoglobinopathies may also play a role in conferring some degree of protection against severe malaria to migrants coming from endemic countries. In many parts of the world, hemoglobin disorders are quite frequent in the general population. Some of them provide some protection against severe malaria by impairing the normal parasite's development in red blood cells. This is particularly the case for sickle cell anemia (hemoglobin S), but it is also the case, to some extent, for α- and β-thalassemia.[42] Studies conducted in various ethnic groups in Britain have shown high prevalence rates of the various hemoglobinopathies. The prevalence of the hemogloblin S trait, homozygote or combined with other hemoglobinopathies such as thalassemia, is 20% to 25% in West Africans and 11% to 14% in African-Caribbeans.[43] This does not mean that carriers do not contract malaria. They can be infected and can develop symptomatic malaria, which will worsen the preexisting anemia.

Nevertheless, physicians should remain cautious and should not consider migrants coming from endemic areas as semi-immune to malaria and at no risk of severe disease. Some authors have found no differences in the clinical presentation of malaria in migrants versus nonimmune travelers.[31,44] In a Swiss ambulatory clinic, there was no difference in the prevalence rates of the clinical signs and laboratory values defining severe malaria between migrants and nonmigrants.[45]

Children born of settled immigrants may be at particularly high risk. As the parents may be unaware of the risk of acquiring malaria when they return to visit relatives, they may bring their nonimmune children (with no chemoprophylaxis) to highly malarious areas. Reports from Britain and the Netherlands already show that an increasing number of children of former immigrants are presenting with malaria[21,29] or fevers from other causes.[46] As illustrated by the Swiss statistics reported previously, these children may develop severe complicated disease with a high risk of fatal outcome.

MALARIA IN MIGRANTS AT THE MEDICAL PRACTICE

Not only specialists in travel and tropical medicine but also family doctors may see more patients of various origins who may present with malaria. While *Plasmodium falciparum* malaria becomes clinically patent usually within a month after the infection and thus soon after the migrant's arrival, doctors may see migrants who present with fever long after they have settled in the host country. *Plasmodium vivax*, *Plasmodium malariae*, and *Plasmodium ovale* can cause a malaria attack months or even years after the initial infective mosquito bite. Family physicians need to understand that even if immigrants or refugees are screened at entry to their new host country or before leaving their country of origin, they may present years later with malaria.[47]

Medical Screening

In North America and in most European coutries, refugees and immigrants undergo some mandatory health assessment or medical screening on arrival. Many immigrants may have had a previous medical examination overseas to obtain a visa for permanent residency. Asylum seekers arriving in the receiving country are most often screened for infectious diseases such as tuberculosis and hepatitis B, and they are immunized according to the national recommendations. In some countries, screening for syphilis, human immunodeficiency virus (HIV) infection, and leprosy is required before entry is granted. The purpose of overseas examination is to identify physical and mental disorders that might prove harmful to the immigrant or to the general population. In most instances there is no routine screening for malaria in asymptomatic immigrants or refugees, even for those coming from hyperendemic areas. There are exceptions, as in 1992, when 402 montagnard refugees from Cambodia were rapidly resettled in North Carolina. After five refugees were diagnosed with malaria, screening of the entire group showed a 58% infection rate with *Plasmodium* species.[48] Coming from a highly endemic area, these refugees had a high prevalence of infection but few manifestations of malarial illness. Because of their partial immunity, reliance on the presence of fever or other symptoms as screening criteria would have resulted in a serious underestimation of the true prevalence of disease.

Recently, innovative enhanced health assessments that screen for parasites in refugees on site before departure for a new country have helped to decrease both the morbidity among refugees and the risk of imported infections.[49] Initial screening of a subset of the refugee population showed that 7% had malarial parasitemia. Mass therapy for intestinal parasites and for malaria (a single dose of sulfadoxine/ pyrimethamine) was given to all Barawan refugees from Somalia, who had fled to

Mombasa, an area with high malaria transmission. Suppressive therapy was given 1 or 2 days before resettlement. Such a prevention program reduces the chances of malarial attacks at the time of arrival, particularly attacks of falciparum malaria, which is predominant in Africa. However, this does not prevent attacks of malaria from other species unless a drug that is active against the liver stages of the parasite (such as primaquine) is used. In the future, atovaquone/proguanil (Malarone) or tafenoquine (not commercialized) could be most valuable in this respect. But routine screening for glucose-6-phosphate dehydrogenase (G6PD) deficiency should be done before administering primaquine or tafenoquine, as both may cause severe hemolysis in G6PD deficiency. G6PD deficiency is prevalent not only in West Africans (up to 20%) and African Caribbeans (12%) but also in people from India (7%), Pakistan (5%), and the Middle East (7%).[42]

Suspected Malaria in Migrants

Any migrant patient presenting with fever should be screened for malaria. However, one should be aware that immigrants and refugees coming from hyperendemic countries may have subclinical infections with almost no symptoms of the classic attack of malaria. Malaria should be looked for in any patient coming from an endemic area who presents with atypical and mild symptoms.

Most physicians will think of malaria in a case of fever, particularly in patients coming from endemic countries. Physicians should also be aware that migrants coming from a non-endemic area may have acquired the infection during their journey, while traveling through malarious regions. This has been recently reported in regard to Chinese migrants arriving in Italy.[50] The detailed histories of the immigrants, who originated in northern China, were difficult to ascertain as none of the patients were able to speak Italian, English, or French. However, their itinerary to Italy included stays in Laos, Myanmar, Bangladesh, Pakistan, and East Africa (personal correspondence from Francesco Castelli and Zeno Bisoffi, communicated on TropNetEurop).

Prompt diagnosis and treatment are the rule. Treatment effective against multidrug-resistant strains of *Plasmodium falciparum* should be chosen according to the region where the infection was acquired. This is particularly relevant for migrants coming from Southeast Asia, where quinine- and mefloquine-resistant strains are frequent. Artemisinin derivatives coupled with a long-acting antimalarial such as artemether/lumefantrine (Riamet) are most effective, as is atovaquone/proguanil (Malarone) in uncomplicated malaria.

Because of their very status, illegal migrants have little access to health services and medical professionals. They are afraid to be denounced to the state authorities, and those who have been smuggled and trafficked may still be under the tight control of local "mafia" networks. Communication difficulties with local medical providers and the absence of insurance coverage are factors that will delay access to adequate treatment in case of an attack of malaria. Physicians should be aware of these possible critical conditions and should try to find ways to ensure and facilitate the full course of malaria therapy.

Prevention

The growing proportion of cases of imported malaria seen in foreign-born residents and immigrants in Europe and North America points to the necessity to extend the efforts to prevent malaria in these new types of travelers. First, there should be a better understanding of why VFRs are at a higher risk of contracting malaria. In this respect, more research should be conducted to identify specific risk factors. Why is it that migrant travelers returning to visit friends and relatives are more exposed to malaria and take fewer preventive measures? Do they have less access to information? Is their perception of risks different from that of other travelers? A better understanding of the factors influencing the health of migrant travelers is necessary to adapt prevention messages and to stress specific considerations according to needs.

New channels for communicating these messages should be explored.[50] For example, migrant travelers could be reached by (a) leaflets on preventive measures, written in the migrants' languages and designed in a culturally sensitive way, taking into account the community's common knowledge and way of expressing messages; or (b) television, radio, and Internet information programs, aimed at specific communities and concentrating on health risks and prevention measures for the most frequent destinations. Embassies and consulates, local associations and clubs, local travel agents, and national airline companies could all play a key role in facilitating access to prevention messages and in reaching specific communities. Religious and community leaders may be sensitized on this subject and can actively participate in the promotion of preventive measures. Hospitals, health services, and schools located in areas where ethnic minorities live could also play a key role in diffusing prevention information and materials. Finally, travel medicine doctors and societies of travel medicine should also participate in the effort to raise migrant travelers' awareness of the necessity of prevention measures when they return to malarious regions.

Of special concern are refugees or migrants returning to their country of origin permanently. Most asylum seekers do not gain refugee status. After several years spent in Europe, those who have not been accepted have to return home. By then, their immunity against malaria has waned, and they may be at high risk of acquiring malaria. Children and pregnant women are at particular risk of severe and complicated malaria. It is essential that returnees to malarious areas be informed about malaria and prevention measures and that they be given adequate chemoprophylaxis or access to drugs for rapid treatment of attacks of the disease. Illegal migrants, who may also have spent years in Europe, may be caught by the police and sent back home. Such forced returns are conducted rapidly, without access to a medical professional to give adequate counseling and provide means of prevention.

PROMOTING CULTURALLY COMPETENT TRAVEL MEDICINE DOCTORS

The increasing movement of travelers, including migrants of various origins and cultural backgrounds, participates in the buildup of more multicultural societies. As medical providers and travel medicine doctors are caring for patients of diverse sociocultural backgrounds, it is essential that the doctors and care providers acquire cultural competence. Patient satisfaction and compliance with medical recommendations and treatment are closely related to the effectiveness of communication and to the quality of the patient-doctor relationship. Physicians need to understand how each patient's sociocultural background affects his or her health beliefs and behavior. Travel medicine doctors and other health professionals need to acquire the appropriate skills to respond to this new demand of culturally adjusted care. Communication difficulties due to the misunderstanding of a complaint or to the lack of access to a common language between patient and provider may delay access to adequate therapy. Access to medical interpreters or mediators can facilitate the work of health professionals. The diseases and illnesses that are associated with travel create challenges for both travel medicine providers and those involved in migration medicine. Closer collaboration between professionals involved in these complementary domains will benefit the health of both the traditional traveler and the migrant. Migrants may be considered global travelers, and their health characteristics, reflecting their geographic origin, can represent a pattern of experience and knowledge for other travelers who may journey in the reverse direction. This wider approach to the health of travelers can increase the scope, coverage, and practice of travel and migration health, within a shared framework of health risk determination and management.[51] Medical providers today face the challenge of caring for patients from many cultures and who have different languages, socioeconomic statuses, and ways of understanding illness and health care. Travel medicine doctors are no exception. They need to acquire more cultural competence to respond to the needs of various types of travelers coming to see them, to provide adequate prevention measures, and also to care for these travelers when they return. To develop cultural competence, medical providers need to integrate health-related beliefs and cultural values, disease incidence and prevalence, and treatment efficacy. To the understanding of the patient model and expectations, an epidemiologic perspective (as illustrated above for refugees and migrants of different origins) should be added. In the case of travel medicine, much emphasis has been put on quantifying the risks of acquiring diseases according to destination, for both preventive and therapeutic measures. How travelers and other mobile populations perceive risk and comply with prophylactic procedures is still largely unknown, as is the degree to which health benefits influence their behavior.

CONCLUSION

This chapter has focused mainly on the characteristics of imported malaria in Europe and North America. Nevertheless, it is important to remember that the vast majority of malaria transmission related to population movement takes place in tropical countries, where access to treatment is often inadequate or absent. Imported malaria in industrialized countries is a justified source of concern but represents a very small proportion of all cases of malaria worldwide. Presently, there is a real concern about the spread of resistant strains of falciparum malaria, the re-introduction of malaria in regions where its transmission has stopped or is under control, and emerging epidemics in nonimmune populations exposed to the disease while moving in endemic areas. Travelers and migrants importing malaria to industrialized countries can be seen as indicators of the overall problem of malaria in the world. They point to the need for strengthened surveillance and monitoring of the global evolution of the epidemiology of this disease. They are also a reminder of the urgent need for concerted action in endemic countries for better control and for improved access to treatment with adequate drugs. Protecting travelers with chemoprophylaxis is no doubt a necessity. Improving migrants' access to information, preventing transmission in migrants returning to their country of origin as VFRs, and providing early detection of malaria in immigrants and refugees arriving in Europe are also essential. Addressing the needs of the majority exposed to malaria worldwide is no doubt beyond the scope of travel medicine alone, but travel medicine should actively participate in this effort. Migrants, as global travelers remind us of this reality every day.

REFERENCES

1. United Nations High Commissioner for Refugees (UNHCR). The state of the world's refugees. Fifty years of humanitarian action. Oxford: Oxford University Press, 2000.
2. World Health Organization. The world health report 1998. Geneva, Switzerland: World Health Organization, 1998.
3. United Nations High Commissioner for Refugees. The state of the world's refugees, 1997–1998. A humanitarian agenda. Oxford: Oxford University Press, 1997.
4. United Nations High Commissioner for Refugees (UNHCR). Refugees by numbers. 2001 Mar. Available from: URL: http://www.unhcr.ch.
5. Gushulak BD, MacPherson DW. Health issues associated with the smuggling and trafficking of migrants. J Immigrant Health 2000;2:67–78.
6. Ghosh B. Huddled masses and uncertain shores. Insight into irregular migration. International Organisation for Migration. The Hague: Martinus Nijhoff Publishers, 1998.
7. Wilson M. Population movements and emerging diseases. J Travel Med 1997;4:183–186.
8. Toole MJ, Waldman RJ. Prevention of excessive mortality in refugee and displaced populations in developing countries. JAMA 1990;263:3296–3302.

9. Seaman J, Mercer AJ, Sondorp E. The epidemic of visceral leishmaniasis in western Upper Nile, southern Sudan: course and impact from 1984 to 1994. Int J Epidemiol 1996;25:862–871.

10. Marfin AA, Moore J, Collins C, et al. Infectious disease surveillance during emergency relief to Bhutanese refugees in Nepal. JAMA 1994;272:377–381.

11. Cruz Marques A. Human migration and the spread of malaria in Brazil. Parasitol Today 1987;3:166–170.

12. Singhasivanon P. Mekong malaria. Malaria, multidrug resistance and economic development in the greater Mekong subregion of Southeast Asia. Southeast Asian J Trop Med Public Health 1999;30 Suppl 4:1–101.

13. Prothero RM. Disease and mobility: a neglected factor in epidemiology. Int J Epidemiol 1977;6:259–276.

14. Prothero RM. Migrants and malaria. London: Longmans, Green and Co. Ltd, 1965.

15. Martens P, Hall L. Malaria on the move: human population movement and malaria transmission. Emerg Infect Dis 2000;6:103–109.

16. Zucker JR. Changing patterns of autochthonous malaria transmission in the United States: a review of recent outbreaks. Emerg Infect Dis 1996;2:37–43.

17. Phillips-Howard PA, Bradley DJ, Blaze M, Hurn M. Malaria in Britain: 1977–86. BMJ 1988;296:245–248.

18. Phillips-Howard PA, Radalowicz A, Mitchell J, Bradley D. Risk of malaria in British residents returning from malarious areas. BMJ 1990;300:499–503.

19. Bradley DJ. Current trends in malaria in Britain. J R Soc Med 1989;82 Suppl 17:8–13.

20. Behrens RH. Travel morbidity in ethnic minority travellers. In: Cook GC. Travel-associated disease. London: Royal College of Physicians of London, 1995.

21. Brabin BJ, Ganley Y. Imported malaria in children in the UK. Arch Dis Child 1997;77:76–81.

22. Swiss Federal Office for Public Health. Infectious diseases in Switzerland. Bull Swiss Federal Office Public Health 2001;Suppl:1–48.

23. Swiss Federal Office for Public Health. Malaria in Switzerland 1995–1996. Bull Swiss Federal Office Public Health 1997;25:9–11.

24. Williams HA, Roberts J, Kachur SP, et al. Malaria surveillance—United States, 1995. MMWR CDC Surveill Summ 1999;48:1–23.

25. Lackritz EM, Lobel HO, Howell BJ, et al. Imported *P. falciparum* malaria in American travellers to Africa. Implications for prevention strategies. JAMA 1991;265:383–385.

26. Legros F, Gay F, Belkaid M, Danis M. Situation du paludisme d'importation en France métropolitaine en 1996. Bull Epidemiol Hebdo 1997;48:213–214.

27. Di Perri G, Solbiati M, Vento S, et al. West African immigrants and new patterns of malaria imported to north eastern Italy. J Travel Med 1994;1:147–151.

28. Mateelli A, Colombini P, Gulletta M, et al. Epidemiological features and case management practices of imported malaria in northern Italy 1991–1995. Trop Med Int Health 1999;4:653–657.

29. Wetsteyn JC, Kager PA, van Gool T. The changing pattern of imported malaria in the Academic Medical Centre, Amsterdam. J Travel Med 1997;4:171–175.

30. Lopez-Velez R, Viana A, Perez-Casas C, et al. Clinico-epidemiological study of imported malaria in travellers and immigrants to Madrid. J Travel Med 1999;6:81–86.

31. Jensenius M, Ronning EJ, Blystad H, et al. Low frequency of complications in imported falciparum malaria: a review of 222 cases in south-eastern Norway. Scand J Infect Dis 1999;31:73–78.

32. Hansmann Y, Staub-Schmidt T, Christmann D. Le paludisme d'importation à Strasbourg: une étude épidémiologique, clinique, biologique et thérapeutique. Trop Med Int Health 1997;2:941–952.

33. Leom M. Enquête épidémiologique sur le paludisme d'importation au secteur nord du CHU de Marseille de 1995 à 1997. Marseille : Thèse de Médecine, 1998.

34. Bourgeade A, Touze JE, Chaudet H, et al. Le paludisme d'importation à *Plasmodium falciparum* dans les hôpitaux de Marseille en 1987. A propos de 104 cas. Bull Soc Pathol Exot 1989;82:101–109.

35. Nüesch R, Scheller M, Gyr N. Hospital admissions for malaria in Basel, Switzerland: an epidemiological review of 150 cases. J Travel Med 2000;7:95–97.

36. Antonini P, Bovier P, Toscani L, Loutan L. Paludisme d'importation à Genève: 1988–1994. Med Hyg 1996;54:1080–1085.

37. Elawad BB, Ong EL. Retrospective study of malaria cases treated in Newcastle General Hospital between 1990 and 1996. J Travel Med 1998;5:193–197.

38. Kain KC, Harrington MA, Tennyson S, Keystone JS. Imported malaria: prospective analysis of problems in diagnosis and management. Clin Infect Dis 1998;27:142–149.

39. Walker E, Brodie C. *Plasmodium falciparum* malaria in Nigerians who live in Britain. BMJ 1982;284:956–957.

40. Deloron P, Chougnet C. Is immunity to malaria really short-lived? Parasitol Today 1992;8:375–378.

41. Chougnet C, Deloron P, Savel J. Persistence of cellular and humoral response to synthetic peptides from defined *Plasmodium falciparum* antigens. Ann Trop Med Parasitol 1991;85:357–363.

42. Molineaux L. The epidemiology of human malaria as an explanation of its distribution, including some implications for its control. In: Wernsdorfer WH, McGregor I. Malaria. Principles and practice of malariology. Edinburgh: Churchill Livingston, 1988.

43. Modell M, Modell B. Genetic screening of ethnic minorities. BMJ 1990;300:1702–1704.

44. Svenson JE, MacLean JD, Gyorkos TW, Keystone J. Imported malaria. Clinical presentation and examination of symptomatic travelers. Arch Inter Med 1995;155:861–868.

45. D'Acremont V, Landry P, Pécoud A, et al. Is clinical presentation of malaria different in migrants than in non-migrants? Proceedings of the annual meeting of the Swiss Society of Tropical Medicine and Parasitology; 1999 Nov 4–5; Solothurn, Switzerland.

46. Klein JL, Millman GC. Prospective, hospital based study of fever in children in the United Kingdom who had recently spent time in the tropics. BMJ 1998;316:1425–1426.

47. Gushulak BD, MacPherson DW. Population mobility and infectious diseases: the diminishing impact of classical infectious diseases and new approaches for the 21st century. Clin Infect Dis 2000;31:776–780.

48. Paxton LA, Slutsker L, Schultz LJ et al. Imported malaria in montagnard refugees settling in North Carolina: implications for prevention and control. Am J Trop Med Hyg 1996;54:54–57.

49. Miller JM, Boyd HA, Ostrowski SR, et al. Malaria, intestinal parasites, and schistosomiasis among Barawan Somali refugees resettling in the United States: a strategy to reduce morbidity and decrease the risk of imported infections. Am J Trop Med Hyg 2000;62:115–121.

50. Loutan L, Ghaznawi H. The migrant as a traveler. In: DuPont HL, Steffen R. Textbook of travel medicine and health. Hamilton, London: BC Decker Inc, 2001.

51. Gushulak B. The migrant as a traveller. Migration Health Newslett 1998;1:1–3.

9.5 Special Groups: Pregnant Women, Infants, and Young Children

Aafje E.C. Rietveld

ABSTRACT

During pregnancy or when traveling with infants and young children, it is preferable to completely avoid travel to areas with chloroquine-resistant *Plasmodium falciparum* malaria. At times, however, that is not possible; in such instances, there are no totally safe and effective preventive measures, and difficult choices have to be made.

This chapter describes why young children and pregnant travelers are at special risk of malaria and lays out the currently available options and safety aspects of chemoprophylaxis and personal protection measures for these high-risk groups. Falciparum malaria in infants, young children, and pregnant women is a medical emergency. The rapid progression of clinical symptoms carries the risk of severe disease, fetal loss, and death. Key practical points for the prevention, early diagnosis, and management of malaria in pregnant travelers and in early childhood are provided.

Key words: breastfeeding; chemoprophylaxis; children; congenital malaria; immigrants; infants; malaria prevention; pregnancy; symptoms; travelers; treatment.

PREGNANT WOMEN

Which pregnant travelers are at risk of clinical malaria? This depends on the risk of exposure to an infective mosquito bite and on the background level of antimalarial immunity in the pregnant woman. Mosquitoes that transmit malaria mainly feed between sunset and sunrise, and pregnant travelers who plan to spend the evening and nighttime hours in areas where malaria transmission is known to occur should be considered at potential risk of infection. Pregnant women who have no antimalarial immunity are at risk of acute and severe clinical disease. This group includes women who have never had significant exposure to the parasite and women who have lost previously acquired immunity, as may occur in immigrant populations originally from endemic countries.

Pregnant travelers are at special risk of malaria because they are more likely to get bitten by malaria-carrying mosquitos. The choice of safe and efficacious drugs for prevention and treament of malaria during pregnancy is limited. Pregnant women with malaria can have a very rapid progression of clinical symptoms and are at risk of fetal loss.

Studies and Case Reports

Published epidemiologic studies on malaria in nonimmune pregnant travelers are very rare because pregnancy status is seldom included in descriptive analyses. In one study of 125 nonimmune female travelers who returned to the Netherlands between 1979 and 1988 with falciparum malaria, 10 women were pregnant. Of the 115 nonpregnant women, 17 (14.8%) developed severe malaria. Of the 10 pregnant patients, 6 (60%) developed severe malaria.[1]

Published case reports of malaria in pregnant travelers are rare and often dramatic, reporting rapid progression of clinical symptoms and fetal distress. Some of the cases occur in tourists; others occur among immigrant populations, sometimes months or even a year or more (in case of *P. vivax* infections) after arrival in the non-endemic country, or in women visiting their home country during the course of pregnancy. Reported complications of *Plasmodium falciparum* infection during pregnancy include severe malaria, emergency cesarian section on account of threatening intrauterine asphyxia, congenital malaria, and maternal death.[1–4]

Data from nonimmune populations living in endemic countries have shown that women of all parities are at risk of severe falciparum malaria and adverse consequences to the fetus. Up to 60% of pregnancies may miscarry as a consequence of *P. falciparum* infection, and maternal mortality rates of up to 10% to 13% have been reported.[5–7]

Even vivax malaria, which is normally considered benign, may lead to adverse consequences during pregnancy, including preterm delivery, low birth weight, maternal anemia, and congenital malaria.[5,7,8] Congenital malaria has also been reported (but much less commonly) from *Plasmodium malariae* and *Plasmodium ovale* infections.[9,10]

Prevention of Mosquito Bites

Protection from mosquito bites is paramount during pregnancy. A recent study in Gambia showed that over the course of a night, pregnant women attract twice the number of *Anopheles* mosquitoes (the vectors for malaria) as did nonpregnant women. Possible causes for this attraction include physiologic changes during pregnancy, such as a higher exhaled-breath volume and higher skin temperature. Pregnant women in the study also left the protection of their bednets twice as frequently as nonpregnant women.[11,12]

The following are practical measures for preventing mosquito bites in infants, young children and pregnant women:

1. Use a mosquito net, with edges tucked in under the mattress or hammock, and ensure that the net is not torn and that there are no mosquitoes inside. Mosquito nets for cots and small beds are available. Keep babies, as much as possible, under insecticide-treated mosquito nets between dusk and dawn. Where

available, pyrethroid-treated mosquito nets are preferred as they provide better personal protection. When leaving the protection of the mosquito net during the night, apply an insect repellent.

2. Apply insect repellent to exposed skin between dusk and dawn, when malaria mosquitoes commonly bite. Choose one containing diethyltoluamide (DEET), IR3535®, or Bayrepel®. Application may be required every 3 to 4 hours, especially in hot and humid climates. The manufacturers' recommendations for use should be strictly adhered to, and dosage must not be exceeded, particularly with small children. Insect repellents should not be sprayed on the face or applied to lips or eyelids. Insect repellents should not be applied to sensitive, sunburned, or damaged skin; to mucous membranes; or to deep skin folds.

3. Treat clothing with permethrin or etofenprox for extra protection, to prevent mosquitoes from biting through clothing. Temporary treatment of clothing with a spray-on repellent may also be useful. Label instructions should be followed to prevent possible damage to certain fabrics.

4. Remain indoors, if possible, in a well-constructed and well-maintained building with air-conditioning or with screens over doors and windows, at times when malaria mosquitoes are biting; if no screens are available, windows and doors should be closed at sunset.

5. Spray indoor sleeping area with aerosol flying-insect killer before bedtime. Use mosquito coils, vaporizing mats, or liquid vaporizers indoors at times when mosquitoes are biting. To supplement the use of insect repellents, outdoor use of mosquito coils may provide additional protection against biting insects when there is little or no air movement.

There is no indication that normal usage of insect repellents containing DEET is harmful during pregnancy.[13,14] As there are many different formulations available, the manufacturer's recommendation for use (on the label and package insert) should be strictly adhered to.

Pyrethroid-treated mosquito nets are safe for use during pregnancy[15] and are most efficacious when they are actually used between dusk and dawn. Pregnant women should take care to apply insect repellent to exposed skin if they have to leave the protection of the mosquito net at night, even for short periods of time.

Drugs for Prevention and Treatment

For ethical and practical reasons, pregnant women are routinely excluded from initial efficacy and safety studies of new antimalarial drugs. The available data on the safety of antimalarial drugs in pregnancy are based on extrapolation of animal study results, on treatment studies of clinical malaria in areas with multidrug-resistant parasites, and on accumulating reports of accidental exposure. As a result, few of the relatively newer drugs can currently be prescribed with confidence throughout a pregnancy. In certain circumstances, the urgent need to use a life-saving drug for treatment of clinical *Plasmodium falciparum* malaria is considered to outweigh a possible risk of side effects. This argument cannot be applied to prophylactic drugs for pregnant travelers.

For women in the first trimester of pregnancy who intend to travel to areas with transmission of *P. falciparum* malaria, there are no safe and highly efficacious drugs for chemoprophylaxis at present, with the exception of chloroquine for Central America and for the island of Hispaniola. For areas with multidrug-resistant *P. falciparum* parasites that are resistant to mefloquine (such as parts of Southeast Asia and the Amazon River basin), there are no safe and highly efficacious chemoprophylaxis options left at present for any trimester of pregnancy.

Chemoprophylaxis

Chloroquine with or without proguanil is safe for chemoprophylaxis during pregnancy and lactation. However, the current spread of antimalarial drug resistance has greatly reduced the usefulness of chloroquine for the prevention of falciparum malaria. *Plasmodium vivax* resistance to chlorquine has also been reported in some areas. Some countries recommend folic acid supplementation for pregnant women taking proguanil prophylaxis, particularly in early pregnancy. Mefloquine prophylaxis can be safely prescribed from the second trimester onward. Early animal studies have documented teratogenic and embryotoxic effects associated with the use of high-dose mefloquine. However, limited data on pregnancy outcomes of women who accidentally took mefloquine prophylaxis during the first trimester of pregnancy are reassuring and do not warrant pregnancy termination.[16,17] Doxycycline is contraindicated throughout pregnancy and during lactation because it impairs skeletal calcification in the fetus, resulting in abnormal osteogenesis and permanent hypoplasia of dental enamel. For safety reasons, pregnancy should be avoided during the period of drug intake and for 3 months after completing mefloquine prophylaxis and 1 week after completing doxycycline prophylaxis.

There are no data on the safety and efficacy of atovaquone/proguanil during pregnancy and lactation,[18] and therefore, its use is not recommended at these times.

Treatment

Chloroquine is safe throughout pregnancy, but in pregnant travelers, it can now only be used for the treatment of the clinical manifestations of *Plasmodium malariae*, *Plasmodium ovale*, and chloroquine-sensitive *Plasmodium vivax* malaria. Data on the safety of amodiaquine during pregnancy are limited. Amodiaquine has little advantage over chloroquine in the treatment of falciparum malaria in pregnant travelers, especially where more efficacious alternatives are available.

Sulfonamides may cause kernicterus in the newborn, even though the risk with doses used for malaria treatment is considered to be very low. The manufacturers therefore recommend that pregnant women at term and nursing mothers should not use sulfadoxine/pyrimethamine. Sulfadoxine/pyrimethamine would not normally be recommended for treatment of falciparum malaria in pregnant travelers when other choices are available.

A retrospective analysis of pregnancy outcomes among women living on the Thailand-Myanmar border showed that mefloquine treatment of *Plasmodium falciparum* malaria during pregnancy was associated with an increased risk of stillbirths, but no definite conclusions could be drawn.[19] Available data on the safety of mefloquine in the first trimester of pregnancy are limited but reassuring (see above).[17] Nevertheless, mefloquine is not normally recommended for treatment of malaria in pregnant travelers when other choices are available.

Tetracycline, like doxycycline, is contraindicated during pregnancy and lactation because it impairs skeletal calcification in the fetus, resulting in abnormal osteogenesis and permanent hypoplasia of dental enamel. Unlike tetracycline and doxycycline, clindamycin has not been reported to cause adverse events in pregnancy or during breastfeeding although experience is limited. It can be used in combination with quinine for the treatment of falciparum malaria acquired in areas with emerging quinine resistance in parts of Southeast Asia and in the Amazon River basin.[20]

Safety and efficacy data on the use of halofantrine and atovaquone/proguanil during pregnancy and lactation are lacking; therefore, these drugs are not recommended.

Based on safety and efficacy considerations, quinine is currently recommended as the drug of choice for emergency standby treatment of suspected falciparum malaria in pregnant travelers. Where available, quinidine may be used for the treatment of confirmed falciparum malaria. Quinidine has antimalarial properties similar to those of quinine but has a greater cardiosuppressant effect; it is used in a similar dosage regimen.

Artemisinin and its derivatives (such as artesunate and artemether) have the advantage over quinine in that they do not induce hypoglycemia, but data on pregnancy outcomes following their use in the first trimester are still limited. Artemisinins are the drugs of choice for severe malaria in the second and third trimester, but they should be used with caution in the first trimester.[21]

Primaquine, the only drug currently used for the treatment of relapsing malaria, may cause hemolysis in persons with glucose-6-phosphate dehydrogenase (G6PD) deficiency. It is contraindicated during pregnancy because of the risk of hemolysis in the fetus. Radical treatment of *Plasmodium vivax* and *Plasmodium ovale* infections with primaquine should thus wait until after delivery. Pregnant travelers who have been diagnosed with *Plasmodium ovale* or chloroquine-sensitive vivax malaria should be treated with chloroquine and covered with weekly chloroquine prophylaxis for the remainder of the pregnancy.

The safety of antimalarial drugs during pregnancy is summarized in Table 9.5–1.

Table 9.5–1. **Safety of Antimalarial Drugs During Pregnancy and Breastfeeding and in Small Children***

Antimalarial Drug	Indication	Pregnancy	Breast Feeding	Small Children
Choroquine	Prophylaxis & treatment	Safe	Safe	Safe
Proguanil	Prophylaxis	Safe	Safe	Safe
Mefloquine	Prophylaxis & treatment	Not recommended in 1st trimester*	Safe	Not recommended under 5 kg body weight*
Doxycycline	Prophylaxis & treatment	Contraindicated	Contraindicated	Contraindicated under 8 years of age
Atovaquone/ proguanil	Prophylaxis & treatment	No data; not recommended	No data; not recommended	Not recommended under 11 kg body weight*
Amodiaquine	Treatment	Apparently safe, but limited data	Apparently safe, but limited data	Safe
Sulfadoxine/ pyrimethamine	Treatment	Safe with caution at term	Safe with caution	Contraindicated under 2 months of age
Quinine	Treatment	Safe	Safe	Safe
Artemisinins	Treatment	Not recommended in 1st trimester*	Safe	Safe
Primaquine	Treatment	Contraindicated	Safe	Contraindicated under 4 years of age
Tetracycline	Treatment	Contraindicated	Contraindicated	Contraindicated under 8 years of age
Clindamycin	Treatment	Apparently safe, but limited data	Apparently safe, but limited data	Apparently safe, but limited data
Halofantrine	Treatment	No data; not recommended	No data; not recommended	Not recommended under 10 kg body weight*

* This table addresses only the safety aspects related to pregnancy, breast feeding, and young children. Each drug also has its own side effects and specific contraindications that should be taken into account.

Rapid Progression of Clinical Symptoms and Risk of Fetal Loss

A pregnant woman with malaria must be diagnosed and treated promptly because pregnancy increases the risk that a *Plasmodium falciparum* infection will develop into severe disease and that the woman will subsequently die of severe malaria. Unfortunately, misdiagnosis on initial contact is common and may contribute to an increased case-fatality rate. In a review of mortality among travelers from the United States, 24 (40%) of 60 fatal malaria cases were initially misdiagnosed.[22] Pregnant women are more likely to develop cerebral and other forms of severe malaria and are particularly susceptible to hypoglycemia and acute pulmonary edema. Falciparum malaria in pregnant women has a mortality two to ten times higher than falciparum malaria in nonpregnant patients.[23]

Falciparum malaria parasites can be abundant in the placenta even when they may not be detectable in the peripheral circulation.[24,25] Fever, anemia, and malarial infection of the placenta increase the risk of abortion, premature delivery, stillbirth, and low birth weight, even in uncomplicated falciparum malaria.[5,26] Malaria may lead to threatened premature labor or may result in established labor despite prompt antimalarial treatment. Once labor has started, fetal or maternal distress may dictate the need to intervene rapidly, and the second stage may need to be shortened with effective obstetric care.

Early Recognition and Management

The symptoms of malaria may be nonspecific and difficult to recognize. As a rule, falciparum malaria must always be suspected in all travelers with a (recent history of) fever, with or without other symptoms, developing at any time between 1 week after the first possible exposure to malaria and 2 months (or even later in rare cases) after the last possible exposure.

Pregnant women should be instructed to seek competent medical help immediately if fever with or without other symptoms of malaria develops, and they should insist on a laboratory examination for malaria. If there is a high clinical suspicion of malaria but the blood smear is negative, then the smear should be repeated at 6-hour intervals while therapy is initiated. Similarly, treatment with a safe and efficacious drug should be started if there is a strong clinical suspicion of malaria but the laboratory results cannot be obtained within 1 to 2 hours. Clinical management of malaria in a pregnant traveler requires close monitoring for the development of severe disease and fetal distress.

Severe Malaria in Pregnant Women

Pregnant women with severe falciparum malaria may present with any of the clinical symptoms of severe malaria normally seen in adults. They are particularly susceptible to hypoglycemia and pulmonary edema. Other dangers include postpartum hemorrhage as well as hyperpyrexia leading to fetal distress. Such patients should be transferred to an intensive care center and managed in close collaboration between specialists in infectious disease, internal medicine, and obstetric care.[23]

Hypoglycemia

Hypoglycemia may be caused by malaria itself and may also be brought on by quinine therapy. Women may stay at risk of hypoglycemia for several days into the postpartum period and after symptoms of malaria have resolved.[27] Hypoglycemia contributes to a high case-fatality rate and should be monitored in all pregnant women with severe malaria by the repeated measuring of blood glucose levels. Because of the risk of quinine-induced hyperinsulinemia and hypoglycemia, artemisinin derivatives are preferable to quinine for treatment of severe malaria in the second and third trimester. For the treatment of severe malaria in the first trimester, the advantages of artemisinin drugs over quinine must be weighed against the fact that there is still limited documentation on pregnancy outcomes following the use of artemisinin drugs.[21]

Hypoglycemia may be asymptomatic for the mother. A deterioration of consciousness and/or fetal distress may be the only signs. Hypoglycemia after quinine therapy may start as abnormal behavior, sweating, and a sudden loss of consciousness.

Symptoms and signs manifest as follows:

- Commonly asymptomatic in the mother, but associated with fetal bradycardia and other signs of fetal distress
- Classic symptoms in conscious patients: anxiety, sweating, dilatation of the pupils, breathlessness, oliguria, feeling of coldness, tachycardia, light-headedness
- Followed by deteriorating consciousness, generalized convulsions, extensor posturing, shock, coma
- Severely ill patients: lactic acidosis and high mortality

Management is as follows:

- If possible, confirm by hypoglycemic biochemical testing.
- If diagnosis is in doubt, give a therapeutic trial with 50% dextrose (20 to 50 mL intravenously) over 5 to 10 minutes.
- Follow with continuous intravenous infusion of 5% or 10% dextrose infusion.
- Continue to monitor blood glucose levels to regulate dextrose infusion.
- Beware of fluid overload, to avoid pulmonary edema.
- If injectable dextrose is not available, give dextrose or sugary solution by nasogastric tube to unconscious patient.

Severe recurrent hypoglycemia may occur despite intravenous glucose therapy. The diagnosis of hypoglycemia may be missed because its clinical symptoms resemble those of severe malaria.

Pulmonary Edema

Pulmonary edema may present at hospital admission or may develop suddenly several days after admission to hospital, at a time when the patient's general condition is improving and peripheral parasitemia is diminishing. It commonly develops in severely anemic women or in women with fluid overload immediately after delivery and separation of the placenta. It may occur at any time in the 1st week post partum.[2,27] Pulmonary edema may occur in vivax malaria.

Pulmonary edema may result from increased pulmonary capillary permeability, resembling adult respiratory distress syndrome (ARDS); it may also be due to fluid overload or to a combination of the two. It is often associated with other complications of severe malaria, including hypoglycemia and metabolic acidosis. Hyperparasitemia and renal failure are predisposing factors.

Symptoms and signs are as follows:

- First indication: increased respiratory rate and dyspnea
- Reduced arterial partial pressure of oxygen (PO_2)

- Features of ARDS
- Hypoxia leading to convulsions and deteriorating consciousness
- Death usually occurs within a few hours

Management is as follows:

- If due to overhydration: stop all intravenous fluids, use hemofiltration immediately. If there is no improvement, withdraw 250 mL blood by venesection into a blood transfusion donor bag.
- General: keep the patient upright; lower the foot of the bed, and raise the head of the bed; give high concentration oxygen by any convenient method, including mechanical ventilation; give diuretic such as 40 mg furosemide intravenously. If no response, increase the dose of furosemide progressively to a maximum of 200 mg.
- Where available: mechanical ventilation with positive end-expiratory pressure (PEEP), vasoactive drugs, and hemodynamic monitoring.

Prevent pulmonary edema by avoiding severe anemia and excessive rehydration.

The clinical management of severe malaria in pregnant travelers is dealt with in two recent World Health Organization (WHO) publications.[23,27]

Summary

Recommendations

The World Health Organization (WHO) advises pregnant women to avoid traveling to areas where chloroquine-resistant *Plasmodium falciparum* occurs. In other words, avoid travel to any country where there is transmission of *P. falciparum*, with the exception of the island of Hispaniola and those parts of Central America where *P. falciparum* is currently still fully sensitive to chloroquine.[23,27]

Falciparum malaria in a pregnant traveler is a medical emergency and carries a high risk of maternal death, neonatal death, miscarriage, and stillbirth. Get medical help immediately, request a laboratory diagnosis if malaria is suspected, and make sure that treatment with an effective and safe antimalarial drug is initiated as soon as possible. Quinine and artemisinin derivatives (second and third trimester) are the drugs of choice for treatment of uncomplicated *P. falciparum* malaria. Artemisinin derivatives are the drugs of choice for treatment of severe malaria in the 2nd and 3rd trimester.

When travel cannot be avoided, it is very important to take effective preventive measures against malaria, even when traveling to areas where there is transmission of vivax malaria only.

Pregnant Women: Main Messages

1. Do not go to a malarious area unless absolutely necessary.

2. Be extra diligent in using measures to protect against mosquito bites, but do not exceed the recommended dosage of insect repellents.
3. Take prophylactic drugs, observing the following:
    - Comply with the recommended regimen. In areas with chloroquine-resistant *Plasmodium falciparum*, chloroquine and proguanil should be taken during the first 3 months of pregnancy; mefloquine prophylaxis may be taken from the 4th month of pregnancy onward.
    - Doxycycline prophylaxis is contraindicated; atovaquone/proguanil prophylaxis is not recommended.
4. Seek medical help immediately if malaria is suspected, and take emergency standby treatment (quinine is the drug of choice) only if medical help is not immediately available. Medical help *must* still be sought as soon as possible after standby treatment.
5. Remember that malaria in a pregnant traveler is a medical emergency. It must be suspected and treated promptly because the disease is more severe, is associated with high parasitemia, and is dangerous for the mother and the fetus.

Malaria in a pregnant woman increases the risk of maternal death, miscarriage, stillbirth, and low birth weight with associated risk of neonatal death.

Women who Might Become Pregnant: Main Messages
1. Both mefloquine and doxycycline prophylaxis may be taken, but pregnancy should be avoided during the period of drug intake and for 3 months after mefloquine prophylaxis is stopped and 1 week after doxycycline prophylaxis is stopped.
2. If pregnancy occurs during antimalarial prophylaxis, the physician should provide information about the possible effects of the drugs on the newborn infant. However, in the case of an unplanned pregnancy, malaria chemoprophylaxis is not considered to be an indication for termination of pregnancy.

CONGENITAL MALARIA

Infants may contract malaria in utero due to transplacental transfer of parasites, or they may contract malaria during delivery. Congenital malaria has been described for all malaria species but has been most often described for *Plasmodium falciparum* and *Plasmodium vivax*. It is more common in infants of nonimmune mothers.[24] The condition is a rare occurrence in non-endemic countries; for instance, only 49 cases were reported in the United States between 1950 and 1991.[10] Nevertheless, it should be considered in all febrile newborns with anemia and splenomegaly who are born to mothers with a history of travel to or immigration from malaria-endemic areas or to mothers whose travel history is unknown.

Congenital malaria can occur in infants of women who have had clinical malaria during pregnancy, but it can also occur in newborns of asymptomatic immigrants from endemic countries. In the latter group, the newborn is typically healthy at birth, and symptoms develop only when maternal antibodies start to wane. Congenital malaria usually occurs within the first 3 months of life. Congenital malaria is caused by the transfer of blood-stage parasites only, and there is no risk of recurrent attacks of vivax or ovale infections.

INFANTS AND YOUNG CHILDREN

Children are especially at risk of malaria infection. Worldwide, almost 40% of the annual 300 million clinical malaria cases and more than 70% of the over 1 million annual malaria deaths are estimated to occur among children under 5 years of age.[28] Travel health authorities recommend against taking young children to endemic areas. Nevertheless, in some non-endemic European countries, pediatric cases account for 10 to 19% of the total malaria burden.[29,30] Immigrant populations may be an important source of pediatric malaria.[30–32] In a hospital series in the Netherlands, the proportion of malaria cases in children under 15 years of age was four times higher among immigrants originally from malarious areas (14 of 66) than among the remainder (18 of 361).[33] Similarly, 86% of 315 pediatric malaria cases in a hospital series in the city of Marseilles originated in Comoros.[30] Malaria may be diagnosed in immigrants who have recently arrived or who have made a family visit to the endemic country. Immigrant families may be more likely to bring small children along when traveling to visit relatives in endemic countries and may stay for longer periods in rural areas with a higher risk of infection. They may also be less aware of effective preventive measures and the need for such measures.

Young children are at special risk of malaria because the choice of safe and efficacious drugs for prevention and treatment of malaria in small children is limited, and it may be difficult to administer oral drugs to a child. Special care should be taken to safely avoid mosquito bites. Children who contract malaria can have a very rapid progression of clinical symptoms, with risk of severe disease and death.

Mosquito Bite Prevention in Small Children: Special Considerations

Safe protection from mosquito bites is particularly important for infants and young children. (See the list under "Prevention of Mosquito Bites," above, for practical measures for preventing mosquito bites in small children.)

Systemic toxic reactions and encephalopathy have been reported in small children after accidental ingestion of DEET and after repeated skin application and spraying.[15] DEET may come into contact with a baby's mouth through heavily sprayed bedding or toys or after it is applied to a baby's hands. There is no indication of a relationship between DEET concentration and the severity of symptoms. However, the risk of serious side effects following the normal use of DEET-containing insect repellents is considered low.[14] Since children appear to be more sensitive to DEET than adults, it has been suggested that their skin exposure should be kept to a minimum and that DEET should be applied to their clothing rather than to their skin.[13] The manufacturers' recommendations for the use of insect repellents (as indicated on labels and package inserts) should be strictly adhered to, and dosage must not be exceeded.

Pyrethroid-treated mosquito nets are safe for use with small children. Small mosquito nets for cots can be obtained. Alternatively, some maneuvering space may be created by placing the entire cot under an adult-size net that reaches the floor, provided that entry of mosquitoes can be prevented. Between dusk and dawn, children should preferably be dressed in long-sleeved pajamas or other protective loose-fitting clothing.

Drugs for Prevention and Treatment

The choice of safe and efficacious drugs for prevention and treatment of malaria in infants and young children is limited.

Chemoprophylaxis

Chloroquine with or without proguanil can be given with confidence to children of all ages; however, these drugs are not very useful in most high-risk areas. Mefloquine prophylaxis can be safely prescribed for babies weighing 5 kg or more. Data on children weighing less than 5 kg are lacking. Accurate dosing at the recommended dose of 5 mg/kg per week for prophylaxis becomes increasingly difficult in smaller children due to the relatively large size of the 250-mg mefloquine base tablets.

Doxycycline is contraindicated in children under 8 years of age because it may produce transient depression of bone growth, permanent discoloration of teeth, and enamel dysplasia.

Data on atovaquone/proguanil in children weighing less than 11 kg are not yet available, and atovaquone/proguanil is therefore not recommended in this group. Data on its use for malaria prophylaxis in international travelers are still very limited. Atovaquone/proguanil may offer a solution as prophylaxis for children with epilepsy who cannot take chloroquine or mefloquine and who are too young to take doxycycline. It can also be prescribed for those rare cases in which a child under 8 years of age has to stay overnight in rural areas with transmission of multidrug-resistant malaria.

Drug regimens for chemoprophylaxis in children are given in Table 9.5–2.

Treatment

Chloroquine is safe for children of all ages, but for travelers, it can now be used only for the treatment of the clinical manifestations of *Plasmodium malariae*, *Plasmodium ovale*, and chloroquine-sensitive *Plasmodium vivax* malaria. Amodiaquine can

Table 9.5–2. **Drug Regimens for Chemoprophylaxis in Children***

Body Weight (kg)	Prophylaxis Regimen	
	Chloroquine† (Tablets/Week)	
	100 mg Base‡	150 mg Base
5–6	0.25	0.25
7–10	0.5	0.5
11–14	0.75	0.5
15–18	1	0.75
19–24	1.25	1
25–35	2	1
36–50	2.5	2
> 50	3	2

Body Weight (kg)	Proguanil Hydrochloride§ 100 mg (Tablets/Day)
5–8	0.25
9–16	0.5
17–24	0.75
25–35	1
36–50	1.5
> 35	2

Body Weight (kg)	Mefloquine‖ 250 mg base (Tablets/Week)
< 5	Not recommended
5–12	0.25
13–24	0.5
25–35	0.75
≥ 35	1

Body Weight (kg)	Doxycycline#** 100 mg Salt (Tablets/Day)
25–35	0.5
36–50	0.75
> 50	1

* Dosage schedules for children must be based on body weight. This table is indicative only.
† 5 mg (base)/kg weekly.
‡ In young children, more precise doses can be obtained with 100 mg (base) tablets.
§ 3 mg/kg daily.
‖ 5 mg/kg weekly.
1.5 mg (salt)/kg daily.
** Doxycycline is contraindicated for children aged < 8 years.

be used in children for the treatment of sensitive strains of nonfalciparum malaria, as a substitute for chloroquine. It has the advantage of tasting better.

Sulfonamides may cause kernicterus in the newborn, even though the risk with the doses used for malaria treatment is considered to be very low. The manufacturers therefore recommend that sulfadoxine/pyrimethamine not be given to infants under 2 months of age. It should also not be given consecutively or concomitantly with sulfa-based antibiotics such as co-trimoxazole. Sulfadoxine/pyrimethamine would not normally be used in the treatment of nonimmune infant travelers with falciparum malaria when alternatives that are more efficacious are available.

Data from the Thailand-Myanmar border show that vomiting is a frequent problem in young children receiving mefloquine for the treatment of uncomplicated falciparum malaria. The risk is inversely proportional to age, and in the study, vomiting was associated with reduced treatment efficacy, even if re-treatment was given. In the same study, young children appeared to be less likely than adults to suffer from the major neuropsychiatric or behavioral side effects of mefloquine treatment.[34]

Quinine is currently recommended as the drug of choice for emergency standby treatment of suspected falciparum malaria in young children. Artemisinin and its derivatives such as artesunate and artemether can be used safely in young children and have the advantages over quinine of an easier dosing schedule, fewer side effects, and a more rapid parasite clearance and relief of clinical symptoms. Suppository formulations are available in some countries.[21] Quinine and the artemisinins are the drugs of choice for treatment of severe malaria in small children.

Tetracycline and doxycycline are contraindicated in children under 8 years of age as these drugs may produce transient depression of bone growth, permanent discoloration of teeth, and enamel dysplasia. Although data are limited, clindamycin is reportedly safe and can be used in combination with quinine for the treatment of falciparum malaria acquired in areas with emerging quinine resistance. It may lead to diarrhea in up to 20% of patients.[20]

Primaquine is contraindicated in children under 4 years of age because of the risk of hemolysis, thus excluding the option of radical treatment of *Plasmodium vivax* and *Plasmodium ovale* infections in this age group. Instead, relapses should be treated symptomatically if and when they occur.

Halofantrine, due to risk of fatal cardiotoxicity, may be used only in well-equipped medical centers and under strict medical supervision. It is not recommended for children weighing less than 10 kg, due to a lack of data for this group. Halofantrine is not normally used in the treatment of falciparum malaria in small children when other alternatives are available.

The safety of antimalarial drugs in infants and young children is summarized in Table 9.5–1.

Administration of Oral Drugs to Young Children

Very few antimalarial drugs are available in pediatric formulations. It is difficult to make young children swallow oral medication. Morever, most antimalarial tablets are notoriously foul tasting. Some tricks that have worked include the following:

- Mix the crushed tablet with a bit of jam, banana, sweetened condensed milk, or similar foods.

- Roll the crushed tablet into a small ball of butter, chocolate paste, or peanut butter, and cover with chocolate sprinkles (P. Phillips-Howard, personal communication Feb. 25, 2001).
- Dissolve the crushed tablet into a small amount of water (≤ 5 mL) and squirt it directly into the mouth with a plastic syringe. Quickly follow this with a little milk or favorite food.[34]

Before departure, parents should ask the pharmacist to pulverize the tablets and to prepare sachets or gelatin capsules with the correct daily or weekly dose for the child, based on body weight.[35]

Sick Children

To reduce the risk of vomiting in sick children, it helps to bring the fever down with paracetamol and tepid sponging before administering oral antimalarial treatment. If a child vomits within 30 minutes of administering an antimalarial drug, the whole dose should be repeated. If the child vomits later but within 1 hour, half the dose should be repeated. A rectal formulation of artesunate can be used as an emergency measure for children who cannot take oral antimalarial treatment.

Keep all antimalarial drugs out of the reach of children and stored in childproof containers. Chloroquine is particularly toxic to children if the recommended dose is exceeded; 300 mg (two tablets) may already be lethal for an infant aged 12 months.[36]

Progression of Clinical Symptoms: Risk of Severe Disease and Death

Children can rapidly die from *Plasmodium falciparum* malaria. Small children can rapidly develop high parasitemias due to their smaller blood volume and red cell mass. Coupled with immunologic immaturity, this may lead to the rapid progression of clinical symptoms and increased risk of severe disease and death.[37] Life-threatening complications can occur within hours of the initial symptoms.[29]

Clinical malaria can occur despite prophylaxis, and any child with a positive travel history and a fever or history of fever must be considered to have malaria until proven otherwise, sometimes repeatedly. If there is a high clinical suspicion of malaria but the blood smear is negative, the smear should be repeated at 6-hour intervals while therapy is initiated.

Early Recognition and Management

Malaria may mimic other diseases, especially in young children. The early symptoms of falciparum malaria are notoriously atypical and difficult to recognize, especially since young children may have fevers from a variety of causes. Initially, a child with malaria may be lethargic, listless, drowsy, irritable, or anorexic. Older children may complain of headache and nausea. They may vomit, cough, or have abdominal pain, anemia, and convulsions.[37] Concurrent infections such as otitis media may mask the early symptoms of malaria.

In a retrospective study involving 20 children admitted to hospital with malaria in the United States (including 5 patients with falciparum malaria), all had had fever for more than 10 days despite oral antibiotic therapy. The initial suspected diagnoses of these children included leukemia and other malignancies, pyelonephritis, and acute appendicitis. This resulted in unnecessary tests and procedures as well as in dangerous delays in initiating adequate antimalarial treatment. Except for the case of two siblings whose mother mentioned the possibility of malaria, it took 4 to 8 days after hospital admission before the correct diagnosis was made.[32]

Fever is a frequent (but not essential) symptom of clinical malaria. It was present in 92% of 315 pediatric malaria cases in a study in France.[30] Malarial fever in young children almost never follows a typical pattern of recurrent fever, and both irregular fever patterns and continued fever may occur.[29, 31]

Clinical falciparum malaria can occur a week after arrival in the endemic area but has also been reported in a child 5 months after return; the first attack of *Plasmodium vivax* infection may occur up to 10 months after return.[30] In a prospective hospital-based study in the United Kingdom, 4 of 31 children admitted with fever and who had been in a tropical country within the previous month were diagnosed with malaria.[38]

Plasmodium vivax infection in young children may result in high fever with convulsions. Anemia is usually more moderate but may become severe with repeated attacks. Death due to a vivax malaria infection is very rare but may occur in children debilitated by other diseases, severe malnutrition, or anemia. Relapses may occur up to 4 years after the initial attack and are often milder and of shorter duration;[37] they can be treated symptomatically with chloroquine or quinine, depending on the drug sensitivity pattern. When the child is older than 4 years of age, radical cure with primaquine can be given. The clinical features of *Plasmodium ovale* infection in young children are similar to those of *Plasmodium vivax* infection.

A clinical attack of *Plasmodium malariae* malaria in young children is rare. It may resemble vivax malaria, but it can occur years after the initial infection. It can be treated with chloroquine or amodiaquine, and there is no risk of relapse. Nephrotic syndrome with severe generalized edema, persistant heavy proteinuria, ascites and severe hypoproteinemia has been described in African children with *Plasmodium malariae* infection; it is reported to respond poorly to treatment.[37]

Severe Malaria in Young Children

The commonest and most important clinical complications of severe *Plasmodium falciparum* malaria in infants and young children are

- cerebral malaria,
- severe anemia,
- respiratory distress (acidosis) with deep breathing, and
- hypoglycemia.[23]

Compared to adults, young children with severe malaria are more likely to experience (or to have a history of) of coughing, convulsions, hypoglycemia on hospital admission, increased cerebrospinal fluid (CSF) opening pressure, respiratory distress (acidosis), and abnormal brain stem reflexes. Pulmonary edema, renal failure, and bleeding and clotting disturbances are less frequent. The history of symptoms preceding coma in small children may be very brief, 1 to 2 days on average, as opposed to 5 to 7 days in adults. Resolution of coma is faster on average (1 to 2 days only). Neurologic sequelae occur in over 10% of children with severe malaria.

If a child is suspected of having severe malaria, do the following immediate tests: a thick and thin blood film, packed-cell volume hematocrit (Ht), finger-prick blood glucose, and lumbar puncture. Take the following emergency measures: (1) insert a nasogastric tube in unconscious children and evacuate stomach contents to minimize the risk of aspiration pneumonia, (2) correct hypoglycemia, (3) restore circulating volume, and (4) treat anemia. In any child with convulsions, exclude hyperpyrexia and hypoglycemia. Hypoglycemia is particularly common in children under 3 years of age and in those with convulsions or hyperparasitemia or in a profound coma. If parasitologic confirmation is likely to take more than 1 hour, start treatment with quinine or an artemisinin derivative before the diagnosis is confirmed. If lumbar puncture is delayed, give antibiotics to cover the possibility of bacterial meningitis.

The details of the clinical management of severe malaria in small children are given in two recent WHO publications, which can be obtained through the WHO Communicable Diseases (CDS) Documentation Centre in Geneva (E-mail address: CDSDOC@who.int.[23,27]

Summary

Recommendations

The World Health Organization advises parents not to take babies or young children to areas with chloroquine-resistant *P. falciparum* transmission. If travel cannot be avoided, the child must be carefully protected against mosquito bites and must be given appropriate chemoprophylactic drugs.

Falciparum malaria in a small child is a medical emergency. Children can rapidly die from malaria. Early symptoms are atypical and are difficult to recognize. Life-threatening complications can occur within hours of the initial symptoms. Always consider the possibility of malaria whenever a child gets a fever within a year of traveling to an endemic area. Immediately request a laboratory diagnosis if malaria is suspected, and make sure that treatment with an effective antimalarial drug is initiated as soon as possible. Quinine and artemisinin derivatives are the drugs of choice.

Children of immigrant families may be at special risk. Any fever in these children should prompt the physician to ask for a travel history. Malaria may occur simultaneously with other obvious causes of fever.

Young Children: Main Messages

1. Do not take babies or young children to a malarious area unless absolutely necessary.
2. Be extra diligent in protecting children against mosquito bites. As much as possible, keep babies under insecticide-treated mosquito nets between dusk and dawn. Follow the manufacturer's instructions on the use of insect repellents, and do not exceed the recommended dosage.
3. Administer prophylactic drugs, observing the following:
   - Give prophylaxis to breastfed babies as well as to bottle-fed babies since they are not protected by the mother's prophylaxis.
   - Dosage schedules for children should be based on body weight.
   - Chloroquine and proguanil are safe for babies and young children; mefloquine may be given from 5 kg of body weight upward.
   - Doxycycline is contraindicated in children below 8 years of age; atovaquone/proguanil is not recommended in children weighing less than 11 kg.
4. Keep all antimalarial drugs out of the reach of children and store in childproof containers. Chloroquine is particularly toxic to children if the recommended dose is exceeded.
5. Seek medical help immediately if a child develops a febrile illness. The symptoms of malaria in children may not be typical, and so malaria should always be suspected, and a laboratory diagnosis should be made. In infants, malaria should be suspected even in nonfebrile illness.
6. Use quinine or artemisinin derivatives as the drugs of choice for the treatment of *Plasmodium falciparum* malaria in small children.

Children can rapidly die from malaria.

BREASTFEEDING MOTHERS AND BREASTFED INFANTS

Tetracycline, doxycycline, halofantrine, and atovaquone/proguanil are contraindicated for breastfeeding mothers (the latter two for lack of data). The manufacturers recommend against using sulfadoxine/pyrimethamine in nursing mothers due to the risk of kernicterus in the newborn; however, the drug is generally considered compatible with breastfeeding for older healthy full-term infants. Even though the other antimalarials are distributed in small amounts into breast milk, the amount of drug consumed by the infant is considered too small to be harmful. The ingested amounts are also too small to provide adequate protection, and breastfed infants still require their own chemoprophylaxis.[39]

As a caution, breastfed infants of mothers taking antimalarial drugs should be monitored for possible side effects such as jaundice and hemolysis, especially if the infant is premature or less than 1 month old. G6PD-deficient infants are at increased risk.[40]

Safety data on antimalarial drugs during breastfeeding are summarized in Table 9.5–1.

ACKNOWLEDGMENTS

The author thanks colleagues from the Roll Back Malaria (RBM) Technical Team and the Communicable Diseases (CDS) Vector Control Team at the World Health Organization, Geneva, for their constructive input and helpful comments. The author also thanks Professor Hugo van de Kaay and Dr. Peter Trigg for critically reviewing the manuscript.

Note: The information in this section is based on the WHO publication *International Travel and Health*—vaccination requirements and health advice, 2001. Geneva: World Health Organization, 2001. p. 67–84. For more recent information, please consult the latest annual edition of *International Travel and Health* or the Web site of the World Health Organization at http://www.who.int/ith.

REFERENCES

1. Wetsteyn JC, de Geus A. Falciparum malaria, imported into The Netherlands, 1979–1988. II. Clinical features. Trop Geogr Med 1995;47:97–102.
2. Subramanian D, Moise KJ Jr, White AC Jr. Imported malaria in pregnancy: report of four cases and review of management. Clin Infect Dis 1992;15:408–413.
3. Hoffmann AL, Ronn AM, Langhoff-Roos J, et al. Malaria og graviditet. Ugeskr Laeger 1992;154:2662–2665.
4. David KP, Petersen JE, Arpi M. *Plasmodium falciparum*-malaria hos en gravid kvinde seks måneder efter ophold i et malariaområde. Ugeskr Laeger 1998;160:4778.
5. Brabin BJ. The risks and severity of malaria in pregnant women. Geneva: World Health Organization; 1991. Applied Field Research in Malaria Reports No.1,TDR/FIELD-MAL/1.
6. Meek SR. Epidemiology of malaria in displaced Khmers on the Thai-Kampuchean border. Southeast Asian J Trop Med Public Health 1988;2:243–252.
7. Singh N, Shukla MM, Sharma VP. Epidemiology of malaria in pregnancy in central India. Bull World Health Organ 1999;77:567–572.
8. Nosten F, McGready R, Simpson JA, et al. Effects of *Plasmodium vivax* malaria in pregnancy. Lancet 1999;354:546–549.
9. Zenz W, Trop M, Kollaritsch H, et al. Konnatale Malaria durch *Plasmodium falciparum* und *Plasmodium malariae*. Wien Klin Wochenschr 2000;112:459–461.
10. Hulbert TV. Congenital malaria in the United States: report of a case and review. Clin Infect Dis 1992;14:922–926.
11. Lindsay S, Ansell J, Selman C, et al. Effect of pregnancy on exposure to malaria mosquitoes. Lancet 2000;355:1972.
12. Martinez-Espinosa F, Alecrim WD, Daniel-Ribeiro C. Attraction of mosquitoes to pregnant women. Lancet 2000;356:685.

13. World Health Organization. Safe use of pesticides, 14th Report of the World Health Organization Expert Committee on Vector Biology and Control. Geneva: World Health Organization, 1991. World Health Organization Technical Report Series: 813.

14. Barnard DR. Repellents and toxicants for personal protection. WHO/CDS/ WHOPES/GCDPP/2000.5. Geneva: World Health Organization, 2000.

15. International Programme on Chemical Safety. INTOX. CD-ROM 2000-1. Geneva: International Programme on Chemical Safety, 2000.

16. Phillips-Howard PA, Steffen R, Kerr L, et al. Safety of mefloquine and other anti-malarial agents in the first trimester of pregnancy. J Travel Med 1998;5:121–126.

17. Schlagenhauf P. Mefloquine for malaria chemoprophylaxis 1992–1998: a review. J Travel Med 1999;6:122–133.

18. Malarone product information. Glaxo Wellcome, July 2000.

19. Nosten F, Vincenti M, Simpson J, et al. The effects of mefloquine treatment in pregnancy. Clin Infect Dis 1999;28:808–815.

20. World Health Organization. Management of uncomplicated malaria and the use of antimalarial drugs for the protection of travelers. Report of an informal consultation; 1995 September 18–21; WHO/MAL/96.1075 Rev.1. Geneva: World Health Organization, 1997.

21. World Health Organization. The use of artemisinin and its derivatives as anti-malarial drugs. Report of a joint CTD/DMP/TDR informal consultation; June 10–12; Geneva. WHO/MAL/98.1086. Geneva: World Health Organization, 1998.

22. Greenberg AE, Lobel HO. Mortality from *Plasmodium falciparum* malaria in travelers from the United States, 1959 to 1987. Ann Intern Med 1990;113:326–327.

23. World Health Organization. Management of severe malaria—a practical handbook. 2nd ed. Geneva: World Health Organization, 2000.

24. Wernsdorfer WH, McGregor I, editors. Malaria—principles and practice of malariology. United Kingdom: Churchill Livingstone, 1988.

25. Rogerson SJ, Beeson JG. The placenta in malaria: infection, disease and foetal morbidity. Ann Trop Med Parasitol 1999;93 Suppl 1:S35–S42.

26. Molyneux M, Fox R. Diagnosis and treatment of malaria in Britain. BMJ 1993;306:1175–1180.

27. World Health Organization/CDS. Severe falciparum malaria. Trans R Soc Trop Med Hyg 2000;94 Suppl1:S18–20 (clinical features in pregnancy),S54–55 (management in pregnancy).

28. World Health Organization. The world health report 1999—making a difference. Geneva: World Health Organization, 1999.

29. Brabin BJ, Ganley Y. Imported malaria in children in the UK. Arch Dis Child 1997;77:76–81.

30. Minodier P, Lanza-Silhol F, Piarroux R, et al. Le paludisme pédiatrique d'importation à Marseille. Arch Pediatr 1999;6:935–943.

31. Cilleruelo Ortega MJ, Mellado Peña MJ, Barreiro Casal G, et al. Paludismo en la edad pediátrica. Communicación de 26 casos. An Esp Pediatr 1988;2:101–104.

32. Emanuel B, Aronson N, Shulman S. Malaria in children in Chicago. Pediatrics 1993;92:83–85.

33. Wetsteyn JC, de Geus A. Falciparum malaria, imported into The Netherlands, 1979–1988. I. Epidemiological aspects. Trop Geogr Med 1995;47(2):53–60.

34. Luxemburger C, Price RN, Nosten F, et al. Mefloquine in infants and young children. Ann Trop Paediatr 1996;16:281–286.

35. Nahlen BL, Parsonnet J, Preblud SR, et al. International travel and the child younger than two years. II. Recommendations for prevention of travelers' diarrhoea and malaria chemoprophylaxis. Pediatr Infect Dis J 1989;8:735–739.

36. Kelly JC, Wasserman GS, Bernard WD, et al. Chloroquine poisoning in a child. Ann Emerg Med 1990;19:47–50.

37. Chongsuphajaisiddhi T. Malaria in paediatric practice. In: Wernsdorfer WH, McGregor I, editors. Malaria—principles and practice of malariology. United Kingdom: Churchill Livingstone, 1988.

38. Klein JL, Millman GC. Prospective, hospital based study of fever in children in the United Kingdom who had recently spent time in the tropics. BMJ 1998;316:1425–1426.

39. Parfitt K, editor. Martindale, the complete drug reference. 32nd ed. London: Pharmaceutical Press, 1999.

40. World Health Organization. Breastfeeding and maternal medication—recommendations for drugs in the 8th World Health Organization Model List of Essential Drugs. WHO/CDR/95.11. Geneva: World Health Organization, 1995.

9.6 Immunocompromised Travelers
Dominique Tessier

ABSTRACT

A significant number of immunocompromised people travel to tropical countries where a risk of malaria is present. Such people represent a heterogeneous group, the possible causes of immunodeficiency being numerous. To advise them properly regarding malaria prevention, it is essential to determine and understand if they are at increased risk of infection or complication from malaria and the possible interactions of chemoprophylaxis for malaria and other medications they may be taking during their trip. Their caregivers must also understand diagnostic and treatment specificity.

Key words: AIDS; HIV; immunosuppression.

IMMUNOSUPPRESSION AND TRAVEL

Nowadays, it is not uncommon to see immunocompromised people preparing for a trip in tropical countries. They do so for pleasure, business, family reasons, or religious considerations. During such trips, they will face important infectious risks, including malaria. It is thus important for the travel medicine advisor to understand the effect of immunosuppression on the risk of malaria acquisition and on possible changes in the presentation and treatment of malaria. Immunocompromised persons represent a heterogeneous group as the underlying cause of immunodeficiency could be a congenital defect, human immunodeficiency virus (HIV) infection, hemopathy, spleen dysfunction, an iatrogenic cause such as chemotherapy for a cancer or secondary to an organ graft, or treatment with high doses of steroids.[1,2] To tell a severely immunosuppressed person not to travel is unrealistic and does not take into consideration that person's own priorities. Fitness for travel is an abstract concept that is greatly influenced by the mental predisposition of the traveler. With very few exceptions, provided that good preparation and counseling is offered and understood, most HIV-infected travelers can undertake their journey safely.

Most experts agree that patients treated for an acute or chronic medical condition or for a cancer and who have not received immunotherapy for at least 3 months are not considered to be immunodeficient. Steroid therapy does not usually induce significant immunosuppression when used for a short term (< 14 days) or when administered topically, by aerosols, or by intra-articular, bursal, or tendon injection. HIV-infected persons with a cluster designation 4 (CD4) count of 500/μL are considered immunocompetent.

Infectious diseases are the leading killers of young people in developing countries; in these countries, infectious diseases are responsible for almost half of the mortality. These deaths occur primarily among the poorest people because such people do not have access to the drugs and commodities necessary for prevention or cure. Approximately half of infectious disease mortality can be attributed to just three diseases—HIV infection, tuberculosis (TB), and malaria. These three diseases cause over 300 million illnesses and more than 5 million deaths each year.[3]

HUMAN IMMUNODEFICIENCY VIRUS INFECTION AND MALARIA

United Nations Program on HIV/AIDS (UNAIDS) and the World Health Organization (WHO) estimated that the number of people living with HIV infection or acquired immunodeficiency syndrome (AIDS) at the end of the year 2000 was 36.1 million. During that year, AIDS killed more than 3 million persons globally, more than any other infectious disease. Malaria is another serious killer, taking the lives of between 2 and 3 million persons annually. Malaria and HIV infections are common, widespread, and overlapping problems in the tropics. In most countries where malaria is endemic, HIV infection is also present with a high incidence. In fact, the large majority of HIV-infected persons in the world live in malaria-endemic areas, namely, African countries, India, and Southeast Asia. It is thus surprising and disappointing to notice that very few studies have looked at the possible impact of malaria on HIV infection and of HIV infection and AIDS on the severity of malaria and on the morbidity associated with malaria.

Compared with those in industrialized countries, people in developing countries have little access to treatment for HIV infection. The majority of critically ill HIV-positive individuals in Africa do not have access to any antiretroviral medications. Such is the cost of these medications that even with significant discounts from the drug companies or with the use of generic drugs made in these countries, few people will have access to treatment without help from the rest of the world. This is unlikely to happen in the near future. As Jeffrey D. Sachs mentioned in the opening ceremony of the 8th Annual Conference on Retroviruses and Opportunistic Infections (CROI) in Chicago in February 2001, "the developed-world help could not have been less."

Studies on drug interactions with antimalarials are generally done in HIV-positive tourists visiting malarious areas or on healthy HIV-negative volunteers. A group large enough to obtain significant numbers is difficult to recruit. The same studies done in Africa would easily recruit a large number of affected individuals, but all drugs would need to be provided to them, thus increasing the cost. Also, it would be unethical to stop all medications at the end of the study.

An association between HIV-1 infection and malaria is expected in theory but has not been convincingly shown in practice. At least one study, by Whitworth and colleagues, showed a relationship between HIV staging and malaria. In that study, clinical malaria was significantly more common at HIV-1–positive visits (55 of 2,788 [2.0%] vs. 26 of 3,688 [0.7%], $p = .0003$), and the odds of having clinical malaria increased with falling CD4 cell counts ($p = .0002$) and advancing clinical stage ($p = .0024$).[4] The risk of clinical malaria tended to increase with falling CD4 cell counts ($p = .052$). This association tends to become more pronounced with advancing immunosuppression and could have important public health implications for sub-Saharan Africa. Coinfection with malaria is associated with a modest immune disturbance.

Sir James Whitworth and colleagues presented evidence that HIV-1 infection leads to increased frequency of symptomatic and symptomless malaria. Among cohorts that were followed up through repeated surveys, they found that malaria parasite density in HIV-1–positive people was higher with advanced immunosuppression, by nearest and previous CD4 cell counts.[5]

It has always been surprising that malaria does not seem to be more common in HIV-infected patients. Watson-Jones and colleagues[6] conducted a prospective study of malaria in pregnant women in Tanzania. Malaria was common but was not associated with HIV-infected status.[7]

The combination of HIV infection and malaria could lead to new epidemics. For example, in Brazil, two outbreaks of both infections occurred at the beginning of the 1990s in the most industrialized state (São Paulo) due to the sharing of needles and syringes by drug users.[8] The authors of the review of the outbreaks caution that new outbreaks of HIV infection and malaria are likely to occur among Brazilian intravenous-drug users (IDUs) and might conceivably contribute to the development of treatment-resistant strains of malaria in this population. Health professionals should be alert to this possibility, which could also eventually occur in IDU networks in developed countries.

Despite the review in the literature, the scientific understanding of the effect that those two infections can have on each other is limited. There is minimal evidence to support an important interaction, other than during pregnancy in multigravid HIV-infected women.[9] It has to be admitted with irony that medicine and science have failed to provide any solutions on how to best address these problems.

HIV-infected people living in developed countries travel quite a lot; they also represent a heterogeneous group. With the use of highly active antiretroviral therapies (HAARTs), many have regained what can be considered a normal immune system. Others have had a more mitigated success, with some degree of immunodeficiency. A large number of HIV-infected persons are either failing therapy or not taking it, with resultant severe immunodeficiency. They represent a challenge for the travel medicine practitioner wishing to advise them on malaria prevention. The same is true for the physician caring for their HIV infection, when faced with fever in the returning immunocompromised traveler.

Health care providers need to be aware of the most important risks and the available preventive measures and should know how to inform the potential traveler about risks and options. Preparing an HIV-infected individual for international travel to a malaria-endemic area requires attention to a number of important issues that are similar to those faced by any immunocompromised traveler for the most part. These considerations include restrictions on crossing international borders, the malaria risk present at the precise destination, the accessibility of specialized health care overseas, and the possible need for medical evacuation home.[10] Counseling on protection from vectors and on self-treatment are even more important for such clients and is briefly described in the following text and in more detail in another chapter.

Many infections encountered by travelers are associated with increased morbidity and mortality in immunocompromised people. One would thus expect malaria to impose additional morbidity and mortality risk to these travelers. These individuals are also more likely to have adverse reactions to drugs used to prevent or treat infections.[10] An increasing number of publications have addressed the subject, but unfortunately, many answers are still to be found.

COUNTRIES WITH ENTRY RESTRICTIONS RELATED TO HUMAN IMMUNODEFICIENCY VIRUS INFECTION

Many countries have restrictions on the entry of individuals infected with HIV. A negative test result may be required from all applicants for permanent residence, students, foreign workers, and intending immigrants, or (in some cases) from all visitors requesting a visa over a certain number of days. Other countries may not request a test result from all travelers but may still limit the entry of HIV-infected individuals. The Laboratory Centre for Disease Control, Health Canada, has prepared informational documents on countries with regulations or restrictions for travelers with HIV infection or AIDS. These documents are not statements of the laws of any country, and it remains the responsibility of travelers to check with the authorities of the country where they wish to travel to determine the requirements with more certainty. (A copy of the Canadian document can be obtained on an individual request basis by telephoning (613) 957-8739 or by faxing (613) 952-8286. The U.S. Web site can be found at URL: http://travel.state.gov/HIVtestingreqs.html.)

TRAVEL COUNSELING

Protection from Vectors

Malaria is a common and infectious disease, transmitted by mosquito bites from dusk to dawn. Counseling about how to reduce mosquito bites should be a priority and should be done by someone knowledgeable about all of the available effective methods for avoiding bites. After all, these methods carry minimal risk and have no interaction with other medication the traveler might be taking. In many endemic areas, a medication that significantly reduces risk should be taken.

Personal protective measures are very effective in reducing the risk of acquiring malaria. All HIV-infected and immunocompromised travelers to endemic areas should be counseled about the use of insect repellent containing diethyltoluamide (DEET) on their exposed skin, the use of bednets, and the wearing of clothing that reduces the amount of exposed skin. An insecticide such as permethrin or deltamethrin on clothes and bednets can further reduce the risk. To allow for a safe needle puncture in the presence of fever (to rule out malaria), travelers should also consider carrying needles and syringes with them in developing countries. The recommended 5 mL syringes with 1.5-inch 21G needles may be difficult to find in pharmacies. At very low cost, physicians can easily prepare envelopes containing five needles and syringes for their clients, with a letter indicating that they are for medical care, to be used in case of emergency. This simple precaution should avoid unnecessary delays at border crossings. An example of such a letter is illustrated in Figure 9.6–1.

Chemoprophylaxis

Many different drugs are currently recommended for the chemoprophylaxis and treatment of malaria. Treatment usually occurs in a controlled environment, with

---

Medical Health Center
Complete address

Date: _____, 200_

Mr./Mrs.

I, _____ , MD, certify that
_____ carries with him/her a medical kit that includes
prescribed medications, syringes, and needles to be used by a doctor, during his/her
trip in case of emergency. These are recommended for personal use only to avoid the
risk of accidental transmission of infectious diseases. They are not to be sold.

_____
Medical Doctor, MD
Medical Director

Figure 9.6–1. Physician's explanatory letter for travelers carrying syringes, needles, and medications.

access to monitoring and possible adjustment or change in therapy should side effects or toxicity occur. Chemoprophylaxis, on the other hand, is given to an individual leaving the country of residence to travel, usually in unfamiliar surroundings, with exposure to numerous other risks. The aim is to prevent a serious and potentially fatal disease. Risk benefit should thus be ascertained carefully. Unfortunately, information on interactions between most antimalarial drugs and the drugs used in the care of HIV-infected people is not available. No studies have explored the interaction of chloroquine, primaquine, or proguanil with anti-HIV drugs.

Mefloquine

Mefloquine is currently recommended as prophylaxis for malaria in most chloroquine-resistant endemic areas. Mefloquine is metabolized at cytochrome P-450 (cyp). The prevailing problem of drug interactions with protease inhibitors or reverse transcriptase inhibitors leads to the question of potential interaction with antimalarials such as mefloquine. Protease inhibitors are metabolized at cytochrome P-450. Some are potent inhibitors of specific sites, as is ritonavir on cyp3A4 and (to a lesser degree) on 2D6, while others are inducers. These processes could result in a slower elimination of drugs such as mefloquine, resulting in an increased risk of side effects and toxicity. Faster metabolization, on the other hand, could result in ineffective blood levels of mefloquine, with a secondary increased risk of malaria. The combination of mefloquine with efavirenz also causes some concerns. The profile of interaction is not known yet, but the most common side effects with efavirenz are neuropsychiatric or related to the skin. At least half of patients will experience serious side effects that tend to decrease in the 1st month of therapy. The more common ones include dizziness (10%), impaired concentration (9%), insomnia (7%), abnormal dreaming (4%), sleepiness, confusion, abnormal thinking, memory loss, agitation, depersonalization, hallucinations, and excitement. It is thus very difficult to imagine safely combining this medication with mefloquine as the two drugs could potentiate their side effects. No information is available on mefloquine and two other non-nucleoside reverse transcriptase inhibitors (nNRTIs), delavirdine and nevirapine.

Atovaquone/Proguanil

Malarone is a new medication recommended for the treatment and prevention of malaria in areas with resistance to chloroquine. One Malarone tablet contains 250 mg of atovaquone, a medication often taken by immunocompromised persons at a daily dose of 1,500 mg. Atovaquone is widely used for the treatment and prevention of *Pneumocystis carinii* pneumonia and occasionally for *Toxoplasma gondii* infection. Interactions of atovaquone with anti-HIV medications have been studied. There are very few data available on Paludrine (proguanil), the other component of Malarone. Atovaquone is known to increase the level of some nucleoside reverse transcriptase inhibitors (NRTIs) like Zerit (stavudine) and to lead to a 35% increase in blood Retrovir (zidovudine [AZT]) levels. This could be associated with mild toxicity for some but not most people. There are no reported effects on atovaquone levels.

Doxycycline

Doxycycline, increasingly used in chloroquine- and mefloquine-resistant areas such as Southeast Asia, can increase the risk of photosensitivity or of a recurrence of candidiasis. For a traveler out of reach of an experienced physician, such a photosensitivity reaction can be difficult to distinguish from a life-threatening reaction to a drug like abacavir. For these reasons, changes in antiretroviral medications should be avoided in the weeks before the trip. Good counseling is mandatory to avoid any life-threatening misunderstandings. In the presence of an antiretroviral regimen, that includes a medication that could induce a potentially lethal rash that would warrant immediate interruption, a malaria chemoprophylaxis drug that does not induce photosensitivity reactions would be preferred.

Azithromycin

Azithromycin is another medication that could be considered as chemoprophylaxis for malaria in special situations, with less than ideal efficacy for individuals with an already complicated therapy or who have experienced severe side effects with previous changes in regimens. Azithromycin is rarely used in practice because of cost and limited efficacy. No dose adjustments are required when azithromycin is used in combination with NRTIs, nNRTIs, and protease inhibitors.

Recommendations

Taking all factors into consideration, doxycycline seems to offer a better profile, with less potential interaction; Malarone would be the next best choice for patients on protease inhibitors. In addition, these drugs have been extensively used in the care of HIV-infected persons.

Side Effects

Interactions of antiretroviral and malaria chemoprophylaxis medications could also be seen in an increased incidence of side effects. Protease inhibitors commonly cause diarrhea, a side effect also associated with drugs such as Malarone and mefloquine.[11] In a tropical area, it could become difficult if not impossible for a traveler taking a combination of these drugs to rapidly identify a potentially serious gastrointestinal infection. A rash is a relatively common sign of toxicity encountered during use of nNRTIs and with abacavir, a potent new NRTI. A significant minority (occurring in up to approximately 5% of patients receiving nNRTIs) of these rashes are severe, and potentially fatal cases of Stevens-Johnson syndrome have been reported. Mild to moderate skin rashes occur in 27% of patients in the first 2 weeks of efavirenz therapy. In most cases, the rash resolves within 1 month, while the patient continues taking efavirenz. The patient should be started on the new regimen at least 1 month before leaving for a malaria-endemic area and adding chemoprophylaxis.

"Drug Holidays" for People Infected with Human Immunodeficiency Virus

The U.S. federal guidelines for the treatment of HIV infection do state that stopping anti-HIV drug therapy could be considered when a patient was no longer deriving any benefits from the drugs and when there were no other options. This certainly has been done for a minority of AIDS patients who have experienced recurrent HIV rebound after having taking many or most of the available drugs in one or more different combinations. "Drug holidays" are increasingly popular among HIV-infected persons who do not fit into those categories. Travel is often mentioned as one of the reasons for considering a drug holiday. All prophylaxis medications should be continued, especially during travel to a tropical or subtropical area where the risk of some opportunistic infections is increased. Malaria chemoprophylaxis should be used as for other travelers and should not be included in the drugs to be stopped during the holiday. Drug holidays are still considered to be very risky.

Immunocompromised Pregnant Women

Malarial infection during pregnancy is often fatal, and prophylaxis against the causative parasite necessitates rational therapeutic intervention. HIV-infected pregnant women traveling to or residing in malaria-endemic areas require protection from malarial infection to avoid placing themselves in double jeopardy. The use of antiretrovirals is recommended for pregnant HIV-infected women to significantly reduce the risk of vertical transmission. AZT alone or in combination with lamivudine and/or nevirapine is the drug most commonly used to reduce mother-to-child transmission of HIV. Women who had already been taking other antiretrovirals when they became pregnant would usually continue on the same regimen during their pregnancy. Various agents have been used for prophylaxis against malaria during pregnancy, including chloroquine, mefloquine, proguanil, pyrimethamine, and pyrimethamine/sulfadoxine. The use of these agents has been based on a risk-benefit criterion, without appropriate toxicologic or teratologic evaluation. Some of the aforementioned prophylactic agents have been shown to alter glutathione levels and may exacerbate the oxidation-reduction imbalance attendant on HIV infection.[12]

Although the potential of most antimalarial agents recommended for pregnant women to cause congenital malformations is low when the agents are used alone, their ability to cause problems when combined with potent antiretroviral therapies has not yet been assessed carefully. Malarone and doxycycline, usually preferred for persons on HAART, are contraindicated for pregnant women. Malaria chemoprophylaxis for a pregnant woman is thus a challenge. Time should be spent with a pregnant woman to ensure that she understands the additional risk imposed by malaria and chemoprophylaxis on herself and the baby she is carrying. HIV infection is associated with a significant increase in the prevalence of malaria in pregnant women of all parities, with the effect apparent from early in gestation.[13]

DIAGNOSIS AND TREATMENT

Malaria can kill any healthy individual in just 3 days. Because immunocompromised persons are more likely to experience fever as a symptom of opportunistic infection, a paludic episode could go unrecognized and could lead to death or severe complications.

Immunocompromised travelers and health care providers alike must consider the diagnosis of malaria in any febrile illness that occurs during or after travel to a malaria-endemic area,[14] even in the presence of other opportunistic infections that could explain the fever.

An antimalarial treatment is sometimes considered for self-administration when fever occurs in travelers and prompt medical attention is unavailable. Although this is not contraindicated for HIV-infected persons, time should be spent with the potential traveler to ensure that he or she understands when and how to use such self-treatment. Medical care should always be sought as soon as possible, even if a self-treatment seems to be effective.

For HIV-infected travelers returning from endemic areas, the symptoms of malaria can go unrecognized for a longer, possibly life-threatening period. Symptoms of malaria are flulike and can include fever, chills, muscle aches, headache, vomiting, diarrhea, and coughing. These symptoms are very common in HIV-associated infections and could be interpreted as side effects of some of the antiretroviral drugs. Unrecognized, malaria can lead to liver and kidney failure, convulsions, and coma. If malaria is suspected, medical diagnosis should be sought immediately and proper treatment should be started without delay. About 2% of patients infected with *Plasmodium falciparum* die, usually because of delayed treatment.[15] HIV infection could thus potentially increase fatality, primarily because of delay in diagnosis and treatment.

Pardridge and colleagues showed that chloroquine has inhibitory effects on HIV-1 replication in human lymphocytes with a median effective dose (ED_{50}) of 15 μM, which approximates the chloroquine plasma concentration generated in the acute treatment of malaria.[16]

Serious and possibly life-threatening interactions could occur if amprenavir is taken with quinidine.

MALARIA AND TESTING FOR HUMAN IMMUNODEFICIENCY VIRUS

Six rapid enzyme immunoassays for the detection of HIV antibody were performed on paired sera from 66 patients with malaria and 9 patients with dengue. Kit specificity ranged from 77% to 100%, demonstrating that more data are needed on cross-reactivity with endemic diseases as the use of rapid HIV tests increases.[17]

Some findings on serology tests could have a serious impact on people requesting immigrant status in countries where HIV testing is done routinely before the delivery of an entry visa. Malaria-positive sera from Papua New Guinean subjects who were presumed to be uninfected with HIV produced a variety of bands (some of intense prominence) to HIV antigen on diagnostic Western blots.[18] The same study indicated that some interactions could also happen with testing for malaria in HIV-positive individuals. The sera from patients from a nonmalarious region who were positive for HIV produced immunoblot bands ranging from 134 kDa to 33 kDa to the *Plasmodium falciparum* antigen.

REFERENCES

1. Mileno MD, Bia FJ. The compromised traveler. Infect Dis Clin North Am 1998; 12:369–412.
2. Delmont J, Igo-Kemenes A, Peyron F, et al. Le voyageur immunocompromis. Med Trop (Mars) 1997;57:452–456.
3. Backgrounder July 2000 HIV, TB MALARIA – MAJOR INFECTIOUS DISEASES THREATS Background G8 discussions Problem Infectious diseases leading killer young people developing countries: Infectious diseases responsible half mortality developing countries. Deaths...modifié: Sunday, October 09, 2000 (10:31) url: http://www.who.int/inf-fs/en/back001.html.
4. Whitworth J, Morgan D, Quigley M, et al. Effect of HIV-1 and increasing immunosuppression on malaria parasitaemia and clinical episodes in adults in rural Uganda: a cohort study. Lancet 2000;356:1051–1056.
5. Verhoef H, Veenemans J, West CE. HIV-1 infection and malaria parasitaemia. Lancet 2000;357:232.
6. Watson-Jones D, Ndokeji SD, Bulmer J, et al. Maternal and placental malaria infection and HIV infection in a prospective cohort, Mwanza Region, Tanzania. Program and abstracts of the 13th International AIDS Conference; 2000 July 9–14; Durban, South Africa. Abstract No.: WePeC4464. Rehovot, Israel: Hebrew University Hadassah Medical School.
7. Maartens G. Management of opportunistic infections in developing countries. HIV-infected patients in developing countries are frequently exposed to opportunistic enteric pathogens. Proccedings of the 13th International AIDS Conference; 2000 July 9–14; Durban, South Africa; Hadassah Medical School.
8. Bastos FI, Barcellos C, Lowndes CM, Friedman SR. Co-infection with malaria and HIV in injecting drug users in Brazil: a new challenge to public health? Addiction 1999;94:1165–1174.

9. French N, Gilks CF. Royal Society of Tropical Medicine and Hygiene meeting at Manson House, London, 18 March 1999. Fresh from the field: some controversies in tropical medicine and hygiene. HIV and malaria, do they interact? Trans R Soc Trop Med Hyg 2000;94:233–237.

10. Health Canada. Statement on travellers and HIV/AIDS. Can Med Assoc J 1995;152:379–380.

11. Ohrt C, Richie TL, Widjaja H, et al. Mefloquine compared with doxycycline for the prophylaxis of malaria in Indonesian soldiers. Ann Intern Med 1997;126:963–972.

12. Okereke CS. Management of HIV-infected pregnant patients in malaria-endemic areas: therapeutic and safety considerations in concomitant use of antiretroviral and antimalarial agents. Clin Ther 1999;21:1456–1496.

13. Verhoef H, Brabin BJ, Hart CA, et al. Increased prevalence of malaria in HIV-infected pregnant women and its implications for malaria control. Trop Med Int Health 1999;4:5–12.

14. Committee to Advise on Tropical Medicine and Travel (CATMAT) 1997 Canadian recommendation for the prevention and treatment of malaria among international travellers. Canada Communicable Disease Report. Ottawa:Health Canada, 1997 Oct. Report No.: 23S5.

15. Preventing malaria in travelers: a guide for travelers to malarious areas. Atlanta: CDC/NCID Brochure Publication, 1995.

16. Partridge WM, Yang J, Diagne A. Chloroquine inhibits HIV-1 replication in human peripheral blood lymphocytes. Immunol Lett 1998;64:45–47.

17. Watt G, Chanbancherd P, Brown AE. Human immunodeficiency virus type 1 test results in patients with malaria and dengue infections. Clin Infect Dis 2000;30:819.

18. Elm J, Desowitz R, Diwan A. Serological cross-reactivities between the retroviruses HIV and HTLV-1 and the malaria parasite *Plasmodium falciparum*. P N G Med J 1998;41:15–22.

Chapter 10

DETERMINATION OF ANTIMALARIAL DRUG LEVELS IN BODY FLUIDS

Yngve Bergqvist

ABSTRACT

This chapter covers analytic methods for determining the body fluid levels of the antimalarials amodiaquine, artemisinin, atovaquone, chloroquine, lumefantrine, mefloquine, proguanil, pyronaridine, pyrimethamine, and sulfadoxine, along with some of their metabolites. Considerable progress has been made in achieving reliable analytic results for clinical studies with antimalarials. The aim of this chapter is to provide information on factors that affect the reliability of the methods used to measure the concentration of antimalarials and their metabolites in biologic fluids. The process of validation is presented; also, some of the preanalytic steps are discussed, and their influence on analytic results is considered. Sampling onto filter paper is discussed, as well as all the available methods for analyzing antimalarial drugs from filter paper samples and some of the preanalytic factors that contribute to the results. The solid-phase extraction method is presented as the first and most important step in isolating antimalarial drugs from the biologic matrix to achieve high selectivity. High-performance liquid chromatography (HPLC) is discussed as the preferred technique by far for the assay of antimalarials in most instances. The importance of harmonization of analytic methods between different laboratories that provide analytic services for clinical studies is presented. The chapter ends with a survey of new technologies that may be suitable for the assay of antimalarial drugs in the future.

Key words: capillary sampling; chromatography; determination; drug assay; filter paper; harmonization; HPLC; new technology; preanalytic; selectivity; solid-phase extraction; specificity; validation.

INTRODUCTION

This chapter covers fundamental developments in the assay of antimalarials and discusses different aspects of validation, solid-phase extraction, and new technologies. Figure 10–1 presents the chemical structures of the antimalarials and some of the important metabolites presented in this chapter. A survey has been done of

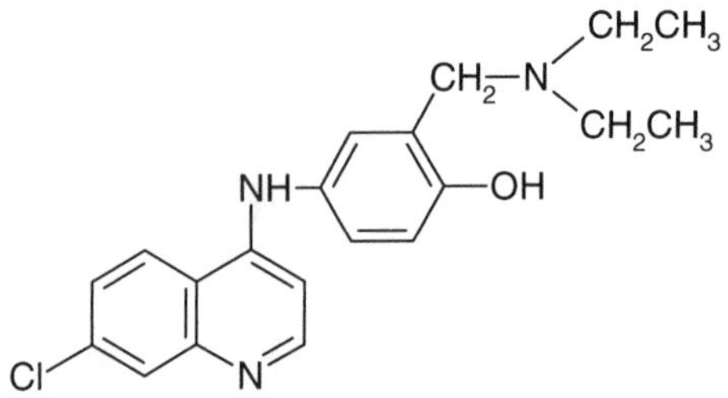

Amodiaquine

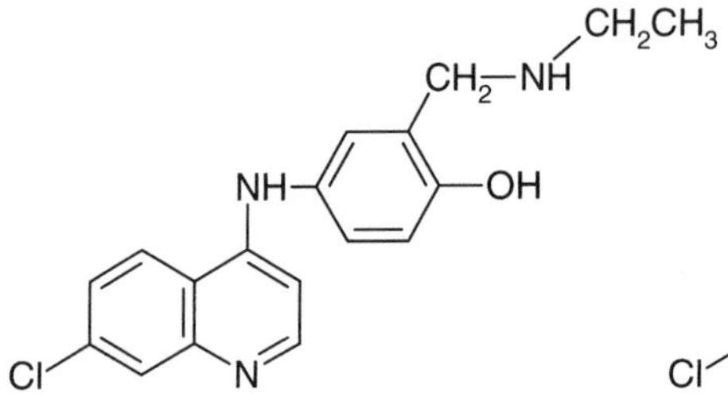

Desethylamodiaquine   **bis-Desethylamodiaquine**

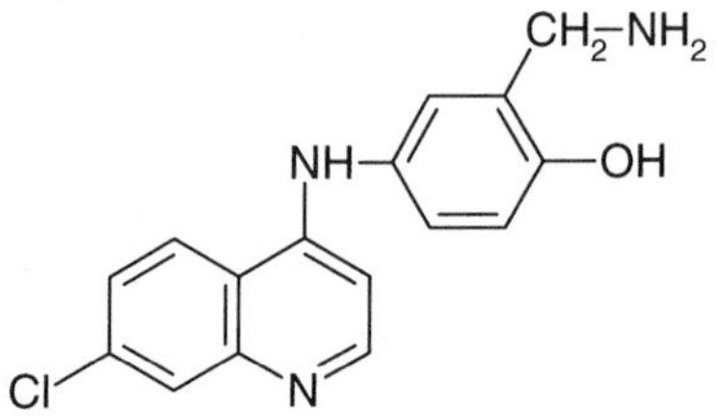

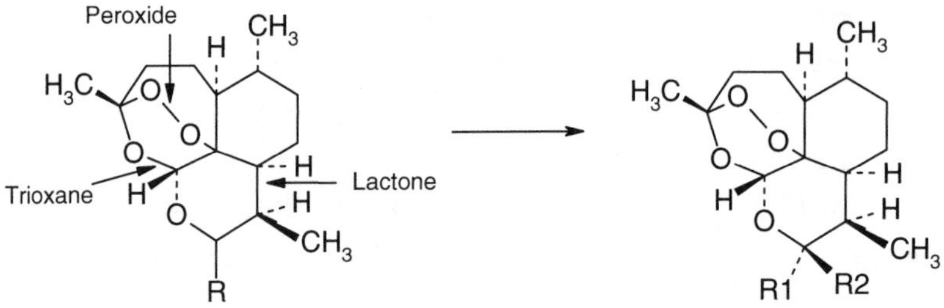

Artemisinin and its derivatives   **Dihydroartemisinin**

-R:		α: R1 = OH; R2 = H
=O	Artemisinin	β: R1 = H; R2 = OH
-OCH₃	Artemether	
-OCH₂CH₃	Arteether	
-OCOCH₂CH₂COONa	Sodium artesunate	
-OCH₂C₆H₄COONa	Sodium artelinate	

-R:
=O   Artemisinin
-OCH$_3$ Artemether
-OCH$_2$CH$_3$ Arteether
-OCOCH$_2$CH$_2$COONa   Sodium artesunate
-OCH$_2$C$_6$H$_4$COONa   Sodium artelinate

α: R1 = OH; R2 = H
β: R1 = H; R2 = OH

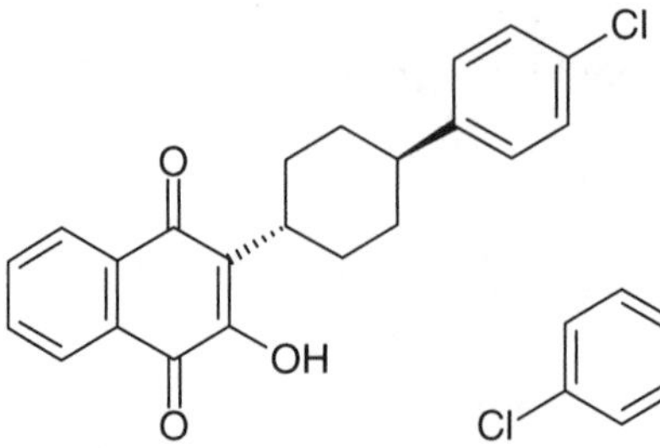

Atovaquone 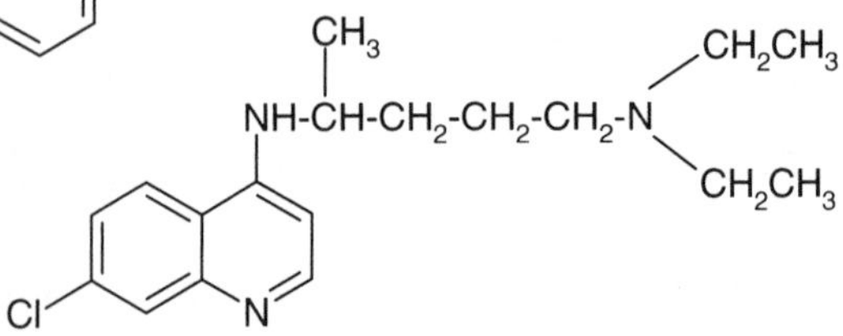   **Chloroquine**

Figure 10–1. Chemical structures.

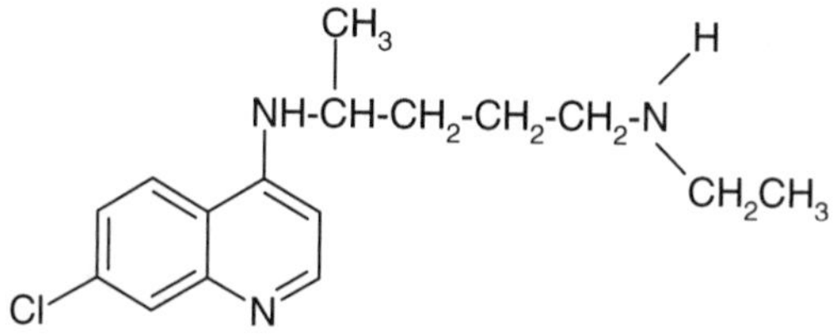

Desethylchloroquine

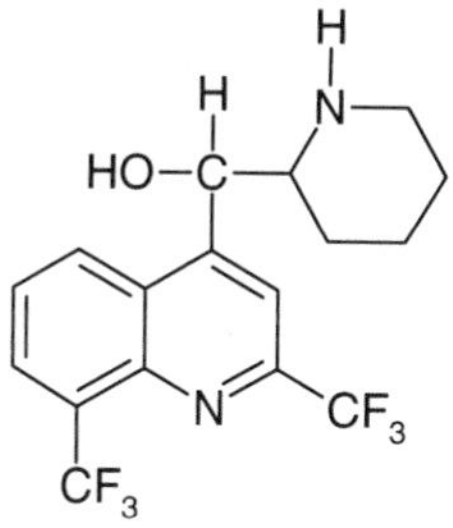

Mefloquine

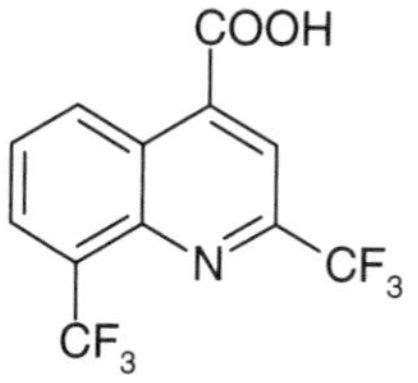

Mefloquine carboxy metabolite

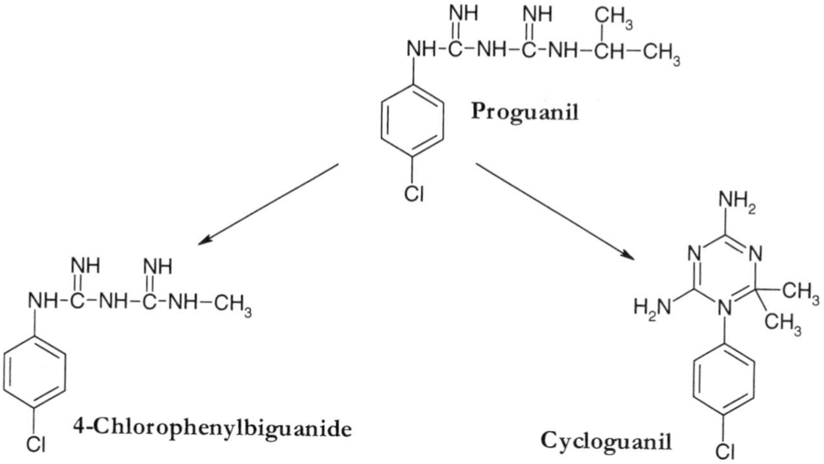

Proguanil

4-Chlorophenylbiguanide

Cycloguanil

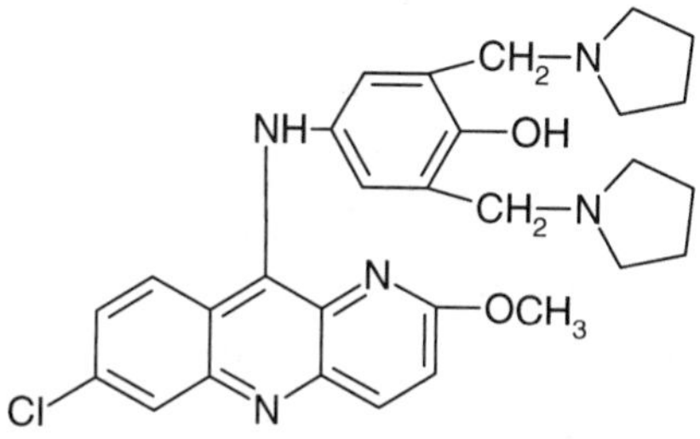

Pyronaridine

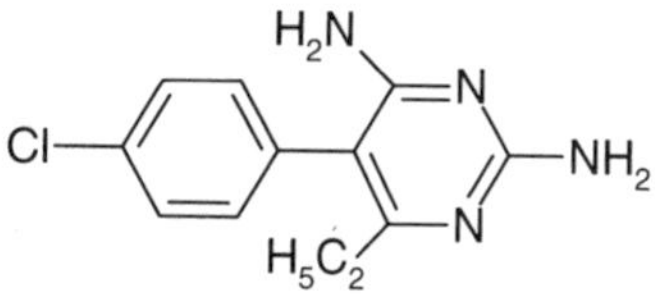

Pyrimethamine

Figure 10–1. Chemical structures continued.

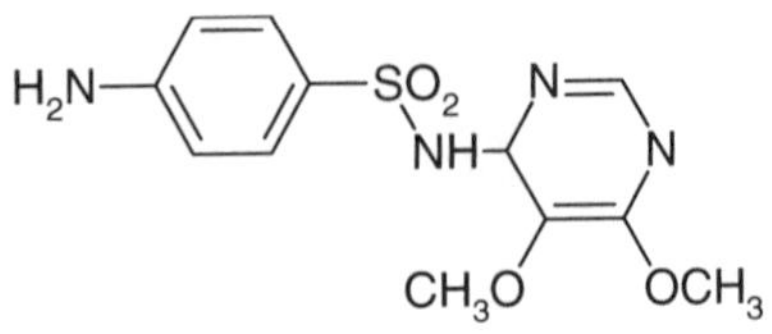

Sulfadoxine

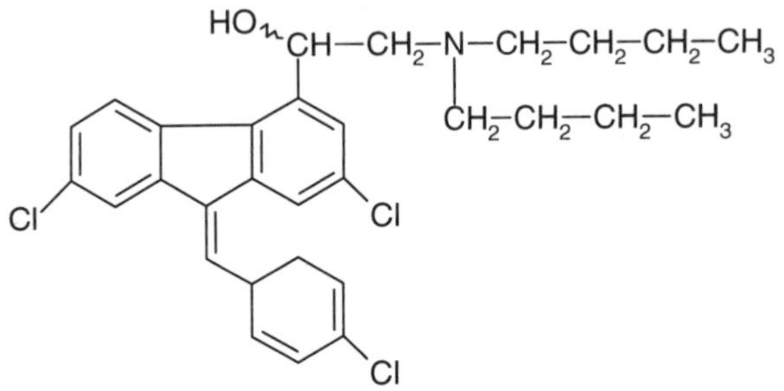

Lumefantrine

Figure 10–1. Chemical structures, continued.

some analytic methodologies for the assay of antimalarial drugs covering publications appearing in Analytical Abstract between January 1986 and June 2000. I have supplemented this with selected research methods of my own. It is not meant to be a comprehensive review. Only publications that I consider significant developments and that are published in English are included.

The pharmacokinetic data (e.g., half-life and protein binding) are taken from Abdi Aden et al., *Handbook of tropical parasitic infections.*[1] Analytic methods for the determination of antimalarials in pharmaceutical dosage forms are not presented in this chapter, nor is the monitoring of drug response in malaria by in vivo and in vitro tests.[2]

In clinical praxis, the determination of drug concentrations is important in the following situations:

- **Prophylaxis.** When symptoms of malaria continue despite stated regular prophylaxis, determination of the concentration of the used antimalarial in biologic fluids is the only way to confirm that the patient really has taken the drug. To evaluate concentrations determined during prophylaxis, one must know the expected concentration during controlled drug intake.
- **Therapy.** Determination of drug concentrations during and after therapy may confirm that the treated subjects have attained anticipated drug concentrations. This would imply that a later treatment failure could not be due to poor patient compliance. When concentrations are determined during therapy, the dose can be adjusted accordingly. This is important with antimalarials that have a narrow therapeutic range and frequent dose-dependent adverse reactions.

- **Adverse reactions.** When symptoms of side effects occur during therapy or prophylaxis, it is important to determine the drug concentration to evaluate whether a high concentration is a possible explanation.
- **Intoxication.** In patients with suspected drug intoxication (not uncommon with chloroquine, mefloquine, and quinine medication), analyses of drug concentration are necessary to confirm or refuse the diagnosis.

Antimalarial concentrations should be measured in the following biologic media:

- **Serum.** For some antimalarial drugs, the concentration in serum is higher than in plasma, due to the release of drug from blood cells during clotting. Chloroquine concentration in serum is twice as high as in plasma.
- **Plasma.** Pharmacokinetic information for antimalarial drugs is most often based on determination in plasma. Plasma samples are less suitable for field studies and almost impossible to obtain in children when repeated sampling is required.
- **Whole blood.** Concentrations in whole blood may more accurately reflect the concentrations acting on the parasite within the erythrocyte since parasitized erythrocytes are present in whole blood but not in serum or plasma.
- **Capillary blood.** Capillary blood is obtained by finger puncture with a lancet. Semi-skilled field workers can perform this after only minimal training. The technique of using blood dried on filter paper is very suitable for field studies because facilities for separating and storing samples are not needed. The filter papers can be sent by ordinary mail to the laboratory for analysis. (Valuable clinical aspects concerning the usefulness of the determination of antimalarials in different biologic matrices are discussed in other sources.[3])

Major advances in many areas of biomedical research have greatly improved the knowledge of the chemotherapy of malaria. One such area is the pharmacokinetics of the drugs. Advances would not have been possible without sensitive and selective analytic methods. Different laboratories must use fully validated analytic methods to obtain reliable and compatible results. Pharmacokinetic data are important in designing rational dosage regimens with optimal clinical efficiency and in avoiding concentration-dependent side effects.

In this chapter, there is a short introduction to each antimalarial drug with respect to chemistry, metabolism, and basic pharmacokinetic parameters. This is important knowledge for the validation of analytic methods for the determination of drug concentrations in different biologic matrices (e.g., serum/plasma, whole blood, and urine).

Combinations of several drugs are now increasingly used for the treatment of malaria (e.g., proguanil combined with atovaquone [Malarone], chlorproguanil with dapsone [Lapdap], and artemether with lumefantrine [Coartem/Riamet]). Combination therapy is used to improve efficacy as well as for preventing the development of parasite resistance. This development calls for analytic methods that can simultaneously determine the individual components of the combinations used.

After its introduction in the late 1960s, HPLC established itself as the leading analytic tool in the pharmaceutical industry. The separation mechanism in HPLC depends on the hydrophobic binding interactions between the analyte (e.g., antimalarial in the mobile phase) and the stationary phase. The stationary phase has a surface of silica with hydrophobic groups of different characters. Dorsey and colleagues[4] produced a very useful and comprehensive survey of the fundamental developments in liquid chromatography during the period of 1995 to 1997. The complexity of HPLC techniques is high but not so high as to require specially trained laboratory technicians to handle the HPLC instruments that run validated assays for determining antimalarials in a biologic matrix. (Two valuable practice-oriented books that contain useful tips on how to handle HPLC systems have recently been published.[5,6] These books are rich in practical information difficult to find in ordinary textbooks.)

According to the Système International d'Unitès (SI) convention, drug concentrations are presented in moles per liter. However, this system is not yet used in all publications. In this chapter, all concentrations are stated in molar units. Molecular weights and pK_a values[7] are given in Table 10–1, as well as the factor for conversion from SI

Table 10–1. **Molecular Weight and pK_a Values of Antimalarials**

Antimalarial	Molecular Weight	pK_a[7]	pK_a Calculated*	Conversion Factor (f)[†]
Amodiaquine	336	—	5.6–9.4–10.9	2.98
Artemisinin	282	—	—	3.55
Dihydroartemisinin	284	—	—	3.52
Artemether	298	—	—	3.36
Artesunate	384	—	—	2.48
Arteether	314	—	—	3.18
Atovaquone	367	—	5.0	2.73
Chloroquine	320	8.4–10.8	6.3–10.5	3.13
Mefloquine	374	8.6	10.1–13.1	2.67
Proguanil	254	2.3–10.4	2.5–11.3	3.94
Pyrimethamine	249	7.3	—	4.02
Pyronaridine	518	—	4.1–8.8–9.6–10.4	1.93
Sulfadoxine	310	6	3.2–7.1	3.23
Lumefantrine	529	—	9	1.89

*Calculated by ACD/Pka DB, Version 1.2. (Advanced Chemistry Developments, Inc.).
[†] Système International (SI) units to mass concentration: nmol/L = f × ng/mL. Opposite conversion: $\frac{nmol/L}{f}$ = ng/mL.

units (nmol/L) to mass concentration (ng/mL). The pK_a values are important when the analytic method is being designed (e.g., solid-phase extraction and HPLC).

VALIDATION

Due to increasing research collaboration among the developing and industrial countries during the last few years, it has become necessary for the results of different analytic methods to be acceptable and comparable internationally. Consequently, to assure a common level of quality, the need for and use of validated methods has increased. The main reason for this is that analytic results are valuable information on which important decisions are often based. Verifying accuracy is one of the basic steps in the process of achieving traceability. To estimate reliable clinical pharmacokinetic data, it is necessary to assay antimalarial concentration in the biologic matrix with a validated analytic method according to an internationally accepted methodology.

A strategy for the validation of chromatographic methods has been formalized in a guide made by the Commission of the Société Francaise des Sciences et Techniques Pharmaceutiques (SFSTP). The SFSTP guide has been produced to help analysts validate their bioanalytic methods.[8,9] The validation strategy in the SFSTP guide comprises two steps: (1) a prevalidation step to select the model for the calibration curve and estimate the limit of determination, the limit of detection, and the recovery; and (2) the actual validation, to confirm the main validation parameters (e.g., precision, accuracy, linearity, and recovery).

The applicability of the SFSTP validation strategy has been tested for the determinations of atenolol in human plasma.[10] The validation of analytic methods for determinations of antimalarial drugs can follow the SFSTP strategy in "part." Another useful document concerning the validation of bioanalytic methods has been presented by Glaxo Wellcome.[11] This document discusses the key analytic parameters: recovery, response function, sensitivity, precision, accuracy, selectivity, and stability. Huber[12] presented an introduction to the determination of a method's robustness for a number of chromatographic parameters that can have an effect on the results. Hartmann and colleagues[13] presented another strategy for the validation of chromatographic methods developed to quantify drugs in biologic material. The main validation steps (such as calibration, precision, accuracy, specificity, assay range, and stability) are discussed and briefly reviewed.

It must be demonstrated that analytic methods are selective for the analyte. The term *selectivity* is often incorrectly used and often confused with the term *specificity*.[14] An analytic method is by definition specific only when it measures the analyte without any kind of interference. It can be helpful to visualize the difference between specificity and selectivity graphically, as illustrated in Figure 10–2.[14] Unfortunately, in many instances, people do not realize and understand that there

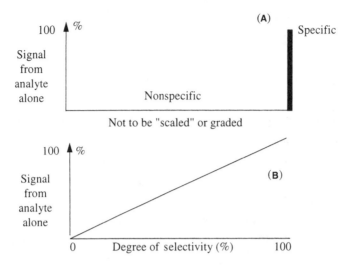

Figure 10–2. Graphic demonstration of selectivity and specificity. The percentage of the measured signal attributable to the analyte alone (on the y-axis) is given as a function of the degree of selectivity (*B*). A perfectly selective method is said to be specific (*A*). (Reproduced with permission from Vessman J. Selectivity or specificity? Validation of analytical methods from the perspective of an analytical chemist in the pharmaceutical industry. J Pharm Biomed Anal 1996;14:867–869.

is a difference between selectivity and specificity. The chromatographic methods used for the assay of antimalarials are not absolute but only relative methods of analysis. Specific analytic methods are very rare, but the use of fluorescent, electrochemical, diode array, and mass spectrometric detectors can enhance method selectivity, leading the analysis toward the specific side, as in Figure 10–2.

A 1989 report from a workshop organized by World Health Organization/Training in Tropical Diseases (WHO/TDR) accurately summarizes the validation of field semiquantitative tests for some antimalarials in body fluids.[15] The objective of the workshop was to carry out, under strictly controlled laboratory conditions, a comparative evaluation of (1) the available chemical, chromatographic, and immunologic tests for determining chloroquine and mefloquine in body fluids and (2) their applicability to field research and malaria control operations. This kind of test is particularly useful in epidemiologic and compliance studies. Since this workshop in 1989, little has been published concerning developments in field analytic methods for antimalarials. Due to the very low selectivity of semiquantitative field tests, paper sampling of capillary blood seems to be a more efficient alternative for field tests.

Most assays of antimalarial drugs are performed by HPLC separations. These are dependent on the properties of packed columns, mobile-phase composition, pH, and other factors. To characterize the properties of packed columns, a variety of test procedures have been described.[16] The majority of the antimalarial drugs are bases, and most HPLC separations are performed at pH levels at which the analytes are ionized. The packing materials in HPLC columns are not stable at a pH > 7 to 8. To achieve good chromatographic performance for particular antimalarial drugs, columns from different manufacturers should be tested to achieve good column efficiency and low silanophilic interactions.[17,18]

Preanalytic Considerations

Preanalytic steps include all the procedures before the assay of an unknown sample: food intake, sampling, handling, storage, and transport to the laboratory.

One can have the most selective method for the determination of antimalarials, but this does not help if even one step in the preanalytic procedure is done incorrectly. Some of these aspects are discussed below.

If the drug is bound to cellular components, there will be a difference in concentration between serum and plasma. Serum is obtained from whole blood after clotting and centrifugation and is enriched with cellular components from the lysed cells (e.g., thrombocytes and leukocytes). The higher drug concentrations in serum than in plasma can thus be explained by the release of the drug from cells during clotting.

Plasma is obtained after sampling in a tube containing an anticoagulant such as ethylenediaminetetraacetic acid (EDTA) or heparin. Anticoagulants inhibit clot formation, and the blood cells are not lysed. A cell-free supernatant is received after centrifugation of the anticoagulated whole blood.

A linear correlation has been shown to exist between serum and plasma concentrations of chloroquine and its main metabolite, as seen in Figure 10–3. Chloroquine and the metabolite have a high concentration inside the blood cells,[19] and the drugs are released from blood cells to the serum during the clotting process. Results from plasma are more representative than those from serum since the serum concentration is highly dependent on the amount of blood cells.

For drugs that are strongly bound to blood cells, the centrifugation speed and time are very important. Centrifugation of whole blood to achieve plasma is normally performed within 30 to 60 minutes after sampling at 2,000 to 3,000 × g for 10 to 15 minutes. If the centrifugation is done after more than 60 minutes and/or at low speed, the content of the drugs inside the thrombocytes will be released, which gives a falsely high plasma drug concentration.[19]

The transfer of the plasma sample to the laboratory freezer is another important preanalytic factor since some antimalarials (e.g., amodiaquine and pyronaridine) are unstable at room temperature. When the determination of concentration of antimalarial drugs in biologic fluids is to be performed, it is very important to contact the analytic laboratory for instructions on handling samples.

Most of the antimalarial drug molecules contain nitrogen, and in physiologic conditions, this nitrogen becomes positively charged and can be adsorbed to glass containers during sampling and extraction. For this reason, it is preferable to use polypropylene tubes during the extraction step and to avoid contact with glass as much as possible during the sampling process.

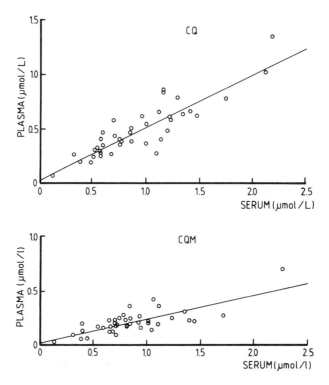

Figure 10–3. Comparison between serum (X) and plasma (Y) from 40 patients on chloroquine therapy for chloroquine (CQ) and desethylchloroquine (CQM). Top graph: Y = 0.50X + 0.024, r = 0.89,
n = 40. Bottom graph: Y = 0.22X + 0.023, r = 0.76, n = 40. (Reproduced with permission from Bergqvist
Y, Domeij-Nyberg B. Distribution of chloroquine and its metabolite desethyl-chloroquine in human
blood cells and its implication for the quantitative determination of these compounds in serum and
plasma. J Chromatogr B 1983;272:137–148.)

Sampling finger-prick capillary blood on filter paper is considered easier to perform, requires less training, is less invasive than conventional venous collection,
and involves little discomfort or risk to the participant (Figure 10–4). Nevertheless,
there is considerable potential for person-dependent sampling variability, which is
often responsible for the discrepancies between finger-prick and venous results.
Finger-prick specimens are subject to dilution by interstitial fluid, giving a lower
drug concentration. Furthermore, the limit of determination is higher, due to low
sample volume (e.g., 100 to 200 μL).

Sampling on filter paper reduces sample handlers' risks of exposure to human
immunodeficiency virus (HIV) and hepatitis. Studies have shown that the drying of
blood reduces the amount of infectious viruses to practically zero.[20] In addition, a
technique using dried blood on filter papers reduces the need to provide facilities for
separating and storing blood samples in the field. Furthermore, dried blood spots can
be conveniently transported without significant risk. However, all contamination on
the filter paper must be avoided. In developing countries, the person who draws

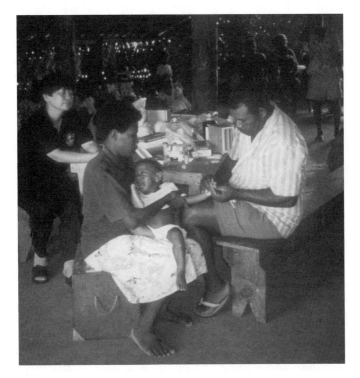

Figure 10–4. Example of capillary blood sampling onto filter paper in the field. (Courtesy of Dr. A. Kaneko.)

blood samples often handles antimalarial tablets, and there is therefore an appreciable risk of contaminating the filter paper with the analytes that are to be measured.[21]

The choice of filter paper is important, especially for rapid drying and for achieving a small-diameter blood spot. Personally, I have found Whatman ET 31 CHR chromatographic paper to be a reliable choice. It is very useful if the calibration of the analytic method can be performed by using of the same type of paper as is used for blood sampling. For proguanil, it has been shown that the recovery is different for different brands of paper.[22]

Another important preanalytic factor that has a strong influence on antimalarial plasma concentration is the intake of food. Lefevre and colleagues[23] found that the concentration of lumefantrine was increased by a factor of 13 when it was taken together with food. Figure 10–5 shows the effect of food on plasma concentrations of artemether and lumefantrine. Similar effects from food intake have been observed with artemether, atovaquone, and mefloquine.[23–25]

Validation and Routine Assay

There are two main steps in the development and validation of an analytic method for assaying antimalarials: (1) the validation process, in which the quality of the assay is defined, and (2) the application of an actual method for the analysis of sam-

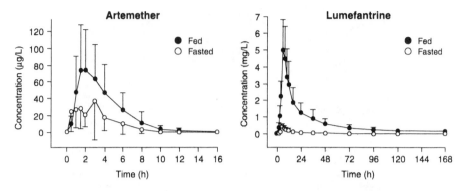

Figure 10–5. Effect of food on plasma concentrations of artemether and lumefantrine in 16 healthy Chinese participants, following a single oral administration of coartemether (80/480 mg) [mean ± SD]. (Reproduced with permission from Lefevre G, Thomsen MS. Clinical pharmacokinetics of artemether and lumefantrine (Riamet®). Clin Drug Invest 1999;18:467–480.)

ples from pharmacokinetic studies by laboratory staff not involved in the validation procedure. The last process consists of running calibration curves and quality control samples to show that the validation parameters and general characteristics of the method are quite similar to the validation results. At least five to six quality control samples should be interspersed with the unknown experimental samples (e.g., at least 20 to 30 unknown samples in one assay run) in the concentration range in which the unknown samples were estimated. The quality control samples should be used to accept or reject the assay run. These quality control samples should be of the same biologic matrix as the unknown samples and spiked with the analyte (e.g., antimalarials) and should cover the concentration range of interest. The rules for the acceptance of the run could be that the run would be rejected if two quality control samples of the same concentration, or more than two quality control samples, deviated more than 20% from the nominal value.

Harmonization of Results between Different Laboratories

Reproducibility between different laboratories could be one of the validation parameters. With regard to accuracy testing, it is very important to analyze the same sample in different laboratories, so that the users can be satisfied that the results are comparable. To facilitate the interpretation of pharmacokinetic results, it is important to estimate and minimize interlaboratory variation.

Laboratories can have large interlaboratory variations due to factors such as different methods, implement applications, and calibration principles. However, a study that compared analyses of mefloquine and its metabolite in an American laboratory and in a European laboratory demonstrated comparable results, with little interlaboratory variation (Figure 10–6).[26]

Analytic assay data from different pharmacokinetic studies can be difficult to interpret, however, which leads to the importance of harmonization among the

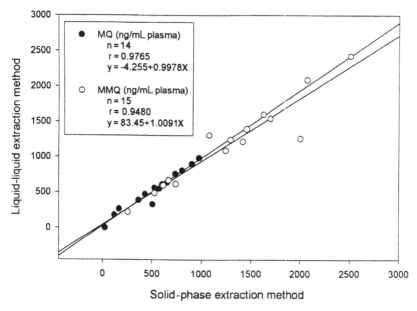

Figure 10–6. Interlaboratory comparison of extraction techniques. (MQ = mefloquine; MMQ = mefloquine metabolite.) (Reproduced with permission from Green MD, Bergqvist Y, Mount DL, et al. Improved validated assay for the determination of mefloquine and its carboxy metabolite in plasma, serum and whole blood using solid-phase extraction and high-performance liquid chromatography. J Chromatogr B 1999;727:159–165.)

biggest institutions analyzing antimalarials for supporting pharmacokinetic studies. Some ideas from the harmonization of routine clinical chemistry results between clinical laboratories can be also applied to antimalarial assays in biologic fluids.[27]

New chemometric procedures that can improve and interpret analytic results and make validation work easier are being developed rapidly. There is a practice-oriented textbook available, which discusses different aspects of statistics (such as regression, calibration, robust methods, quality control during routine assay, and treatment of outliers) and gives an introduction to experimental design.[28]

SOLID-PHASE EXTRACTION

Even with the use of sophisticated analytic instrumentation for the determination of antimalarials in a biologic matrix, there must be an isolation and extraction step before chromatographic separation and quantitation. Sample preparation generally represents at least 50% to 60% of the total time required for the analysis of antimalarials. For a long time, the traditional method for sample isolation before the chromatography step was liquid-liquid extraction with various organic solvents. However, there is continuous pressure to decrease the use of organic solvents in analytic laboratories due to health and environmental concerns.

Solid-phase extraction (SPE) has existed in its modern form for more than 15 years. The technique has shown slow but steady growth. Today, SPE is the most popular sample preparation method. The field of separation science is very active in the marketplace, and more than 50 companies make products for SPE.[29] One reason for the growing interest in SPE techniques is the large choice of sorbents, from polar to nonpolar sorbents, which closely resemble those used in HPLC. SPE is also an active area of research, as shown by the increasing number of publications describing new and more selective sorbents and procedures. SPE considerably reduces variability, compared to liquid-liquid extraction, especially if an automatic SPE robot performs the extraction. It is clear that the more selective the SPE step is, the more selectivity is obtained in the final chromatographic separation and determination of antimalarials. Selectivity may be enhanced if an SPE sorbent that is different from the HPLC column sorbent is used. A typical SPE procedure that involves six main steps for the extraction of an antimalarial is shown in Figure 10–7. This SPE procedure is the most commonly used mode and consists of the following six steps:

1. Sample pretreatment
2. SPE column solvation
3. SPE column equilibration
4. Sample loading
5. Interference elution
6. Analyte elution

The SPE procedure allows not only the isolation of the antimalarial from the biologic matrix but also its preconcentration, which allows a low limit of determination. After the elution step, the eluate is injected into a chromatographic system (e.g., HPLC).

To understand the isolation process, it is necessary to have a knowledge of the interactions between the antimalarial and the SPE sorbent. Reviews and a comprehensive book have been published during the last 3 years.[29–31] In these references, sorbents and related techniques are discussed, as well as recent trends in SPE and applications in the determination of drugs. One example is the use of medium polar CN sorbents for the isolation of polar antimalarial proguanil[32,33] in determination of its concentration in a biologic matrix.

Artemisinin derivatives have been extracted by SPE using phenyl as the sorbent,[34] with a very good recovery of 96% by the addition of acetate buffer to the sample before extraction. Mixed-mode sorbents containing both nonpolar and cation or anion exchange groups have been used for the extraction of basic drugs.[30] Restricted-access-material (RAM) sorbents combine size-exclusion and nonpolar sorbents. These sorbents could be well suited for the isolation of antimalarials. Determination of artemisinin has been presented with an on-line RAM sorbent with HPLC.[35]

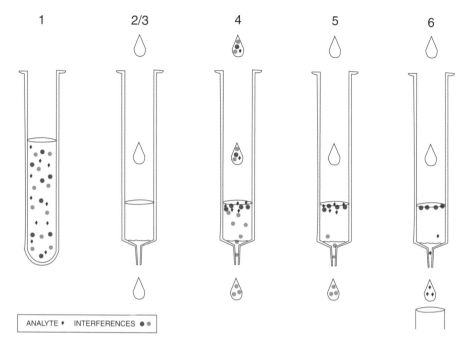

1   2/3   4   5   6

ANALYTE ♦   INTERFERENCES ● ●

Figure 10–7. Solid-phase extraction steps for isolation of an antimalarial from the biologic matrix. (Reproduced with permission from International Sorbent Technology.) (See Color Plates)

Empore® extraction disks consist of a silica or silica-based bonded phase embedded in a stable inert matrix web of polytetrafluoroethylene (PTFE) fibrils. Extraction disks are able to adsorb analytes more efficiently from a biologic matrix because of their smaller particle size. Figure 10–8 shows an example of the use of extraction disks in the determination of mefloquine and its acid metabolite.[26] Recovery is about 75% for mefloquine and about 92% for the acid metabolite in plasma and whole blood. This is a good example of the simultaneous extraction of a base (mefloquine) and an acid metabolite with SPE techniques and illustrates the usefulness of SPE technology for determining antimalarial drugs.

DETERMINATION OF SPECIFIC ANTIMALARIAL DRUGS

Amodiaquine

Amodiaquine (AQ), 7-chloro-4-(3'-diethylamino-methyl-4'-hydroxyanilino)-quinoline (see Figure 10–1), has been used since around 1940 for the prophylaxis and treatment of malaria. It is structurally similar to chloroquine. The use of AQ has increased in the last 20 years because of widespread chloroquine resistance.

After oral administration, AQ is rapidly and almost completely metabolized, in contrast to chloroquine. Three main metabolites have been discovered: desethyl-amodiaquine (AQM-1), bis-desethylamodiaquine (AQM-2), and 2-hydroxy-desethylamodiaquine.[36] In vitro studies of AQ and these metabolites suggest that

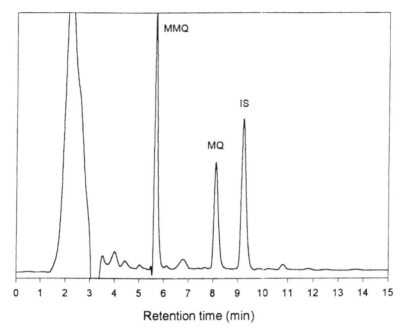

Figure 10–8. Typical chromatogram of extracted spiked whole blood. Mefloquine (MQ) and mefloquine metabolite (MMQ) concentration = 1,000 ng/mL, using the SymmetryShield column. (IS = internal standard.) (Reproduced with permission from Green MD, Bergqvist Y, Mount DL, et al. Improved validated assay for the determination of mefloquine and its carboxy metabolite in plasma, serum and whole blood using solid-phase extraction and high-performance liquid chromatography. J Chromatogr B 1999;727:159–165.)

AQM-1 is mainly responsible for the antimalarial activity. The elimination half-life of AQM-1 is about 98 hours.[37] After an oral dose of 306 mg of AQ, C_{max} (maximum concentration) in plasma was 24 nmol/L for AQ and AQM-2 and 182 nmol/L for AQM-1. In whole blood, the concentration of AQ and AQM-2 was below the limit of determination (< 30 nmol/L), and the concentration of AQM-1 was 292 nmol/L.[37] AQM-1 (but not AQ) appears to be concentrated in blood cells, and the concentration ratio of whole blood to plasma was > 3.[38] AQ is very sensitive to light, and its stability at room temperature is low due to oxidation of the hydroxyl group.

HPLC methods for the determination of AQ and its metabolites in a biologic matrix have been developed. Most of them include liquid-liquid extraction with organic solvents. Winstanley and colleagues used HPLC with ultraviolet (UV) detection at 340 nm and achieved a limit of determination of 15 nmol/L in 1 mL of plasma and whole blood.[38] The most sensitive assay of AQ and its three known metabolites used HPLC with electrochemical detection in oxidative mode. This method has a limit of determination of 3 nmol/L for AQ, AQM-1, and AQM-2 and 10 nmol/L for 2-hydroxy-desethylamodiaquine in whole blood, using a 1-mL sample.[39] A method used by Pussard and colleagues[40] quantifies chloroquine, desethylchloroquine, AQ, and AQM-1 simultaneously in body fluids, with a limit of determination of 10 nmol/L for each of the analytes, using 1-mL samples. This method is a good example of the simultaneous determination of two commonly used antimalarial drugs and their metabolites. No method is presently available for the determination of AQ and its main metabolites from capillary blood applied to filter paper.

Artemisinin

Artemisinin (ART) (qinghaosu) (see Figure 10–1) is a sesquiterpene lactone extracted from the Chinese medicinal plant *Artemisia annua L.* and represents a class of antimalarials that have been used for the treatment of malaria in countries with multidrug-resistant *Plasmodium falciparum*. Unlike current antimalarial drugs, which have a nitrogen-containing heterocyclic ring system, ART has a tetracyclic structure with a trioxane ring and a lactone ring. The trioxane ring contains a peroxide bridge (see Figure 10–1).

The peroxide group is essential for the antimalarial activity of the drug and generates free radicals, which kill the parasite.[41] The hemin-rich internal environment of the *Plasmodium* parasites is assumed to be responsible for the apparent toxicity of artemisinin to parasites. The peroxide bridge configuration of ART has a unique mode of action that is unrelated to that of other antimalarials. ARTs are also well tolerated and the most potent of all antimalarial drugs.[42] ART and its derivatives are all metabolized to the active metabolite dihydroartemisinin, which exists as two isomers, α and β. This biotransformation occurs very rapidly. The ART derivatives are strongly bound to erythrocytes,[43] and it is extremely difficult to assay the drug concentration in whole blood. Hydrolysis of ART derivatives to dihydroartemisinin may occur if whole blood is not centrifuged within 1 hour after sampling and after separating plasma from blood cells. ART is bound to plasma proteins to about 60%,[44] and a half-life of between 1 to 10 and 5 to 21 hours has been estimated for dihydroartemisinin.

The determination of ART and its derivatives in biologic samples is difficult due to the lack of chromophore groups and ART's lack of functional groups suitable for derivatization reactions. A number of HPLC methods have been published, but the selectivity of some of these methods is generally unsatisfactory. The endoperoxide configuration of ART has been used as a detection mode both in electrochemical detection in reductive mode and in luminescence detection in HPLC methods.

Postcolumn derivatization has been used to enhance absorptivity. Many publications have determined ART concentrations by an HPLC postcolumn on-line derivatization and UV detection at 289 nm.[45] The eluate from the analytic column is mixed with an alkaline stream at high temperature to achieve UV-absorbing derivatives of ART. The limit of determination is approximately 35 nmol/L. This postcolumn method has been used in different pharmacokinetic studies.[46,47]

By using hemin as a catalyst to generate a free radical from ART, chemoluminescent light can be detected in the presence of luminol.[48]

A previously developed HPLC method with UV detection and postcolumn derivatization and a column-switching system for the analysis of ART coupled to alkyl-diol silica (ADS) as a precolumn, allowing direct injection of plasma samples, has been described.[35] This precolumn material is cold RAM and excludes macromolecules such as plasma proteins without causing their denaturation, while small hydrophobic molecules (e.g., ART) are retained. The limit of determination after directly injecting 100 µL of plasma was 35 nmol/L.[35] High sample volume in the precolumn can be used to concentrate the sample before injections are made into the analytic column.

The peroxide structure of the ART groups is reduced at the working electrode in the electrochemical detector, and the resulting signal is used for detection. The drawbacks to the use of electrochemical detector technology are that it requires rigorously controlled anaerobic conditions and deoxygenation of biologic samples and that a mobile phase is needed. This system needs trained and experienced personnel to handle the HPLC electrochemical system. Conventional deoxygenation, which involves purging an inert gas through the sample and mobile-phase solution, is difficult to handle in an automated HPLC system. Numerous publications on the determination of ART and its derivatives were presented during the 1990s.[49–51] The limit of determination is about 18 nmol/L for most of these methods.

One alternative deoxygenation technique is to use semipermeable-membrane deoxygenation.[52] This technique seems to be more efficient than other techniques. The sample and the mobile phase can be deoxygenated simultaneously by a commercial on-line deoxygenator. The detection limit is about 18 to 28 nmol/L.

A selective gas chromatography–mass spectrometry–selected ion monitoring method has been developed for the determination of artemether and dihydroartemisinin, with a limit of determination in plasma of 18 nmol/L.[53]

No method is presently available for the determination of ART and its derivatives from capillary blood samples on filter paper.

Atovaquone

Atovaquone (ATQ), trans-2-[4-(4-chlorophenyl)cyclohexyl]-3-hydroxy-1,4-naphthoquinone, is a hydroxynaphthoquinone (see Figure 10–1). ATQ is a highly lipophilic antimalarial compound and is difficult to handle because of its physiochemical properties. It is poorly soluble in a variety of organic solvents, and its solubility in aqueous solvent is very limited (< 270 nmol/L).[54] The compound has received great interest in a number of trials because of its synergistic activity against *Plasmodium falciparum* in vitro when combined with another antimalarial compound, proguanil.[55,56] ATQ is more than 99.9% bound to plasma protein and has a plasma half-life of 2 to 3 days.[57] Administration with dietary fat greatly increases ATQ's bioavailability.

Traditionally, the extraction of ATQ from plasma is performed by liquid-liquid extraction[58–60] or by protein precipitation.[61] A combination of protein precipitation with acetonitrile followed by an automated SPE on C8 column was recently reported.[62] The automated SPE-HPLC method shows very good precision and is rapid and simple. The lower limit of determination in plasma and whole blood was 150 nmol/L from a 500-μL sample volume, with an intra-assay precision of less than 15%. A protein precipitation step was necessary to increase the recovery from plasma since atovaquone has a very high affinity to plasma proteins. A method of capillary sampling onto filter paper is available for ATQ,[63] with a limit of determination of about 1,000 nmol/L in a 100-μL sample.

Chloroquine

Chloroquine (CQ) 7-chloro-4-(4'-diethylamino-1'-methylbutylamino) quinoline and its principle metabolite, desethylchloroquine (CQM), are shown in Figure 10–1. CQ is a cheap, well-tolerated, and readily available antimalarial drug. It is a chiral drug with one asymmetric carbon and exists as two enantiomers, (+)–CQ and (−)–CQ. One study reported that the (−)–CQ enantiomer is less active than the (+)–CQ enantiomer against CQ-resistant strains.[64] CQM is less active in vitro against CQ-resistant strains than against CQ-sensitive strains of *Plasmodium falciparum*.[65] Despite reports of the *Plasmodium falciparum* parasite's resistance to CQ, the drug is still useful for treating acute uncomplicated malaria in many endemic areas, particularly in Africa. During the last 10 to 15 years, the pharmacokinetics of CQ have been re-investigated with selective chromatographic methods. By the use of improved analytic methods that permit a very low limit of determination (e.g., 0.5 nmol/L for CQ and CQM[66]), the terminal half-life has been estimated. The half-life can vary in different studies, from several days up to about 50 to 60 days.[67]

The analysis of chloroquine in blood is complicated due to the pronounced accumulation of the drug in the platelets since the concentration of the drug in plasma is only about 15% of that in whole blood.[68,69] Determination of plasma concentrations is unreliable unless strictly standardized centrifugation conditions are used for the removal of blood cells. For this reason, it is often preferable to determine CQ and CQM concentrations in whole blood. In whole blood, CQ and CQM concentration is seven to eight times higher than in plasma, due to the high concentration in the blood cells. Whole blood concentrations might also be more relevant when relating drug concentrations to the antiparasitic effect.

At the beginning of the 1980s, the first selective HPLC methods for the simultaneous determination of CQ and its main metabolite, CQM, were developed.[69,70] These methods have been used in different pharmacokinetic studies.[71,72]

Walker and colleagues presented a cost-effective modification of an HPLC method for the determination of CQ and CQM in biologic fluids, with a limit of determination of 65 nmol/L for CQ and CQM.[73] Simple and selective HPLC methods for the determination of CQ and CQM in capillary blood samples on filter paper have been described.[74,75] With fluorescence detection, it is possible to achieve a limit of determination of 20 nmol/L for CQ and CQM, using a 100-μL sample. Stalcup and colleagues presented a chiral separation of CQ enantiomers using heparin as a chiral selector.[76] Two immunologic methods for the simultaneous determination of chloroquine and its main metabolites in biologic samples, radioimmunoassay (RIA) and enzyme-linked immunosorbent assay (ELISA), have been described.[77] The limit of determination of chloroquine in 10 μL of plasma is 10 to 15 nmol/L with the RIA method. Both methods cross-react with metabolites and are therefore suitable only for controlling compliance and in epidemiologic studies.

Lumefantrine

Lumefantrine (known formerly as benflumetol), 2-dibutylamino-1-[2,7-dichloro-9-(4-chloroenzylidene)-9H-fluren-4-yl]-ethanol (see Figure 10–1), was synthesized in the 1970s in China. Lumefantrine has one asymmetric carbon atom and exists in two enantiomeric forms, (+)– and (–)–lumefantrine. The drug is very poorly soluble in water. After a single oral dose of 480 mg, the C_{max} is about 950 nmol/L in fasting subjects.[23] Lumefantrine is highly bound (> 99%) to high-density lipoproteins[78] and to erythrocytes (8%).[23] The half-life is about 33 hours.[79] Coartem/Riamet is a new oral dose combination of artemether and lumefantrine that has been highly effective in the treatment of multidrug-resistant *Plasmodium falciparum*.[80] The bioavailability of lumefantrine was increased by a factor of 16 when the drug was taken with a high-fat meal, compared to its bioavailability in a fasting subject.[23] There was no difference in lumefantrine concentration between capillary and venous blood plasma.[81]

Two HPLC methods are available for the determination of lumefantrine.[82,83] Both have a limit of determination of about 95 nmol/L. No method is presently available for the determination of lumefantrine from capillary blood sampling onto filter paper.

Mefloquine

Mefloquine (MQ), (±) erythro-α-(2-piperidyl)-2,8-bis(trifluoromethyl)-4-quinolinemethanol, is a quinoline methanol structurally similar to quinine (see Figure 10–1). It is used both for prophylaxis and for the treatment of multidrug-resistant *Plasmodium falciparum* malaria. The main metabolite, 2,8-bis (trifluoromethyl)-4-quinoline-carboxylic acid (MMQ) (see Figure 10–1), has no antimalarial effect. The therapeutic levels of MQ and MMQ in plasma are 1 to 4 μmol/L and 2 to 6 μmol/L, respectively. MQ is highly (98%) bound to plasma proteins.[84] The half-life is about 15 to 27 days, and the plasma and whole blood concentrations are similar in healthy volunteers.[85,86] However, MMQ concentrations are about two times higher in serum than in whole blood.[87] MQ is a chiral drug with two asymmetric carbon atoms and may exist in four isomeric forms: two erythroisomers (RS-MQ and SR-MQ) and two threoisomers (RR-MQ and SS-MQ). The available preparation is a racemate of the (+) RS-MQ and (–) SR-MQ enantiomers in equal proportions. Both enantiomers are active against *Plasmodium falciparum* in vitro[88] although a slightly higher activity for (+) RS-MQ has been reported.[89] The MQ enantiomers differ extensively in their kinetics; (–) SR-MQ has a half-life of 430 hours, compared to 172 hours for (+) RS-MQ in plasma.[90] In a healthy adult during steady state, the concentration ratio between –SR–MQ and +RS–MQ is 7.9 in plasma and about 5.0 in whole blood.[91]

Two publications describing selective simultaneous determination of MQ and its main carboxyl metabolite (MMQ) exist.[92,93] One of these methods[93] permits determination down to 100 nmol/L of MQ and MMQ. One method can determine MQ and MMQ by using 100 μL of capillary blood dried on filter paper.[94] The limit of determination in 100 μL of capillary blood is 500 nmol/L for MQ and 250 nmol/L for MMQ. Capillary sampling onto filter paper collected in the field is very attractive due to several advantages: small sample volume, ease of performing the finger-prick sampling, good acceptance for repeated sampling, and the lack of the need for freezing facilities in the field. Figure 10–9 shows examples from an HPLC method for the determination of MQ and MMQ from capillary blood samples on filter paper. The stability of MQ and MMQ in dried form on filter paper is

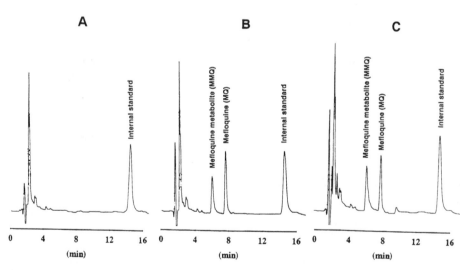

Figure 10–9. (*A*), Chromatogram of drug-free human capillary blood spotted on chromatography paper. (*B*), Chromatogram obtained following injection of MQ (2.5 μmol/L) and MMQ (2.5 μmol/L) in the mobile phase. (*C*), Chromatogram of blood from a patient who received 250 mg of MQ as oral dose, followed by capillary sampling onto paper 12 hours after dosing and analyzed by the present method. Concentrations: MQ, 1.9 μmol/L; MMQ, 2.5 μmol/L. Retention times: MMQ, 6.1 min; MQ, 7.8 min; internal standard, 14.6 min. (Reproduced with permission from Bergqvist Y, Al Kabbani J, Krysen B, et al. High-performance liquid chromatographic method for the simultaneous determination of mefloquine and its carboxyl metabolite in 100-μL capillary blood samples dried on paper. J Chromatogr B 1993;615:297–302.)

good. Concentrations are unaltered for at least 50 days, both at room temperature and at higher temperature (+37°C).[94]

HPLC is now one of the most frequently used techniques for the determination of drug enantiomers. Chiral separations can be done as direct and indirect methods. The indirect method involves precolumn derivatization of enantiomers with a homochiral reagent to obtain a pair of diastereoisomers. These diastereomers can be baseline-separated on a conventional column for HPLC. In direct separation, the enantiomers react with a chiral selector in the mobile phase or in the stationary phase.

HPLC methods are available for the determination of MQ enantiomers.[95,96] One of these methods[96] can be used for the determination of MQ enantiomers after capillary sampling onto filter paper. The capillary blood sampling method[96] is an indirect precolumn derivatization method with the (1)-1-(9-fluorenyl) ethyl chloroformate ((–)–FLEC) reagent, which has a very high fluorescence. Due to the fluorescent properties of the derivatives, a limit of determination down to 125 nmol/L for both enantiomers can be achieved in 100 μL of capillary blood.

Proguanil

Proguanil (PG), N_1-(3,4-dichlorophenyl)-N_5-iso-propyldiguanide (see Figure 10–1), is a biguanide that was synthesized in 1945. It is metabolized in the liver to the active triazine metabolite[97] cycloguanil (CG) (see Figure 10–1). This metabolite has been shown to have a much higher in vitro activity against *Plasmodium falciparum* blood stages than the parent compound or the other PG metabolite, 4-chlorophenylbiguanide (4-CPB)[98] (see Figure 10–1). The plasma protein binding of PG is approximately 75%, and the half-life of PG is about 16 hours. PG is partly metabolized by the enzyme CYP2C19 to the active metabolite CG. Results from Watkins and colleagues[99] indicate that the activity against *Plasmodium falciparum* is due entirely to the action of the active metabolite CG. Recently, however, studies have indicated that PG also has antimalarial activity.[100,101] There are large interindividual differences in the ability to metabolize PG to CG.[102] This is mediated by the enzyme CYP2C19, which shows genetic polymorphism.[103] The resulting large interindividual differences in plasma concentrations of the active metabolite CG between extensive and poor metabolizers are probably of clinical importance for malaria prophylaxis.

Analytic methods for the determination of PG should also be able to detect CG at low concentrations (< 50 nmol/L) to give an indication of poor metabolism.[104] Selective HPLC with SPE methods have been described for the determination of PG and its metabolites.[32,105,106] HPLC methods with SPE for the determination of PG, CG, and 4-CPB in 100 μL of capillary blood dried on filter paper are available.[33,107] The limit of determination was 50 nmol/L for CG and 4-CPB and 125 nmol/L for PG. Different kinds of sampling paper were tested. Due to very hard binding of the analytes to the cellulose matrix, the paper had to be pretreated with a quaternary ammonium compound to reduce binding of the analytes before the sampling. Venous and capillary blood concentrations of PG and its metabolites were found to be similar. No decrease in the concentration of the analytes on the filter paper occurred during a storage period of at least 30 days at 37°C.[33]

Pyronaridine

Pyronaridine, 2-methoxy-6-chloro-9[3,5-bis(1-pyrrolidinylmethyl)-4-hydroxy] anilino-1-aza-acridine (see Figure 10–1), is a schizonticidal drug active against the erythrocytic stages of malaria parasites. The drug was developed in China at the end of the 1970s. It is a derivative of benzonaphthyridine, with a ring system similar to that of mepacrine and a side chain similar to amodiaquine. Pyronaridine has both acidic and basic functional groups and cannot be obtained in uncharged form. In a study with semi-immune children in Africa, it was shown that pyronaridine was highly effective in treating acute uncomplicated falciparum malaria,[108] and Dutta and colleagues showed that pyronaridine is an effective antimalarial against multidrug-resistant malaria.[109]

No reliable information is available on the pharmacokinetics of pyronaridine in humans. The half-life is about 60 hours in both rabbits and humans, after various routes of administration.[110] Pyronaridine has very low stability in both refrigerated and frozen whole blood samples. After 8 weeks, pyronaridine in refrigerated samples decreases by 13% to 21%.[111]

A selective HPLC method using electrochemical detection for monitoring pyronaridine concentration in biologic samples was described in 1990. Blood analysis includes liquid-liquid extraction and subsequent SPE that removes an interferent present in blood. The method uses an analogue of amodiaquine as an internal standard.[111] The native fluorescence properties of pyronaridine have been used for detection in an HPLC system.[112] This method uses liquid-liquid extraction, an HPLC with a C18 column and fluorescence detector with $\lambda ex = 267$ nm, $\lambda em = 443$ nm (λex = extinction, λem = emission). The limit of determination is about 19 nmol/L in 250 µL of sample. A weak cation exchanger as SPE sorbent was recently presented for the determination of pyronaridine by HPLC and UV detector in plasma.[113] The limit of determination, using 500 µL of plasma, was about 100 nmol/L. No method is presently available for the determination of pyronaridine from capillary blood samples on filter paper.

Pyrimethamine and Sulfadoxine

Pyrimethamine (2,4-diamino-5-p-chlorophenyl-6-ethylpyrimidine) (see Figure 10–1), is a diaminopyrimidine. The mechanism of action is inhibition of dihydrofolic reductase necessary for folic acid synthesis in the parasite. When the drug is combined with sulfadoxine, the effect of pyrimethamine is potentiated. Pyrimethamine is 80% protein bound in plasma, and its half-life is around 4 days.

Sulfadoxine, N'-(5,6-dimethoxy-4-pyrimidinyl)-sulfanilamide (see Figure 10–1), is a sulfonamide. Malaria parasites synthesise their folate cofactors and cannot use dietary folic acid as the human host can. Sulfonamides compete with para-amonobenzoic acid (PABA) for binding to the enzyme dihydropteroate synthetase in the synthesis of dihydropterotes.[114]

Only a small proportion (< 10%) of sulfadoxine is metabolized to the main metabolite N_4-acetyl-metabolite. The ratio of sulfadoxine concentration between whole blood and plasma is 0.56[115] and is due to the fact that about 90% of the sulfadoxine is bound to albumin. The rest is distributed in plasma (about 6%) and erythrocytes (about 4%).[116] The half-life is between 7 and 9 days.

For assay in biologic fluids, it is useful if both pyrimethamine and sulfadoxine can be determine simultaneously. However, the plasma concentration of pyrimethamine is about 0.2% of that of sulfadoxine, as seen in Figure 10–10.[117]

There are a numerous reported methods for the simultaneous determination of sulfadoxine and pyrimethamine in biologic fluids. A simple and selective HPLC method for the simultaneous determination of sulfadoxine and pyrimethamine in plasma is available.[115,118] The acetylsulfadoxine metabolite could be separated and quantified. The limit of determination is 5 μmol/L for sulfadoxine and about 40 nmol/L for pyrimethamine. Two other methods have been reported for the selective quantification of sulfadoxine and the N_4-acetyl-metabolite of sulfadoxine and pyrimethamine[119,120] in body fluids. One method uses an automated SPE technique for the simultaneous determination of sulfadoxine and pyrimethamine in plasma.[121]

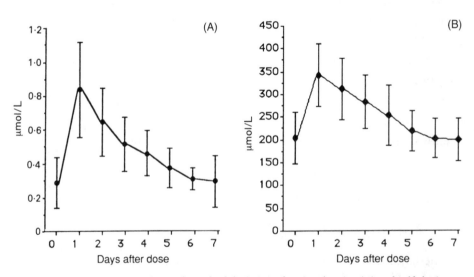

Figure 10–10. Mean concentration and standard deviation of pyrimethamine (A) and sulfadoxine (B) in plasma during prolonged weekly prophylaxis with 500 mg sulfadoxine and 25 mg pyrimethamine (n = 11). (Reproduced with permission from Hellgren U, Angel VH, Bergqvist Y, et al. Plasma concentrations of sulfadoxine-pyrimethamine and of mefloquine during regular long term malaria prophylaxis. Trans R Soc Trop Med Hyg 1990;84:46–49.)

Green and colleagues[122] presented a very simple HPLC-validated calorimetric SPE method for the determination of sulfadoxine in 100 μL of whole blood. The method uses sodium dodecyl sulfate for extraction of sulfadoxine from whole blood and to enhance the calorimetric reaction produced by p-dimethylaminocinnamaldehyde.

An HPLC method for the determination of sulfadoxine in capillary blood dried on filter paper has been published.[123] The technique was validated by comparing the sulfadoxine concentration in simultaneously collected capillary blood, dried on filter paper, and conventional venous whole blood samples ($r = 0.99$). Using 100 μL of capillary blood, the method has a limit of determination of 25 μmol/L, with a precision of 3% to 5% in the concentration range of 50 to 400 μmol/L. Sulfadoxine was stable on the dried filter papers for at least 15 weeks at 37°C. Due to a very low concentration in blood, no method is presently available for the determination of pyrimethamine from capillary blood samples on filter paper.

NEW TECHNOLOGIES FOR THE ASSAY OF ANTIMALARIAL DRUGS

Solid-Phase Extraction

Several new patented sorbents have been introduced onto the market recently. They are all presented as the "universal" extraction sorbents since they are capable of extracting acidic, basic, and neutral compounds, whether polar or nonpolar.[26] One example of these universal SPE sorbents is Oasis HLB from Waters, which has both hydrophilic and lipophilic properties in the same sorbent. This sorbent is a co-polymer and does not need to be conditioned with a wetting solvent as with the reversed-phase silica sorbents.

Stationary Phases for High-Performance Liquid Chromatography

Different studies have shown that the combination of antimalarial drugs is important in investigating possible synergistic, additive, or antagonistic effects. Atovaquone/proguanil and artemether/lumefantrine are examples of drug combinations that have shown synergistic activity. For all new combinations, there should be new pharmacokinetic studies as the drugs may interact with each other and change pharmacokinetic properties. Developing new methods for the simultaneous determination of these drugs is a challenge.

One recent development in stationary phases for improved column separation is mixed-mode columns. This is a mixture of a cation exchange for the interaction with the polar compound (e.g., proguanil) and a hydrophobic stationary phase for the lipophilic atovaquone. An example of separation with a commercially available mixed column is the simultaneous separation of the components of Malarone, atovaquone and proguanil,[124] which have significant differences in their chemical properties. The separation is shown in Figure 10–11.

Another improvement in the stationary phase is the introduction of shield groups to protect the analytes from the negatively charged silanol groups in the stationary phase. Most of the antimalarial drugs contain nitrogen, and they become positively charged at a pH of < 7. Waters SymmetryShield is one example, and an illustration of this effect for the assay of mefloquine and its acid metabolite is presented in the 1999 report by Green and colleagues.[26]

Liquid Chromatography–Mass Spectrometry

Liquid chromatography–mass spectrometry (LC-MS) functions very efficiently as the detector in a chromatographic system for the assay of analytes. The inlets to LC-MS can be used for HPLC or capillary electrophoresis (CE). Detection can be achieved by single-ion monitoring (SIM). Effective use of SIM requires prior knowledge about the characteristics of the analyte of interest. Therefore, SIM can be used only for quantification and for monitoring a known chromatographically separated peak. The mass spectrometry (MS) technique improves selectivity and is very useful when other detection techniques give very low selectivity and limits of determination (e.g., for artemisinin derivatives). Ortelli and colleagues[125] presented an analysis of dihydroartemisinin by LC-MS. The limit of determination was 35 nmol/L

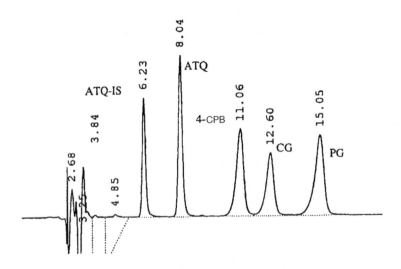

Figure 10–11. High-performance liquid chromatography (HPLC) profiles for the separation of analytes. Column: C18/SCX Hypersil Cation Duet. Mobile phase: acetonitrile-phosphate buffer pH 6.8 (60:40 v/v), 65 mmoL l^{-1} K⁺. Figures on the top of the peaks are retention times in minutes. (ATQ = atovaquone; CG = cycloguanil; IS = internal standard; PG = proguanil; 4-CPB = 4-chlorophenylbiguanide.) (Reproduced with permission from Bergqvist Y, Hopstadius C. Simultaneous separation of atovaquone, proguanil and its metabolites on a mixed mode high-performance liquid chromatographic column. J Chromatogr B 2000;741:189–193.)

with a coefficient of variant (CV) of about 15% to 16%. Another LC-MS method is available for analysis in the nanogram range in crude biologic samples.[126]

In the future, MS detectors in HPLC could be one of the detectors that replace UV and other detectors in the assay of antimalarials because of their much better selectivity and reliability.

Capillary Electrophoresis

Capillary electrophoresis developed in the early 1980s is a highly efficient means of separation for the analysis of complex mixtures with extremely small sample volumes. The relatively short separation times, simple instrumentation, and low operational costs make it an attractive alternative to HPLC for the assay of antimalarial drugs. Currently, UV-absorbance detectors are employed in commercial CE instruments.

Chemoluminescence (CL) is one of the less developed detection systems for CE. CL detection systems are characterized by simple and cheap optical systems requiring no light sources.[127] The combination of CE and CL would be a very useful instrument for the assay of artemisinin derivatives. The light emitted in such a CL system is directly proportional to the concentration of the endoperoxide moiety in artemisinin derivatives. A detection limit of 10^{-9} to 10^{-10} mol/L has been achieved in CL systems.[127]

Several antimalarial drugs as well as a variety of other drugs were analyzed by capillary zone electrophoresis (CZE). Chou and colleagues presented a rapid and simple CZE method for the determination of atovaquone, with a limit of determination of 8 μmol/L.[128] CZE was used as the chiral stationary phase, with heparin as a chiral mobile-phase additive, for separation of chloroquine, primaquine, mefloquine, and halofantrine.[129] Separation of the chiral antimalarial drugs seems to be important for studies of the individual antimalarial activity of the chiral isomers.

Chiral Separations

Following the guidelines in different countries, single enantiomers of chiral drugs should be brought to the market wherever possible. The enantiomers must be separated, and the pharmacologic effects must be studied separately for each enantiomer. Examples of chiral drugs in antimalarials are chloroquine, mefloquine, halofantrine, and quinine. Koppenhoeffer and colleagues reported on selected reviews that present the enantioselective separation of 86 chiral drugs by CZE with cyclodextrins as a chiral selector.[130] In this review, chiral separations of chloroquine and mefloquine are presented.[130]

Detectors and Light-Scattering Detectors

The search for sensitive and specific detection systems for antimalarials continues to be an important analytic goal. Avery and colleagues presented evaporative light-scattering detection (ELSD), a technique for detecting compounds without chromophore groups (e.g., artemisinin derivatives).[131] The detection limit was about 10 to 11 μmol/L, not enough for the assay of artemisinin in plasma. Koropchak and colleagues presented condensation nucleation scattering detection (CNLSD), a development of the ELSD technique with much lower limits of detection.[132] The limit of detection with CNLSD was improved by a factor of 1,000, compared to ELSD.

SUMMARY

Considerable progress has been made during recent years in increasing the range of available techniques for both extraction and isolation with SPE in regard to the chromatographic separation, detection, and quantification of antimalarials. Selectivity has increased for the analysis of antimalarials from the biologic matrix, and new antimalarial metabolites have been detected and determined (e.g., artemisinin). The simultaneous determination of antimalarials during combination therapy is still complex and seems to increase the difficulties of achieving high selectivity in extraction and chromatography.

Precise measurements depend largely on good laboratory practices. These include the consistent use of standard operating procedures and the establishment of, and adherence to, carefully designed protocols for specific analytic processes. Good laboratory practices also include the consistent use of qualified and closely supervised personnel, reliable and well-maintained equipment, and appropriate calibrations and standards. Every analytic system contains sources of inaccuracy and imprecision that have variable components; thus, a strategy for minimizing errors is needed.

It is often useful to apply various methods when conducting a clinical study in malaria-endemic areas. Field-adapted methods for the analysis of urine samples can be applied at the study site for screening, and corresponding blood samples (e.g., finger-prick samples applied to filter paper) can be preserved for subsequent analysis in the laboratory. Selecting samples for laboratory analysis is based on clinical, parasitologic, and field assay data.

ACKNOWLEDGMENTS

I am very grateful to my colleagues Urban Hellgren, Lars Funding, Mike Green, and Jamie Stevenson for constructive comments and to Daniel Blessborn for drawing the chemical structures.

REFERENCES

1. Abdi Aden Y, Gustavsson LL, Ericsson Ö, Hellgren U. Handbook of tropical parasitic infections. London: Taylor & Francis, 1995.

2. Advances in malaria chemotherapy. Geneva: World Health Organization, 1984. Technical Report Series 711.

3. Hellgren U. Drug concentrations during antimalarial treatment and prophylaxis—relation to in vivo outcome and in vitro susceptibility. Stockholm: Karolinska Institute, 1990.

4. Dorsey JG, Cooper WT, Siles BA, et al. Liquid chromatography: theory and methodology. Anal Chem 1998;70:591R–644R.

5. Kromidas S. Practical problem solving in HPLC. Wiley-Vch Verlag GmbH, 2000.

6. Meyer VR. Pitfalls and errors of HPLC in pictures. Heidelberg: Hüthig Verlag, 2000.

7. Kristensen S, Orsteen A-L, Sande SA, et al. Photoreactivity of biologically active compounds. VII. Interaction of antimalarial drugs with melanin in vitro as part of phototoxicity screening. Photochem Photobiol 1994;26:87–95.

8. Caporal-Gautier J, Nivet JM, Algranti P, et al. Guide de validation analytiue. Rapport d'une commission SFSTP. I Méthodologie. S.T.P Pharma Pratiques 1992;2:205–226.

9. Hubert PH, Chiap P, Crommen J, et al. The SFSTP guide on the validation of chromatographic methods for drug analysis: from the Washington Conference to the laboratory. Anal Chim Acta 1999;391:135–148.

10. Chiap P, Hubert PH, Boulanger B, Crommen J. Validation of an automated method for the liquid chromatographic determination of atenolol in plasma: application of a new validation protocol. Anal Chim Acta 1999;391:227–238.

11. Caisson R. Validation of chromatographic methods in biomedical analysis. Viewpoint and discussion. J Chromatogr B 1997;689:175–180.

12. Huber L. Validation of analytical methods: review and strategy. LC-GC Int 1998;February:96–105.

13. Hartman C, Smeyers-Verbeke J, Massart DL, McDowall RD. Validation of bioanalytical chromatographic methods. J Pharm Biomed Anal 1998;17:193–218.

14. Vessman J. Selectivity or specificity? Validation of analytical methods from the perspective of an analytical chemist in the pharmaceutical industry. J Pharm Biomed Anal 1996;14:867–869.

15. The validation of chemical and immunological tests for antimalarials in body fluids. International Monograph Series no 3. World Health Organization. Syarikat Jasmin: Pulau Pinang; 1990.

16. Claessens HA. Characterization of stationary phases for reversed-phase liquid chromatography [thesis]. Netherlands: Technische Universiteit Eindhoven, 1999.

17. Engelhardt M, Arangio M, Lobert T. A chromatographic test procedure for reversed-phase HPLC column evaluation. LC-GC International 1997;Dec:803–812.

18. Engelhardt M, Grüner R. Characterization of reversed-phase columns for efficiency, retention and silanophilic activity. LC-GC Int 1999;Sep;34–42.

19. Bergqvist Y, Domeij-Nyberg B. Distribution of chloroquine and its metabolite desethyl-chloroquine in human blood cells and its implication for the quantitative determination of these compounds in serum and plasma. J Chromatogr B 1983;272:137–148.

20. Knudsen RC, Slazyk WE, Richmond JY, et al. Guidelines for the shipment of dried blood spot specimens. Infant Screen 1993;16:1–5.

21. Bergqvist Y, Ericsson Ô, Rais M. Determination of chloroquine in dried blood spots on filter paper: importance of sample handling. Ther Drug Monit 1986;8:211–213.

22. Bergqvist Y, Funding L, Kaneko A, et al. Improved method for the simultaneous determination of proguanil and its metabolites by high-performance liquid chromatography and solid-phase extraction of 100 µL capillary blood samples dried on sampling paper. J Chromatogr B 1998;719:141–149.

23. Lefevre G, Thomsen MS. Clinical pharmacokinetics of artemether and lumefantrine (Riamet®). Clin Drug Invest 1999;18:467–480.

24. Rolan PE, Mercher AJ, Weatherley BC, et al. Examination of some factors responsible for a food induced increase in absorption of atovaquone. Br J Clin Pharmacol 1994;37:13–20.

25. Hans Lobel, Centers for Disease Control (CDC), Atlanta (GA). Personal communication.

26. Green MD, Bergqvist Y, Mount DL, et al. Improved validated assay for the determination of mefloquine and its carboxy metabolite in plasma, serum and whole blood using solid-phase extraction and high-performance liquid chromatography. J Chromatogr B 1999;727:159–165.

27. Baadenhuijsen H, Scholten R, Willems HL, et al. A model for harmonization of routine clinical chemistry results between clinical laboratories. Ann Clin Biochem 2000;37:330–337.

28. Miller N, Miller JC. Statistics and chemometrics for analytical chemistry. Chichester: Ellis Horwood Ltd., 1998.

29. Majors RE. A review of modern solid-phase extraction. LC-GC, Current Trends and Development in Sample Preparation 1998;May:8–15.

30. Thurman EM, Mills MS. Solid-phase extraction—principles and practice. New York: John Wiley & Sons Inc., 1998.

31. Hennion M-C. Solid-phase extraction: method development, sorbents, and coupling with liquid chromatography. J Chromatogr A 1999;856:3–54.

32. Bergqvist Y, Funding F, Krysen B, et al. Improved validated assay for the determination of proguanil and its metabolites in plasma, whole blood and urine using solid-phase extraction and high-performance liquid chromatography. Ther Drug Monit 1998;20:325–330.

33. Bergqvist Y, Funding L, Kaneko A, et al. Improved method for the simultaneous determination of proguanil and its metabolites by high-performance liquid chromatography and solid-phase extraction of 100 µL capillary blood samples dried on sampling paper. J Chromatogr B 1998;719:141–149.

34. Taylor RB, Awad MI, Reid RG, Moody RR. Determination of sodium artesunate in plasma using ion-pairing high-performance liquid chromatography. J Chromatogr B 2000;744:415–421.

35. Gordi T, Nielsen E, Yu Z, et al. Direct analysis of artemisinin in plasma and saliva using coupled-column high-performance liquid chromatography with a restricted-access material pre-column. J Chromatogr B 2000;742:155–162.

36. Churchill FC, Mount DL, Patchen LC. Isolation, characterisation and standardisation of a major metabolite of amodiaquine by chromatographic and spectroscopic methods. J Chromatogr B 1986;377:307–318.

37. Laurent F, Saivin S, Chretien P, et al. Pharmacokinetic and pharmacodynamic study of amodiaquine and its two metabolites after a single oral dose. Arzneimittelforschung 1993;43:612–616.

38. Winstanley P, Edwards G, Orme M, et al. The disposition of amodiaquine in man after oral administration. Br J Clin Pharmacol 1987;23:1–7.

39. Mount DL, Patchen LC, Nguyen-Dinh P, et al. Sensitive analysis of blood for amodiaquine and three metabolites by high-performance liquid chromatography with electrochemical detection. J Chromatogr B 1986;383:375–386.

40. Pussard E, Verdier F, Blayo MC. Simultaneous determination of chloroquine, amodiaquine and their metabolites in human plasma, red blood cells, whole blood and urine by column liquid chromatography. J Chromatogr B 1986;374:111–118.

41. Meshnick S. The mode of action of antimalarial endoperoxides. Trans R Soc Trop Med Hyg 1994;88 Suppl 1:31–32.

42. White NJ. Preventing antimalarial drug resistance through combinations. Drug Resist Updates 1998;1:3–9.

43. Colussi D, Parisot C, Legay F, Lefevre G. Binding of artemether and lumefantrine to plasma proteins and erythrocytes. Eur J Pharm Sci 1999;9:9–16.

44. Luo XD, Shen CC. The chemistry, pharmacology and clinical applications of qinghaosu (artemisinin) and its derivatives. Med Res Rev 1987;7:29–52.

45. Edlund PO, Westerlund D, Carlqvist J, et al. Determination of arsenate and dihydroartemisinin in plasma by liquid chromatography with post-column derivatization and UV detection. Acta Pharm Suec 1984;21:223–234.

46. Svensson USH. Pharmacokinetics drug metabolism and clinical effect of the antimalarial artemisinin. Acta Univ Ups 2000;224.

47. Alin MH. Artemisinin and its derivatives in the treatment of faliciparum malaria. Acta Univ Ups 1995;140.

48. Green MD, Mount DL, Todd GD, et al. Chemiluminescent detection of artemisinin. Novel endoperoxide analysis using luminol without hydrogen peroxide. J Chromatogr B 1995;695:237–242.

49. Navaratnam V, Mordi MN, Mansor SM. Simultaneous determination of artesunic acid and dihydroartemisinin in blood plasma by high-performance liquid chromatography for application in clinical pharmacological studies. J Chromatogr B 1997;669:157–162.

50. van Agtmael MA, Butter JJ, Portier EJ, et al. Validation of an improved reversed-phase high-performance liquid chromatographic assay with reductive electrochemical detection for the determination of artemisinin derivatives in man. Ther Drug Monit 1998;20:109–116.

51. Na-Bangchang K, Congpuong K, Hung LN, et al. Simple high-performance liquid chromatographic method with electrochemical detection for the simultaneous determination of artesunate and dihydroartemisinin in biological fluids. J Chromatogr B 1998;708:201–207.

52. Jastrebova J, Nyholm L, Markides KE, Bergqvist Y. On-line deoxygenation for reductive electrochemical detection of artemisinin and dihydroartemisinin in liquid chromatography. Analyst 1998;123:313–317.

53. Mohamed SS, Khalid SA, Ward SA, et al. Simultaneous determination of artemether and its major metabolite dihydroartemisinin in plasma by gas chromatography-mass spectrometry-selected ion monitoring. J Chromatogr B 1999;731:251–260.

54. Canfield CJ, Pudney M, Gutteridge WE. Interactions of atovaquone with other antimalarial drugs against *Plasmodium faliciparum* in vitro. Exp Parasitol 1995;80:373–381.

55. Looareesuwan S, Viravan C, Webster HK, et al. Clinical studies of atovaquone alone or in combination with other antimalarial drugs for treatment of acute uncomplicated malaria in Thailand. Am J Trop Med Hyg 1996;54:62–66.

56. Sabchareon A, Attanath P, Phanuaksook P, et al. Efficacy and pharmacokinetics of ato-vaquone and proguanil in children with multidrug resistant *Plasmodium falciparum* malaria. Trans R Soc Trop Med Hyg 1998;92:201–206.

57. Artymowicz RJ, James VE. Atovaquone: a new antipneumocystis agent. Clin Pharm 1993;12:563–570.

58. DeAngelis DV, Long JD, Kanics LL, et al. High-performance liquid-chromatographic assay for the measurement of atovaquone in plasma. J Chromatogr B 1994;652:211–219.

59. Hannan SL, Ridout GA, Jones AE. Determination of the potent antiprotozoal compound atovaquone in plasma using liquid-liquid extraction followed by reversed-phase high-performance liquid chromatography with ultraviolet detection. J Chromatogr B 1996;678:297–302.

60. Studenberg SD, Long JD, Woolf J, et al. A robotics-based liquid chromatographic assay for the measurement of atovaquone in plasma. J Pharm Biomed Anal 1995;13:1383–1393.

61. Hansson AG, Mitchell S, Jatlow P, et al. Rapid high-performance liquid chromatographic assay for atovaquone. J Chromatogr B 1996:675:180–182.

62. Lindegårdh N, Bergqvist Y. Automated solid-phase extraction method for the determination of atovaquone in plasma and whole blood by rapid high-performance liquid chromatography. J Chromatogr B 2000;744:9–17.

63. Lindegårdh N, Bergqvist Y. Automated solid-phase extraction method for the determination of atovaquone in plasma and whole blood by rapid high-performance liquid chromatography. J Chromatogr B 2000;744:9–17.

64. Fu S, Björkman A, Wåhlin B, et al. In vitro activity of chloroquine, the enantiomers of chloroquine, desethylchloroquine and pyronaridine against *Plasmodium falciparum*. Br J Clin Pharmacol 1986;22:93–96.

65. Verdier F, Le Bras J, Clavier F, Hatin I. Blood levels and in vitro activity of desethylchloroquine against *Plasmodium falciparum* [letter]. Lancet 1984;1:1186–1187.

66. Bergqvist Y, Domeij-Nyberg B. Distribution of chloroquine and its metabolite desethylchloroquine in human blood cells and its implication for the quantitative determination of these compounds in serum and plasma. J Chromatogr B 1983;272:137–148.

67. Gustavsson LL, Rombo L, Alvan G, et al. The disposition of chloroquine in man after single intravenous and oral doses. Br J Clin Pharmacol 1983;15:471–479.

68. Rombo L, Ericsson Ô, Lindström B, et al. Chloroquine and desethylchloroquine in plasma, serum and whole blood. Problems in assay and handling of samples. Ther Drug Monit 1985;7:211–215.

69. Bergqvist Y, Frisk-Holmberg M. Sensitive method for the determination and its metabolite desethylchloroquine in human plasma and urine by high performance liquid chromatography. J Chromatogr B 1980;221:119–127.

70. Alvan G, Ekman L, Lindström B. Determination of chloroquine and its desethyl metabolite in plasma red blood cells and urine by liquid chromatography. J Chromatogr B 1982;229:241–247.

71. Frisk-Holmberg M, Bergqvist Y, Termond E, Domeij-Nyberg B. The single dose kinetics of chloroquine and its major metabolite desethylchloroquine in healthy subjects. Eur J Clin Pharmacol 1984;26:521–530.

72. Alvan G, Ekman L, Lindström B, et al. Chloroquine and desethyl-chloroquine concentrations during regular long term prophylaxis. Bull World Health Organ 1987;65:879–883.

73. Walker O, Ademowo G. A rapid cost-effective liquid chromatographic method for the determination of chloroquine and desethylchloroquine in biological fluids. Ther Drug Monit 1996;18:92–96.

74. Patchen LC, Mount DL, Schwartz IK, Churchill FC. Analysis of filter-paper-absorbed finger-stick blood samples for chloroquine and its major metabolite using high performance liquid chromatography with fluorescence detection. J Chromatogr B 1983;278:81–89.

75. Lindström B, Ericsson Ö, Alvan G, et al. Determination of chloroquine and its desethyl metabolite in whole blood. An application for samples collected in capillary tubes dried on filter paper. Ther Drug Monit 1985;7:207–210.

76. Stalcup AM, Gahm KH, Baldueza M. Chiral separation of chloroquine using heparin as a chiral selector in high-performance liquid chromatography. Anal Chem 1996;68:2248–2250.

77. Escande C, Chevalier P, Verdier F, Bourdon R. Sensitive radioimmunoassay and enzyme-linked immunosorbent assay for the simultaneous determination of chloroquine and its metabolites in biological fluids. J Pharm Sci 1990;79:23–27.

78. van Vugt M. Artemether-lumefantrine. Universiteit van Amsterdam, 1994.

79. White J, van Vugt M, Ezzet F. Clinical pharmacokinetics and pharmacodynamics of artemether-lumefantrine. Clin Pharmacokinet 1999;37:105–125.

80. Looareesuwan S, Krudsood S, Silachamroon U, et al. Efficacy and tolerability of a six-dose regimen of Coartem® (artemether/lumefantrine) in the treatment of multi-drug resistant falciparum malaria [abstract]. Proceedings of the 15th International Congress for Tropical Medicine and Malaria; 2000 Aug 20–25; Cartagena, Columbia.

81. van Vugt M, Ezzet F, Phaipun L, et al. The relationship between capillary and venous concentration of lumefantrine (benflumetol). Trans R Soc Trop Med Hyg 1998;92:564–565.

82. Zeng MY, Lu ZL, Yang SC, et al. Determination of benflumetol in human plasma by reversed-phase high-performance liquid chromatography with ultraviolet detection. J Chromatogr B 1966;681:299–306.

83. Mansor SM, Navaratnam V, Yahaya N, et al. Determination of a new antimalarial drug, benflumetol, in blood plasma by high-performance liquid chromatography. J Chromatogr B 1996;682:321–325.

84. Mu JY, Israil ZH, Dayton PG. Studies of the disposition and metabolism of mefloquine HCl (WR 142,490), a quinolinemethanol antimalarial, in the rat. Limited studies with an analogue WR 30,090. Drug Metab Dispos 1975;3:198–210.

85. Franssen G, Rouveix B, Le Bras J, et al. Divided dose kinetics of mefloquine in man. Br J Clin Pharmacol 1989;28:179–184.

86. Hellgren U, Angel VH, Bergqvist Y, et al. Plasma concentrations of sulfadoxine-pyrimethamine and of mefloquine during long term malaria prophylaxis. Trans R Soc Trop Med Hyg 1990;84:46–49.

87. Todd GD, Hopperus-Buma APCC, Green MD, et al. Comparison of whole blood and serum levels of mefloquine and its carboxylic acid metabolite. Am J Trop Med Hyg 1997;57:399–402.

88. Basco LK, Gillotin C, Gimenez F, et al. In vitro activity of the enantiomers of mefloquine, halofantrine and enpiroline against Plasmodium falciparum. Br J Clin Pharmacol 1992;33:517–520.

89. Karle JM, Olmeda R, Gerena L, Milhous WK. *Plasmodium falciparum*: role of absolute stereochemistry in the antimalarial activity of synthetic amino alcohol antimalarial agents. Exp Parasitol 1993;76:345–351.

90. Gimenez F, Pennie RA, Koren G, et al. Stereoselective pharmacokinetics of mefloquine enantiomers in healthy Caucasians after multiple dose. J Pharm Sci 1994;83:824–827.

91. Hellgren U, Jastrebova J, Jerling M, et al. Comparison between concentrations of racemic mefloquine, its separate enantiomers and the carboxylic acid metabolite in whole blood serum and plasma. Eur J Clin Pharmacol 1996;51:171–173.

92. Arnold PJ, Stetten OV. High-performance liquid chromatographic analysis of mefloquine and its main metabolite by direct plasma injection with pre-column enrichment and column switching techniques. J Chromatogr B 1986;353:193–200.

93. Bergqvist Y, Hellgren U, Churchill FC. High-performance liquid chromatographic assay for the simultaneous monitoring of mefloquine and its acid metabolite in biological samples using protein precipitation and ion-pair extraction. J Chromatogr B 1988;432:253–263.

94. Bergqvist Y, Al Kabbani J, Krysen B, et al. High-performance liquid chromatographic method for the simultaneous determination of mefloquine and its carboxyl metabolite in 100-µL capillary blood samples dried on paper. J Chromatogr B 1993;615:297–302.

95. Souri E, Farsam H, Jamali F. Stereospecific determination of mefloquine in biological fluids by high-performance liquid chromatography J Chromatogr B 1997;700:215–222.

96. Bergqvist Y, Al Kabbani J, Krysen B, et al. High-performance liquid chromatographic determination of (SR)- and (RS)-enantiomers of mefloquine in plasma and capillary blood samples on paper after derivatisation with (-)-1-(9-fluorenyl) ethyl chloroformate. J Chromatogr B 1994;652:73–81.

97. Carrington HC, Crowther AF, Davey DG, et al. A metabolite of "paludrine" with high antimalarial activity. Nature 1951;168:1080.

98. Funck-Brentano C, Becquemont L, Leneveu A, et al. Inhibition by omeprazole of proguanil metabolism: mechanism of the interaction in vitro and prediction of in vivo experiments. J Pharmacol Exp Ther 1997;280:730–738.

99. Watkins WM, Sixsmith DG, Chulay JD. The activity of proguanil and its metabolites, cycloguanil and p-chlorophenylbiguanide, against *Plasmodium falciparum* in vitro. Ann Trop Med Parasitol 1984;78:273–278.

100. Kaneko A, Bergqvist Y, Takechi M, et al. Intrinsic efficacy of proguanil against falciparum and vivax malaria independent of the metabolite cycloguanil. J Infect Dis 1999;179:974–979.

101. Fidock DA, Nomura T, Wellems TE. Cycloguanil and its parent compound proguanil demonstrate distinct activities against *Plasmodium falciparum* malaria parasites transformed with human dihydrofolate reductase. Mol Pharmacol 1998;54:1140–1147.

102. Ward SA, Watkins WM, Mberu E, et al. Inter-subject variability in the metabolism of proguanil to the active metabolite cycloguanil in man. Br J Clin Pharmacol 1989;27:781–787.

103. Helsby NA, Ward SA, Edwards G, et al. In vitro metabolism of the biguanide antimalarials in human liver microsomes; evidence for a role of the mephenytoin hydroxylase (P450 MP) enzyme. Br J Clin Pharmacol 1990;30:287–291.

104. Kaneko A, Bergqvist Y, Taleo G, et al. Proguanil disposition and toxicity in malaria patients from Vanuatu with high frequencies of CYP2C19 mutations. Pharmacogenetics 1999;9:317–326.

105. Taylor RB, Behrens R, Moddy RR, et al. Assay method for the simultaneous determination of proguanil, chloroquine and their main metabolites in biological fluids. J Chromatogr B 1990;527:490–497.

106. Chaulet JF, Grelaud G, Bellemin-Maigniot P, et al. Simultaneous determination of chloroquine, proguanil and their metabolites in human biological fluids by high-performance liquid chromatography. J Pharm Biomed Anal 1994;12:111–117.

107. Kolawole JA, Taylor RB, Moody RR. Determination of proguanil and metabolites in small sample volumes of whole blood stored on filter paper by high-performance liquid chromatography. J Chromatogr B 1995;674:149–154.

108. Ringwald P, Bickii J, Basco LK. Efficacy of oral pyronaridine for the treatment of acute uncomplicated falciparum malaria in African children. Clin Infect Dis 1998;26:946–953.

109. Dutta GP, Puri SK, Awasthi A, et al. Pyronaridine—an effective antimalarial against multidrug-resistant malaria. Life Sci 2000;67:759–764.

110. Feng Z, Wu ZF, Wang CY, et al. Pharmacokinetics of pyronaridine in malaria patients. Acta Pharm Sin 1988;8:543–546.

111. Wages SA, Patchen LC, Churchill FC. Analysis of blood and urine samples from *Macaca mulata* for pyronaridine by high-performance liquid chromatography with electrochemical detection. J Chromatogr B 1990;527:115–126.

112. Jayaraman SD, Ismail S, Nair NK, Navaratnam V. Determination of pyronaridine in blood plasma by high-performance liquid chromatography for application in clinical pharmacological studies. J Chromatogr B 1997;690:253–257.

113. Blessborn D, Bergqvist Y, Ericsson Ö. Determination of pyronaridine by solid phase extraction with cation exchange sorbent and HPLC [abstract]. Proceedings of the 15th International Congress for Tropical Medicine and Malaria; 2000 Aug 20–25; Cartagena.

114. Wernsdorfer WH, Trigg PI. The biology of malaria parasites. Geneva: World Health Organisation, 1987. Technical Report Series No. 743.

115. Bergqvist Y, Eriksson M. Simultaneous determination of pyrimethamine and sulphadoxine in human plasma by high-performance liquid chromatography. Trans R Soc Trop Med Hyg 1985;79:297–301.

116. Berneis K, Boguth W. Distribution of sulfonamides and sulfonamide potentiators between red blood cells, proteins and aqueous phases of the blood of different species. Chemotherapy 1976;22:390–409.

117. Hellgren U, Angel VH, Bergqvist Y, et al. Plasma concentrations of sulfadoxine-pyrimethamine and of mefloquine during regular long term malaria prophylaxis. Trans R Soc Trop Med Hyg 1990;84:46–49.

118. Edstein MD, Lika ID, Chongsuphajaisiddhi T, et al. Quantitation of Fansimef components (mefloquine + sulfadoxine + pyrimethamine) in human plasma by two high-performance liquid chromatographic methods. Ther Drug Monit 1991;13:146–151.

119. Midskov C. High-performance liquid chromatographic assay of pyrimethamine, sulfadoxine and its N4-acteyl metabolite is serum and urine after ingestion of Suldox. J Chromatogr B 1984;308:217–227.

120. Edstein M. Simultaneous measurement of sulfadoxine, N_4-acetylsulfadoxine and pyrimethamine in human plasma. J Chromatogr B 1984;305:502–507.

121. Astier H, Renard C, Cheminel V, et al. Simultaneous determination of pyrimethamine and sulphadoxine in human plasma by high-performance liquid chromatography after automated liquid-solid extraction. J Chromatogr B 1997;698:217–223.

122. Green MD, Dwight LM, Todd GD. Determination of sulfadoxine concentrations in whole blood using C_{18} solid-phase extraction, sodium dodecyl sulfate and dimethylaminocinnamaldehyde. Analyst 1995;120:2623–2626.

123. Bergqvist Y, Hjelm E, Rombo L. Sulfadoxine assay using capillary samples dried on filter paper—suitable for monitoring of blood concentrations in the field. Ther Drug Monit 1987;9:203–207.

124. Bergqvist Y, Hopstadius C. Simultaneous separation of atovaquone, proguanil and its metabolites on a mixed mode high-performance liquid chromatographic column. J Chromatogr B 2000;741:189–193.

125. Ortelli D, Rudaz S, Cognard EW, et al. Analysis of dihydroartemisinin in plasma by liquid chromatography-mass spectrometry [abstract]. Basel: PBA, 2000.

126. Sahai P, Vishwakarma RA, Bharel S, et al. HPLC-electrospray ionization mass spectrometric analysis of antimalarial drug artemisinin. Anal Chem 1998;70:3084–3087.

127. Huang XJ, Fang ZL. Chemiluminescence detection in capillary electrophoresis. Anal Chim Acta 2000;414:1–14.

128. Chou C-C, Brown MP, Merritt KA. Capillary zone electrophoresis for the determination of atovaquone in serum. J Chromatogr B 2000;742:441–445.

129. Stalcup AM, Agyel NM. Heparin: a chiral mobile-phase additive for capillary zone electrophoresis. Anal Chem 1999;66:3054–3059.

130. Koppenhoefer B, Zhu X, Jakob A, et al. Separation of drug enantiomers by capillary electrophoresis in the presence of neutral cyclodextrins. J Chromatogr B 2000;857:135–161.

131. Avery BA, Venkatesh KK, Avery MA. Rapid determination of artemisinin and related analogues using high-performance liquid chromatography and an evaporate light scattering detector. J Chromatogr B 1999;730:71–80.

132. Koropchak JA, Sadain S, Yang X, et al. Nanoparticle detection technology for chemical analysis. Anal Chem 1999;71:386A–394A.

Chapter 11

CLINICAL FEATURES OF MALARIA IN RETURNING TRAVELERS AND MIGRANTS

Blaise Genton and Valérie D'Acremont

ABSTRACT

The level of immunity of the host will condition the clinical features of malaria. Travelers have no immunity against the parasite and are therefore prone to severe disease and death if rapid action is not taken to reduce parasite growth and multiplication. The clinical manifestations of malaria are nonspecific; they include fever (97% of cases), chills (79%), headache (70%), sweats (64%), myalgia (36%), and nausea and vomiting (27%), the latter being more frequent in children. These features resemble those of influenza or any other viral infection, which often leads to misdiagnosis or delay in diagnosis in non-endemic areas. Clinical and laboratory predictors for a diagnosis of malaria include sweating, no abdominal pain, enlarged spleen, poor general condition , temperature > 38°C, thrombocytopenia, anemia, and absence of leukocytosis. Pooled data from the most relevant studies of imported malaria show a mean rate of 5% for severe malaria. Cerebral malaria is the most common presenting feature in severe malaria followed by acute renal failure, severe anemia, and pulmonary edema. Multiorgan failure often occurs in such situations, which explains the relatively high fatality rate (1% to 2%) of malaria in nonimmune travelers, in spite of the availability of intensive care. Since delay in diagnosis is the main reason for an adverse outcome, the traveler must be well informed prior to the journey, and the physician must have a high index of suspicion and take prompt action, including possibly the administration of a presumptive treatment

Key words: children; clinical features; complication; falciparum; laboratory; malaria; mortality; nonimmune; predictor; severe; travel.

INTRODUCTION

The level of immunity of the host will condition the clinical features of malaria. Travelers have no immunity against the parasite or the disease. Also, migrants from malaria-endemic areas who then live in a temperate country lose their immunity to parasites and hence the protection they have acquired against the disease. Both populations are therefore prone to severe disease and death if no rapid action is taken to reduce parasite growth and multiplication. The clinical manifestations of malaria are nonspecific and resemble those of influenza or any other viral infection. This similarity often leads to misdiagnosis or delay in diagnosis in countries where physicians are not used to the clinical presentation of malaria or simply do not think of it. Unfortunately, delay in diagnosis often leads to an adverse outcome. The parasites may reach most of the vital organs before appropriate treatment is started. Multiorgan failure is one of the characteristics of malaria in nonimmune travelers and contributes to malaria's relatively high fatality rate. A high index of suspicion by physicians, along with prompt action and possibly presumptive treatment, can save lives.

This chapter will review some aspects of the history, symptoms, signs, and laboratory parameters of malaria in travelers and migrants, so that physicians or medical personnel can identify, early enough for treatment, patients suspected of having malaria. As a rule, any traveler or migrant with fever or malaise who is returning from an endemic area should be considered as potentially having contracted malaria unless proven otherwise.

Although useful as background information, most of the literature on diseases in returning travelers is flawed by the lack of reliable epidemiologic indicators such as denominators (total number of travelers), case definition of severe malaria, patients serving as comparators, etc. Also, almost all published studies are retrospective, dealing with hospitalized patients or with patients who attended a university center specializing in tropical medicine. Thus, published descriptions are certainly biased toward increased severity. It is likely that a study that would include the whole cohort of travelers coming back with fever would give a different epidemiologic and clinical picture than do those in the literature.

EPIDEMIOLOGIC CONSIDERATIONS

The epidemiology of malaria in nonimmune travelers is covered in another chapter of the present book. The following considerations on demographic and travel characteristics are discussed here because they are relevant to establishing the level of probability for a diagnosis of malaria in a returning traveler or migrant with fever.

Demographics

Most studies on imported malaria report a predominance of males over females.[1-6]Since there is no reliable denominator on the sex of travelers from world tourism statistics, it is not known whether the imbalance is a genuine difference in susceptibility to malaria or the reflection of a higher number of men traveling to endemic areas. Some authors have argued that men are less likely to adhere to preventive measures and are therefore at increased risk of disease. In a case-control study of fever in returning travelers (case: documented malaria; control: no documented malaria), we did not find major differences between men and women in terms of the use of protective measures and compliance to chemoprophylaxis, but we still retrieved this increased susceptibility of males to malaria when all other potential confounding factors were taken into account.[6]

An increasing proportion of malaria cases is observed in immigrants revisiting their country of origin. Although highly relevant for suspecting malaria, the traveler, being from an endemic country for malaria, is not in itself a risk factor for the disease, when compared to the case of the average traveler returning from the tropics. The major determinant for a diagnosis of malaria is the migrant's use or nonuse of preventive measures when visiting friends or relatives abroad.

Travel Destinations

Depending on where the given paper originates, the published literature mentions the Solomon Islands, Papua New Guinea, sub-Saharan Africa, and India as the main destinations where travelers get malaria. Australia reports a high proportion of imported malaria from the islands of the Pacific;[2] France, Switzerland, Germany, and Italy, from sub-Saharan Africa;[7-10] and the United Kingdom and Singapore, from India.[11,12] Travel destination determines the degree of risk of catching the disease and also the species of *Plasmodium* most likely to be acquired: *Plasmodium falciparum* in sub-Saharan Africa and *Plasmodium vivax* in the Far East.[13] A traveler returning from one of those areas and complaining of fever is always highly suspect of having malaria.

Protective Measures and Chemoprophylaxis

The efficacy of repellents or bednets in reducing the risk of acquiring malaria has not been thoroughly assessed in travelers. Only one study has shown that the use of bednets protected against the disease.[14] On the contrary, several authors reported a protective effect of chemoprophylaxis.[6,15,16] Retrospective studies on imported malaria invariably show that infected individuals never use, or do not comply with, drug regimens.[9,10,17,18] Non-existent or inadequate chemoprophylaxis therefore represents one of the major predictors of malaria in a returning traveler with fever.[6]

Time Frame

Precise data on the duration of the pre-patent period (time from sporozoite inoc-ulation to the first positive blood film) and the incubation period (time from sporozoite inoculation to the first symptom) derive from the detailed studies of malaria therapy for syphilis and from the many artificial infection experiments in nonimmune volunteers.[19] The shortest incubation period ever documented was reported in a sailor who docked briefly in West Africa and developed malaria 3 days later.[20] The story still remains to be proven, and it is likely that a minimum of 6 days is required after inoculation for the parasite to appear in the blood and pro-voke symptoms. Studies on imported malaria show that most of the infections due to *Plasmodium falciparum* become apparent in the month following the traveler's return. The median time from return to the first symptoms (which does not cor-respond to the definition of the incubation period) is approximately 10 days for *P. falciparum* and 50 days for *Plasmodium vivax*.[13] It is likely to be even more for *Plasmodium ovale* and *Plasmodium malariae* [7] because these parasites are better adapted to humans.

The duration of the incubation period is strongly influenced by chemoprophy-laxis and by the level of immunity (i.e., previous exposure). Both reduce effective multiplication, which prolongs the pre-patent and incubation periods. Interesting-ly, in populations living in endemic areas, the pre-patent period is usually shorter than the incubation period because of some degree of tolerance to the parasite whereas in nonimmune individuals such as travelers, the incubation period is short-er since the parasite density threshold at which the symptoms occur is lower. This means that in a nonimmune traveler, the first microscopic examination may be neg-ative and that only the second or third blood slide will be positive for *Plasmodium* parasites. This peculiarity is important to take into account when deciding the appropriateness of giving presumptive treatment. The type of chemoprophylaxis also affects both the pre-patent and incubation periods. Day and Behrens[21] showed that chemoprophylaxis with mefloquine, which is a drug with a long half-life (14 to 28 days), led to a delay in the onset of symptoms. The question remains as to why some long-term residents never experience a malaria episode when living in endem-ic areas but suffer from an attack as soon as they come back to temperate countries. This may be linked to the interruption of an efficacious chemosuppression, but often this population does not use it. An alternative explanation may be that the stress or the cold triggers the multiplication of the circulating parasites or the release of the hypnozoite from the liver through hormonal changes.

A long period between the individual's return from an endemic area and the onset of fever should not exclude a diagnosis of malaria. Two of the longest incu-bation periods documented are 4 years for *Plasmodium falciparum*[22] and 30 years for *Plasmodium vivax*. Without chemoprophylaxis, a primary attack of *P. vivax* is usually symptomatic, and a relapse is therefore easy to diagnose. On the contrary, if an effective drug suppresses a primary episode, only the relapse may become symptomatic, which may confound the establishment of a correct diagnosis. The time interval between a primary attack and a relapse depends on the parasite strain involved, clones originating from cooler regions being characterized by a longer cycle than those from tropical areas. The rhythm of parasite relapses is probably programmed genetically; however, environmental factors may also trigger the reappearance of the parasites, as mentioned earlier. A report from a couple who suffered repeated simultaneous attacks of *Plasmodium falciparum* and *Plasmodium vivax*, the last attacks being during winter holidays in the snow, illustrates well the contribution of genetics and environment.[23]

CLINICAL FEATURES OF UNCOMPLICATED MALARIA

Symptoms

The clinical features of uncomplicated malaria are common to all four species of *Plasmodium* although there is a suggestion that *Plasmodium vivax*, which tends to synchronize rapidly, may cause more severe symptoms early in the course of infection.[19] The onset of *Plasmodium falciparum* may be gradual (as are the onsets of *Plasmodium ovale* and *Plasmodium malariae*) or fulminant. At the beginning, the symptoms are nonspecific and resemble those of influenza, which is one of the main reasons for delay in diagnosis in temperate countries, especially during the winter. Malaise, headache, and muscular aches usually precede fever by up to 2 days. The patient then experiences mild chills and raised temperature sometimes accompanied by abdominal discomfort, especially in children. At first, recovery between fever attacks is almost complete, and the patient can continue his or her daily activities. After some days of erratic fever peaks, the classic pattern of rhythmic fever appears, with a 2-day cycle for *Plasmodium vivax* and *Plasmodium ovale* (tertian fever) and a 3-day pattern for *Plasmodium malariae* (quartan fever). However, some studies suggest that this typical feature is rather rare in nonimmune people.[7] *Plasmodium falciparum* episodes are characterized by a rather unpredictable pattern of fever. In a paroxysm, the patient will experience rapidly rising temperature (up to 39° to 41°C) associated with shaking limbs and a strong headache. The classic teeth-chattering rigors and profuse sweating are relatively rare nowadays since symptomatic episodes are treated rather early. Rigor lasts about a half hour; then, profuse sweating breaks out. Vasodilatation often occurs, resulting in low blood pressure. A period of intense fatigue follows. There is not much documentation on the natural course of falciparum malaria in nonimmune patients, but it is likely that in the absence of treatment, the parasites continue to multiply, resulting in severe disease and death. This may not be so when other species are involved although severe malaria associated with *Plasmodium vivax* has been reported on numerous occasions.[4,24,25]

When travelers are under chemosuppression, the typical clinical picture can turn into a mild and prolonged course of atypical symptoms, with low-grade fever and, for example, vague abdominal complaints or a slight cough.

The prevalence rates of imported malaria cases presenting with a particular symptom are listed in Table 11–1. Frequencies are estimated by using pooled data from all studies that mentioned a list of symptoms and their respective occurrences. Fever is obviously the cardinal symptom, but it should be stressed that in most studies, there were 2% to 4% of patients who did not complain of any fever. Chills, headache, sweating, and myalgia are the other common symptoms. Gastrointestinal complaints are rather rare except in children.

Signs

The clinical examination is rather unspecific or even completely unremarkable and thus does not contribute much to the diagnosis of uncomplicated malaria. Raised temperature (> 38°C) is common but is also encountered in patients suffering from other infectious diseases. An enlarged spleen is the only sign that strongly suggests a diagnosis of malaria. Depending on the correspondence between the time of the consultation and the time of the last fever peak, the general condition of the patient may be either poor (with pallor, hypotension, and raised respiratory rate) or surprisingly good, with no obvious abnormality.

The prevalence rates of uncomplicated malaria cases presenting with a particular sign are presented in Table 11–2, using data from the same studies used for Table 11–1. Raised temperature was the most common sign, followed by splenomegaly.[6]

Table 11–1. **Prevalence Rates of Symptoms in Imported Malaria Cases**

Symptom	Total Patients Assessed	% of Patients Affected (95% CI)*
Fever	1,032	97 (96–98)
Chills	1,243	79 (76–81)
Headache	1,234	70 (67–73)
Sweating	801	64 (60–67)
Myalgia	826	36 (32–39)
Nausea	777	27 (24–30)
Vomiting	678	27 (23–30)
Diarrhea	1,234	16 (14–18)
Cough	681	13 (10–16)
Abdominal pain	1,120	12 (10–14)
Blood in stool	441	3 (1–5)

CI = confidence interval.
*57% of the patients were semi-immune.
Data from Svenson et al.,[4] Hansmann et al.,[7] Jelinek et al.,[9] Oh et al.,[12] Wiselka et al.,[17] Jensenius et al.,[31] and D'Acremont and Genton (unpublished data).

Table 11–2. **Prevalence Rates of Signs in Imported Malaria Cases**

Sign	Total Patients Assessed	% of Patients Affected (95% CI)*	
Temperature > 38°C	926	81	(78–83)
Splenomegaly	1,061	26	(23–29)
Hepatomegaly	1,056	14	(12–17)
Pallor	487	12	(10–16)
Icterus	1,049	8	(6–9)
Dehydration	323	6	(3–9)

CI = confidence interval.
*64% of the patients were semi-immune.
Data from Svenson et al.,[4] Hansmann et al.,[7] Oh et al.,[12] Wiselka et al.,[17] Jensenius et al.,[31] and D'Acremont and Genton (unpublished data).

Predictive Values of Clinical Features

Since the symptoms and signs of uncomplicated malaria are unspecific and since most of them are also encountered in diseases such as dengue fever, hepatitis, typhoid fever, and influenza, it is important to estimate their respective rates of occurrence both in malaria and in other diseases that can cause fever in returning travelers. We conducted a prospective study of all returning travelers or migrants presenting to our outpatient clinic with a complaint of malaise or fever. We compared the prevalence rates of symptoms and signs in malaria cases and in fevers due to other causes. Results are presented in Table 11–3. We used a case-control approach to identify significant predictors of *Plasmodium* parasitemia in terms of symptoms and signs; sweating, abdominal pain, temperature ≥ 38°C, poor general health, and enlarged spleen remained significantly associated with malaria in the final multivariate logistic regression model. We then estimated the test performance of each parameter in diagnosing malaria (Table 11–4). The presence of an enlarged spleen had the best likelihood rate for a positive test.

LABORATORY FINDINGS

When malaria is suspected on clinical grounds, simple laboratory investigations should be performed so that (1) the probability of making a correct diagnosis is increased and (2) the level of severity of the disease can be fully assessed and appropriate management initiated.

Hematology and Biochemistry

Thrombocytopenia (< 150 × 10³ platelets/μL) is the most frequent abnormality observed on the hemogram and is present in about 60% of the cases (Table 11–5). Normochromic normocytic anemia (generally defined as < 12 g/dL) is less com-

Table 11–3. **Prevalence Rate of Symptoms and Signs in Nonmalaria Cases and Imported Malaria Cases**

Symptom or Sign	Imported Malaria (% of Patients Affected)* N = 116	Non-malaria (% of Patients Affected)* N = 468
Fever	97	82
Headache	81	61
Chills	78	51
Myalgia	71	48
Sweating	65	44
Nausea	37	31
Diarrhea	22	36
Vomiting	21	15
Abdominal pain	18	31
Blood in stool	3	4
Temperature > 38°C	59	25
Pallor	26	11
Splenomegaly	19	2
Dehydration	16	6
Jaundice	9	3
Hepatomegaly	4	3

*42% of the patients were semi-immune.
Data from D'Acremont V and Genton B (unpublished).

mon and depends on the duration of infection; it occurs in about 30% of cases. The white cell count is usually within the normal range. Hyperleukocytosis is predominately observed in severe malaria and should always alert the clinician for a possible associated bacterial infection. Absence of eosinophilia is typical of malaria; eosinophilia very rarely exceeds 5% during the acute phase.[6]

Total and conjugated bilirubin concentration is elevated in about 40% of cases of mild malaria, as are hepatic liver enzymes (serum glutamic-oxaloacetic transaminase

Table 11–4. **Test Performance of Health Conditions Associated with Malaria**

Condition	Sensitivity (%)	Specificity (%)	PPV (%)	NPV (%)	Efficiency (%)
Enlarged spleen	23	98	85	76	76
Poor general health	30	92	59	76	74
Temperature ≥ 38°C	57	75	48	81	70
Sweating	68	54	37	81	58
No abdominal pain	81	32	33	81	46

NPV = negative predictive value; PPV = positive predictive value.

Table 11–5. **Prevalence Rates of Laboratory Findings in Imported Malaria Cases**

Laboratory Findings	Total Patients Assessed	% of Patients Affected (95% CI)*
Thrombocytopenia	1,111	61 (58–63)
Hyperbilirubinemia	750	43 (39–46)
Anemia	1,263	30 (27–32)
Transaminases↑	847	30 (27–33)
Leukopenia	1,262	26 (24–29)
Creatinine↑ (>110)	444	18 (15–22)
Hypoglycemia	573	1 (1–3)

*64% of the patients were semi-immune.
Data from Svenson et al.,[4] Hansmann et al.,[7] Oh et al.,[12] Wiselka et al.,[17] Jensenius et al.,[31] and D'Acremont and Genton (unpublished data).

[SGOT] and serum glutamate pyruvate transaminase [SGPT]) (see Table 11–5). It must be stressed that these parameters are measured only in a small proportion of cases, which obviously leads to biased estimates. Creatininemia may be slightly raised. Glycemia is usually within the normal range, at least in adults. There may be mild hyponatremia, especially in children.[26] C-reactive protein (CRP) is almost invariably elevated in the acute phase. One study that measured the lipid concentrations showed that 62% of the patients with imported malaria had hypertriglyceridemia and that 81% had hypocholesterolemia.[7] These abnormalities have not been assessed in other studies of imported malaria or of fever due to other causes and therefore need to be validated before being used as diagnostic tools for malaria.

Again, the values mentioned above are only indicative. Prevalence rates of abnormal values may be much higher in studies that included only hospitalized cases. The more severe the malaria is, the more extreme the values are. One study divided the severe cases from the mild ones, and the differences were quite obvious, with, for example, a mean platelet count of $71 \times 10^3/\mu L$ in the severe cases versus $127 \times 10^3/\mu L$ in the uncomplicated ones, a raised total bilirubin in 87% of severe cases versus 48% of mild cases, and raised liver enzymes in 60% of severe cases versus 36% of mild cases.[7]

Predictive Values of Laboratory Parameters

Doherty and colleagues[27] showed that thrombocytopenia associated with a raised total bilirubin had a positive predictive value of 95% for diagnosing malaria. This was the first attempt to estimate the performance of laboratory tests in guiding the clinician in the differential diagnosis of a fever in a returning traveler. Such calculations are necessary since it is of little value to know that 97% of patients with imported malaria have an elevated CRP without knowing what the percentage is in patients with other diagnoses such as dengue fever or hepatitis. In our study (described above),[6] we investigated the sensitivity, specificity, and predictive values of standard laboratory tests. The results for the variables (which were retained in the final logistic regression mode because they were associated with parasitemia) are shown in Table 11–6. Thrombocytopenia had by far the best test efficiency, with a positive predictive value of 82% and a negative predictive value of 85%. Quick screening of patients with simple and rapid laboratory tests is important; all patients should have a full blood cell count and perhaps a measurement of bilirubin concentration. The results should always be regarded with caution and put in a clinical context; indeed, a study on imported dengue fever showed that almost half of the patients also had thrombocytopenia.[28]

SEVERE MALARIA

Epidemiology

Nonimmune travelers and migrants living in non-endemic areas are at increased risk of severe malaria since they do not have immunity against the multiplying parasites. Most of the burden is related to falciparum malaria, but there are numerous reports of complications[5,24] and even deaths due to *Plasmodium vivax* infections.[4]

The true rates of severe malaria and death in nonimmune or almost nonimmune populations are not known. Even if the old standardized World Health Organization (WHO) definition of severe malaria was used in most of the studies,[29] there are still several other parameters that may influence the rates, namely, the ratio of nonimmune cases to migrant cases, the ratio of *Plasmodium falciparum* to other species, and the ratio of patients using adequate chemoprophylaxis to patients using inappropriate prophylaxis or no prophylaxis. Also, the nature of the institutions where the studies were conducted can lead to biased estimates of mortality rates or severity; for example, specialized centers do not cover the whole spectrum of the clinical disease, in the sense that they tend to see patients with more severe disease. When all studies that reported the rate of severe malaria (as defined by the old WHO definition) were considered,[29] the prevalence ranged between 1% and 38%, with a mean of 5.5%, and the case-fatality rate was between 0% and 8%, with a mean of 1.0% (Table 11–7). The lowest estimates derived from studies that

Table 11–6. **Test Performance of Laboratory Parameters Associated with Malaria**

Parameter	Sensitivity (%)	Specificity (%)	PPV (%)	NPV (%)	Efficiency (%)
Platelets < 150×10^3/μL	60	95	82	85	85
Hemoglobin < 12 g/dL	16	97	65	74	73
Leukocytes < 10×10^3/μL	97	27	35	96	47
Eosinophils < 5%	95	12	31	85	36

NPV = negative predictive value; PPV = positive predictive value.

Table 11–7. Number of Cases and Overall Prevalence Rates (in pooled data) of Severe Manifestations of *Plasmodium falciparum* Malaria in Nonimmune Travelers or Migrants

	Matteelli 1999	Gauzere 1997	Wetsteyn 1995	Calleri 1998	Svenson 1995	Jensenius 1999	D'Acremont 2001	Kain 1998	Wiselka 1990	Khoo 1998	Nuesch 2000	Pooled Data N/Total (%)
Total number of patients	551	486	361	194	182	222	79	44	37	37	150	2,343
WHO criteria (1990 definition)												
Cerebral malaria (coma)	13	0	10	11	4	1	0	0	2	0	4	45/2,343 (1.9)
Acute renal failure (creatinine > 265 μmol/L)	8	4	6	3	2	4	0	0	2	9	6	44/2,343 (1.9)
Severe anemia (Hb < 50 g/L)	5	0	15	0	0	4	0	0	3	0	3	30/2,343 (1.3)
ARDS or pulmonary edema	7	3	3	4	3	1	0	1	0	3	1	26/2,343 (1.1)
Hypotension (syst < 70 mm Hg) or shock	0	1	0	0	4	0	0	0	0	0	3	8/2,343 (0.3)
Repeated convulsions	0	0	3	0	0	0	0	0	0	2	0	5/2,343 (0.2)
Bleeding or DIC	0	0	1	4	0	0	0	0	0	0	1	6/2,343 (0.3)
Hypoglycemia (< 2.2 mmol/L)	1	0	0	0	0	0	0	0	1	0	0	2/2,343 (0.1)
Acidemia (pH < 7.25)	1	0	0	0	0	0	0	0	0	0	0	1/2,343 (0.04)
Hemoglobinuria	0	0	1	0	0	1	0	0	0	0	1	3/2,343 (0.1)
Total number of patients with 1 or more 1990 WHO criteria (%)*	26 (4.7)	5 (1.0)	—	17 (8.8)	9 (4.9)	8 (3.6)	0	1 (2.3)	13 (35.1)	14 (37.9)	16 (10.7)	109/1982 (5.5)†

Continued on next page.

Table 11–7. Number of Cases and Overall Prevalence Rates (in pooled data) of Severe Manifestations of *Plasmodium falciparum* Malaria in Nonimmune Travelers or Migrants, continued

	Matteelli 1999	Gauzere 1997	Wetsteyn 1995	Calleri 1998	Svenson 1995	Jensenius 1999	D'Acremont 2001	Kain 1998	Wiselka 1990	Khoo 1998	Nuesch 2000	Pooled Data N/Total (%)
Total number of patients	551	486	361	194	182	222	79	44	37	37	150	2,343
Added WHO criteria (2000 definition)												
Impairment of consciousness	—	4	—	—	—	—	2	0	—	3	4	13/796 (1.6)
Prostration or weakness	—	0	—	—	—	—	0	0	—	0	0	0
Hyperparasitemia (> 5%)	—	4	31	—	2	18	0	2	—	9	15	66/1,561 (4.2)
Jaundice (> 50)	—	2	14	—	—	—	1	0	—	15	1	33/1,157 (2.9)
Total number of patients with 1 or more 2000 WHO criteria (%)‡	—	5 (1.0)	52 (14.4)	—	11 (6.0)	20 (9.0)	3 (3.8)	3 (6.8)	—	20 (54.1)	20 (13.3)	134/1,561 (8.6)§
Deaths (%)	8(1.5)	3(0.6)	1(0.3)	3(1.5)	0	0	0	0	1(2.7)	3(8.1)	4(2.7)	23/2,343(1.0)‖

ARDS = adult respiratory distress syndrome; DIC = disseminated intravascular coagulation; Hb = hemoglobin; syst = systolic pressure; WHO = World Health Organization.
*Data from Warrell DA, Molyreux ME, Beales PF. Severe and complicated malaria. Trans R Soc Trop Med Hyg 1990;84:1–65.
† 95% confidence interval (CI) 4.6–6.6.
‡ Data from World Health Organization. Severe falciparum malaria. Trans R Soc Trop Med Hyg 2000;94 Suppl 1: S1–31.
§ 95% CI 7.3–10.1.
‖95% CI 0.6–1.5.

include nonimmune travelers and migrants attending outpatient clinics and having any species of malaria;[4,6] the highest estimates came from studies that considered only nonimmune travelers hospitalized in specialized centers.[24]

Risk factors for severe malaria and death included older age,[24,30–32] female sex[4,30] (especially when related to pregnancy),[7,33] totally "naive" nonimmune individuals (nonimmigrants),[32,34] comorbidity (alcohol consumption, human immunodeficiency virus [HIV] infection),[35] no chemoprophylaxis,[31,33,36] delay in initiating treatment,[30,31] and coma on admission.[8]

The frequency of the clinical features defining severe malaria in travelers or migrants are shown in Table 11–7. Cerebral malaria is the most common presenting criterion, followed by acute renal failure, severe anemia, and pulmonary edema. The clinical picture resembles that found in children living in areas with a moderate level of transmission[37] and where cerebral involvement outreaches anemia, suggesting that malaria in naive nonimmune subjects with mature immune systems results in this presentation. Multiorgan failure often occurs in nonimmune patients because they have no tolerance to the parasites. The parasites multiply rapidly in the absence of immunity and alter the function of vital organs such as the brain, the kidneys, and the liver.

As mentioned above, severe malaria can be strictly defined with rather stringent criteria to assist clinical and epidemiologic descriptions.[29] In clinical practice, the patient must be assessed for any symptom or sign that would suggest that he or she is at an increased risk of developing complications and must be immediately treated accordingly, irrespective of laboratory results that will be obtained later. Since the purpose of attempting to describe and define severe malaria is to alert physicians to the symptoms and signs that are associated with progression to life-threatening disease, WHO experts recently proposed a broader definition of severe malaria, one that includes clinical manifestations or laboratory findings that are associated with a bad prognostic value in children or adults in endemic areas (Table 11–8).[38]

Clinical Features

Cerebral Malaria

In most published studies of imported malaria, a diagnosis of cerebral malaria was made when the patient had any sign of impaired consciousness. It is clear that some patients were wrongly classified since it is known, for example, that high fever alone can produce mild impairment of consciousness without direct involvement of the central nervous system, but this conservative definition fits with the idea of identifying those needing immediate serious care. The strict definition, at least in adults, requires the presence of unrousable coma (after the exclusion of other encephalopathies) and the finding of asexual forms of *Plasmodium* in the peripheral blood film.[38]

Table 11–8. **Severe Manifestations of *Plasmodium falciparum* Malaria and Prognostic Values in Nonimmune Travelers or Migrants**

Clinical Manifestation	Prognostic Value*	Laboratory Finding	Prognostic Value*
Prostration	+	Severe anemia	+
Impaired consciousness	+++	Hypoglycemia	+
Respiratory distress	+++	Acidosis	+++
Multiple convulsions	++	Hyperlactemia	+++
Circulatory collapse	+++	Hyperparasitemia	+++
Pulmonary edema	+++	Renal impairment	++
Abnormal bleeding	++		
Jaundice	+		
Hemoglobinuria	+		

*Empiric assessment of prognostic value (inferred from observations in young children in endemic regions who lack immunity to malaria).
Adapted from World Health Organization. Severe falciparum malaria. Trans R Soc Trop Med Hyg 2000;94 Suppl 1:1–31.

The onset of coma in cerebral malaria may be sudden, often preceded by a generalized seizure (especially in children), or gradual, with initial drowsiness, confusion, disorientation, delirium, or agitation, followed by unconsciousness.[19] The prodromal history can be as short as 6 to 12 hours in nonimmune patients and almost invariably includes strong headache, which can be the only symptom (personal observation). On examination, there should be no sign of meningeal irritation, nor should there be any petechiae. Signs of bleeding are infrequent. The patient is usually warm and well perfused peripherally. Sustained hyperventilation indicates a poor prognosis since it reflects metabolic acidosis if the chest is clear and associated lung infection or edema if it is not. Jaundice is frequent. The neurologic features are those of a diffuse symmetric encephalopathy. Focal signs are unusual. The depth of coma is assessed by the response to standard painful or vocal stimuli. The gaze is usually normal or divergent, but there is no evidence of extraocular paresis. Corneal and pupillary reflexes are usually retained. Papilledema is rare, but retinal hemorrhages are common (up to 20% of cases). There may be forced jaw closure with bruxism (grinding of teeth). Cranial nerve impairment is unusual. Tone and reflexes may be normal, increased, or decreased. Abdominal reflexes are invariably absent, and the plantar responses are extensor in about half of the patients. Children, in particular, can sometimes present with extensor posturing of the decorticate (arm flexed, legs extended) or (more usually) decerebrate (arms and legs extended) types.[19] Spontaneous movement implies a lighter coma and therefore a better prognosis than no movement at all. Generalized or sometimes focal seizures may occur.

The duration of coma varies from 2 hours to several days but is usually shorter in children than in adults. Although well studied in patients living in endemic areas, the case-fatality rates and the incidence of sequelae in cerebral malaria cases are not known in nonimmune persons, due to the small number of patients. Also, patients usually do not present with pure cerebral malaria but with a combined syndrome involving several vital organs such as the lungs, kidneys, and liver. Aspiration pneumonia or associated septicemia often occur and worsen the prognosis.

The differential diagnoses of returning travelers or migrants with impaired consciousness include hyperpyrexia due to other causes, bacterial meningitis, viral encephalitis prevalent at the journey destination, and any other cause of cerebral dysfunction.

Respiratory Distress

Respiratory distress has been recognized recently as one of the major features of severe malaria in African children.[39] This complication is often missed, at least at the beginning of symptoms. In nonimmune travelers, physicians should be aware that a cough associated with a positive blood slide is an "alert" sign that requires thorough investigation and prompt treatment. In tachypnea related to high fever, breathing is shallow compared with the labored hyperventilation associated with metabolic acidosis, pulmonary edema, or pneumonia.[19] Acute respiratory distress syndrome can develop at any time during the course of falciparum malaria. It is mostly found in patients who have cerebral malaria initially or in elderly patients and is often complicated with bacteremia. Physicians must be aware that respiratory distress, like other features of severe malaria, frequently occurs when parasitemia has resolved.[40] Such patients should thus be closely monitored. Chest radiography can show the classic picture of pneumonia or pulmonary edema; the accompanying signs (fever or high venous central pressure, respectively) will then guide the diagnosis and the treatment. The types of abnormalities seen on the chest radiographs are diverse, ranging from confluent nodules to bilateral bibasilar infiltrates; they can be observed even in the absence of any sign of infection or fluid overload. Since they bear a bad prognostic value, they all require appropriate treatment.

Acute Renal Failure

The fulminant form of renal failure is usually observed on admission, with severe acute oliguria and (usually) with other manifestations of severe malaria. In this situation, there is a high incidence of associated impairment of hepatic function and metabolic acidosis, pulmonary edema being the terminal event. More often, renal dysfunction becomes evident when the patient recovers from the acute phase of severe malaria and bears a much better prognosis. The patient may be oliguric or sometimes polyuric. The serum creatinine rises over some days, and hyperkalemia or uremic complications may require dialysis. Similarly to other complications of severe malaria, acute renal failure may develop once the parasitemia has been cleared.

The bad reputation of blackwater fever comes from the high mortality documented in Europeans and Asians working in Africa in the first decades of the century.[19] Today, the observed dark urine, resulting from massive hemolysis, is usually transient and resolves without complications. In severe cases, renal failure may develop, behaving as acute tubular necrosis.

Hypotension and Shock

Patients with severe malaria often have hyperpyrexia, with high cardiac output, low peripheral vascular resistance, and consequent low blood pressure. Severe hypotension (< 80 mm Hg) with features of circulatory failure can develop suddenly, usually with pulmonary edema, metabolic acidosis, and gram-negative septicemia or after massive gastrointestinal hemorrhage or splenic rupture. In recent large studies of severe malaria in malaria-endemic areas, the frequency of shock was 8% in Vietnamese adults[41] and 0.4% in African children.[39] A study of imported malaria in European adults showed that 14 of 50 (28%) patients with severe disease had evidence of shock.[42] This high rate was likely partially due to selection bias (referrals, etc.) but may well have reflected a genuine higher incidence in naive subjects. Seven of these patients underwent pulmonary artery catheterization, which found peripheral vasodilatation in all, associated with an elevated cardiac output in five. Seven among these 14 patients had proven bacteremia and five of these died. On the basis of these results, the authors recommended standard treatment for septic shock, with investigation of hemodynamics in the most severe cases.[42] Circulatory collapse was found also to be the main feature of severe imported vivax malaria.[24]

Anemia

Unlike the anemia reported by studies of severe malaria in children in highly endemic areas (where anemia is the number one cause of death) anemia is not a major contributor to fatality in nonimmune travelers, probably because signs of severe disease in this group appear at a lower parasite density. Also, the episode is usually unique in travelers whereas in African children, anemia builds up from repeated and chronic *Plasmodium* infections. Also, in developed countries, blood transfusions are always available in hospitals; this is not the case in sub-Saharan Africa. Severe anemia is still found to be the most frequent complication in some studies of imported malaria;[5,10,33] since it may cause circulatory collapse, it needs to be closely monitored.

Jaundice

Mild jaundice may result from hemolysis alone whereas a very high bilirubin concentration indicates hepatic dysfunction. Mild hyperbilirubinemia was found to be an excellent predictor of malaria in one study on fever in returning travelers.[27] Tender enlargement of the liver and spleen is frequent in all human malaria forms, particularly in nonimmune individuals. Jaundice was the most common defining criterion for severe malaria in two studies on imported malaria.[24,33] This complication is often accompanied by acute renal failure or other signs of severe malaria.[38]

Bleeding

Although thrombocytopenia is a common feature of falciparum and vivax malaria, evident bleeding is rather uncommon in cases of imported malaria. The lack of obvious hemorrhage is related to the fact that thrombocytopenia, even when profound, is usually not associated with abnormalities of other parameters of coagulation. However, disseminated intravascular coagulation, a different phenomenon, does occur and is usually associated with other complications. Gastrointestinal hemorrhage is the most frequent source of bleeding.

Complicating and Associated Infections

Studies on severe malaria in African children have shown that bacteremia is a frequent occurrence, with an incidence that reaches 30% in children aged less than 30 months.[43] It is likely that septicemia is one of the common complications of severe malaria in nonimmune travelers, but its true incidence cannot be estimated since broad-spectrum antibiotics are often given prophylactically, which is certainly a life-saving measure in many instances. Septicemia can result from aspiration pneumonia in patients who have had generalized seizures, from other respiratory infection following emergency intubation, and from urinary tract infection associated with indwelling urethral catheters. Gram-negative septicemia usually originates from the intestines. An associated infection must always be considered when the clinical condition worsens, especially when hypotension develops, and the infection must be treated if its source has not been clearly identified.

Hypoglycemia

Hypoglycemia is a well-recognized complication of malaria and its treatment with quinine in African children and pregnant women. It is very rare in nonimmune travelers (constituting 0.1% of all malaria cases and 2.0% of the severe cases). However, close monitoring of early symptoms and signs, as well as glycemia, should be performed in all malaria cases, particularly those treated with quinine.

Hyperpyrexia and Hyperparasitemia

The patient's temperature and parasite count should be considered together since they are interdependent. A patient presenting on admission without a raised temperature but with a parasite density of 2% may well have 10-fold more circulating parasites when sampled during a febrile peak. Whereas there is no association between the degree of fever and the likelihood of developing severe malaria, a parasite count of more than 4% in the peripheral blood is definitely a bad prognostic factor in nonimmune or almost nonimmune patients.[44] The prognostic value of parasite density can be improved considerably by assessing the stage of parasite development in the peripheral blood film; at any given parasite density, the prognosis worsens if there is a predominance of more mature stages (i.e., late trophozoites or schizonts [containing visible pigments]).[38]

IMPORTED MALARIA IN SPECIFIC GROUPS

Pregnant Women

Traveling in endemic areas during pregnancy is not advisable because of the increased susceptibility of the mother to malaria and severe disease and because of the possible deleterious effect of the parasites on the outcome of pregnancy. However, some women have no choice, either because they live in endemic areas (nonimmune expatriates) or because they have recently migrated in temperate countries. Other women consider traveling necessary for their well-being, which is also respectable. The scant documentation of imported malaria in pregnant women tends to confirm both the high risk of developing severe disease during this condition and the detrimental effect of the infection on the fetus. Six of 10 pregnant women in one study[33] and 2 of 5 in another suffered from complicated malaria. In the latter study, 3 of the 5 women lost their babies.[7] Although sparse, these data reinforce the importance of pretravel advice for this group of travelers; chemoprophylaxis with an effective drug is of major importance if potential exposure to infection is unavoidable.

Children

Although malaria in children has been extensively studied in endemic areas, little is known about the clinical presentation and outcome of pediatric malaria in temperate countries. The two main reasons for this lack of reports are the low number of cases and the fact that the clinical picture is likely to be quite similar to the adult one because of the absence of preexisting immunity in all age groups. The low incidence of disease may be related to better compliance with chemoprophylaxis regimens in children than in adults, at least in short-term travelers.

Few studies have been published on imported pediatric malaria.[18,26,45–48] Children often present after school holidays. A recent history of a malaria episode in another member of the family has been reported in up to 25% of the cases.[48] The clinical presentation is usually nonspecific, which often leads to misdiagnosis and delay in initiating adequate treatment.[26,48] Fever is the commonest symptom, as in adults. On the other hand, gastrointestinal symptoms are much more frequent in children than in adults, with up to 75% of affected children complaining of abdominal pain, diarrhea, or vomiting.[45] These symptoms can be quite misleading, especially in temperate countries where physicians do not often think of malaria. In a French study, two patients even underwent surgery due to a wrong diagnosis of appendicitis for one and intussusception for the other.[45] Splenomegaly can be detected in more than two-thirds of the children,[18,48] as can hepatomegaly.[26] Anemia is the most common abnormal finding on the hemogram, with up to 100% of patients having a hemoglobin level of < 10 g/dL,[46] followed by thrombocytopenia, found in up to 70% of patients.[48]

Most of the clinical episodes are mild, perhaps because parents consult a health care worker quickly with their febrile child. Precise prevalence rates of the diverse complications are difficult to estimate, due to the low number of severe pediatric malaria cases. As in endemic areas, severe anemia predominates. Complications such as true cerebral malaria, renal failure, and pulmonary edema are rare.

One study[18] described three children with congenital malaria diagnosed at an age ranging from 19 to 60 days. Two children presented with fever and were admitted for possible sepsis, and a third one presented with pallor and sweats. All three had hepatosplenomegaly and positive slides for *Plasmodium vivax*. Very similar findings were reported in a study from Canada.[48] Blood smears for malaria parasites should be part of the evaluation of a febrile newborn whose mother emigrated from a malaria-endemic area during pregnancy.

Migrants

During the last decade, the number of imported malaria cases has increased considerably in some European countries.[49,50] This trend is likely to be associated with recent waves of immigration from countries where malaria is endemic. It is common sense to state that malaria episodes in migrants are milder than in nonmigrants because of a certain level of residual immunity. A lower incidence of severe disease and a lower case-fatality rate among migrants has been observed in several studies.[32,34] Matteelli and colleagues[34] reported an incidence of severe diseases of 1.3% (4 of 312 malaria cases) in migrants versus 9.2% (22 of 239 cases) in nonimmune travelers; 8 deaths were recorded, all in the latter category. This difference is unlikely to be due to the confounding effect of chemoprophylaxis since all studies report a much lower drug intake in migrants than in nonimmune travelers. The same study showed that fever clearance time after treatment was also shorter in migrants than in nonmigrants. Hansmann and colleagues[7] reported lower temperature and reduced prevalence rates of hepatomegaly and splenomegaly in migrants.

In studies looking at a broader spectrum of the disease (i.e., in hospitalized and ambulatory patients), the difference between migrants and nonmigrants was much less striking. Neither Svenson and colleagues[4] nor Jensenius and colleagues[31] could find differences in the clinical presentation. In our sample of imported malaria, which included primarily mild disease since the study was done in an outpatient clinic, only the prevalences of diarrhea and splenomegaly were significantly different between the two groups of patients. Symptoms, signs, or laboratory values defining severe malaria were equally balanced between migrants and nonmigrants, after adjustment for age, sex, travel destination, use of protective measures, and chemoprophylaxis.

Comparisons between studies must always be considered with caution due to differences in the definitions used (e.g., for migrant, severe malaria, etc.), the level of severity of the cases included, the main travel destinations, and the ratio of falciparum to nonfalciparum species. However, it is likely that migrants originating from endemic areas have a lower risk of dying than totally naive patients, even if a long period had elapsed since the migrants left their country of origin. Indeed, a certain degree of immunity remains even in the absence of natural exposure, probably for life.[51] One possible reason for the lower case-fatality rate in migrants is that they usually present earlier in the course of the disease since they know the symptoms of malaria. Also, physicians are alerted by the patient's origin and tend to forget less about the likelihood of malaria in the differential diagnosis. Since migrants know about this disease's presentation, physicians should systematically give presumptive treatment for malaria (after excluding any other obvious diagnoses) if a migrant states, "I have malaria."

CONCLUSION

Documentation of *Plasmodium* parasitemia is the "gold standard" for a diagnosis of malaria. In nonimmune travelers, symptoms appear early in the course of parasite multiplication. The results of the first microscopic examination may therefore be normal. Repeated microscopic examinations should be made every 12 to 24 hours, coupled (if possible) with a rapid antigen test to increase the sensitivity of the investigation. Also, doctors should be encouraged to look, themselves, for parasites on the blood film. When the clinical constellation strongly suggests malaria, it is justified to administer presumptive antimalarial treatment. There is no danger in giving an antimalarial drug to a nonmalaria patient whereas it can be fatal to wait for a clear documentation of parasitemia. Nevertheless, an alternative diagnosis should always be considered in this context; typhoid fever, which can be equally dangerous if left untreated, should be especially considered.

REFERENCES

1. Phillips-Howard PA, Bradley DJ, Blaze M, Hurn M. Malaria in Britain: 1977–86. BMJ 1988;296:245–248.
2. Boreham RE, Relf WA. Imported malaria in Australia. Med J Aust 1991;155:754–757.
3. Calleri G, Macor A, Leo G, Caramello P. Imported malaria in Italy: epidemiologic and clinical studies. J Travel Med 1994;1:231–234.
4. Svenson JE, MacLean JD, Gyorkos TW, Keystone J. Imported malaria. Clinical presentation and examination of symptomatic travelers. Arch Intern Med 1995;155:861–868.
5. Lopez-Velez R, Viana A, Perez-Casas C, et al. Clinicoepidemiological study of imported malaria in travelers and immigrants to Madrid. J Travel Med 1999;6:81–86.
6. D'Acremont V, Landry P, Mueller I, et al. Clinical and laboratory predictors of imported malaria—a case-control study. Ann Intern Med 2000 [submitted].
7. Hansmann Y, Staub-Schmidt T, Christmann D. [Malaria brought into Strasbourg: an epidemiological, clinical, biological and therapeutic study (published erratum appears in Trop Med Int Health 1997;2(11):1110)]. Trop Med Int Health 1997;2:941–952.

8. Nuesch R, Scheller M, Gyr N. Hospital admissions for malaria in Basel, Switzerland: an epidemiological review of 150 cases. J Travel Med 2000;7:95–97.

9. Jelinek T, Nothdurft HD, Loscher T. Malaria in nonimmune travelers: a synopsis of history, symptoms, and treatment in 160 patients. J Travel Med 1994;1:199–202.

10. Raglio A, Parea M, Lorenzi N, et al. Ten-year experience with imported malaria in Bergamo, Italy. J Travel Med 1994;1:152–155.

11. Phillips-Howard PA, Radalowicz A, Mitchell J, Bradley DJ. Risk of malaria in British residents returning from malarious areas. BMJ 1990;300:499–503.

12. Oh HM, Kong PM, Snodgrass I. Imported malaria in a Singapore hospital: clinical presentation and outcome. Int J Infect Dis 1999;3:136–139.

13. Dan M, Costin C, Slater PE. Malaria imported by travelers: the Israeli experience. J Travel Med 1996;3:182–185.

14. Behrens RH, Barrett J, Everret T. The benefits of permethrin impregnated bednets in preventing malaria. Proceedings of the IV International Conference on Travel Medicine; 1995 April 23–27. Acapulco, Mexico. p. 90.

15. Steffen R, Fuchs E, Schildknecht J, et al. Mefloquine compared with other malaria chemo-prophylactic regimens in tourists visiting east Africa. Lancet 1993;341:1299–1303.

16. Gyorkos TW, Svenson JE, MacLean JD, et al. Compliance with antimalarial chemo-prophylaxis and the subsequent development of malaria: a matched case-control study. Am J Trop Med Hyg 1995;53:511–517.

17. Wiselka MJ, Kent J, Nicholson KG. Malaria in Leicester 1983–1988: a review of 114 cases. J Infect 1990;20:103–110.

18. Rivera-Matos IR, Atkins JT, Doerr CA, White AC Jr. Pediatric malaria in Houston, Texas. Am J Trop Med Hyg 1997;57:560–563.

19. White NJ. Malaria. In: Cook GC, editor. Manson's tropical diseases. London: Saunders 1996. p. 1107–1118.

20. Shute PG. Malaria. BMJ 1951;11:1280.

21. Day JH, Behrens RH. Delay in onset of malaria with mefloquine prophylaxis [letter]. Lancet 1995;345:398.

22. Manson-Bahr PEC, Bell DR, editor. Manson's tropical diseases. London: Baillier Tindal, 1987.

23. Genton B, Dickson R, Alpers MP. A couple with simultaneous fevers due to falciparum and vivax malaria. J Travel Med 1996;3:235–236.

24. Khoo KL, Tan WL, Eng P, Ong YY. Malaria requiring intensive care. Ann Acad Med Singapore 1998;27:353–357.

25. Blum J, Tichelli A, Hatz C. [Diagnostic and therapeutic difficulties with malaria ter-tiana]. Schweiz Rundsch Med Prax 1999;88:985–991.

26. Viani RM, Bromberg K. Pediatric imported malaria in New York: delayed diagnosis. Clin Pediatr (Phila) 1999;38:333–337.

27. Doherty JF, Grant AD, Bryceson AD. Fever as the presenting complaint of travellers returning from the tropics. QJM 1995;88:277–281.

28. Shirtcliffe P, Cameron E, Nicholson KG, Wiselka MJ. Don't forget dengue! Clinical features of dengue fever in returning travellers. J R Coll Phys Lond 1998;32:235–237.

29. Warrell DA, Molyreux ME, Beales PF. Severe and complicated malaria. Trans R Soc Trop Med Hyg 1990;84:1–65.

30. Greenberg AE, Lobel HO. Mortality from *Plasmodium falciparum* malaria in travelers from the United States, 1959 to 1987. Ann Intern Med 1990;113:326–327.

31. Jensenius M, Ronning EJ, Blystad H, et al. Low frequency of complications in imported falciparum malaria: a review of 222 cases in south-eastern Norway. Scand J Infect Dis 1999;31:73–78.

32. Calleri G, Lipani F, Macor A, et al. Severe and complicated falciparum malaria in Italian travelers. J Travel Med 1998;5:39–41.

33. Wetsteyn JC, de Geus A. Falciparum malaria, imported into the Netherlands, 1979–1988. II. Clinical features. Trop Geogr Med 1995;47:97–102.

34. Matteelli A, Colombini P, Gulletta M, et al. Epidemiological features and case management practices of imported malaria in northern Italy 1991–1995. Trop Med Int Health 1999;4:653–657.

35. Gauzere BA, Roblin X, Blanc P, et al. [Importation of *Plasmodium falciparum* malaria, in Reunion Island, from 1993 to 1996: epidemiology and clinical aspects of severe forms.] Bull Soc Pathol Exot 1998;91:95–98.

36. Lewis SJ, Davidson RN, Ross EJ, Hall AP. Severity of imported falciparum malaria: effect of taking antimalarial prophylaxis. BMJ 1992;305:741–743.

37. Snow RW, Omumbo JA, Lowe B, et al. Relation between severe malaria morbidity in children and level of *Plasmodium falciparum* transmission in Africa. Lancet 1997;349:1650–1654.

38. World Health Organization. Severe falciparum malaria. Trans R Soc Trop Med Hyg 2000;94 Suppl 1:S1–31.

39. Marsh K, Forster D, Waruiru C, et al. Indicators of life-threatening malaria in African children. N Engl J Med 1995;332:1399–1404.

40. Asiedu DK, Sherman CB. Adult respiratory distress syndrome complicating *Plasmodium falciparum* malaria. Heart Lung 2000;29:294–297.

41. Day NP, Phu NH, Bethell DP, et al. The effects of dopamine and adrenaline infusions on acid-base balance and systemic haemodynamics in severe infection [published erratum appears in Lancet 1996;348(9031):902]. Lancet 1996;348:219–223.

42. Bruneel F, Gachot B, Timsit JF, et al. Shock complicating severe falciparum malaria in European adults. Intensive Care Med 1997;23:698–701.

43. Berkley J, Mwarumba S, Bramham K, et al. Bacteraemia complicating severe malaria in children. Trans R Soc Trop Med Hyg 1999;93:283–286.

44. Luxemburger C, Nosten F, Raimond SD, et al. Oral artesunate in the treatment of uncomplicated hyperparasitemic falciparum malaria. Am J Trop Med Hyg 1995;53:522–525.

45. Begue P, Ayivi B, Quinet B, Ter Sakarian M. [Malaria of importation in the child: epidemiological, clinical and therapeutic analysis. Apropos of 70 cases observed in a pediatric hospital in Paris.] Bull Soc Pathol Exot 1991;84:154–163.

46. Emanuel B, Aronson N, Shulman S. Malaria in children in Chicago. Pediatrics 1993;92:83–85.

47. McCaslin RI, Pikis A, Rodriguez WJ. Pediatric *Plasmodium falciparium* malaria: a ten-year experience from Washington, DC. Pediatr Infect Dis J 1994;13:709–715.

48. Lynk A, Gold R. Review of 40 children with imported malaria. Pediatr Infect Dis J 1989;8:745–750.

49. Sabatinelli G, Majori G, D'Ancona F, Romi R. Malaria epidemiological trends in Italy. Eur J Epidemiol 1994;10:399–403.

50. Castelli F, Matteelli A, Caligaris S, et al. Malaria in migrants. Parassitologia 1999;41:261–265.

51. Nguyen-Dinh P, Deloron PL, Barber AM, Collins WE. *Plasmodium* fragile: detection of a ring-infected erythrocyte surface antigen (RESA). Exp Parasitol 1988;65:119–124.

Chapter 12

DIAGNOSIS OF MALARIA IN RETURNED TRAVELERS

Martin P. Grobusch and Gerd-Dieter Burchard

ABSTRACT

Malaria must be given priority in the differential diagnosis of travelers returning febrile from endemic areas. Patients can present with a wide range of nonspecific symptoms and signs.

Microscopy of thick and thin blood smears remains the standard laboratory method for the diagnosis of malaria, allowing not only species identification and quantification of parasitemia but also assessment of additional features with relevance for prognosis in falciparum malaria, that is, presence of schizonts, gametocytes, or malaria pigment. The major drawback of conventional blood film microscopy particularly in non-endemic areas is that continuous training in examining blood films is required. Various modifications to conventional microscopy have been investigated. Fluorescent microscopy requires uncomplicated staining techniques but expensive fluorescence equipment, and sensitivities in various studies are below those of thick-film microscopy. The quantitative buffy coat technique (QBC), combining fluorescent staining with cytoconcentration, yields satisfying sensitivities. However, difficulty with species identification, quantification of parasitemia, and technical problems have been identified as the main drawbacks with this method.

Flow cytometric automated blood cell differentiation by multiangle polarized scatter separation of leukocytes is in use for routine blood count preparations in many affluent countries, most of which are non-endemic for malaria. It has been shown recently to carry some potential as an adjuvant diagnostic tool, possibly of use for detecting patients with imported malaria whose diagnosis might otherwise be missed due to a lack of clinical suspicion.

Polymerase chain reaction (PCR) has become an important diagnostic and research technique in malaria. Although sensitive and specific, it is a time-consuming procedure that requires specialized and costly equipment. Therefore, the role of PCR for the diagnosis of acute disease is limited to very few indications.

Antibody detection tests are of value for a retrospective diagnosis of malaria. They are of no value for the diagnosis of acute malaria.

Key words: antibody detection; flow cytometry; fluorescent microscopy; light microscopy; malaria diagnosis; polymerase chain reaction (PCR); QBC®; travelers.

INTRODUCTION

In travelers returning from malaria-endemic areas, malaria must be considered in the differential diagnosis of any fever. Malaria can present with a wide range of nonspecific symptoms and signs. It also has to be considered that individuals originating from malaria-endemic countries may have acquired some resistance to local plasmodial strains, modifying the clinical picture of the disease. Correct diagnosis of malaria, including parasite species and density, is the key to effective disease management.

CLINICAL DIAGNOSIS

The nonspecific clinical presentation of a returning traveler may be independent of whether he is nonimmune or semi-immune. The earlier the patient presents after onset of symptoms, the less specific they are. Even if the natural course of the disease has not been "disturbed" by (self-)medication with antipyretics, antibiotics, or other drugs, fever may not follow a typical pattern. This applies particularly to falciparum malaria. Signs and symptoms predominantly consist of fever and chills, headache, musculoskeletal pain, and fatigue, accompanied to a varying extent by a wide range of complaints such as abdominal discomfort, nausea and vomiting (predominantly in semi-immune individuals), or diarrhea (predominantly in nonimmune travelers). Hepatosplenomegaly, pallor (a sign of anemia), low urinary output, dyspnea, and impaired level of consciousness indicate a prolonged course of disease prior to presentation and herald complicated (falciparum) malaria. Blood pressure, heartbeat frequency, body temperature, breathing rate, and state of consciousness are all important but nonspecific parameters at baseline.

Diagnostic problems arise from the nonspecific presentation, which may resemble that of other tropical conditions, from rickettsiosis or dengue fever to viral hemorrhagic fevers.[1–3] If clinical features cannot be explained adequately by the diagnosis of malaria alone, additional conditions (infectious and noninfectious, e.g., hyperthyroidism) should be considered.

In nonfalciparum malaria, the first bout of disease (and relapses in benign tertian malaria) can be delayed for years or even decades.[4,5] In semi-immune travelers, even falciparum malaria may occur years after they have left endemic areas. Malaria may even be acquired in regions now considered to be malaria free.[6] The term "odyssean malaria" applies to forms of malaria, in non-endemic areas, acquired from the bites of imported mosquitoes.[7] In this manner, new foci can develop in areas that were previously malaria free.[8]

Malaria has to be considered in all travelers returning from endemic areas who have been exposed 5 days to 3 months prior to clinical onset of disease, and in any cases of relapsing fever, particularly with a 48- or 72-hour rhythm, even years after visits to endemic areas. For a more detailed description, please refer to Chapter 11, "Clinical Features of Malaria in Nonimmune Travelers."

MICROSCOPIC DIAGNOSIS: CONVENTIONAL LIGHT MICROSCOPY

Microscopy of Giemsa- or Field-stained thick and thin blood smears is the standard laboratory method for the diagnosis of malaria (Figures 12–1 to 12–15). Smears are preferably prepared from fresh blood obtained by finger prick or venipuncture, but later preparation from an ethylenediamenetetraacetic acid (EDTA)–preserved sample is also possible. Thick films are best to screen blood for the presence of *Plasmodium*. Thin smears are preferred for identification of species (including those of double infections) and further prognostic factors, that is, schizonts, gametocytes, and malaria pigment (hemozoin). Preparation of thick and thin films and staining methods have been well described.[9]

Accuracy

The number of necessary fields per thick film to be examined in routine use and clinical studies to determine a sample to be free of parasites is currently in dispute, and "standards" in various studies differ from 30 to 500.[10–12] Thick-film examinations of 100 fields or less may not detect even those infections with considerable parasite density.[13–16] However, results of as many as 200 visual fields yielded sensitivities of only 80% to 90% when re-examined extensively by microscopy or PCR analysis.[14–16] Even in a research study, extensive re-examination of 100 fields in thick films revealed that 64 of 309 (20.7%) malaria cases were

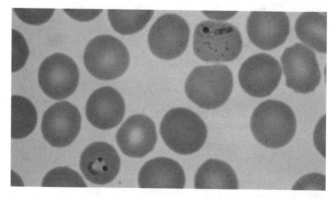

Figure 12–1. Plasmodium vivax. Thin blood film (Giemsa stain, oil immersion). One infected red blood cell contains a young trophozoite showing a double chromatin dot; this cell is not enlarged. The other infected erythrocyte is enlarged and Schüffner's stippling is evident; the organism within already is ameboid and has increased in size. (Courtesy of L.R. Ash and T.C. Orihel. Human parasitology, teaching slide set. ASCP Press, 1990.) (See Color Plates)

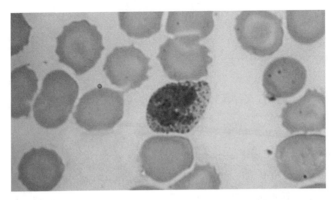

Figure 12–2. Plasmodium vivax. Thin blood film (Giemsa stain, oil immersion). An enlarged red blood cell with pronounced Schüffner's stippling contains a mature, ameboid trophozoite. Note brown pigment grains within the parasite. (Courtesy of L.R. Ash and T.C. Orihel. Human parasitology, teaching slide set. ASCP Press, 1990.) (See Color Plates)

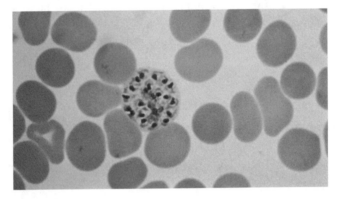

Figure 12–3. Plasmodium vivax. Thin blood film (Giemsa stain, oil immersion). A mature schizont fills this enlarged red blood cell. As is typical for this stage in *P. vivax,* there are approximately 20 merozoites. Brown pigment grains have coalesced in the center of the schizont. (Courtesy of L.R. Ash and T.C. Orihel. Human parasitology, teaching slide set. ASCP Press, 1990.) (See Color Plates)

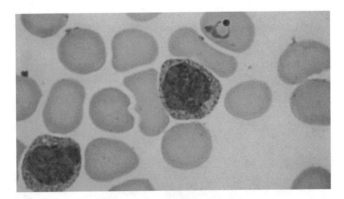

Figure 12–4. Plasmodium vivax. Thin blood film (Giemsa stain, oil immersion). Two mature female gametocytes (macrogametocytes) are present. In one, the compact red chromatin mass lies at the periphery of the enlarged, stippled red blood cell, and in the other, it is central in position. Dark pigment grains are scattered in the cytoplasm. A young trophozoite is present in a red blood cell, which is neither enlarged nor contains Schüffner's stippling. (Courtesy of L.R. Ash and T.C. Orihel. Human parasitology, teaching slide set. ASCP Press, 1990.) (See Color Plates)

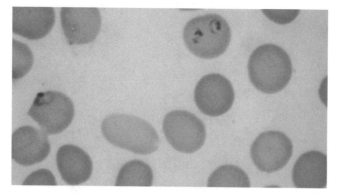

Figure 12–5. *Plasmodium falciparum.* Thin blood film (Giemsa stain, oil, immersion). In one of the two infected red blood cells, a young trophozoite is seen at the margin (often called an appliqué or accolé form). The other red blood cell is infected with two young trophozoites, one of which has a double chromatin dot. Note that the infected red cells are normal in size and lack any stippling. (Courtesy of L.R. Ash and T.C. Orihel. Human parasitology, teaching slide set. ASCP Press, 1990.) (See Color Plates)

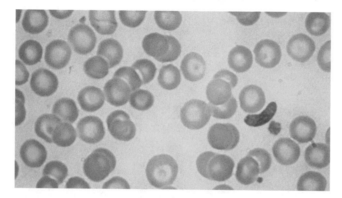

Figure 12–6. *Plasmodium falciparum.* Thin blood film (Giemsa stain, oil immersion). A mature macrogametocyte has the typical "banana" shape with compact chromatin and dark pigment granules. This organism is within a red blood cell, but the erythrocyte membrane cannot be seen. (Courtesy of L.R. Ash and T.C. Orihel. Human parasitology, teaching slide set. ASCP Press, 1990.) (See Color Plates)

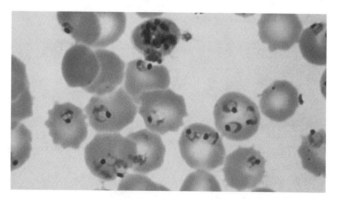

Figure 12–7. *Plasmodium falciparum.* Thin blood film (Giemsa stain, oil immersion). The presence of many infected red blood cells, which may contain one to several ring forms, schizonts, and gametocytes, is a characteristic feature of overwhelming *P. falciparum* infection. This field shows a red blood cell containing a schizont and many red cells with one or more ring stages. Only rarely are stages other than rings and gametocytes found in blood films of individuals with this infection. (Courtesy of L.R. Ash and T.C. Orihel. Human parasitology, teaching slide set. ASCP Press, 1990.) (See Color Plates)

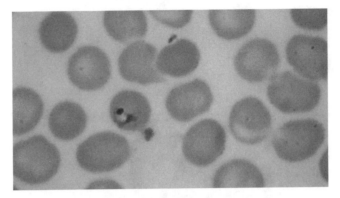

Figure 12–8. Plasmodium malariae. Thin blood film (Giemsa stain, oil immersion). Ring forms of this species have a single large chromatin dot and a more prominent circle of cytoplasm. The infected red blood cells are not enlarged and stippling is rarely seen. (Courtesy of L.R. Ash and T.C. Orihel. Human parasitology, teaching slide set. ASCP Press, 1990.) (See Color Plates)

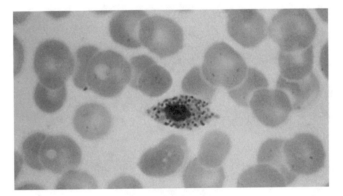

Figure 12–9. Plasmodium malariae. Thin blood film (Giemsa stain, oil immersion). A growing trophozoite in the characteristic "band form" is seen in this infected, normal-sized red blood cell. The red chromatin mass is elongated and some brown pigment grains can be seen at the periphery of the cytoplasm. (Courtesy of L.R. Ash and T.C. Orihel. Human parasitology, teaching slide set. ASCP Press, 1990.) (See Color Plates)

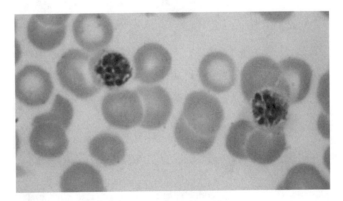

Figure 12–10. Plasmodium malariae. Thin blood film (Giemsa stain, oil immersion). Two mature schizonts are present in normal-sized, infected red blood cells. Mature schizonts of this species will usually contain 6 to 12 merozoites. (Courtesy of L.R. Ash and T.C. Orihel. Human parasitology, teaching slide set. ASCP Press, 1990.) (See Color Plates)

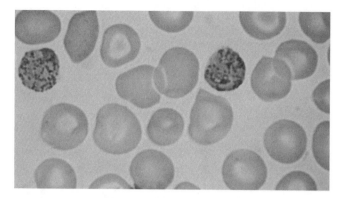

Figure 12–11. *Plasmodium malariae.* Thin blood film (Giemsa stain, oil immersion). Mature male and female gametocytes. The diffuse chromatin of the microgametocyte (male) is purplish-red, compared with the compact chromatin mass of the macrogametocyte. Brown pigment grains are scattered throughout the cytoplasm of the parasites. (Courtesy of L.R. Ash and T.C. Orihel. Human parasitology, teaching slide set. ASCP Press, 1990.) (See Color Plates)

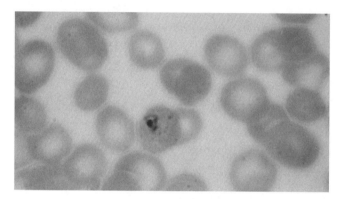

Figure 12–12. *Plasmodium ovale.* Thin blood film (Giemsa stain, oil immersion). A typical ring form is seen in this enlarged, infected red blood cell; note that the red cell contains some stippling. (Courtesy of L.R. Ash and T.C. Orihel. Human parasitology, teaching slide set. ASCP Press, 1990.) (See Color Plates)

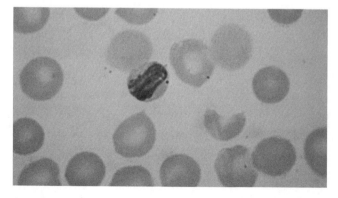

Figure 12–13. *Plasmodium ovale.* Thin blood film (Giemsa stain, oil immersion). The growing trophozoite seen here occupies an enlarged, fimbriated red blood cell. Note the presence of coarse stippling. (Courtesy of L.R. Ash and T.C. Orihel. Human parasitology, teaching slide set. ASCP Press, 1990.) (See Color Plates)

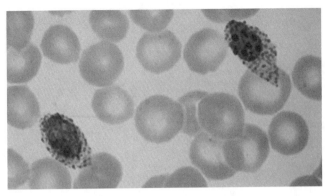

Figure 12–14. *Plasmodium ovale.* Thin blood film (Giemsa stain, oil immersion). Two schizonts, one immature and the other mature, are seen here. A mature schizont of this species typically contains eight merozoites. The red cells are enlarged, elongate, and stippled. Pigment grains are prominent in the cytoplasm of the parasites. (Courtesy of L.R. Ash and T.C. Orihel. Human parasitology, teaching slide set. ASCP Press, 1990.) (See Color Plates)

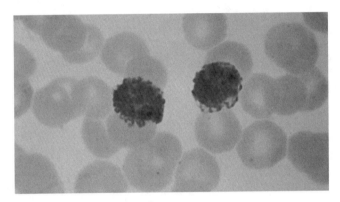

Figure 12–15. *Plasmodium ovale.* Thin blood film (Giemsa stain, oil immersion). Two female gametocytes (macrogametocytes) are shown here. In each, the chromatin masses are compact and brown pigment grains are scattered in the cytoplasm. (Courtesy of L.R. Ash and T.C. Orihel. Human parasitology, teaching slide set. ASCP Press, 1990.) (See Color Plates)

initially missed.[13] In 100 fields of thick films, approximately 0.25 μL of blood are examined, whereas in 100 fields of thin films, only 0.005 μL can be screened. Based on volume alone, the sensitivity of thick films compared to thin films should be 50 times better. However, since as many as 60% to 80% of parasites can get lost during thick-film staining,[17] the detection limit of 5 to 20 parasites/μL is estimated to be on average 10 times lower than in thin films.[18,19] In summary, at least 200 visual fields should be examined before reporting a negative result.[20]

Parasite Densities

In nonimmune travelers, any parasitemia is relevant. Several methods to quantify malaria parasites in thick and thin blood smears have been described. One method consists of counting the number of parasites and leukocytes in a thick film until several hundred leukocytes have been enumerated. The ratio of parasites to leukocytes gives the number of parasites per microliter of blood. Another possibility is to calculate the percentage of erythrocytes that are parasitized.[21] Whereas in benign tertian and quartan malaria, parasite rates rarely exceed 2% to 3% of erythrocytes, they can be high in falciparum malaria. In endemic areas, parasitemia below a density of 5,000 to 10,000/μL is often asymptomatic.[22] Whichever method is employed, parasitemia expressed as a percentage or parasite count/μL both correlate well with clinical features and prognosis[23] and are considered useful indicators of severity.[24] A hyperparasitemia of >5% is considered a serious prognostic sign.[25] However, in falciparum malaria, a patient late in the infection with many sequestered parasites may have a body burden more than 100 times that of a recently infected individual with comparable "visible" parasitemia.[24] In these patients, with only moderate parasitemia but a poorer prognosis due to progressed disease, malaria might be identified microscopically by the indicators of more advanced disease (late trophozoites, schizonts, and gametocytes) in peripheral blood smears.[26] In patients with falciparum malaria, the bulk of parasites is sequestered in tissue capillaries and may not always be present in the peripheral blood; hence an infection might not be detected unless blood samples are repeated several times.[27]

Malaria Pigment

Another marker of disease severity seems to be the amount of malaria pigment in neutrophils and monocytes. A study of Vietnamese patients showed that those who died of malaria had higher proportions of malaria-containing neutrophils on admission than did survivors.[28] Similar studies of tourists need to be performed.

Summary

In summary, major drawbacks of conventional light microscopy, particularly in non-endemic areas, are that continous training in examining blood films is required[29] and sufficient samples need to be examined to allow correct exclusion of infection. This requires considerable time, as even an expert takes approximately 3 minutes to read 100 fields in a thick film.[21] A thin-film reading of 30 minutes is considered comparable. An institution may not have sufficient numbers of staff with microscopy expertise available during on-call hours;[30] a U.K. study showed that more than 10% of positive slides were not identified.[31] Mixed infections often are diagnosed incorrectly.[31] A lesser problem is that initiation of therapy might blur the clarity of species identification at follow-up examinations, as parasites might appear "damaged" due to therapy, and yet still be present in the blood stream. An advantage of light microscopy is that costs of laboratory equipment (a high-quality light microscope and staining bench) and consumables are low.

MICROSCOPIC DIAGNOSIS: FURTHER MICROSCOPIC TECHNIQUES

Various refined methods have been described to improve and facilitate conventional microscopy: darkfield microscopy, fluorescent microscopy, and quantitative buffy coat technique (QBC).

Darkfield Microscopy

The birefringent (doubly refractive) properties of hemozoin (malaria pigment) were tested in a darkfield microscopy technique, but parasite detection not only required special microscopic equipment but was less sensitive than in thick-film microscopy.[32] However, these optical properties are now being exploited in flow cytometric methods of malaria detection.

Fluorescent Microscopy

Malaria parasites contain (deoxy-)ribonucleic acids (DNA/RNA), but erythrocytes (except reticulocytes) do not. Therefore, fluorescent dyes, usually acridine orange[33] or rhodamine-123, are used to test for the presence of DNA/RNA.[34] In some studies, comparable sensitivities were found with fluorescent stains and thick-film microscopy.[35–37] Craig and Sharp[14] examined 600 fields of acridine orange–stained thin and thick films and found sensitivities of 82% and 93%, respectively, compared to 600 thick films in standard technique. In another study,[38] a sensitivity of 85% was reported. Makler et al.[39] circumvented the problem of co-staining viable leukocytes by using benzothiocarboxypurine with another fluorescent microscopy device.

In summary, although staining techniques are uncomplicated, since expensive fluorescence equipment is needed and sensitivities are less than those of thick-film microscopy, the effort does not seem justified.

Quantitative Buffy Coat Technique

A heparinized capillary tube precoated with acridine orange is filled with 50 to 100 μL of blood, centrifuged, and viewed under a fluorescent microscope.[40] Malaria trophozoites can be seen in the nonfluorescent erythrocyte layer underneath the buffy coat, while gametocytes are present in the fluorescent white cell layer. Whereas early studies reported a sharp increase in sensitivity compared to that of standard microscopy,[41–43] later studies found sensitivities in the range of 70% to 100%.[44]

Long et al.[45] found that parasites in infected individuals were detected 1 to 3 days earlier in 47% of individuals tested with QBC compared to standard thick-film microscopy. Laboratory technicians were able to perform QBC and routine microscopy equally well,[46] and time saving was considered advantageous by several investigators.[47,48] However, several major drawbacks have been identified. Identification of the species and quantification of parasite density are difficult; thus, a subsequent Giemsa smear preparation is required.[21,44,49] Some feel the technique is too complicated and the training too time consuming. In addition, the samples cannot be stored for later reference.[38]

AUTOMATED BLOOD CELL DIFFERENTIATION

Microscopy, rapid diagnostic tests (Chapter 13), or PCR (p. 74) are performed only on the grounds of a clinical suspicion. Malaria is not always immediately included in the differential diagnosis of the febrile returning traveler, particularly in non-endemic areas; however, a serious delay in establishing the correct diagnosis may occur. With automated differential counting systems, laboratories theoretically could diagnose malaria even in the absence of an initial clinical suspicion.[50]

Examinations by Coulter counters can show abnormalities of the leukocytes (called large unstained cells [LUCs]) and thrombocytopenia, but these findings can occur in several diseases.[51–53]

Anecdotal experience working with flow cytometric multiangle polarized scatter separation (MAPSS) has revealed that samples from malaria patients display a characteristic granularity/lobularity scattergram profile independent of the infecting *Plasmodium* species. In brief, this phenomenon seems to be due to the detection of malaria pigment (hemozoin), which has birefringent optical properties. One such instrument, the CellDyn 3500® (Abbott Diagnostics, Santa Clara, CA), uses a helium-neon laser and detects the scattered laser light of a focused stream of leukocytes [WBCs] at four different angles to generate a WBC differential (Figure 12–16, *A* and *B*). Up to 10,000 cells are evaluated for size (0°), nucleus-to-cytoplasm ratio (10°), nuclear lobularity (90°), and the presence of depolarizing cytoplasmic granules (90° depolarized). The result is a depiction of eosinophils in a granularity/lobularity plot, presented as green dots above a threshold line, below which the monocyte (purple dots), lymphocyte (blue dots), and neutrophil (yellow dots) populations are represented. When samples of patients with malaria were processed for full blood counts, abnormal lobularity/granularity plots were noticed, with appearance of purple dots (representing monocytes) in the eosinophil area and an abnormally distributed and widely scattered eosinophil population. Both phenomena seem to be due to the presence of birefringent depolarizing malaria pigment in monocytes and neutrophils.[54] The instrument seems to classify monocytes correctly, but due to the optical properties of hemozoin, they are included in the eosinophil area. As malaria pigment–containing neutrophils share many discriminating characteristics with eosinophils (size, nucleus-to-cytoplasm ratio, lobularity), they are probably misclassified by the instrument as eosinophils. However, slight differences in their nuclei (lobularity, 90°) and degree of depolarization caused by the malaria pigment (granularity, 90° depolarized) may cause their abnormal distribution as compared with a normal eosinophil population.

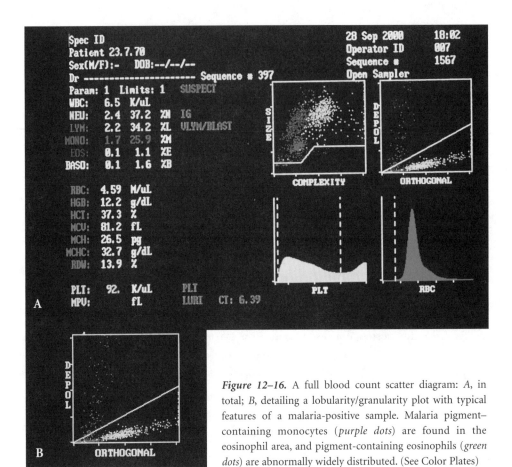

Figure 12–16. A full blood count scatter diagram: *A*, in total; *B*, detailing a lobularity/granularity plot with typical features of a malaria-positive sample. Malaria pigment–containing monocytes (*purple dots*) are found in the eosinophil area, and pigment-containing eosinophils (*green dots*) are abnormally widely distributed. (See Color Plates)

In a first study of the phenomenon in South Africa,[54] 224 samples of suspected cases of malaria were investigated (95 positive, 129 negative; definite diagnosis established by microscopy and antigen detection). Using a CellDyn 3500® instrument, sensitivity and specificity reached 72% and 96%, respectively (positive predictive value [PPV] 93%, negative predictive value [NPV] 82%). In a Portuguese study using a CellDyn 3500® instrument, 174 samples were analyzed. The sensitivity was 95% and the specificity was 88% compared with microscopy. Five false-positive samples all stemmed from patients presenting for follow-up examinations 5 to 21 days after clinical and microscopic cure of malaria. The vast majority of patients were immigrants from malaria-endemic countries.

The large variation in sensitivities within the studies is due, to a certain extent, to the differences in the patient populations, as the percentage of semi-immune individuals is correlated with the sensitivity. A possible explanation for this correlation is that the pyrogenic threshold of semi-immune patients is reached only after a longer asymptomatic period, therefore allowing more time for hemozoin production than in nonimmune persons. As kinetic studies show that malaria pigment–containing leukocytes may persist for up to 3 weeks in the circulation after parasite eradication, this method does not appear to be of use for follow-up investigations after chemotherapy.

Currently, several further developments of this technique are possible. Whereas specificity appears to be acceptable, sensitivity of the method is limited by the standard software, which is tailored toward the needs of routine full blood counts, therefore limiting the number of analyzed gated events to a maximum of 10,000 leukocytes per count. Modified software facilitating analysis of nonhemolyzed erythrocytes in which pigment-containing parasites can also be detected would enhance the usefulness of this technique. Moreover, other instruments use an argon ion laser, which facilitates detection of parasitic nucleic acid by fluorescent dye detection,[57] and a combination of the two approaches is possible.

Whereas this technique is far too expensive for use in less developed countries, the knowledge of this phenomenon might be helpful in affluent countries—where MAPSS technology is routinely used—to detect cases of imported malaria that might otherwise be missed.

DIAGNOSIS BY POLYMERASE CHAIN REACTION

Principle

The molecules that have been predominantly exploited in new diagnostic assays to date are DNA and protein, although other methods involving RNA, excretory factors, and fatty acid typing, for example, have also been explored. The advantage of DNA-based detection methods is that the genome of an organism is normally a stable and constant entity throughout its life cycle, whereas proteins and RNA are variable. Thus, DNA probes can be obtained and tested on stages that are most easily cultured in the laboratory or isolated from the host. The simplest DNA-based approach is to examine differences in restriction enzyme patterns obtained when the whole genome is cut and fractionated by gel electrophoresis. More recently, specific DNA sequences have been detected by hybridization of a radioactive or nonradioactive probe to a target sequence in the parasite. For *Plasmodium falciparum*, the diagnostic probes were based mainly on an imperfectly repeated 21 bp sequence, present in many thousands of copies.[58,59] These probes were at best only as sensitive as microscopic evaluation of thick blood smears.[60] Better results were obtained by using probes based on ribosomal DNA.[61]

Eventually, the exploitation of molecular biologic techniques culminated in the use of the PCR.[62] In PCR-based techniques, two oligonucleotide primers flanking the target sequence, and a polymerase, are used in successive cycles of DNA denaturation and extension to generate billions of copies of the target sequence. The amplified target sequence is then detected by internal probes or analyzed by gel electrophoresis. PCR thus potentially represents the most sensitive method for the detection of a particular DNA sequence in a given sample, since, theoretically, only one copy of the target sequence needs to be present in the sample for successful amplification.

During the past few years, PCR has become a major diagnostic and research technique in malaria. PCR has been used not only to detect human *Plasmodium* species in diagnostic probes, but also to study parasite diversity, recombination rates, multiplicity of infections, and the development and frequency of drug resistance.

Polymerase Chain Reaction Methods

A number of efficient PCR-based protocols have been devised and validated. Often used as the target for PCR amplification is the gene coding for the small subunit ribosomal RNA (ssrRNA). These genes consist of regions whose sequence is conserved in the different species, interspersed with regions containing sequences specific of each of the species.[63,64] Normally, a nested PCR with a second set of primers is used to overcome nonspecific amplification problems.[65]

Briefly, in an initial amplification reaction (nest 1), DNA purified from the sample to be analyzed is used as a template for the amplification of a large portion of the plasmodial ssrRNA genes. The oligonucleotide primer pairs used for this reaction are genus specific and will therefore amplify the target from the four species. To determine which of the parasite species is present in the sample, four separate amplification reactions (nest 2) must be performed for the detection of each of the four species. The template for these reactions is a small proportion of the amplification product obtained following the nest 1 reaction. The detection of the amplification product is then achieved through ethidium bromide staining following electrophoresis in an agarose gel.[63] In a modified protocol better suited for screening examinations, genus-specific primers in the initial PCR (nest 1) and either genus- or species-specific primers for the nest 2 amplification are used.[66]

Apart from the gene encoding for the small subunit ribosomal RNA, many others have been used for amplification by PCR and specific detection. PCR primers and probes that are specific for sections of the *Plasmodium* genes encoding their circumsporozoite (CS) proteins have been developed.[67–70] Probes are also derived from the dihydrofolate reductase–thymidylate synthase gene of *P. falciparum*.[65,71–73] Repetitive genomic DNA has been used for DNA probes.[74,75] Primers complementary to sequences in the gene encoding the Pf155/ring-infected erythrocyte surface antigen (RESA) of *P. falciparum* have been developed.[10,71]

Different methods for the detection of amplified DNA have also been studied. Many non-isotopic colorimetric PCR-based assays have been developed,[76] for example, microtiter plate hybridization using specific probes that are immobilized on plate wells allowing visualization of biotinylated PCR products.[73]

Quantification of parasites by PCR is also possible. This is achieved by coamplification of the RNA in the sample with one modified in vitro RNA as a competitor.[77] During recent years, reverse transcriptase PCR and in situ amplification techniques have been described. Such approaches could possibly identify gameto-cyte-positive infections, for example,[78] and the expression of particular parasite proteins or antigens.

Sample Preparation

PCR can be performed from fresh blood samples and is unaffected by citrate and EDTA but somewhat inhibited by heparin.[79] Blood can be collected on solid support as well. Many types of paper or glass filters are available. The blood can be stored for long periods of time; however, repeated thawing results in loss of sensitivity.

Simple procedures for the diagnosis of malaria using PCR directly on dried blood spots transported to the laboratory have been described.[80] The sensitivity of this technique in the 1-to-100/μL range is 94%. PCR can also be performed from Giemsa-stained thin blood smears.[81,82]

Accuracy

The sensitivity and specificity of PCR-based methods, estimated using microscop-ic examination of blood smears as the "gold standard," are both >90%.[83] A speci-ficity of 100% in infections with 5 parasites/μL has been described.[84] Using nested PCR, 1 *P. falciparum* parasite/μL of blood can be detected.[85]

False-negative results can occur. Samples identified by microscopy as containing *P. falciparum* at a fairly high density were not similarly recognized by the PCR method.[75,86] In 3 out of 695 patients studied in Nigeria, parasites were found by microscopy but not by PCR.[87] Reasons for these false-negative results include dele-tion or variation of the targeted gene sequences, or mutations in the primer-annealing sites. False-positive results can occur after treatment.[88]

Two problems concerning PCR-based diagnosis of malaria remain unsolved:

- It is not known whether PCR can be positive in travelers taking (sufficient) pro-phylaxis with drugs that act on erythrocytic forms of the parasite (e.g., chloro-quine, mefloquine). False-positive reactions seem to be possible because the parasites released from the liver circulate for some time in the blood stream before they are killed by the drugs.
- In rodent malaria infection, no parasite DNA has been detected by PCR 48 hours after the injection of killed parasites.[89] In man, however, it is not known how long PCR can remain positive after treatment. Thus, it is not clear whether a semiquantitative PCR can be used to monitor early treatment failures.[90,91]

Applications

PCR is sensitive and specific. It is, however, a time-consuming procedure that requires specialized and costly equipment. Therefore, PCR is indicated in the fol-lowing special situations only:

- In donors for blood transfusion or organ transplantation,[92] since the microscopic and immunologic methods in current use for malaria diagnosis are unsatisfactory for low levels of parasitemia in blood donations
- In congenital malaria, which may have low levels of parasitemia[93]
- In advanced postmortem to confirm diagnosis of malaria, since autolytic processes and putrefaction may thwart traditional diagnostic procedures[94]
- In cases of clinically suspected malaria with repeatedly negative blood films, since symptomatic malaria can occur in nonimmune travelers at parasite densities that are below the detection threshold of microscopy and rapid immunochromatographic tests
- By reference laboratories that survey imported malaria cases[95]

Genotyping

In *P. falciparum* infections, a complex mix of parasite populations is found. This has been shown by isoenzyme analysis, with monoclonal antibodies, and by PCR.[96–98] Genotyping by PCR is possible because of the high polymorphism in some loci of the haploid genome of the parasite. Genetic markers often used are the merozoite surface protein 1 (MSP 1), the merozoite surface protein 2 (MSP 2), and the glutamate-rich protein (GLURP). This genotyping has no role in the routine diagnosis of malaria.

Detection of Drug Resistance

In practice, drug resistance is suspected when acute cases of *P. falciparum* malaria do not fully and rapidly respond to standard regimens. In vitro tests that measure the inhibition of schizont maturation have been described but are not useful for diagnosis of drug resistance in the individual patient. Since drug resistance is genetically determined, PCR can be used for detection—if the responsible mutation is known.

Pyrimethamine and proguanil (cycloguanil) are dihydrofolate reductase (DHFR) inhibitors. Point mutations in the active site of the DHFR enzyme, such as a change from serine to asparagine at position 108, reduce the binding of pyrimethamine. These mutations can be detected by PCR.[99–102] Several genes seem to be involved in chloroquine resistance, which has been mapped to a locus on chromosome 7.[103] Here, a highly polymorphic protein (cg2) or a digestive vacuole transmembrane protein (PfCRT) might be resistance mediators.[104,105] An association between the PfCRT mutation resulting in the substitution of threonine (Thr-76) for lysine at position 76 and the development of chloroquine resistance during the treatment of malaria has recently been demonstrated.[106] Single point mutations in the gene encoding a cytochrome confer resistance to atovaquone.[107] The overexpression of multiple drug resistance genes—encoding proteins that excrete drugs from the cells—seems to play a role in resistance development against chloroquine, mefloquine, quinine, halofantrine, and artemisinin,[108–110] but diagnosis of resistance in the individual patient remains elusive. In summary, PCR does not play any role in routine management but can be used in special situations to diagnose drug resistance.

COMPARISON OF METHODS

The Gold Standard: Microscopy

The classic method of diagnosing malaria is to demonstrate circulating forms in peripheral blood, using a high-powered microscope. A highly experienced microscopist can detect one parasite in 0.5×10^6 erythrocytes (10 parasites/µL of blood), equivalent to a parasitemia of 0.00002%, although a figure of 0.002% is normally taken as a more practical limit.

Microscopy versus Rapid Diagnostic Tests

Rapid diagnostic tests (RDTs) are based on the detection of antigens derived from malaria parasites in lysed blood, using immunochromatographic methods (see Chapter 13). Most frequently they employ a dipstick or test strip bearing monoclonal antibodies against the target parasite antigens.[111] Many studies comparing RDTs with microscopy have been performed in malaria-endemic areas; only a few have been done in nonimmune travelers.[112,113] Studies on returning febrile travelers, comparing the results obtained with RDTs and expert microscopy, found that both sensitivity and specificity were in general above 90%[115–120] (Table 12–1).

In summary, sensitivity and specificity of RDTs are good; however, since the RDTs do not establish the degree of parasitemia, they complement rather than replace the blood film. Of some concern is the fact that in nonimmune individuals, symptomatic malaria can occur at parasite densities that are below the detection threshold of currently available RDTs. However, these cases also are difficult to detect by microscopy. Of more concern is the fact that false-negative results with RDTs have been reported in patients with high parasitemias.[120,121] False-positive RDTs have been reported in patients with rheumatoid factor.[122]

Table 12–1. **Comparison of RDTs with Expert Microscopy in Malaria Diagnosis in Travelers**

RDT	Year	Location	Sensitivity	Specificity
ParaSight F[115]	1996	U.K.	92	98
ParaSight F[116]	1997	France	93	98
ParaSight F[117]	1998	France	86.4	100
ParaSight F[118]	1988	Belgium	95	90
ParaSight F[119]	2000	U.K.	93.3	98.3
ICT P.f[116]	1997	France	96	98
ICT P.f[118]	1998	Belgium	95	89
OptiMAL[120]	2000	Italy	83	—

RDT = rapid diagnosic test.

Microscopy versus Polymerase Chain Reaction

Compared with blood smears, sensitivity and specificity of PCR are >90%. False-negative results in PCR can occur, probably caused by mutations in primer-annealing sites (see page 407). Many studies have demonstrated, however, that PCR can detect lower parasitemias than microscopy. In endemic areas of Vietnam, the PCR method was shown to detect more cases with low parasitemia than did microscopy (63% vs. 10%).[92] In epidemiologic studies in Nigeria, the parasite rate found by microscopy was 48.8%, but parasite rate by PCR was 68%, indicating a high percentage of submicroscopic infections.[87] Similarly, studies in the Sudan revealed a substantial group of asymptomatic, submicroscopically patent infections.[123] Microscopy seems to be especially weak in detecting double or mixed infections when compared to PCR.[67,124] These results pose the question of whether PCR should now become the reference method for the detection of malaria parasites.

Rapid Diagnostic Tests versus Polymerase Chain Reaction

A few studies have been performed that compare RDTs and PCR.[125–128] Some studies have been done in travelers. An evaluation of the ParaSight test for the detection of *P. falciparum* infection in 151 febrile travelers was performed in Toronto. Compared with PCR, the dipstick test had a sensitivity of 88% and a specificity of 97%. The ability of the dipstick test to detect *P. falciparum* was similar to that of microscopy (88% vs. 83%), which did not detect the species of *Plasmodium* in 14 of 133 malaria-infected patients, due to low parasite numbers.[11]

A comparison of the ParaSight test and the ICT test for the detection of *P. falciparum* infection was performed in 200 febrile travelers in Toronto. As determined by PCR and microscopy, 148 travelers had malaria. Compared to PCR, the ParaSight F and ICT Malaria P.f tests showed initial sensitivities of 94% and 90% and specificities of 95% and 97%, respectively.[129]

In Germany, specimens from 231 patients were screened; samples from 53 patients (22.9%) were positive for *P. falciparum* by microscopy and/or PCR. While the test kit based on the detection of histidine-rich protein 2 (HRP-2) performed with a sensitivity of 92.5% and a specificity of 98.3%, the kit for the detection of parasite-specific lactate dehydrogenase (pLDH) showed a sensitivity of 88.5% and a specificity of 99.4%.[130]

Summary

Advantages and disadvantages of each of the above diagnostic methods are outlined in Table 12–2. Microscopy remains the mainstay of malaria diagnosis.

IMMUNODIAGNOSTICS

Antibodies that are useful for diagnosis are produced by the erythrocytic forms of the parasite. The persistence of these antibodies is dependent on the duration and level of parasitemia, on the characteristics of the plasmodial strain, and on the immune status of the patient.

Antigens

Homologous antigens that can be used are derived from *Plasmodium* from in vitro cultures, infected monkeys, or human erythrocytes. The use of cultured parasites offers the most convenient and stable source of antigens. Because cultivation of *P. vivax* and *P. malariae* is difficult, and because human infections with these species are rare, heterologous antigens from *Plasmodium* monkeys are also used: *P. fieldi* cross-reacts with *P. vivax*, and *P. brasilianum* cross-reacts with *P. malariae*.

A number of antibodies against molecularly defined antigens also have been used, for example, the C-terminal 19-kDa fragment of MSP 1,[131] variants of the polymorphic N-terminal fragment of MSP 1,[132] MSP 2,[133] *P. falciparum* erythrocyte membrane protein 1 (PfEMP 1),[134] or circumsporozoite protein (CSP).[135,136] In general, measurement of these antibodies is more important in epidemiologic studies than in routine diagnostics. Thus, antibodies against the NANP epitope of the CSP have been reported to reflect the degree of exposure to sporozoite-infected mosquitoes,[137–140] although no significant relationship between entomological inoculation rate and either CS-antibody prevalence or concentration has been found in a hyperendemic area in Papua New Guinea.[141] Antibodies against several

Table 12–2. **Advantages and Disadvantages of Methods of Malaria Diagnosis**

Method	Advantages	Disadvantages
Microscopy	Identification of the species by visual examination is possible Determination of stage of development is possible Evaluation of level of anemia is possible Detection of other parasites in the blood is possible Method is comparatively cheap	Reliable analysis of very-low-level parasitemias is time consuming or sometimes impossible Species identification is problematic with low levels of parasitemia or those of mixed infections Common lack of familiarity with the appearances of malaria parasites exists in laboratories in affluent countries *Babesia* and *Bartonella* infections may be mistaken for malaria
RDTs	Simple to perform and interpret No special equipment or training required Kits can be stored under ambient conditions	False-negative results are possible in patients with high parasitemias False-positive results can occur in patients with rheumatoid factor Not quantitative Indicate positive results for up to 2 weeks after chemotherapy
PCR	Ability to detect infection in patients with low parasitemias	Labor-intensive and expensive due to high cost of enzymes and primers used Involves multiple steps, taking several hours Cannot be used to distinguish between viable and nonviable organisms

RDT = rapid diagnostic test; PCR = polymerase chain reaction.

defined antigens have been evaluated regarding the level of parasitemia,[142] the development of clinical symptoms,[143] and immunity. A protective role of antibodies against ring-infected erythrocyte surface antigen,[142] glutamate-rich protein,[144] MSP 1,[145-147] and MSP 2[133,147] has been postulated but could not be confirmed by other authors.[149] In summary, it is not clear which antibodies are important in conferring clinical immunity.

Immune Reactions

The indirect immunofluorescence antibody test (IFAT) is still the method of choice. In the IFAT procedure, the antigen consists of a film of infected blood on a microscope slide. The slide is covered first with the test serum and then with a solution of anti–human globulin labeled with fluorescein isothiocyanate. After washing and drying, the slides are evaluated under the fluorescent microscope. The IFAT method is advantageous because it gives a visual picture of the parasites used as the antigen.[150]

The enzyme-linked immunosorbent assay (ELISA) also has been employed in antigen detection. Using antigen from late stages of *P. falciparum*, results have been comparable to indirect immunofluorescence.[151] The ELISA technique is suited for evaluation of large numbers of samples on microtiter plates, and it is often used with defined antigens.

The indirect hemagglutination test (IHA) also has been used for malaria diagnosis. It is useful as a field test, as it does not require a fluorescent microscope. In this test, glutaraldehyde-stabilized tanned sheep cells are sensitized with the specific soluble antigen. Test sera are then added, and the presence of malaria antibodies is indicated by agglutination. This test is used for epidemiologic studies, but sensitivity and specificity are insufficient for individual diagnosis.

Interpretation of Test Results

High titers of antibodies in the IFAT (≥ 1.320) suggest recent infection. In primary infection, species differentiation is possible by the use of an appropriate antigen; in further infections, however, cross-reacting antibodies are produced.[152] Antibodies in median ranges (1:80 to 1:160 in IFAT) can be found in infections with low parasitemias or in past infections. Low antibody titers suggest past infection, but they also can be found after (sufficient) chemoprophylaxis.[153] When interpreting test results, one must bear in mind that in very severe complicated malaria, antibody production can be reduced.[154]

The time of appearance of antibodies is dependent on the parasitemia. The early treatment of malaria in a nonimmune traveler produces a low level of antibody for a few weeks. In severe infections, antibodies appear on days 2 to 4, and in less severe infections, between days 6 and 10. The plateau is reached at about 2 weeks in *P. falciparum* and *P. vivax* infections but only after several weeks in

P. malariae infection. Antibody titers begin to decline between 3 and 30 weeks after primary infection; however, the decline is retarded in re-infections.[155-158]

False-positive test results can occur in hman immunodeficiency virus (HIV)–positive patients, because of a cross-reactivity of antiplasmodial antibodies and HIV tests.[159-160]

Summary

Serologic tests are of value in providing a retrospective confirmation of malaria or a history thereof.[161] They are of no value as a guide to treatment and management. Serology has been used to exclude malaria in the diagnosis of patients with anemia, hepatosplenomegaly, or nephrotic syndrome in the absence of any parasites in the blood by microscopy; however, PCR is currently the method of choice in such situations.

REFERENCES

1. Winters RA, Murray HW. Malaria—the mime revisited: fifteen more years of experience at a New York City teaching hospital. Am J Med 1992;93:243–246.
2. Magill AJ. Fever in the returned traveler. Infect Dis Clin North Am 1998; 12:445–469.
3. Dorsey G, Gandhi M, Oyugi JH, Rosenthal PJ. Difficulties in the prevention, diagnosis, and treatment of imported malaria. Arch Intern Med 2000;160:2505–2510.
4. Grobusch MP, Wiese A, Teichmann D. Delayed primary attack of vivax malaria. J Travel Med 2000;7:104–105.
5. Tsuchida H, Yamaguchi K, Yamamoto S, Ebisawa I. Quartan malaria following splenectomy 36 years after infection. Am J Trop Med Hyg 1982;31:163–165.
6. Vinetz JM, Li J, McCutchan TF, Kaslow DC. *Plasmodium malariae* infection in an asymptomatic 74-year-old Greek woman with splenomegaly. N Engl J Med 1998;338:367–371.
7. Frean I. African malaria vectors in European aircraft. Lancet 2001;357:235.
8. Jelinek T, Corchan M, Grobusch M, et al. Falciparum malaria in European tourists to the Dominican Republic. Emerg Infect Dis 2000;6:537–538.
9. World Health Organization. Basic malaria microscopy. Part I: Learner's guide. Geneva: WHO, 1991.
10. Seesod N, Nopparat P, Hedrum A, et al. An integrated system using immunomagnetic separation, polymerase chain reaction, and colorimetric detection for diagnosis of *Plasmodium falciparum*. Am J Trop Med Hyg 1997;56:322–328.
11. Humar A, Ohrt C, Harrington MA, et al. Parasight F test compared with the polymerase chain reaction and microscopy for the diagnosis of *Plasmodium falciparum* malaria in travelers. Am J Trop Med Hyg 1997;56:44–48.
12. Hanscheid T, Valadas E. Malaria diagnosis. Am J Trop Med Hyg 1999;61:179.
13. Caraballo A, Ache A. The evaluation of a dipstick test for *Plasmodium falciparum* in mining areas of Venezuela. Am J Trop Med Hyg 1996;55:482–484.
14. Craig MH, Sharp BL. Comparative evaluation of four techniques for the diagnosis of *Plasmodium falciparum* infections. Trans R Soc Trop Med Hyg 1997;91:279–282.

15. Di Perri G, Olliaro P, Nardi S, et al. The ParaSight-F rapid dipstick antigen capture assay for monitoring parasite clearance after drug treatment of *Plasmodium falciparum* malaria. Trans R Soc Trop Med Hyg 1997;91:403–405.

16. Kodisinghe HM, Perera KL, Premawansa S, et al. The ParaSight-F dipstick test as a routine diagnostic tool for malaria in Sri Lanka. Trans R Soc Trop Med Hyg 1997;91:398–402.

17. Dowling MA, Shute GT. A comparative study of thick and thin blood films in the diagnosis of scanty malaria parasitaemia. Bull World Health Organ 1966;34: 249–267.

18. Pam Menter MD. Techniques for the diagnosis of malaria. S Afr Med J 1988;74: 55–57.

19. Hanscheid T. Diagnosis of malaria: a review of alternatives to conventional microscopy. Clin Lab Haematol 1999;21:235–245.

20. Bain B, Chiodini P, England J, Bailey J. The laboratory diagnosis of malaria. Clin Lab Haematol 1997;19:165–170.

21. Warhurst DC, Williams JE. ACP Broadsheet No. 148. July 1996. Laboratory diagnosis of malaria. J Clin Pathol 1996;49:533–538.

22. Armstrong-Schellenberg JRM, Smith T, Alonso PL, Hayes RJ. What is clinical malaria? Finding case definitions for field research in highly endemic areas. Parasitol Today 1994;10:439–442.

23. Field JW. Blood examination and prognosis in acute falciparum malaria. Trans R Soc Trop Med Hyg 1949;43:33–48.

24. White NJ, Krishna S. Treatment of malaria: some considerations and limitations of the current methods of assessment. Trans R Soc Trop Med Hyg 1989;83:767–777.

25. World Health Organization. Severe falciparum malaria. Trans R Soc Trop Med Hyg 2000;94 Suppl 1.

26. Silamut K, White NJ. Relation of the stage of parasite development in the peripheral blood to prognosis in severe falciparum malaria. Trans R Soc Trop Med Hyg 1993;87:436–443.

27. Moody AH, Chiodini PL. Methods for the detection of blood parasites. Clin Lab Haematol 2000;22:189–201.

28. Phu NH, Day N, Diep PT, et al. Intraleukocytic malaria pigment and prognosis in severe malaria. Trans R Soc Trop Med Hyg 1995;89:200–204.

29. Payne D. Use and limitations of light microscopy for diagnosing malaria at the primary health care level. Bull World Health Organ 1988;66:621–626.

30. Chiodini PL. Non-microscopic methods for diagnosis of malaria. Lancet 1998;351:80–81.

31. Milne LM, Kyi MS, Chiodini PL, Warhurst DC. Accuracy of routine laboratory diagnosis of malaria in the United Kingdom. J Clin Pathol 1994;47:740–742.

32. Jamjoom GA. Improvement in dark field microscopy for the rapid detection of malaria parasites and its adaptation to field conditions. Trans R Soc Trop Med Hyg 1991;85:38–39.

33. Kawamoto F. Rapid diagnosis of malaria by fluorescence microscopy with light microscope and interference filter. Lancet 1991;337:200–202.

34. Srinavasan S, Moody AH, Chiodini PL. Comparison of blood-film microscopy, the OptiMAL™ dipstick, rhodamine-123 fluorescence staining and PCR, for monitoring antimalarial treatment. Ann Trop Med Parasitol 2000;94:227–232.

35. Wongsrichanalai C, Chuanak N, Webster HK, Prasittisuk M. Practical uses of acridine orange fluorescence microscopy of centrifuged blood (QBC Malaria Test) and the QBCII Hematology System in patients attending malaria clinics in Thailand. Southeast Asian J Trop Med Public Health 1992;23:406–413.

36. Gay F, Traore B, Zanoni J, et al. Direct acridine orange fluorescence examination of blood slides compared to current techniques for malaria diagnosis. Trans R Soc Trop Med Hyg 1996;90:516–518.

37. Kong HH, Chung DI. Comparison of acridine orange and Giemsa stains for malaria diagnosis. Korean J Parasitol 1995;33:391–394.

38. Delacollette C, van der Struyft P. Direct acridine orange staining is not a 'miracle' solution to the problem of malaria diagnosis in the field. Trans R Soc Trop Med Hyg 1994;88:187–188.

39. Makler MT, Ries LK, Ries J, et al. Detection of *Plasmodium falciparum* infection with the fluorescent dye, benzothiocarboxypurine. Am J Trop Med Hyg 1991;44:11–16.

40. Levine R, Wardlaw S, Patton C. Detection of haematoparasites using quantitative buffy coat analysis tubes. Parasitol Today 1989;5:132–134.

41. White N, Silamut K. Rapid diagnosis of malaria. Lancet 1989;8635:435.

42. Levine RA, Wardlaw SC. QBC malaria diagnosis. Lancet 1992;339:1354.

43. Perrone JB, Popper C. QBC malaria diagnosis. Lancet 1992;339:1354–1355.

44. Wongsrichanalai C, Namsiripongpun V, Pornsilapatip J, et al. Sensitivity of QBC malaria test. Lancet 1992;340:792–793.

45. Long G, Jones T, Rickman L, et al. Acridine orange diagnosis of *Plasmodium falciparum*: evaluation after experimental infection. Am J Trop Med Hyg 1994;51:613–616.

46. Clendennen TE III, Long GW, Baird JK. QBC and Giemsa-stained thick blood films: diagnostic performance of laboratory technologists. Trans R Soc Trop Med Hyg 1995;89:183–184.

47. Benito A, Roche J, Molina R, et al. Application and evaluation of QBC malaria diagnosis in a holoendemic area. Appl Parasitol 1994;35:266–272.

48. Bosch I, Bracho C, Perez HA. Diagnosis of malaria by acridine orange fluorescent microscopy in an endemic area of Venezuela. Mem Inst Oswaldo Cruz 1996;91:83–86.

49. Lowe BS, Jeffa NK, New L, et al. Acridine orange fluorescence techniques as alternatives to traditional Giemsa staining for the diagnosis of malaria in developing countries. Trans R Soc Trop Med Hyg 1996;90:34–36.

50. Hanscheid T, Valadas E, Grobusch MP. Automated malaria diagnosis using pigment detection. Parasitol Today 2000;16:549–551.

51. Fialon P, Macaigne F, Becker M, et al. Aspects hematologiques du paludisme d'importation. Intérêt diagnostique dans les formes pauci-parasitaires. Pathol Biol (Paris) 1991;39:122–125.

52. Giacomini T, Lusina D, Foubard S, et al. Diagnostic biologique du paludisme: dangers de l'automatisation de la formule sanguine. Bull Soc Pathol Exot 1991; 84:330–337.

53. Bunyaratvej A, Butthep P, Bunyaratvej P. Cytometric analysis of blood cells from malaria-infected patients and in vitro infected blood. Cytometry 1993;14:81–85.

54. Metzger WG, Mordmuller BG, Kremsner PG. Malaria pigment in leucocytes. Trans R Soc Trop Med Hyg 1995;89:637–638.

55. Mendelow BV, Lyons C, Nhlangothi P, et al. Automated malaria detection by depolarization of laser light. Br J Haematol 1999;104:499–503.

56. Hänscheid T, Christino J, Pointo BG. Automated detection of malaria pigment in white blood cells for the diagnosis of malaria in Portugal. 2001. [In press]

57. Hoffmann JJ, Pennings JM. Pseudo-reticulocytosis as a result of malaria parasites. Clin Lab Haematol 1999;21:257–260.

58. McLaughlin GL, Ruth JL, Jablonski E, et al. Use of enzyme-linked synthetic DNA in diagnosis of falciparum malaria. Lancet 1987;8535:714–716.

59. Sethabutr O, Brown AE, Gingrich J, et al. A comparative field study of radiolabeled and enzyme-conjugated synthetic DNA probes for the diagnosis of falciparum malaria. Am J Trop Med Hyg 1988;39:227–231.

60. Lanar DE, McLaughlin GL, Wirth DF, et al. Comparison of thick films, in vitro culture and DNA hybridization probes for detecting *Plasmodium falciparum* malaria. Am J Trop Med Hyg 1989;40:3–6.

61. Waters AP, McCutchan TF. Rapid, sensitive diagnosis of malaria based on ribosomal RNA. Lancet 1989;1:1343–1346.

62. Jaureguiberry G, Hatin I, d'Auriol L, Galibert G. PCR detection of *Plasmodium falciparum* by oligonucleotide probes. Mol Cell Probes 1990;4:409–414.

63. Snounou G. Detection and identification of the four malaria parasite species infecting humans by PCR amplification. In: Clapp JP, editor. Methods in molecular biology. Species diagnostics protocols: PCR and other nucleic acid methods. Vol. 50. Humana Press: 263291.

64. Snounou G, Viriyakosol S, Zhu XP, et al. High sensitivity of detection of human malaria parasites by the use of nested polymerase chain reaction. Mol Biochem Parasitol 1993;61:315–320.

65. Arai M, Mizukoshi C, Kubochi F, et al. Detection of *Plasmodium falciparum* in human blood by a nested polymerase chain reaction. Am J Trop Med Hyg 1994;51:617–626.

66. Singh B, Bobogare A, Cox-Singh J, et al. A genus- and species-specific nested polymerase chain reaction malaria detection assay for epidemiologic studies. Am J Trop Med Hyg 1999;60:687–692.

67. Brown AE, Kain KC, Pipithkul J, Webster HK. Demonstration by the polymerase chain reaction of mixed *Plasmodium falciparum* and *P. vivax* infections undetected by conventional microscopy. Trans R Soc Trop Med Hyg 1992;86:609–612.

68. Kain KC, Brown AE, Mirabelli L, Webster HK. Detection of *Plasmodium vivax* by polymerase chain reaction in a field study. J Infect Dis 1993;168:1323–1326.

69. Tahar R, Ringwald P, Basco LK. Diagnosis of *Plasmodium malariae* infection by the polymerase chain reaction. Trans R Soc Trop Med Hyg 1997;91:410–411.

70. Han GD, Zhang XJ, Zhang HH, et al. Use of PCR/DNA probes to identify circumsporozoite genotype of *Plasmodium vivax* in China. Southeast Asian J Trop Med Public Health 1999;30:20–23.

71. Holmberg M, Wahlberg J, Lundeberg J, et al. Colorimetric detection of *Plasmodium falciparum* and direct sequencing of amplified gene fragments using a solid phase method. Mol Cell Probes 1992;6:201–208.

72. Wataya Y, Arai M, Kubochi F, et al. DNA diagnosis of falciparum malaria using a double PCR technique: a field trial in the Solomon Islands. Mol Biochem Parasitol 1993;58:165–167.

73. Kimura M, Miyake H, Kim HS, et al. Species-specific PCR detection of malaria parasites by microtiter plate hybridization: clinical study with malaria patients. J Clin Microbiol 1995;33:2342–2346.

74. Tirasophon W, Ponglikitmongkol M, Wilairat P, et al. A novel detection of a single *Plasmodium falciparum* in infected blood. Biochem Biophys Res Commun 1991;175:179–184.

75. Barker R Jr, Banchongaksorn T, Courval JM, et al. A simple method to detect *Plasmodium falciparum* directly from blood samples using the polymerase chain reaction. Am J Trop Med Hyg 1992;46:416–426.

76. Zhong KJ, Kain KC. Evaluation of a colorimetric PCR-based assay to diagnose *Plasmodium falciparum* malaria in travelers. J Clin Microbiol 1999;37:339–341.

77. Schoone GJ, Oskam L, Kroon NC, et al. Detection and quantification of *Plasmodium falciparum* in blood samples using quantitative nucleic acid sequence-based amplification. J Clin Microbiol 2000;38:4072–4075.

78. Babiker HA, Abdel-Wahab A, Ahmed S, et al. Detection of low level *Plasmodium falciparum* gametocytes using reverse transcriptase polymerase chain reaction. Mol Biochem Parasitol 1999;99:143–148.

79. Farnert A, Arez AP, Correia AT, et al. Sampling and storage of blood and the detection of malaria parasites by polymerase chain reaction. Trans R Soc Trop Med Hyg 1999;93:50–53.

80. Long GW, Fries L, Watt GH, Hoffman SL. Polymerase chain reaction amplification from *Plasmodium falciparum* on dried blood spots. Am J Trop Med Hyg 1995;52:344–346.

81. Kimura M, Kaneko O, Inoue A, et al. Amplification by polymerase chain reaction of *Plasmodium falciparum* DNA from Giemsa-stained thin blood smears. Mol Biochem Parasitol 1995;70:193–197.

82. Edoh D, Steiger S, Genton B, Beck HP. PCR amplification of DNA from malaria parasites on fixed and stained thick and thin blood films. Trans R Soc Trop Med Hyg 1997;91:361–363.

83. Makler MT, Palmer CJ, Ager AL. A review of practical techniques for the diagnosis of malaria. Ann Trop Med Parasitol 1998;92:419–433.

84. Kawamoto F, Miyake H, Kaneko O, et al. Sequence variation in the 18S rRNA gene, a target for PCR-based malaria diagnosis, in *Plasmodium ovale* from southern Vietnam. J Clin Microbiol 1996;34:2287–2289.

85. Cox-Singh J, Mahayet S, Abdullah MS, Singh B. Increased sensitivity of malaria detection by nested polymerase chain reaction using simple sampling and DNA extraction. Int J Parasitol 1997;27:1575–1577.

86. Barker R, Banchongaksorn T, Courval JM, et al. *Plasmodium falciparum* and *P. vivax*: factors affecting sensitivity and specificity of PCR-based diagnosis of malaria. Exp Parasitol 1994;79:41–49.

87. May J, Mockenhaupt FP, Ademowo OG, et al. High rate of mixed and subpatent malarial infection in southwest Nigeria. Am J Trop Med Hyg 1999;61:339–343.

88. Miyake H, Kimura M, Wataya Y. PCR diagnosis of malaria at convalescent stage post-treatment. J Travel Med 1996;3:119–121.

89. Jarra W, Snounou G. Only viable parasites are detected by PCR following clearance of rodent malarial infections by drug treatment or immune responses. Infect Immun 1998;66:3783–3787.

90. Kain KC, Kyle DE, Wongsrichanalai C, et al. Qualitative and semiquantitative polymerase chain reaction to predict *Plasmodium falciparum* treatment failure. J Infect Dis 1994;170:1626–1630.

91. Ciceron L, Jaureguiberry G, Gay F, Danis M. Development of a *Plasmodium* PCR for monitoring efficacy of antimalarial treatment. J Clin Microbiol 1999;37:35–38.

92. Vu TT, Tran VB, Phan NT, et al. Screening donor blood for malaria by polymerase chain reaction. Trans R Soc Trop Med Hyg 1995;89:44–47.

93. Rubio JM, Roche J, Berzosa PJ, et al. The potential utility of the Semi-Nested Multiplex PCR technique for the diagnosis and investigation of congenital malaria. Diagn Microbiol Infect Dis 2000;38:233–236.

94. Becker K, Ortmann C, Bajanowski T, et al. Use of polymerase chain reaction for postmortem diagnosis of malaria. Diagn Mol Pathol 1999;8:211–215.

95. Rubio JM, Benito A, Berzosa PJ, et al. Usefulness of seminested multiplex PCR in surveillance of imported malaria in Spain. J Clin Microbiol 1999;37:3260–3264.

96. Babiker HA, Creasey AM, Bayoumi RA, et al. Genetic diversity of *Plasmodium falciparum* in a village in eastern Sudan. 2. Drug resistance, molecular karyotypes and the mdr1 genotype of recent isolates. Trans R Soc Trop Med Hyg 1991;85:578–583.

97. Mercereau-Puijalon O, Jacquemot C, Sarthou JL. A study of the genomic diversity of *Plasmodium falciparum* in Senegal. 1. Typing by Southern blot analysis. Acta Trop 1991;49:281–292.

98. Mercereau-Puijalon O, Fandeur T, Bonnefoy S, et al. A study of the genomic diversity of *Plasmodium falciparum* in Senegal. 2. Typing by the use of the polymerase chain reaction. Acta Trop 1991;49:293–304.

99. Jelinek T, Ronn AM, Lemnge MM, et al. Polymorphisms in the dihydrofolate reductase (DHFR) and dihydropteroate synthetase (DHPS) genes of *Plasmodium falciparum* and in vivo resistance to sulphadoxine/pyrimethamine in isolates from Tanzania. Trop Med Int Health 1998;3:605–609.

100. Duraisingh MT, Curtis J, Warhurst DC. *Plasmodium falciparum*: detection of polymorphisms in the dihydrofolate reductase and dihydropteroate synthetase genes by PCR and restriction digestion. Exp Parasitol 1998;89:1–8.

101. Basco LK, Ringwald P. Molecular epidemiology of malaria in Yaoundé, Cameroon. I. Analysis of point mutations in the dihydrofolate reductase-thymidylate synthase gene of *Plasmodium falciparum*. Am J Trop Med Hyg 1998;58:369–373.

102. Basco LK, Ringwald P. Molecular epidemiology of malaria in Yaoundé, Cameroon. II. Baseline frequency of point mutations in the dihydropteroate synthase gene of *Plasmodium falciparum*. Am J Trop Med Hyg 1998;58:374–377.

103. Su X, Kirkman LA, Fujioka H, Wellems TE. Complex polymorphisms in an approximately 330 kDa protein are linked to chloroquine-resistant *P. falciparum* in Southeast Asia and Africa. Cell 1997;91:593–603.

104. McCutcheon KR, Freese JA, Frean JA, et al. Chloroquine-resistant isolates of *Plasmodium falciparum* with alternative CG2 omega repeat length polymorphisms. Am J Trop Med Hyg 2000;62:190–192.

105. Fidock DA, Nomura T, Talley AK, et al. Mutations in the *P. falciparum* digestive vacuole transmembrane protein PfCRT and evidence for their role in chloroquine resistance. Mol Cell 2000;6:861–871.

106. Djimde A, Doumbo OK, Cortese JF, et al. A molecular marker for chloroquine-resistant falciparum malaria. N Engl J Med 2001;344:257–263.

107. Korsinczky M, Chen N, Kotecka B, et al. Mutations in *Plasmodium falciparum* cytochrome b that are associated with atovaquone resistance are located at a putative drug-binding site. Antimicrob Agents Chemother 2000;44:2100–2108.

108. Grobusch MP, Adagu IS, Kremsner PG, Warhurst DC. *Plasmodium falciparum*: in vitro chloroquine susceptibility and allele-specific PCR detection of Pfmdr1 Asn86Tyr polymorphism in Lambaréné, Gabon. Parasitology 1998;116:211–217.

109. Duraisingh MT, Jones P, Sambou I, et al. The tyrosine-86 allele of the pfmdr1 gene of *Plasmodium falciparum* is associated with increased sensitivity to the anti-malarials mefloquine and artemisinin. Mol Biochem Parasitol 2000;108:13–23.

110. Reed MB, Saliba KJ, Caruana SR, et al. Pgh1 modulates sensitivity and resistance to multiple antimalarials in *Plasmodium falciparum*. Nature 2000;403:906–909.

111. World Health Organization. Malaria diagnosis—new perspectives. Geneva: WHO, 2000.

112. Burchard GD. Malariaschnelltests. Bundesgesundheitsblatt 1999;42:643–649.

113. Jelinek T, Grobusch M, Nothdurft H. Use of dipstick tests for the rapid diagnosis of malaria in nonimmune travelers. J Travel Med 2000;7:175–179.

114. Chiodini PL, Hunt Cooke A, Moody AH, et al. Medical Devices Agency evaluation of the Becton Dickinson ParaSight F test for the diagnosis of *Plasmodium falciparum*. MDA/96/33. London: Her Majesty's Stationery Office, 1996.

115. Cavallo JD, Hernandez E, Gerome P, et al. Antigénémie HRP-2 et paludisme d'importaion à *Plasmodium falciparum*: comparaison du ParaSight-F et de l'ICT P.f. Med Trop (Mars) 1997;57:353–356.

116. Bellagra N, Ajana F, Caillaux M. Apport du ParaSight F dans le diagnostic du paludisme à *Plasmodium falciparum*. Pathol Biol (Paris) 1998;46:301–306.

117. Van den Ende J, Vervoort T, Van Gompel A, Lynen L. Evaluation of two tests based on the detection of histidine rich protein 2 for the diagnosis of imported *Plasmodium falciparum* malaria. Trans R Soc Trop Med Hyg 1998;92:285–288.

118. Cropley IM, Lockwood DN, Mack D, et al. Rapid diagnosis of falciparum malaria by using the ParaSight F test in travellers returning to the United Kingdom: prospective study. BMJ 2000;321:484–485.

119. Ricci L, Viani I, Piccolo G, et al. Evaluation of OptiMAL assay test to detect imported malaria in Italy. New Microbiol 2000;23:391–398.

120. Beadle C, Long GW, Weiss WR, et al. Diagnosis of malaria by detection of *Plasmodium falciparum* HRP-2 antigen with a rapid dipstick antigen-capture assay. Lancet 1994;343:564–568.

121. Wongsrichanalai C, Chuanak N, Tulyayon S, et al. Comparison of a rapid field immunochromatographic test to expert microscopy for the detection of *Plasmodium falciparum* asexual parasitemia in Thailand. Acta Trop 1999;73:263–273.

122. Grobusch MP, Alpermann U, Schwenke S, et al. False-positive rapid tests for malaria in patients with rheumatoid factor. Lancet 1999;353:297.

123. Roper C, Elhassan IM, Hviid L, et al. Detection of very low level *Plasmodium falciparum* infections using the nested polymerase chain reaction and a reassessment of the epidemiology of unstable malaria in Sudan. Am J Trop Med Hyg 1996;54:325–331.

124. Snounou G, Viriyakosol S, Jarra W, et al. Identification of the four human malaria parasite species in field samples by the polymerase chain reaction and detection of a high prevalence of mixed infections. Mol Biochem Parasitol 1993;58:283–292.

125. Banchongaksorn T, Yomokgul P, Panyim S, et al. A field trial of the ParaSight-F test for the diagnosis of *Plasmodium falciparum* infection. Trans R Soc Trop Med Hyg 1996;90:244–245.

126. Quintana M, Piper R, Boling HL, et al. Malaria diagnosis by dipstick assay in a Honduran population with coendemic *Plasmodium falciparum* and *Plasmodium vivax*. Am J Trop Med Hyg 1998;59:868–871.

127. Iqbal J, Sher A, Hira PR, Al-Owaish R. Comparison of the OptiMAL test with PCR for diagnosis of malaria in immigrants. J Clin Microbiol 1999;37:3644–3646.

128. Lee MA, Aw LT, Singh M. A comparison of antigen dipstick assays with polymerase chain reaction (PCR) technique and blood film examination in the rapid diagnosis of malaria. Ann Acad Med Singapore 1999;28:498–501.

129. Pieroni P, Mills CD, Ohrt C, et al. Comparison of the ParaSight-F test and the ICT Malaria Pf test with the polymerase chain reaction for the diagnosis of *Plasmodium falciparum* malaria in travellers. Trans R Soc Trop Med Hyg 1998;92:166–169.

130. Jelinek T, Grobusch MP, Schwenke S, et al. Sensitivity and specificity of dipstick tests for rapid diagnosis of malaria in nonimmune travelers. J Clin Microbiol 1999;37:721–723.

131. Hirunpetcharat C, Tian JH, Kaslow DC, et al. Complete protective immunity induced in mice by immunization with the 19-kilodalton carboxyl-terminal fragment of the merozoite surface protein-1 (MSP1[19]) of *Plasmodium yoelii* expressed in *Saccharomyces cerevisiae*: correlation of protection with antigen-specific antibody titer, but not with effector CD4+ T cells. J Immunol 1997;159:3400–3411.

132. Cavanagh DR, Elhassan IM, Roper C, et al. A longitudinal study of type-specific antibody responses to *Plasmodium falciparum* merozoite surface protein-1 in an area of unstable malaria in Sudan. J Immunol 1998;161:347–359.

133. Taylor RR, Allen SJ, Greenwood BM, Riley EM. IgG3 antibodies to *Plasmodium falciparum* merozoite surface protein 2 (MSP2): increasing prevalence with age and association with clinical immunity to malaria. Am J Trop Med Hyg 1998; 58:406–413.

134. Bull PC, Lowe BS, Kortok M, et al. Parasite antigens on the infected red cell surface are targets for naturally acquired immunity to malaria. Nat Med 1998;4:358–360.

135. Marussig M, Renia L, Motard A, et al. Linear and multiple antigen peptides containing defined T and B epitopes of the *Plasmodium yoelii* circumsporozoite protein: antibody-mediated protection and boosting by sporozoite infection. Int Immunol 1997;9:1817–1824.

136. Shi YP, Hasnain SE, Sacci JB, et al. Immunogenicity and in vitro protective efficacy of a recombinant multistage *Plasmodium falciparum* candidate vaccine. Proc Natl Acad Sci U S A 1999;96:1615–1620.

137. Esposito F, Lombardi S, Modiano D, et al. Immunity to *Plasmodium* sporozoites: recent advances and applications to field research. Parassitologia 1986;28:101–105.

138. Esposito F, Lombardi S, Modiano D, et al. Prevalence and levels of antibodies to the circumsporozoite protein of *Plasmodium falciparum* in an endemic area and their relationship to resistance against malaria infection. Trans R Soc Trop Med Hyg 1988;82:827–832.

139. Druilhe P, Pradier O, Marc JP, et al. Levels of antibodies to *Plasmodium falciparum* sporozoite surface antigens reflect malaria transmission rates and are persistent in the absence of reinfection. Infect Immun 1986;53:393–397.

140. Teuscher T. Household-based malaria control in a highly endemic area of Africa (Tanzania): determinants of transmission and disease and indicators for monitoring—Kilombero Malaria Project. Mem Inst Oswaldo Cruz 1992;3:121–130.

141. Burkot TR, Graves PM, Wirtz RA, et al. Differential antibody responses to *Plasmodium falciparum* and *P. vivax* circumsporozoite proteins in a human population. J Clin Microbiol 1989;27:1346–1351.

142. Bjorkman A, Lebbad M, Perlmann H, et al. Longitudinal study of seroreactivities to Pf155/RESA and its repetitive sequences in small children from a holoendemic area of Liberia. Parasite Immunol 1991;13:301–311.

143. Carlson J, Helmby H, Hill AV, et al. Human cerebral malaria: association with erythrocyte rosetting and lack of anti-rosetting antibodies. Lancet 1990;336:1457–1460.

144. Hogh B, Petersen E, Dziegiel M, et al. Antibodies to a recombinant glutamate-rich *Plasmodium falciparum* protein: evidence for protection of individuals living in a holoendemic area of Liberia. Am J Trop Med Hyg 1992;46:307–313.

145. Riley EM, Allen SJ, Wheeler JG, et al. Naturally acquired cellular and humoral immune responses to the major merozoite surface antigen (PfMSP1) of *Plasmodium falciparum* are associated with reduced malaria morbidity. Parasite Immunol 1992;14:321–337.

146. Egan AF, Morris J, Barnish G, et al. Clinical immunity to *Plasmodium falciparum* malaria is associated with serum antibodies to the 19-kDa C-terminal fragment of the merozoite surface antigen, PfMSP-1. J Infect Dis 1996;173:765–769.

147. Branch OH, Udhayakumar V, Hightower AW, et al. A longitudinal investigation of IgG and IgM antibody responses to the merozoite surface protein-1 19-kiloDalton domain of *Plasmodium falciparum* in pregnant women and infants: associations with febrile illness, parasitemia, and anemia. Am J Trop Med Hyg 1998;58:211–219.

148. al-Yaman F, Genton B, Anders RF, et al. Relationship between humoral response to *Plasmodium falciparum* merozoite surface antigen-2 and malaria morbidity in a highly endemic area of Papua New Guinea. Am J Trop Med Hyg 1994;51:593–602.

149. Dodoo D, Theander TG, Kurtzhals JA, et al. Levels of antibody to conserved parts of *Plasmodium falciparum* merozoite surface protein 1 in Ghanaian children are not associated with protection from clinical malaria. Infect Immun 1999;67:2131–2137.

150. Sulzer AJ, Wilson M. The fluorescent antibody test for malaria. CRC Crit Rev Clin Lab Sci 1971;2:601–619.

151. Schapira A, Fogh S, Jepsen S, Pedersen NS. Detection of antibodies to malaria: comparison of results with ELISA, IFAT, and crossed immunoelectrophoresis. Acta Pathol Microbiol Immunol Scand [B] 1984;92:299–304.

152. Mannweiler E. Immundiagnostik der Malaria. Mikrobiologi 1997;7:3–10.

153. Leibovitz A, Freeborn RF, Lillie HJ, et al. The prevalence of malarial fluorescent antibodies in Vietnam returnees with no history of overt malaria. Mil Med 1969;134:1344–1347.

154. Brasseur P, Ballet JJ, Druilhe P. Impairment of *Plasmodium falciparum*–specific antibody response in severe malaria. J Clin Microbiol 1990;28:265–268.

155. Collins WE, Jeffery GM, Skinner JC. Fluorescent antibody studies in human malaria. II. Development and persistence of antibodies to *Plasmodium falciparum*. Am J Trop Med Hyg 1964;13:256–260.

156. Tobie JE, Abele DC, Hill GJD, et al. Fluorescent antibody studies on the immune response in sporozoite-induced and blood-induced vivax malaria and the relationship of antibody production to parasitemia. Am J Trop Med Hyg 1966;15:676–683.

157. Collins WE, Skinner JC, Jeffery GM. Studies on the persistence of malarial antibody response. Am J Epidemiol 1968;87:592–598.

158. Mannweiler E, Mohr W, zum Felde I, et al. Zur Serodiagnostik der malaria. Münch Med Wochenschr 1976;118:1139–1144.

159. Elm J, Desowitz R, Diwan A. Serological cross-reactivities between the retroviruses HIV and HTLV-1 and the malaria parasite *Plasmodium falciparum*. P N G Med J 1998;41:15–22.

160. Fonseca MO, Pang L, de Avila SDL, et al. Cross-reactivity of anti–*Plasmodium falciparum* antibodies and HIV tests. Trans R Soc Trop Med Hyg 2000;94:171–172.

161. Draper CC, Sirr SS. Serological investigations in retrospective diagnosis of malaria. BMJ 1980;280:1575–1576.

Chapter 13

Use of Rapid Malaria Tests for and by Travelers

Hans D. Nothdurft and Tomas Jelinek

ABSTRACT

Accurate and timely diagnosis and treatment of falciparum malaria in non-endemic areas is frequently complicated by lack of experience of involved laboratory personnel. Diagnostic tools based on the dipstick principle for the detection of plasmodial histidine-rich protein 2 (HRP-2) and parasite-specific lactate dehydrogenase (pLDH), respectively, have become available for the qualitative detection of falciparum malaria.

All dipstick tests have the potential to enhance speed and accuracy of the diagnosis of falciparum malaria, especially if the tests must be performed by nonspecialized laboratories. However, microscopic testing remains mandatory in every patient with the possible diagnosis of malaria, because occasionally, even high parasitemias are not detected by the rapid diagnostic test (RDT).

Nonfalciparum malaria is not reliably detected by the available RDTs, especially in patients with low parasitemias. Major modifications and improvements must be done before RDTs are able to diagnose tertian or quartan malaria.

Self-use of dipstick tests for malaria diagnosis by travelers should not be recommended routinely, as accuracy of test performance and interpretation of results by the traveler are uncertain. These tests should only be recommended to travelers for specific situations (i.e., long-term stay; far from medical assistance; expedition-type travel) and after appropriate instruction and training, including a successful performance of the test procedure.

Key words: dipstick tests for malaria; HRP-2; nonmicroscopic diagnosis of malaria; pLDH; rapid diagnostic tests; RDT.

Health facilities in areas not endemic for malaria increasingly face the challenge to diagnose and treat imported malaria rapidly and competently. Numbers of international travelers to malarious areas continue to rise. It has been estimated that 90% of infected travelers do not develop symptoms until after returning home.[1] Accurate and timely treatment of imported malaria requires fast and reliable diagnosis. Microscopic examination of stained blood films still remains the mainstay of diagnostic methods. However, correct interpretation of blood films requires considerable expertise that is not necessarily available at peripheral medical centers in non-endemic countries.[2] Thus, the availability of a simple and accurate test could greatly aid the diagnosis of malaria in nonimmune travelers.

Fast and simple dipstick tests for the rapid diagnosis of malaria (RDTs) are available. These immunochromatographic kits detect circulating parasite antigen by use of specific antibodies that are bound to a membrane: ICT Malaria Pf ® (ICT Diagnostics, Sydney, Australia) and ParaSight F® (Beckton-Dickinson, Franklin Lakes, U.S.A.) target histidine-rich protein 2 (HRP-2) of *Plasmodium falciparum*; OptiMAL® (Flow Inc., Portland, OR) detects parasite-specific lactate dehydrogenase (pLDH). Recently, a test kit capable of detecting antigen of *P. falciparum* and *P. vivax* has been introduced—ICT Malaria P.f/P.v® (ICT Diagnostics, Sydney, Australia). The principles and procedural steps of RDTs are shown in Figure 13–1.

SENSITIVITY AND SPECIFICITY OF RAPID DIAGNOSTIC TESTS IN DIFFERENT POPULATIONS

By the end of 2000, there were more than 40 studies published evaluating different RDTs in various populations.[3,4] Some of these studies compared RDTs by using light microscopy as the "gold standard" for diagnosis (Table 13–1).[5–11] The sensitivity for detecting symptomatic *P. falciparum* infections was high for all RDTs used and ranged between 90% and 100% compared to light microscopy results. In some cases, a positive RDT result was obtained before parasite detection by microscopic examination. However, at low parasitemias, the sensitivity of all tests decreased and was only 50% to 70% for parasitemias of less than 100/μL.[3,12]

Some studies showed a fair number of false-negative results of RDT testing even in patients with high parasitemias.[13,14] One possible explanation is that in some *P. falciparum* strains, the expression of the parasitic antigen is missing or decreased; therefore, the test could not detect that antigen. In the case of a false-negative ICT test in a patient with a parasitemia of 30%, the dilution of the blood sample by 1:10 produced a positive RDT result. This result could be explained as a prozone phenomenon in a blood sample with a high antigen concentration.[13]

Most studies showed a specificity between 90% and 100%; however, false-positive results are possible in all RDTs used, particularly in patients with rheumatoid factor[15–17] (Table 13–2).

Only a limited number of studies have evaluated the use of RDTs detecting nonfalciparum infections. In detecting *P. vivax* infections, the OptiMAL test achieved in several studies a sensitivity and specificity of more than 90%.[9,18,19] The ICT P.f/P.v test was comparable in terms of specificity (> 90%); in terms of sensitivity, however, it was 72% to 75%.[20,21] A new study using a second-generation ICT

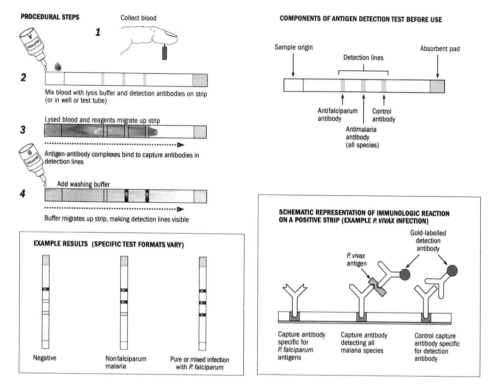

PROCEDURAL STEPS   Collect blood

1

2

Mix blood with lysis buffer and detection antibodies on strip
(or in well or test tube)

Lysed blood and reagents migrate up strip

3

Antigen-antibody complexes bind to capture antibodies in
detection lines

Add washing buffer

4

Buffer migrates up strip, making detection lines visible

EXAMPLE RESULTS (SPECIFIC TEST FORMATS VARY)

Negative   Nonfalciparum malaria   Pure or mixed infection with P. falciparum

COMPONENTS OF ANTIGEN DETECTION TEST BEFORE USE

Sample origin   Absorbent pad

Detection lines

Antifalciparum antibody   Control antibody

Antimalaria antibody (all species)

SCHEMATIC REPRESENTATION OF IMMUNOLOGIC REACTION ON A POSITIVE STRIP (EXAMPLE P. VIVAX INFECTION)

Gold-labelled detection antibody

P. vivax antigen

Capture antibody specific for P. falciparum antigens   Capture antibody detecting all malaria species   Control capture antibody specific for detection antibody

Figure 13–1. Principles and procedures of dipstick tests. (Reproduced with permission from World Health Organization. New perspectives—malaria diagnosis. Report of a joint workshop WHO/USAID informal consultation, 25–27 October 1999. Geneva: WHO, 2000.)

combined test in 19 European travelers infected with *P. vivax* found a sensitivity of 88% and a specificity of 99%.[22]

A commonality of all tests is that low parasitemias (< 500 parasites/µL)—common in patients with vivax malaria—produce a much lower sensitivity and are therefore inferior to microscopic diagnosis.[9,11,23]

No valid evaluations are available for RDTs detecting *P. ovale* and *P. malariae* infections. There are several reports on false-negative RDT results, in patients with microscopically confirmed infection with either *P. ovale* or *P. malariae*, for the OptiMAL and the ICT P.f/P.v tests.[12,24,25] The parasitemias of these infections are usually very low and seem to deter the diagnostic value of the currently available RDTs. In addition, no RDTs can accurately discriminate between *P. vivax*, *P. ovale*, and *P. malariae*, nor can they establish the diagnosis of a mixed infection of two or more *Plasmodium* spp.

SELF-USE OF RAPID DIAGNOSTIC TESTS BY TRAVELERS

Following the introduction of RDTs that can be performed without any laboratory equipment or complicated procedures, it was thought that the availability of a simple and accurate test could greatly aid the diagnosis of malaria in nonimmune travelers.

Table 13–1. **Comparative Studies on Sensitivity and Specificity of Rapid Diagnostic Tests**

Country	Year	Population*	Gold Standard†	ParaSight F		ICT		OptiMAL		Reference
				Sensitivity (%)	Specificity (%)	Sensitivity (%)	Specificity (%)	Sensitivity (%)	Specificity (%)	
Uganda	1997	OPD	Mic‡	71–97§	96	71–100§	92	—	—	5
France	1997	RT	Mic	93	98	96	98	—	—	6
Senegal	1998	OPD	Mic	88	87	89	100	—	—	7
Belgium	1998	RT	Mic	95	90	95	89	—	—	8
Honduras	1998	OPD||	Mic	65	—	65	—	88||	99||	9
Canada	1998	RT	PCR	94	95	90	97	—	—	10
Germany	1999	RT	Mic/PCR	—	—	92.5	98.3	88.5||	99.4||	11

* OPD = outpatients with malaria-like symptoms; RT = returning traveler with malaria-like symptoms.
† Mic = light microscopy of a thick and thin blood film; PCR = detection of plasmodia-specific deoxyribonucleic acid (DNA) after amplification with polymerase chain reaction (PCR).
‡ Microscopy by village workers.
§ Sensitivity according to parasitemias from 1–100/µL to 5,000/µL.
|| During a malaria outbreak.
Modified from Milne L, Kyi M, Chiodini P. Accuracy of routine laboratory diagnosis of malaria in the United Kingdom. J Clin Pathol 1994;47:740–742.

Table 13–2. **False-Positive Results of Rapid Diagnostic Tests in Patients with Rheumatoid Factor**

Type of Malaria RDT	False-Positive Results/No. Investigated Patients* (%)	
ParaSight F	15/92	(16.3)
ICT Malaria P.f	6/91	(6.6)
OptiMAL	3/91	(3.3)

RDT = rapid diagnostic test.
*Patients with positive rheumatoid factor and no history or signs of malaria.
Data from Grobusch MP, Alpermann U, Schwenke S, et al. False-positive rapid tests for malaria in patients with rheumatoid factor. Lancet 1999;353:297.

A febrile traveler who had a test kit could perform the test and then decide whether to take antimalarial treatment or not. A negative test result for malaria could prevent the traveler from taking unnecessary or even potentially harmful antimalarials.

The reliability and practicability of self-use of RDTs have been evaluated in several studies (Table 13–3). One hundred sixty healthy Swiss travelers were asked, prior to travel, to perform the ParaSight F test, following oral instructions. Only 75% of the individuals performed the test correctly; after more thorough written and oral instruction, the performance rate increased to 90%. However, the interpretation of results was still unsatisfactory (70.6% correct interpretations, with 14.1% false-negative results).[26] A comparative study (N = 98) of healthy volunteers who evaluated the ParaSight F test and ICT P.f test did not show any difference in the performance of either test, with a high level of interpretation and technical problems in both. The readings and interpretations at higher parasitemias (0.1% to 2%) were better in the ICT test (96% vs. 92% correct interpretations). At lower parasitemias (< 0.1%) the ParaSight F results were superior but still unsatisfactory (52% vs. 11%).[27]

Table 13–3. **Self-Use of Rapid Diagnostic Tests by Travelers**

Setting	Test Used	Main Findings
Healthy Swiss travelers—dry run prior to travel (Trachsler et al.)	ParaSight F (N = 160)	• 75% success after oral instruction; 90% success after additional oral/written instruction • 14% false-negative interpretation of pre-prepared test • Major technical modifications recommended
Healthy Swiss travelers—dry run prior to travel (Funk et al.)	ParaSight F, ICT P.f (N = 98)	• Interpretation problems at low parasitemias (< 0.1%) • High level of false-negative interpretations • Technical improvement and instruction required
Febrile travelers (Kenya) (Jelinek et al.)	ICT P.f (N = 98)	• 68% success with manufacturer's instructions only • Only 1 of 11 patients with confirmed falciparum malaria tested successfully • Intensive training/instruction required
Febrile returning travelers (London) (Behrens and Whitty)	ICT P.f (N = 153)	• 91% success after intensive instruction and assistance obtaining sample • In 22 patients with confirmed falciparum malaria: 100% success, sensitivity 95%, specificity 97%

A study from London used a different setting: febrile patients returning from malaria-endemic areas were asked to perform the ICT P.f test themselves and to interpret the results. The patients had detailed instructions on how to perform the test and were given assistance with problems obtaining the blood samples. Of 153 patients included in this study, 91% were able to perform the test correctly. All 22 patients with confirmed falciparum malaria interpreted the test results correctly. The calculated rates for sensitivity and specificity were 95% and 97%, respectively.[28]

Ninety-eight European tourists with fever were investigated in Kenya to see how well they performed the ICT P.f test by themselves.[29] While waiting for the microscopy results, patients were asked to perform and interpret the test, with only the instructions given by the test manufacturer. Only 68% of the patients performed the test correctly[30] (Table 13–4). More important, 10 of 11 patients with confirmed falciparum malaria did not achieve the diagnosis of malaria by using the RDT. When tested by the attending physician, all patients were clearly positive in the RDT.

Table 13–4. **Self-Use of Malaria Rapid Diagnostic Tests by Tourists: Reasons for Performance Problems***

Problem	n	%
Unable to draw blood (finger prick)	22	71.0
Unable to place the blood drop appropriately on the test kit	8	25.8
No adherence to the recommended waiting period (8 min)	12	38.7
Unable to identify the bands indicating the test result	18	58.1
Unable to interpret the result	27	87.1

*N = 31; multiple entries are possible.
Data from Jelinek T, Grobusch MP, Nothdurft HD. Use of dipstick tests for the rapid diagnosis of malaria in non-immune travelers. J Travel Med 2000;7:175–179.

REFERENCES

1. Molyneux M, Fox R. Diagnosis and treatment of malaria in Britain. BMJ 1993;306:1175–1180.
2. Milne L, Kyi M, Chiodini P. Accuracy of routine laboratory diagnosis of malaria in the United Kingdom. J Clin Pathol 1994;47:740–742.
3. Burchard GD. Malariaschnelltests. Bundegesundheitsbl Gesundheitsforsch Gesundheitsschutz 1999;42:643–649.
4. World Health Organization. New perspectives—malaria diagnosis. Report of a joint workshop WHO/USAID informal consultation, 25–27 October 1999. Geneva: WHO, 2000.
5. Kilian AH, Mughusu EB, Kabagambe G, von Sonnenburg F. Comparison of two rapid, HRP2-based diagnostic tests for *Plasmodium falciparum*. Trans R Soc Trop Med Hyg 1997;91:666–667.
6. Cavallo JD, Hernandez E, Gerome P, et al. Antigenemie HRP-2 et paludisme d'importation à *Plasmodium falciparum*: comparaison du ParaSight F et de'l lCT P.f. Med Trop (Mars) 1997;57:353–356.

7. Gaye O, Diouf M, Dansokho EF, et al. Diagnosis of *Plasmodium falciparum* using ParaSight F, ICT malaria PF and malaria IgG CELISA assays. Parasite 1998;5:189–192.
8. Van den Ende J, Vervoort T, Van Gompel A, Lynen L. Evaluation of two tests based on the detection of histidine rich protein 2 for the diagnosis of imported *Plasmodium falciparum* malaria. Trans R Soc Trop Med Hyg 1998;92:285–288.
9. Palmer CJ, Lindo JF, Klaskala WI, et al. Evaluation of the OptiMAL test for rapid diagnosis of *Plasmodium vivax* and *Plasmodium falciparum* malaria. J Clin Microbiol 1998;36:203–206.
10. Pieroni P, Mills CD, Ohrt C, et al. Comparison of the ParaSight-F test and the ICT Malaria Pf test with the polymerase chain reaction for the diagnosis of *Plasmodium falciparum* malaria in travellers. Trans R Soc Trop Med Hyg 1998;92:166–169.
11. Jelinek T, Grobusch MP, Schwenke S, et al. Sensitivity and specificity of dipstick tests for rapid diagnosis of malaria in nonimmune travelers. J Clin Microbiol 1999;37:721–723.
12. Dyer ME, Tjitra E, Currie BJ, Anstey NM. Failure of the 'pan-malarial' antibody of the ICT Malaria P.f/P.v immunochromatographic test to detect symptomatic *Plasmodium malariae* infection. Trans R Soc Trop Med Hyg 2000;94:518.
13. Risch L, Bader M, Huber AR. Self-use of rapid tests for malaria diagnosis. Lancet 2000;355:237.
14. Stow NW, Torrens JK, Walker J. An assessment of the accuracy of clinical diagnosis, local microscopy and a rapid immunochromatographic card test in comparison with expert microscopy in the diagnosis of malaria in rural Kenya. Trans R Soc Trop Med Hyg 1999;93:519–520.
15. Grobusch MP, Alpermann U, Schwenke S, et al. False-positive rapid tests for malaria in patients with rheumatoid factor. Lancet 1999;353:297.
16. Iqbal J, Sher A, Rab A. *Plasmodium falciparum* histidine-rich protein 2–based immunocapture diagnostic assay for malaria: cross-reactivity with rheumatoid factors. J Clin Microbiol 2000;38:1184–1186.
17. Laferl H, Kandel K, Pichler H. False positive dipstick test for malaria. N Engl J Med 1997;337:1635–1636.
18. Lee MA, Aw LT, Singh M. A comparison of antigen dipstick assays with polymerase chain reaction (PCR) technique and blood film examination in the rapid diagnosis of malaria. Ann Acad Med Singapore 1999;28:498–501.
19. Moody A, Hunt-Cooke A, Gabbett E, Chiodini P. Performance of the OptiMAL malaria antigen capture dipstick for malaria diagnosis and treatment monitoring at the Hospital for Tropical Diseases, London. Br J Haematol 2000;109:891–894.
20. Singh N, Saxena A, Valecha N. Field evaluation of the ICT malaria P.f/P.v immunochromatographic test for diagnosis of *Plasmodium falciparum* and *P. vivax* infection in forest villages of Chhindwara, central India. Trop Med Int Health 2000;5:765–770.
21. Tjitra E, Suprianto S, Dyer M, et al. Field evaluation of the ICT malaria P.f/P.v immunochromatographic test for detection of *Plasmodium falciparum* and *Plasmodium vivax* in patients with a presumptive clinical diagnosis of malaria in eastern Indonesia. J Clin Microbiol 1999;37:2412–2417.
22. Jelinek T, Grobusch MP, Harms G. Evaluation of a dipstick test for the rapid diagnosis of imported malaria among patients presenting within the network TropNetEurop. Scand J Infect Dis 2001. [In press]
23. Iqbal J, Sher A, Hira PR, Al-Owaish R. Comparison of the OptiMAL test with PCR for diagnosis of malaria in immigrants. J Clin Microbiol 1999;37:3644–3646.

24. Cooke AH, Chiodini PL, Doherty T, et al. Comparison of a parasite lactate dehydroge-nase–based immunochromatographic antigen detection assay (OptiMAL) with microscopy for the detection of malaria parasites in human blood samples. Am J Trop Med Hyg 1999;60:173–176.

25. John SM, Sudarsanam A, Sitaram U, Moody AH. Evaluation of OptiMAL, a dipstick test for the diagnosis of malaria. Ann Trop Med Parasitol 1998;92:621–622.

26. Trachsler M, Schlagenhauf P, Steffen R. Feasibility of a rapid dipstick antigen-capture assay for self-testing of travellers' malaria. Trop Med Int Health 1999;4:442–447.

27. Funk M, Schlagenhauf P, Tschopp A, Steffen R. MalaQuick versus ParaSight F as a diagnostic aid in travellers' malaria. Trans R Soc Trop Med Hyg 1999; 93:268–272.

28. Behrens RH, Whitty CJ. Self-use of rapid tests for malaria diagnosis. Lancet 2000; 355:237.

29. Jelinek T, Amsler L, Grobusch MP, Nothdurft HD. Self-use of rapid tests for malaria diagnosis by tourists. Lancet 1999;354:1609.

30. Jelinek T, Grobusch MP, Nothdurft HD. Use of dipstick tests for the rapid diagnosis of malaria in nonimmune travelers. J Travel Med 2000;7:175–179.

Chapter 14

CLINICAL TREATMENT OF MALARIA IN RETURNED TRAVELERS

Christoph Hatz

ABSTRACT

Millions of travelers are exposed to malaria each year. The infection can be cured with appropriate treatment. If the diagnosis is not made in time, the disease often has a fatal outcome. Three main classes of drugs used in industrialized countries are the quinoline-related compounds (quinine, quinidine, chloroquine, amodiaquine, mefloquine, halofantrine, and primaquine), the antifol drugs (proguanil, chlorproguanil, pyrimethamine, and trimethoprim), and the artemisinin derivatives. Vivax malaria is usually treated with chloroquine whereas this drug remains active against falciparum malaria in only a few places. Multidrug resistance of falciparum malaria is an increasing problem. This may result in reduced rates of parasite clearance in travelers, but it does not affect mortality. Management of severe malaria requires special attention. Fast-acting drugs achieve rapid parasite reduction. Other antimalarials with longer half-lives are required to eradicate the parasites in a second phase of treatment. Combination therapy is thus recommended in most cases of falciparum malaria to prevent recrudescence of infection.

Key words: malaria; management; nonimmune; antimalarial drugs.

INTRODUCTION

Early travelers, the Fathers of the Society of Jesus, brought the longest-known antimalarial drug across the Atlantic in the early 1600s. The Jesuits' bark was successfully promoted in Europe despite a polemic carried on for over 200 years on the merits of the medicament, long before the alkaloid quinine was isolated from the cinchona bark and before the malaria parasites were identified. On the other side of the universe, extracts of the qinghao plant had been used in China to treat fever. The antimalarial properties of the wormwood *Artemisia annua* were rediscovered 2,000 years later and are now entering the pharmacopeia of industrialized countries. Many of the antimalarial drugs developed and introduced in the 20th century were tied to warfare as armies fighting in tropical and subtropical countries lost "more men to malaria than bullets."[1] Mepacrine, dihydrofolate reductase inhibitors, and chloroquine are products of research in the middle of the last century. The development of resistance, mainly against falciparum malaria, resulted in new efforts during the wars in Asia, leading to the compounds mefloquine and halofantrine. In the absence of newly developed drugs, the 1990s saw a new effort to overcome the increasing resistance to almost all antimalarials. Combination therapies including established drugs and new derivatives such as atovaquone plus proguanil and artemether plus lumefantrine were successfully tested in endemic areas and are now becoming available in many countries worldwide.

The choice of treatment depends on the following points: (1) the age of the patients, (2) their level of immunity (including pregnancy), (3) the drug's adverse events profile, (4) intolerance reactions, (5) interactions with other drugs, (6) cost, (7) the severity of disease, (8) the presence of concomitant diseases, and (9) the assessment of potential resistance.[2] In industrialized countries, the efficacy and the adverse events profile are considered the most important factors. The therapeutic ratio of two of the major groups, quinoline-related compounds (quinine, quinidine, chloroquine, amodiaquine, mefloquine, halofantrine, primaquine) and antifol antimalarials (proguanil, chlorproguanil, pyrimethamine, trimethoprim), is narrow. Although these drugs are therefore considered more toxic than antibiotics, serious adverse events are rare.[3] The third major group of antimalarials in general use, the artemisinin derivatives, have the broadest time window of action on the asexual malarial parasites, and they produce the fastest parasite clearance.[4]

All imported cases should be treated with the best available drug with the lowest risk of adverse events. It is recommended that all drugs be dosed according to the recipient's weight.[5,6] Adults weighing between 60 and 90 kg are usually treated with fixed standard doses. Treatment in patients weighing < 60 kg or > 90 kg receive dosages according to their weight. The same dosages should be used irrespectively of both the duration of the patient's stay in endemic areas and the genetic background of the patient. Reduced doses are not appropriate as experience shows that the potential semi-immune status of African migrants may not always prevent these patients from developing severe disease and dying.[7] Reasons include the loss of immunity due to prolonged absence from an endemic country, previous low exposure, and concomitant diseases (personal observations). All antimalarials should be given with or after food, for better tolerance and therapeutic blood levels.

Falciparum malaria parasites that are resistant to chloroquine and to sulfadoxine/pyrimethamine have spread to most endemic areas. Whereas the development of chloroquine resistance was relatively slow,[8] resistance to the combination sulfadoxine/pyrimethamine occurred more rapidly, mainly due to the genetic determinants of point mutations in dihydrofolate reductase (DHFR).[9,10] Cross-resistance among quinolines is not fully understood and is somewhat puzzling; it exists between mefloquine and halofantrine,[11] but there is also evidence that increasing mefloquine resistance is associated with increased susceptibility to chloroquine.[12]

One factor for chloroquine resistance is drug pressure. Sensitivity may return if the drug pressure is removed; but in the absence of hard evidence, there is no place for recommending chloroquine to treat nonimmune patients with falciparum malaria in areas where chloroquine resistance has been previously established.

CURRENT THERAPY FOR UNCOMPLICATED MALARIA IN TRAVEL MEDICINE

Table 14–1 lists drugs currently registered in industrialized countries. Chloroquine, quinine, mefloquine, and halofantrine are used as monotherapies. Sulfadoxine/

Table 14–1. **Drugs for Malaria Treatment in Industrialized Countries**

Drug	Therapy	Plasmodia Treated	Advantages	Disadvantages
Chloroquine	M	Po, Pm, Pv, Pf (acute attacks in areas with full sensitivity)	Safety	Resistance (Pf, Pv)
Quinine	M/C	All	Efficacy; safety; switch to parenteral use in severe cases	AE; some resistance; often insufficient to clear all parasites
Mefloquine	M (C)	All	Efficacy; well documented	AE; some resistance
Halofantrine	M	All	Activity	(Fatal) AE; oral bioavailability; drug interaction (quinolines)
Sulfadoxine/ pyrimethamine	Fixed C	Pf (areas with full sensitivity) activity against Pv	Synergistic combination; tolerability intrinsically poor	Resistance (Pf); AE (especially in HIV-positive patients);
Atovaquone/ proguanil	Fixed C	Pf, Pv; (Po, Pm)	Efficacy against multi-drug-resistant parasites; safety; synergistic combination	Poor documentation in nonimmunes; risk of resistance development
Artemether/ lumefantrine	Fixed C	Pf, Pv; (Po, Pm)	Efficacy against multi-drug-resistant parasites; safety; synergistic combination; rapid action; low risk of resistance development	Availability; poor documentation in nonimmunes
Tetracycline, doxycycline	C with quinine	All	No resistance	Slow action
Clindamycin	C with quinine	Pf	Safety in children and pregnant women	Only in combination with quinine or quinidine
Primaquine	M	Liver stages of Pv and Po	Efficacy against hypnozoites	Risk of hemolysis (G6PD)

AE = adverse effects; C = combination; G6PD = glucose-6-phosphate dehydrogenase; HIV = human immunodeficiency virus; M = monotherapy; Pf = *Plasmodium falciparum*; Pm = *Plasmodium malariae*; Po = *Plasmodium ovale*; Pv = *Plasmodium vivax*.

pyrimethamine, atovaquone/proguanil and artemether/lumefantrine are fixed combinations. Tetracyclines (doxycycline) and clindamycin are usually combined with quinine. Some of these drugs are not registered in all countries.

Patients suffering from malaria due to *Plasmodium vivax*, *Plasmodium ovale*, and *Plasmodium malariae* are usually treated as outpatients. Treatment of uncomplicated falciparum malaria at home is an option under specific conditions in some countries whereas hospital treatment is always practiced in other countries. Table 14–2 summarizes a decision tree that has been adopted in Switzerland. Clinical and social factors (e.g., living alone) govern the recommendations for practical use, which are based on experience in this particular health system. Outpatient treat-

Table 14–2. **Decision Process Summary for Treatment of Falciparum Malaria in Industrialized Countries**

Signs of Uncomplicated Malaria	*Clinical Manifestations Suspicious of Developing Severe (=Complicated) Malaria**		*Clinical Manifestations of Severe Malaria (Poor Prognosis)*

Fever, rigors
Headache
Body and joint aches
Myalgia
Abdominal pain, diarrhea
Nausea, vomiting
Dry cough
	Poor health status
	Any neurologic sign with or
	  without high fever
	Repeated vomiting
	Oliguria
	Biochemical features[†]
			(*Impaired consciousness*)
			(*Respiratory distress*)
			Pulmonary edema
			Prostration
			(*Circulatory collapse*)
			(*Multiple convulsions*)
			Jaundice
			Severe anemia
			(*Bleeding*)
			Biochemical and hematologic
			  features[‡]

Lab: thin and thick smear	Lab: thin and thick smear;
	  blood glucose
			Lab: thin and thick smear;
			  blood glucose; biochemical
			  and hematologic features[‡]

Decision	*Decision*		*Decision*
Outpatient treatment[§] or hospitalization: oral mefloquine, quinine with tetracycline or clindamycin, atovaquone/proguanil, artemether/lumefantrine; halofantrine, chloroquine, sulfadoxine/pyrimethamine in areas with known sensitivity to the drug	Hospitalization;[∥] quinine (oral)	Hospitalization; parenteral quinine	Hospitalization mandatory; parenteral quinine

* Recommendations for practical use, not proven by studies.
† Hypoglycemia (glucose < 2.2 mmol/L); parasitemia > 2%.
‡ Renal impairment (serum creatinine > 250 mol/L); acidosis (plasma bicarbonate < 15 mmol/L); jaundice (serum total bilirubin > 43 mol/L); elevated aminotransferase levels > 3 times normal; hyperlactatemia (venous lactate > 5 mmol/L); hypoglycemia (glucose < 2.2 mmol/L); parasitemia > 5%; > 5% of neutrophils contain malaria pigment.
§ Treatment at home: assurance that (1) patient can reach the doctor at any time, (2) patient is looked after for 48 hours at home, (3) transport to nearest hospital can be organized in case of deterioration of health status, and (4) clinical assessment including laboratory parameters is performed within 24 hours after initial treatment.
∥ Risk of aggravation at home.

ment may be considered if (1) the patient has no neurologic signs, (2) close monitoring is possible at home, and (3) medical help is assured in case problems arise.

If hospitalized patients with uncomplicated malaria have an uneventful course over the first 24 to 48 hours, it appears to be safe to discharge them.

Vivax, Ovale, Malariae, and Sensitive Falciparum Malaria

Chloroquine is the drug of choice for infections due to *Plasmodium ovale*, *Plasmodium malariae*, *Plasmodium vivax* (except for infections from Papua New Guinea, Sumatra, Irian Jaya, Burma, Vanuatu, India, and the Amazon region of Brazil), and *Plasmodium falciparum* (originating from Central America north of the Panama Canal, Haiti, Egypt, scattered parts of Asia, and South America) (Tables 14–3 and 14–4). Coadministrations with the "resistance-reversing" antihistamine chlorpheniramine[13] or promethazine are poorly documented and are not recommended for travelers.

Mefloquine or one of the new combination drugs (see Table 14–3) is the option in case of suspected resistance to chloroquine in vivax malaria.[14] Sulfadoxine/pyrimethamine is not recommended because *Plasmodium vivax* is intrinsically insensitive to this medication.[15]

Table 14–3. **Oral Dosage Regimens for Treatment of Malariae and Vivax/Ovale Malaria Infections**

Infection	Drug of Choice (Doses)	Second-Line Drug (Doses)
P. malariae	Chloroquine 25 mg base (10 mg/kg initial dose; 5 mg/kg each at 6, 24, 48 h)	Mefloquine 25 mg base (12.5 mg/kg initial dose; 8.3 mg/kg at 6–8 h and 4.2 mg/kg at 16 h)
Uncomplicated *P. vivax* and *P. ovale*, originating from chloroquine-sensitive areas	Chloroquine 25 mg base (10 mg/kg initial dose; 5 mg/kg each at 6, 24, 48 h)	Mefloquine 25 mg base (12.5 mg/kg initial dose; 8.3 mg/kg at 6–8 h and 4.2 mg/kg at 16 h)
Uncomplicated *P. vivax* and *P. ovale*, originating from Papua New Guinea, Sumatra, Irian Jaya, Burma, Vanuatu, India, and Amazon region in Brazil	Mefloquine 25 mg base (12.5 mg/kg initial dose; 8.3 mg/kg at 6–8 h and 4.2 mg/kg at 16 h)	Artemether/lumefantrine 8 mg/kg Ar, 48 mg/kg L (1.3 mg/kg Ar plus 8 mg/kg L at 0, 8, 24, 36, 48, 60 h) Atovaquone/proguanil 50 mg/kg At, 20 mg/kg P (16.7 mg/kg At plus 6.7 mg/kg P at 0, 24, 48 h)
Hypnozoites of *P. vivax* and *P. ovale*	Primaquine phosphate* 3.5 mg (base)/kg (0.25 mg [base]/kg daily for 14 d)	None available
Hypnozoites of *P. vivax* and *P. ovale* in Oceania and Southeast Asia	Primaquine phosphate* 4.6 mg (base)/kg (0.33 mg [base]/kg daily for 14–21 days)	None available

Ar = artemether; At = atovaquone; L = lumefantrine; P = proguanil; *P.* = *Plasmodium*.
* Primaquine: 26.3 mg of the salt equals 15 mg of the base.

Table 14–4. **Dosage Regimens for Treatment of Falciparum Malaria**

Type; Region of Origin	Drug of Choice* (Doses)	Second-Line Drug* (Doses)
Uncomplicated; Central America north of Panama Canal, Haiti, Egypt, scattered parts of Asia and South America	Chloroquine 25 mg base (10 mg/kg initial dose; 5 mg/kg each at 6, 24, 48 h)	Mefloquine 25 mg (base)/kg; sulfadoxine 20 mg/kg and pyrimethamine 1 mg/kg in a single oral dose
Uncomplicated, parasitemia < 2%; sub-Saharan Africa, South America, Asia (except areas with multidrug resistance [see below])	Mefloquine 25 mg base (12.5 mg/kg initial dose; 8.3 mg/kg mg at 6–8 h and 4.2 mg/kg at 16 h)	Artemether/lumefantrine 8 mg/kg Ar, 48 mg/kg L (1.3 mg/kg Ar plus 8 mg/kg L at 0, 8, 24, 36, 48, 60 h). Atovaquone/proguanil 50 mg/kg At; 20 mg/kg P (16.7 mg/kg At plus 6.7 mg/kg P at 0, 24, 48 h). Halofantrine 2 × 24 mg/kg (8 mg/kg each at 0, 6, 12 h;[†] repeat the dose 1 week later).
Uncomplicated, parasitemia < 2%; Thailand, Cambodia, Burma, Vietnam (Laos)	Quinine 210 mg (salt)/kg (10 mg [salt]/kg tid for 7 days) plus doxycycline 21 mg/kg (3 mg/kg od for 7 days) or clindamycin 140 mg/kg (10 mg/kg bid for 7 days).	Artemether/lumefantrine, atovaquone/proguanil; as above
Uncomplicated, but suspicious of developing severe malaria, parasitemia < 5%; any endemic region IV treatment preferred	Quinine 210 mg (salt)/kg (10 mg [salt]/kg tid for 7 d) plus doxycycline 21 mg/kg (3 mg/kg od for 7 days) or clindamycin 140 mg/kg (10 mg/kg bid for 7 days)	None available

Ar = artemether; At = atovaquone; L = lumefantrine; od = once daily; P = proguanil; tid = three times daily.
* Caution: not all drugs mentioned are available in all countries.
† Patients treated with halofantrine should be hospitalized. Halofantrine should not be given to patients with pre-existing cardiac conduction defects, those who have a long Q-Tc interval, those who have received mefloquine within the previous 28 days (chemoprophylaxis), and those who take drugs known to prolong the Q-Tc interval (quinine, quinidine, chloroquine, tricyclic antidepressants, neuroleptic drugs, terfenadine, and astemizole).

Prior to starting an eradication treatment of hypnozoites to prevent relapses of vivax and ovale malaria, a deficiency of the enzyme glucose-6-phosphate dehydrogenase (G6PD) must be ruled out. Oxydant hemolysis is a serious threat when primaquine is administered in patients with this enzyme deficiency. A time lapse between chloroquine and primaquine treatments does not bear the risk of a relapse of vivax malaria since it usually takes a few weeks for relapses to occur after the initial attack. The dosage and the duration of primaquine therapy may be increased according to the origin of the vivax malaria. Some experts recommend giving a standard dose of 15 mg of adult dose per day for 21 to 28 days or 30 mg of adult dose per day for 14 days for vivax malaria from Asian and South American areas where primaquine failures have been reported.

Chloroquine causes gastrointestinal adverse effects, transient accommodation disturbance, and (rarely) neuropsychologic effects (dysphoria, cerebellar dysfunction, and transient neuropsychiatric syndrome). Pruritus is an unpleasant event in dark-skinned patients.

Primaquine also causes gastrointestinal disturbances if it is taken on an empty stomach, but hemolysis is the crucial problem with this drug.

Sulfadoxine/pyrimethamine has been associated with hepatitis, blood dyscrasias, and exfoliative dermatitis.

Chloroquine-Resistant *Plasmodium falciparum*

There are a number of options for treating chloroquine-resistant uncomplicated falciparum malaria (see Table 14–4). Mefloquine is the best-documented drug and has been registered in industrialized countries for more than 15 years.[16] Its long elimination half-life of 2 to 3 weeks does not allow adjusted treatment if adverse events occur.[17] Although relatively well tolerated, mefloquine may cause self-limiting neuropsychologic reactions in up to 0.5% to 1% of treated travelers.[18,19] The drug is contraindicated in patients with a history of seizures and psychiatric disorders. Giddiness, clouding of consciousness, and nightmares are regularly reported by patients as very disturbing side effects of treatment or chemoprophylaxis.

Mefloquine (split dose of 15 and 10 mg/kg on days 2 and 3) in combination with artesunate (4 mg/kg each on days 1, 2, and 3) has been the standard treatment of uncomplicated multidrug-resistant falciparum malaria in Thailand for more than 5 years.[20] This medication is not registered in industrialized countries. Therefore, oral quinine in combination with tetracyclines or clindamycin (for children < 8 years old and for pregnant women)[21] are among the recommended treatments for infections from areas with multidrug-resistant falciparum malaria in those countries. Quinine and quinidine (registered in the United States) are efficacious and safe although their therapeutic ratio is narrow; they are always given in combination with tetracyclines or clindamycin, which may be started after the initial dose of quinine or quinidine. The possibility of switching from oral to parenteral administration in case the patient's clinical condition deteriorates is an advantage over other antimalarials registered in industrialized countries. The main disadvantage is that neither drug is well tolerated. The bitter taste and cinchonism (nausea, dysphoria, tinnitus, and deafness to high tones) often lead to poor compliance with the recommended 7-day regimen. Tetracyclines and clindamycin cause mainly mild gastrointestinal disturbances, photosensitivity, and allergic (skin) reactions.

Halofantrine is better tolerated than mefloquine,[22] but its oral bioavailability is poor if the drug is not taken with a fatty meal. Atrioventricular conduction problems and ventricular repolarization disturbances may cause fatal arrhythmia, which is why halofantrine may only be given under close supervision (i.e., in a hospital). It must not be given to patients with an abnormally long corrected Q-T interval or to those who take drugs that may prolong the Q-T interval.[23]

Two combination medicaments are registered in some industrialized countries. Atovaquone/proguanil and artemether/lumefantrine are highly efficacious blood schizonticides against multidrug-resistant falciparum malaria and have a good safety profile among patients in endemic areas of Africa and Asia.[24,25] The risk of developing point mutation atovaquone resistance may affect the use of the synergistic atovaquone/proguanil if it is being used on a large scale.[26] Artemether/lumefantrine possibly clears the parasites faster. Both combinations are still poorly documented in nonimmune patients.

Adverse events that are mainly mild include (in order of frequency) abdominal pain, headaches, diarrhea, and vomiting for atovaquone/proguanil, and headaches, anorexia, abdominal pain, dizziness, and sleeping disturbances for artemether/lumefantrine. Neurotoxicity (brain stem nuclei damage) has been reported after parenteral artemether administration in animals but not after oral administration.[27,28] There has been no report on such toxicity in humans.[29] There is also no evidence of cardiotoxicity during antimalarial treatment with artemether/lumefantrine,[30] a suspicion raised by the relationship of the chemical structures of lumefantrine and halofantrine. Careful monitoring for rare but serious potential adverse events will tell how safe the two new combination drugs are.

Most drugs are safe for use in children > 5 kg in body weight. Antimalarials are generally well tolerated, but vomiting occurs more often, suggesting that antiemetics be administered. Drug interactions (e.g., metoclopramide and atovaquone) must be considered, though. If vomiting occurs within 1 hour, the full dose is repeated (for vomiting of mefloquine between 30 and 60 minutes, give a half dose). If vomiting occurs later, it is not necessary to re-administer the drugs.[17] Fever reduction is achieved with physical measures and antipyretics (caution is advised with paracetamol/acetaminophen because of liver toxicity).

The following drugs can be administered to pregnant women: chloroquine, sulfadoxine/pyrimethamine (second trimester), quinine, quinidine, and mefloquine (second and third trimesters). No data exist on artemisinin derivatives in pregnancy. Except for halofantrine and primaquine, all antimalarial drugs may be given to women who are breastfeeding.

Therapeutic Response

Assessment of the therapeutic response depends on the severity of the disease. In severe falciparum malaria, a rise in parasitemia within 12 to 24 hours has been reported, but rising parasitemia beyond 36 to 48 hours after the start of treatment with an antimalarial may indicate treatment failure.[31] In uncomplicated falciparum malaria, parasite clearance is usually achieved within 3 days. The classic assessment of three grades of resistance is still valid for malaria in nonimmune patients.[32] New criteria for assessing clinical response (adequate clinical response; early and late failures) have been designed for patients in endemic areas and do not appear to be appropriate for assessing the therapeutic response in nonimmune travelers.[33]

Antimalarial Drug Interactions

Mefloquine, halofantrine, quinine, and quinidine are structurally similar and may compete for blood- and tissue-binding sites. Cardiotoxicity of these drugs is assumed to be additive. Combined quinine and mefloquine therapy, however, did not produce significant adverse cardiovascular events[34] in uncomplicated malaria. Quinine may therefore be safely administered in patients who have previously taken mefloquine for malaria chemoprophylaxis.

Drug interactions of antimalarials with antiretrovirals and medicaments against opportunistic infections need careful consideration in travelers who are positive for human immunodeficiency virus (HIV).[35]

Breakthrough Malaria

An estimated 75% of travelers take an irregular chemoprophylactic regimen or no chemoprophylactic regimen.[36] Malaria attacks are therefore to be expected among this group. Few travelers who take regular chemoprophylaxis suffer from a confirmed malaria attack. Such breakthrough malaria occurs in the presence of nontherapeutic blood levels of the drug. Although the same drug used for prophylaxis could often be administered in therapeutic dosages, switching to another drug is generally recommended in such cases. However, if mefloquine is the chemoprophylactic drug, halofantrine must not be given as treatment, due to the increased risk of fatal cardiac arrhythmia.

Recrudescent Infections

Patients treated with any antimalarial drug should be cautioned that a symptomatic recrudescence of parasitemia may occur after 1 or several weeks. In such cases, treatment with an alternative medication against potential multidrug-resistant parasites is administered, and the parasitemia is subsequently followed until clearance. In vitro testing is not routinely recommended.

MANAGEMENT OF SEVERE MALARIA

Initial Treatment

Parenteral treatment with quinine should be started as quickly as possible in severe malaria (Table 14–5). Due to the risk of drug resistance, chloroquine has no place in treating severe falciparum malaria in nonimmune travelers The only drugs for parenteral use in industrialized countries are quinine and quinidine. Whereas quinine is used in most countries, quinidine is in use in the United States because of its wide availability. Quinidine-treated patients should be monitored electrocardiographically because of a fourfold greater effect on the heart. Patients treated with parenteral quinine do not routinely need such monitoring. The main adverse

Table 14–5. **Parenteral Treatment of Severe (Complicated) Falciparum Malaria**

Drug of Choice (Doses)	*Second-Line Drug (Doses)*
Quinine dihydrochloride* salt by intravenous infusion: total dose of 160–190 mg/kg over 7 days (7 mg [salt]/kg loading dose over 30 min, or 20 mg [salt]/kg loading dose infused over 4 h, followed by 10 mg/kg salt infused over 4 h every 8 h for at least 3 days; subsequently, a dose reduction by 30% to 50% is appropriate) plus doxycycline 21 mg/kg (3 mg/kg od over 30 min for 7 days) or clindamycin 140 mg/kg (10 mg/kg bid over 30 min for 7 days)[‡]	Quinidine[†] 10 mg (base)/kg infused at a constant rate over 1 h, followed by 0.02 mg/kg/min
	Electrocardiographic monitoring

bid = twice daily; od = once daily.
* Not available in the United States.
[†] Currently recommended in the United States.
[‡] 1. No loading dose if mefloquine was previously given.
  2. Monitoring of dosage if possible: therapeutic level at 20–40 mol/L (8–15 mg/L).
  3. No reduction of initial two dosages in patients with renal failure; no increase in dosage when dialysis is performed.
  4. Oral treatment should be substituted as the patient can take tablets by mouth (earliest after 24 h IV treatment).

event of parenterally given quinine and quinidine is hypoglycemia, which is caused by both drug-induced hyperinsulinemia (usually after at least 24 hours of treatment) and malaria itself.[37] Pregnant women are most prone to this problem.[38]

The pharmacokinetic properties of quinine-related drugs are influenced by malaria, with a reduced volume of distribution and a reduction in clearance that is proportional to the severity of disease.[39] Doses should therefore be reduced by 30% to 50% after the 3rd day of treatment to avoid accumulation of the drugs in patients who remain seriously ill.[17] Binding to plasma proteins is increased in malaria, explaining the different occurrences of severe adverse events in subjects with and without malaria.

Parenterally administered quinine and artemether show an equal effect in mortality rates but indicate a trend toward greater effectiveness of artemether in regions with recognized quinine resistance.[40] Parenteral artemisinin drugs are not yet marketed in industrialized countries.

If a severe course of malaria is suspected or confirmed (see Table 14–2) and no parenteral treatment is available within 2 hours, treatment should be started before the patient is transferred to the highest possible level of care. Preferentially, an antiemetic applied rectally or orally should be given, followed by oral quinine if the patient can swallow. Mefloquine and halofantrine are not generally recommended if a co-medication with cardioactive drugs exists. The measures taken by the primary care physician are documented and communicated to the hospital. The fear of subsequent problems arising from drug interaction should not interfere with this decision. Potential drug interactions can be handled at the intensive care unit as long as the potential of problems is acknowledged.

Intensive Care

The management of a patient with severe malaria is described in a special publication[41] that states the detailed principles of intensive care. A lumbar puncture (to rule out concomitant bacterial meningitis) and blood cultures are recommended in cases of severe malaria.[42] Acute renal failure, jaundice, and pulmonary edema were found to be more common among adults than children in endemic areas. Special attention is given to the hydration status because of the risk of pulmonary edema resulting from fluid overload or increased capillary permeability. Monitoring of central venous pressure (0 to 5 cm), a balanced fluid intake, and a propped-upright position help to prevent pulmonary edema. Once pulmonary edema is established, oxygen and further reduction of central venous pressure (best done by venesection) is required. Correction of hypoglycemia, metabolic acidosis, and coagulation problems must be assured. Skeletal-muscle damage increases during initial therapy, thus contributing to the risk of impaired renal function.[43] Hemodialysis is useful in oliguric and nonoliguric acute renal failure in patients with severe malaria, particularly when initiated early in the course of illness.[44]

Recommended supportive treatments include antipyretics such as paracetamol/acetaminophen (caution: liver toxicity in long-term use) or ibuprofen. The latter is less safe in case of bleeding diathesis but may lower the temperature more efficiently.[45] Anticonvulsants are currently recommended in case of any epileptic sign, but their prophylactic use is still in dispute.[41]

Exchange Blood Transfusion

The benefits of exchange blood transfusion (EBT) have not been documented in randomized controlled trials. It is known that nonimmune patients with high parasitemia have been cured with drug treatment only.[46] However, EBT is worth considering because it can achieve (1) the removal of rigid, nondeformable, parasitized, and unparasitized red blood cells; (2) the rapid reduction of parasite burden, antigen load, and parasite-derived toxins; and (3) the replenishment of healthy and unparasitized cells with normal mechanical properties. Fluid overload, transfusion-related infections, and transfusion reactions can be avoided or managed in well-equipped intensive care units (ICUs) of hospitals in industrialized countries. Suggested indications for EBT for hyperparasitemia in cases of imported falciparum malaria include (1) a parasitemia > 30% in the absence of clinical complication, (2) a parasitemia > 10% in the presence of severe disease, and (3) a parasitemia > 10% and poor prognostic factors (e.g., elderly patient, late-stage parasites in the peripheral blood, pigment in leukocytes).[41]

Red cell exchange (erythrocytapheresis) has been suggested as an alternative measure, using an automated cell separator. The risk of hemodynamic disturbance is thus reduced, but the method will not remove the parasite-derived toxins.[47]

DOUBTFUL ANCILLARY TREATMENTS

The following ancillary treatments are not recommended because they have not been shown to be beneficial in cerebral malaria:[41]

- Corticosteroids
- Other anti-inflammatory/antiedema agents
- Hyperimmune serum
- Iron-chelating agents (desferrioxamine B)
- Adrenaline
- Prostacyclin; cyclosporin A
- Oxypentifylline
- Low-molecular-weight dextran
- Anti–tumor necrosis factor antibodies
- Hyperbaric oxygen
- Heparin
- Dichloracetate

CONCLUSION

Effective drugs are currently available to treat all cases of malaria in nonimmune patients, provided that the patient is referred in time. In the future, the increasing resistance of malaria parasites may be managed by new drug combinations and (it is hoped) by newly detected or developed antimalarials.

ACKNOWLEDGMENTS

The author wishes to thank Drs. B. Genton, K. Markwalder, J. Blum, and B. Beck for critically reviewing the manuscript.

REFERENCES

1. Melville CH. The prevention of malaria in war. In: Ross R, editor. The prevention of malaria. 2nd ed. London: Murray, 1911.
2. Newton P, White NJ. Malaria: new developments in treatment and prevention. Annu Rev Med 1999;50:179–192.
3. White NJ. Drug treatment and prevention of malaria. Eur J Clin Pharmacol 1988;34:1–14.
4. ter Kuile F, White NJ, Holloway P, et al. *Plasmodium falciparum*: in vitro studies of the pharmacodynamic properties of drugs used for the treatment of severe malaria. Exp Parasitol 1993;76:85–95.
5. Corachan M, Gascon J. Malaria chemoprophylaxis and traveller's weight. Lancet 1988;2:791–792.

6. Schwartz E, Regev-Yochay G, Kurnik D. Short report: a consideration of primaquine dose adjustment for radical cure of *Plasmodium vivax* malaria. Am J Trop Med Hyg 2000;62:393–395.

7. Schönberg I, Apitzsch L, Rasch G. Malariaerkrankungen und Sterbefälle in Deutschland, 1993–1997. Gesundheitswesen 1998;60:755–761.

8. Moore DV, Lanier JE. Observations on two *Plasmodium falciparum* infections with abnormal response to chloroquine. Am J Trop Med Hyg 1961;10:5–9.

9. Peterson DS, Walliker D, Wellems T. Evidence that a point mutation in dihydrofolate reductase-thymidylate synthase confers resistance to pyrimethamine in falciparum malaria. Proc Natl Acad Sci U S A 1988;85:9114–9118.

10. Basco LK, Tahir R, Keundjian, Ringwald P. Sequence variations in the genes encoding dihydropteroate synthase and dihydrofolate reductase and clinical response to sulfadoxine-pyrimethamine in patients with acute uncomplicated falciparum malaria. J Infect Dis 2000;182:624–628.

11. Cowman AF, Galatis D, Thompson JK. Selection for mefloquine resistance in *Plasmodium falciparum* is linked to amplification of the pfmdr1 gene and cross-resistance to halofantrine and quinine. Proc Natl Acad Sci U S A 1994;91:1143–1147.

12. Brasseur P, Kouamouo J, Brandicourt O. Patterns of in-vitro resistance to chloroquine, quinine, and mefloquine of *Plasmodium falciparum* in Cameroon 1985–1986. Am J Trop Med Hyg 1988;39:166–172.

13. Sowumni A, Oduola AMJ, Ogundahunsi OAT, Salako LA. Comparative efficacy of chloroquine plus chlorpheniramine and pyrimethamine/sulfadoxine in acute uncomplicated falciparum malaria in Nigerian children. Trans R Soc Trop Med Hyg 1998;92:77–81.

14. Blum J, Tichelli A, Hatz C. [Diagnostic and therapeutic difficulties with tertian malaria.] Schweiz Rundsch Med Prax 1999;88:985–991.

15. Laing ABG. Hospital and field trials of sulphormethoxine with primaquine against Malaysian strains of *P. falciparum* and *P. vivax*. Med J Malaysia 1968;23:15–19.

16. Markwalder K, Hatz C. Malaria-Therapie 1998. Schweiz Med Wochenschr 1998; 128:1313–1327.

17. White NJ. The treatment of malaria. New Engl J Med 1996;335:800–806.

18. Weinke T, Trautmann M, Held T. Neuropsychiatric side effects after the use of mefloquine. Am J Trop Med Hyg 1991;45:86–91.

19. Phillips-Howard PA, ter Kuile FO. CNS adverse events associated with antimalarial agents: fact or fiction? Drug Saf 1995;12:370–383.

20. Price RN, Nosten F, Luxemburger C, et al. Artesunate/mefloquine treatment of multidrug resistant falciparum malaria. Trans R Soc Trop Med Hyg 1997;91:574–577.

21. Pukrittayakamee S, Chantra A, Vanijanonta S, et al. Therapeutic responses to quinine and clindamycin in multidrug resistant falciparum malaria. Antimicrob Agents Chemother 2000;44:2395–2398.

22. ter Kuile FO, Dolan G, Nosten F, at al. Halofantrine versus mefloquine in treatment of multidrug-resistant falciparum malaria. Lancet 1993;341:1044–1049.

23. Nosten F, ter Kuile FO, Luxemburger C, et al. Cardiac effects of antimalarial treatment with halofantrine. Lancet 1993;341:1054–1056.

24. Hatz C, Abdulla S, Mull R, et al. Efficacy and safety of CGP 56697 (artemether and benflumetol) compared with chloroquine to treat falciparum malaria in Tanzanian children aged 1–5 years. Trop Med Int Health 1998;3:498–504.

25. Looareesuwan S, Chulay JD, Canfield CJ, et al. Malarone™ (atovaquone and proguanil hydrochloride): a review of its clinical development for treatment of malaria. Am J Trop Med Hyg 1999;60:533–541.

26. Korsinczky M, Chen N, Kotecka B, et al. Mutations in *Plasmodium falciparum* cytochrome b that are associated with atovaquone resistance are located at a putative drug-binding site. Antimicrob Agents Chemother 2000;44:2100–2108.

27. Brewer TG, Peggins JO, Grate SJ, et al. Neurotoxicity in animals due to arteether and artemether. Trans R Soc Trop Med Hyg 1994;88 Suppl 1:S33–S36.

28. Nontprasert A, Pukrittayakamee S, Nosten-Bertrand M, et al. Studies of the neurotoxicity of oral artemisinin derivatives in mice. Am J Trop Med Hyg 2000;62:409–412.

29. Bakshi R, Hermeling-Fritz I, Gathmann I, Alteri E. An integrated assessment of the clinical safety of artemether-lumefantrine: a new oral fixed-dose combination antimalarial drug. Trans R Soc Trop Med Hyg 2000;94:419–424.

30. Van Vugt M, Ezzet F, Nosten F, et al. No evidence of cardiotoxicity during antimalarial treatment with artemether-lumefantrine. Am J Trop Med Hyg 1999;61:964–967.

31. Watt G, Shanks GD, Phintuyothin P. Prognostic significance of rises in parasitaemia during treatment of falciparum malaria. Trans R Soc Trop Med Hyg 1992;86:359–360.

32. World Health Organization. Chemotherapy of malaria and resistance to antimalarials. Report of a WHO Scientific Group. World Health Organ Tech Rep Ser 1973;529:30–35.

33. World Health Organization. Assessment of therapeutic efficacy of antimalarial drugs for uncomplicated falciparum malaria in areas with intense transmission. WHO/MAL/1996.

34. Supanaroanond W, Suputtamonkol Y, Davis TM, et al. Lack of significant adverse cardiovascular effect of combined quinine and mefloquine therapy for uncomplicated malaria. Trans R Soc Trop Med Hyg 1997;91:694–696.

35. Oehler T, Büchel B, Hatz C, Furrer HJ. Beratung HIV-Infizierter vor Reisen in tropische und subtropische Gebiete. Schweiz Med Wochenschr 2000;130:1041–1050.

36. Dorsey G, Gandhi M, Oyugi JH, Rosenthal PJ. Difficulties in the prevention, diagnosis, and treatment of imported malaria. Arch Intern Med 2000;160:2505–2510.

37. White NJ, Warrell DA, Chanthanavich P, et al. Severe hypoglycemia and hyperinsulinemia in falciparum malaria. N Engl J Med 1983;309:61–66.

38. Looareesuwan S, Phillips RE, White NJ, et al. Quinine and severe malaria in late pregnancy. Lancet 1985;2:4–8.

39. White NJ, Looareesuwan S, Warrell DA, et al. Quinine pharmacokinetics and toxicity in cerebral and uncomplicated falciparum malaria. Am J Med 1982;73:564–572.

40. Pittler MH, Ernst E. Artemether for severe malaria: a meta-analysis of randomized clinical trials. Clin Infect Dis 1999;28:597–601.

41. World Health Organization. Severe falciparum malaria. Trans R Soc Trop Med Hyg 2000;94 Suppl 1:110.

42. Berkley J, Mwarumba S, Bramham K, et al. Bacteraemia complicating severe malaria in children. Trans R Soc Trop Med Hyg 1999;93:283–286.

43. Davis TM, Supanaranond W, Pukrittayakamee S, et al. Progression of skeletal muscle damage during treatment of severe falciparum malaria. Acta Trop 2000;76:271–276.

44. Wilairatana P, Westerlund EK, Aursudkij B, et al. Treatment of malarial acute renal failure by hemodialysis. Am J Trop Med Hyg 1999;60:233–237.

45. Krishna S, Pukrittayakamee S, Supanaranond W, et al. Fever in uncomplicated *Plasmodium falciparum* malaria: randomized double-"blind" comparison of ibuprofen and paracetamol treatment. Trans R Soc Trop Med Hyg 1995;89:507–509.

46. Burchard GD, Kröger J, Knobloch J, et al. Exchange blood transfusion in severe falciparum malaria: retrospective evaluation of 61 patients treated with, compared to 63 patients treated without, exchange transfusion. Trop Med Int Health 1997;8:733–740.

47. Macallan DC, Pockock M, Robinson GT, et al. Red cell exchange, erythrocytapheresis, in the treatment of malaria with high parasitaemia in returning travellers. Trans R Soc Trop Med Hyg 2000;94:353–356.

Chapter 15

STANDBY EMERGENCY TREATMENT BY TRAVELERS

Patricia Schlagenhauf

ABSTRACT

Whereas prophylaxis remains the safest choice for most travelers to areas of high malaria transmission when their stay in the area is longer than 1 week, standby emergency treatment (SBET) is an option for clearly defined situations. Care should be taken in recommending an SBET strategy, and antimosquito measures should be stressed. Concise advice is necessary for travelers, along with stress on the importance of medical consultation at the first sign of illness. Travelers' behavior and the difficulty of defining simple diagnostic guidelines are delimiting factors in this strategy. In choosing a suitable SBET agent, the following must be considered: (1) level of malaria transmission at the destination, (2) type and intensity of resistance, (3) efficacy and toxicity of available options, (4) prophylactic agent used (if applicable), and (5) ease of administration of the standby therapy. There is no worldwide consensus as to the choice and use of SBET, and some countries are very restrictive in their SBET recommendations. The future points to the use of newer combination therapies for this indication, assuming that the cumulative experience of such therapies in nonimmune subjects is favorable. Simple diagnostic tests would mitigate the most negative aspect of the SBET strategy, namely, the self-diagnosis of malaria; but to date, travelers have experienced major problems in the performance and interpretation of these tests.

Key words: atovaquone/proguanil; artemether/lumefantrine; malaria; rapid tests; standby emergency self-treatment; travelers.

INTRODUCTION

Self-treatment of malaria on the basis of indicative symptoms is by no means a modern concept. Indeed, this response to fever preceded the identification of plasmodia and the science of malariology. Cinchona bark was the 17th-century febrifuge, and the Chinese medicinal herb qinghaosu (*Artemisia annua L)* (Figure 15–1) was recommended for the treatment of fever in a pharmacopeia of emergency prescriptions from A.D. 341.[1]

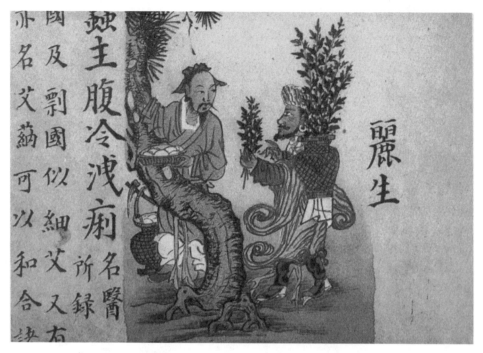

Figure 15–1. *Artemisia annua L,* Chinese febrifuge herb. (See Color Plates)

DEFINITION, RATIONALE, AND GUIDELINES FOR USE

SBET is described by the World Health Organization (WHO) as the self-administration of antimalarial drugs when malaria is suspected and when prompt medical attention is unavailable within 24 hours of the onset of symptoms.[2] Presumptive self-treatment is thus indicated only in emergency situations and must be followed by medical consultation as soon as possible. This concept has been reviewed recently.[3] The rationale for SBET is based on a risk-benefit analysis. Prophylactic drugs have traditionally been recommended to those at risk of acquiring malaria. The goal of prophylaxis is to prevent symptomatic malarial infection; however, prophylaxis carries a risk of adverse events (AEs). Most of these events are mild, but serious AEs have been reported.

A risk-benefit analysis (AEs vs. avoided infections) is necessary for travelers minimally exposed to malarial infection. For low-risk malaria-endemic areas of Asia and South America, the risk of toxicity from chemoprophylactic drugs actually outweighs the benefit of avoided infection; here, SBET offers an alternative. Furthermore, it is recognized that no antimalarial prophylactic regimen gives complete protection, and this is especially true in areas of high transmission of resistant *Plasmodium falciparum.* Additional protection against breakthrough malaria can be afforded by the availability of a standby therapy. Thus, SBET has a place, whether used alone or in combination with a chemoprophylactic regimen.

Criteria for Recommendation

A traveler visiting a malaria-endemic area once only and for less than 1 week does not require SBET because even if he or she is bitten by an infected mosquito, a minimal period of 6 to 7 days will elapse before malaria symptoms develop, by which time the traveler will already be back in the home country. Other factors relevant to deciding on the need for standby medication include frequent or long-term travel, intended prophylactic cover, risk of falciparum malaria, and probable access to prompt diagnosis and treatment. Optimal chemoprophylactic regimens may not be chosen because of drug intolerance, concomitant use of interacting medications, or other contraindications. Chemoprophylactic regimens might not be advised for travelers who intend to visit resorts or cities without malaria risk; in these situations, however, deviations from the itinerary can place travelers at risk, and standby therapy may be warranted. In summary, SBET may be required by travelers who

- use suboptimal or no chemoprophylaxis and who may visit a remote malarious area far from health service facilities;
- have changing itineraries and who thus possibly visit foci of multidrug resistance not adequately covered by their prophylactic regimen;
- have contraindications to priority antimalarials and are therefore prescribed suboptimal or no chemoprophylaxis;
- are abroad for many months and who are at high risk of infection because of high exposure and poor compliance (e.g., backpackers); or
- frequently travel to malarious areas for short periods (e.g., aircrews,[4] businesspersons).

Individually targeted information on SBET is needed for expatriates, young children, pregnant women, and travelers with chronic illnesses.

Guidelines for Use

The traveler should be provided with simple written guidelines for the use of SBET. Indications for SBET are as follows:

1. The traveler is unwell, with fever (> 37.5°C) and/or other symptoms such as malaise, headache, myalgia, gastrointestinal-tract symptoms, or shivering.
2. Medical attention is unavailable within 24 hours of the onset of symptoms.
3. A minimal period of at least 6 days has elapsed since the traveler entered the malaria-endemic area.

Under such conditions, the traveler is advised to take the following steps:

1. Reduce fever (with tepid sponging and paracetamol).
2. Administer SBET with adequate fluids.

3. Seek medical attention at the first opportunity.

The traveler should be aware that the symptoms of malaria may often be mild and that fever is absent in some cases. WHO emphasizes that the important factors determining the survival of patients with falciparum malaria are early diagnosis and appropriate treatment. It should be stressed that malarial symptoms often occur after departure from endemic areas and that malaria must be considered in the differential diagnosis of any fever in anyone who has visited a malaria-endemic area within the previous year. If SBET is necessary, the traveler should be aware of the need to seek medical attention as soon as possible to check the presumptive diagnosis and to receive further advice and/or treatment.

International opinions differ on the role of presumptive treatment, as shown by varying Swiss,[5] U.K.,[6] and Centers for Disease Control and Prevention (CDC)[7] guidelines. The Swiss have a liberal approach and recommend carrying SBET rather than using chemoprophylaxis in areas with a very low risk of malaria.[5] The following SBET agents are recommended in Switzerland: chloroquine, mefloquine, sulfadoxine/pyrimethamine (Fansidar), artemether/lumefantrine (Riamet), and atovaquone/proguanil (Malarone). The U.K. list includes chloroquine, sulfadoxine/pyrimethamine (Fansidar), mefloquine, quinine plus sulfadoxine/pyrimethamine (Fansidar), and quinine plus doxycycline. CDC recommends sulfadoxine/pyrimethamine (Fansidar) and atovaquone/proguanil (Malarone) only. WHO recommends the use of several agents as possible SBET (Table 15–1). Halofantrine has been dropped from WHO guidelines for this indication, following reports that it can result in the prolongation of Q-Tc intervals and in ventricular dysrhythmias in susceptible individuals.

THERAPEUTIC EFFICACY AND TOXICITY OF SPECIFIC AGENTS

Available data suggest good to excellent effectiveness for the agents currently recommended as SBET. It is, however, unclear how closely the therapeutic potency of malarial treatments used for semi-immune populations can be correlated with the potency of similar regimens used by nonimmune subjects, but in many cases, this is the only currently available information on which to base recommendations.

Generalizations are further complicated by the evolution and changing epidemiology of drug-resistant strains. Areas of multidrug resistance pose a particular problem for SBET. Regions such as the northwestern and eastern border regions (respectively adjacent to Myanmar and Cambodia) of Thailand are areas of multidrug resistance (although these areas lie off the usual tourist trail). Travelers to areas of multidrug resistance must be aware that their emergency malarial treatment in such areas will most likely act as a short-term febrifuge and symptom suppressant rather than be a total cure, and that prompt medical attention is imperative.

Table 15–1. **Available Options for Standby Emergency Treatment**

Generic Name	Trade Name(s)	Amount per Dosage	SBET Dosage (Adult)
Chloroquine	Aralen, Avlochlor, Nivaquine, Resochin	Tablet: 100 or 150 mg (base); syrups available	600 mg on days 1 and 2, followed by 300 mg on day 3
Sulfadoxine/ pyrimethamine	Fansidar	Tablet: 500 mg/25 mg	3 tablets in a single dose
Sulfadoxine/ pyrimethamine/ mefloquine	Fansimef	Tablet: 500 mg/25 mg/250 mg	3 tablets in a single dose
Sulfalene/ pyrimethamine/	Metakelfin	Tablet: 500 mg/25 mg	3 tablets in a single dose
Mefloquine	Lariam, Mephaquin	Tablet: 250 mg (U.S., 228 mg)	5–6 tablets in divided doses,* depending on body weight
Quinine (sulfate, bisulfate, dihydrochloride, hydrochloride)		Tablet: 300 mg (salt)	600 mg (2 tablets) t.i.d. for 7 days (total of 42 tablets)
Atovaquone/ proguanil	Malarone	Tablet: 250 mg/100 mg	4 tablets daily as a single dose on 3 consecutive days (total of 12 tablets)
Artemether/ proguanil[†]	Riamet	Tablet: 20 mg/120 mg	4 tablets initially on day 1, followed by a further 4 tablets 8 hours later; 4 tablets twice daily on days 2 and 3 (total of 24 tablets)

SBET = standby emergency treatment; t.i.d. = three times daily; WHO =World Health Organization.
* Manufacturer's recommendation: 25 mg/kg for nonimmunes. WHO recommendation: 15 mg/kg (25 mg/kg for areas on Thailand border).
[†] There is a paucity of data regarding the efficacy and tolerability of these newer combinations in nonimmune travelers.
Note: halofantrine is no longer on the WHO-recommended list; for use under medical supervision only.

AEs also pose a problem because SBET may expose people to a significant drug risk, and this is a major factor in the treatment of "possible" malarias. With mefloquine, serious neurotoxicity is approximately 60 times more probable after treatment than with prophylactic use of the agent.[8] Halofantrine has been associated with fatal electrocardiographic changes, namely, prolongation of the Q-Tc interval.[9a,9b]

Chloroquine

Chloroquine was once the favored treatment for susceptible malaria; however, only *Plasmodium malariae* and *Plasmodium ovale* now remain fully sensitive to chloroquine. Resistant *Plasmodium vivax* has been reported.[10,11] The use of chloroquine as a possible SBET is currently limited due to widespread chloroquine-resistant *Plasmodium falciparum* (CRPF). It has been reported that over 90% of isolates in some parts of Southeast Asia are now resistant to chloroquine. The drug, however, remains effective on the island of Hispaniola, in Central America, and in the Near East.

Quinine

Quinine is effective against most CRPF although sensitivity to this agent is also diminishing in certain areas (notably Thailand and Vietnam). Quinine is associated with a spectrum of AEs including nausea, vomiting, headache, tinnitus, and cardiovascular side effects. This factor, together with its complicated dosage regimen, detracts from its usefulness as an SBET agent. Combination treatment regimens of quinine plus tetracycline have proven successful in areas of quinine resistance, but the complexity of such a combination regimen over a prolonged period (7 days) makes it a questionable option for SBET because of projected poor compliance. Rather, this treatment option is for malaria cases that are under a physician's supervision. On the plus side, quinine is an SBET agent that is considered safe for pregnant women,[2,8] who should nevertheless seek urgent medical attention for all febrile episodes.

Antifolate/Sulfa-Drug Combinations (Fansidar, Metakelfin)

The problem of resistance has been further compounded by the increasing prevalence of parasites resistant to the antifolate and sulfa-drug combinations, particularly in Southeast Asia (especially Thailand and Myanmar) and in South America (Amazon basin). The pyrimethamine/sulfadoxine (Fansidar) combination remains effective in parts of Africa (especially West Africa) and southern Asia. In individuals without a known intolerance to sulfonamides, the risk of severe cutaneous side effects (Stevens-Johnson syndrome and toxic epidermal necrolysis) with SBET appears to be lower than that reported with systematic repetitive dosages in a prophylactic setting. However, at least one serious adverse AE has been reported after SBET with pyrimethamine/sulfadoxine (Fansidar).[12]

Mefloquine

Multidrug-resistant strains of plasmodia remain largely sensitive to mefloquine, except in the notorious border regions of Thailand, which contain the most drug-resistant parasites in the world and which show mefloquine cure rates of only 41%[13] or lower. In vitro studies in both West Africa and Southeast Asia indicated the presence of resistant parasites prior to the use of the drug in those particular areas, suggesting that emerging resistance is a function of drug pressure. Despite the threat of a relentless rise in resistance, mefloquine satisfies many of the criteria for standby treatment, with a relatively simple dosage regimen over a short time period. Split dosage should reduce the incidence of AEs (especially vomiting, which occurs frequently at the levels of drug used for therapy). AEs, especially nausea and dizziness, have been observed, and cases of neuropsychiatric disturbances have been reported, including sporadic episodes of seizures, hallucinations, depression, and acute psychosis. Although the incidence of serious neuropsychiatric events in a prophylactic setting is relatively rare, neurotoxicity appears to be more probable after treatment

(1 in 216 cases) than with prophylactic use of mefloquine.[5] The mechanism of serious neurotoxicity is unknown and may be dose related[14] although serious AEs have occurred at relatively low plasma mefloquine concentrations. The drug has a long and variable mean terminal half-life, with interindividual variation ranging from 6 to 33 days; thus, for those using mefloquine prophylaxis, malaria treatment with mefloquine or quinine should be administered only under close medical supervision because of the possibility of added toxicity. There are promising reports of the use of an oral mefloquine/artesunate combination treatment, which may be a future possibility for the traveler. Luxemburger and colleagues[15] compared the therapeutic efficacy and toxicity of a combination of low-dose mefloquine (15 mg/kg) and artesunate (10 mg/kg) with that of the standard 25-mg/kg mefloquine dose in 552 patients with uncomplicated falciparum malaria on the Thailand-Myanmar border and found that the combination gave faster clinical and parasitologic responses and prevented early treatment failure.

For nonimmune adult travelers, the curative dose of mefloquine (6 tablets in 1 day) can be split into three doses taken at 6- to 8-hour intervals (e.g., $3 + 2 + 1$ or $2 + 2 + 2$), with the objective of reducing the incidence or severity of AEs. More data are required, especially with regard to compliance with the split dose used in an SBET setting. WHO[2] recommends a total mefloquine dose of 15 mg/kg or 1,000 mg (whichever is lower) except in Thailand border areas of multidrug resistance, where a total dose of 25 mg/kg (or 1,500 mg) is recommended (as an initial dose of 15 mg/kg, followed 6 to 8 hours later by 10 mg/kg).

Fansimef is a triple combination drug (tablets contain mefloquine [250 mg], sulfadoxine [500 mg], and pyrimethamine [25 mg]) that was developed to delay the development of mefloquine resistance,[16] a strategy that did not hinder the emergence of resistant strains. WHO does not include Fansimef in its list of recommended SBETs due to the concern that adding sulfadoxine/pyrimethamine (Fansidar) to mefloquine increases the risk of toxicity, with little benefit.

Halofantrine

Clinical trials have confirmed the efficacy of this phenanthrene methanol in the treatment of falciparum malaria in areas of chloroquine and sulfonamide/pyrimethamine resistance. In the eastern areas of Thailand, the efficacy of halofantrine is quite low (29%). Some failures of halofantrine have been attributed to its poor and variable absorption. The efficacy and tolerability of this agent have also been assessed in the treatment of acute malaria in returned nonimmune travelers,[17] when the malaria was imported from areas with drug-resistant *Plasmodium falciparum* (mainly in Africa). The breakthrough rate after the recommended single dose was 12%, but an efficacy rate of 100% was observed in patients (n = 29) who received an additional therapeutic dose 1 week after the initial treatment. Only mild AEs were observed in this study. Other reported AEs include a transient rise in liver enzymes, coughing, minor gastrointestinal-tract symptoms, headache, occasional pruritus, and rash.[18] There is, however, considerable anxiety regarding the arrhythmogenic potential of this agent, which can be fatal; 8 patients are known to have experienced cardiac arrest (6 patients died),[6] and a recent report from the CDC details the sudden death of a 22-year-old traveler in Togo following halofantrine administration.[9b] As a result of reports describing ventricular dysrhythmias and prolongation of Q-Tc intervals, halofantrine is no longer recommended by WHO for self-treatment. These cardiac changes may be accentuated if halofantrine is taken with other antimalarial drugs that can decrease myocardial conduction.[2,6] Nevertheless, some countries continue to recommend halofantrine as SBET when other agents are contraindicated, but only for those persons known to have a normal Q-Tc interval. A recent paper suggests that pretreatment electrocardiography (ECG) is poorly predictive of lengthening Q-Tc intervals during therapy.[19]

The manufacturer has expanded the list of contraindications to include personal or family history of heart disease that causes Q-T interval prolongation, concurrent use of a medication that may lengthen the interval, electrolyte imbalance, and thiamine deficiency. Halofantrine should not be given with food, and the dose should not exceed 24 mg/kg (given as 8 mg/kg in three doses at 6-hour intervals).

Artemisinin Derivatives

Artemisinin is derived from *Artemisia annua L,* which, has been used in Chinese traditional medicine for over 2,000 years. Artemisinin is a compound with a peculiar structure, low toxicity, and high efficacy even in severe CRPF malaria. This important antimalarial group (which includes artemether, arteether, and artesunate) is available in several dosage forms, including artesunate in tablet form. One disadvantage is a commonly reported recrudescence that can be avoided by combining the drug with a longer-acting antimalarial. As previously mentioned, a single day's treatment with artesunate augments the antimalarial efficacy of mefloquine[15] and provides a rapid initial therapeutic response followed by the sustained action of the longer-acting mefloquine. These agents are generally well tolerated, but there are worries regarding the neurotoxicity observed in animal studies.[20] Until recently, the use of these agents (alone or in combination) was limited to use in endemic populations because the artemisinin derivatives had to meet stringent Western safety standards before they could be approved. In early 1999, a new oral fixed-combination tablet containing artemether was registered in Switzerland for treatment and SBET of acute uncomplicated *Plasmodium falciparum* infection or mixed malarial infections (see "New Combinations of Agents," below).

Primaquine and Radical Cure

To achieve a radical cure (i.e., elimination of exoerythrocytic stages of *Plasmodium vivax* and *Plasmodium ovale* only), a follow-up course of primaquine is necessary (contraindicated for patients with glucose-6-phosphate dehydrogenase [G6PD] deficiency). The presumptive use of primaquine is rarely indicated for regular travelers but could be considered for such groups as volunteers or missionaries returning home after extensive periods of exposure in areas where *Plasmodium vivax* and *Plasmodium ovale* are endemic. It may also be indicated for refugee groups.[21]

Summary: Choice of Agent

Theoretically, there are several available medications that could be used as presumptive treatment in emergency situations. The choice of SBET will depend on the expected parasite type and level of drug resistance, the traveler's medical history, the availability of medication in the country of prescription, the prophylactic agent used (if applicable), and finally, the ease of administering the SBET under consideration. The range of options available are outlined in Table 15–1. Ideally, an SBET should be easily administered, and correct dosage and compliance should be easy to ensure. (In this regard, the simple therapy regimens have the advantage of easy administration.)

USE IN CHILDREN

Infants and young children are at special risk of malaria and should avoid endemic areas, especially those where CRPF is widespread. Impregnated mosquito nets should be used meticulously, and prophylaxis should be administered if appropriate. In cases of fever, every attempt must be made to seek prompt medical attention. Recommendations regarding pediatric doses for SBET are particularly difficult to formulate, and practical administration is further complicated by a paucity of pediatric formulations (Table 15–2). Chloroquine is available in syrup form, and halofantrine is available as a suspension (Halfan S). Otherwise, appropriate fractions of antimalarials can be crushed and mixed into jam. The approximate fractions of antimalarial dosages for children are given in Table 15–2.

EXPERIENCE TO DATE

Aircrews

Aircrews make up a group of frequently exposed travelers that has provided data on the use of emergency presumptive therapy. Continuous chemoprophylaxis was optional for Swissair crews after 1985, and a therapeutic approach was favored for all tropical Swissair stations in the Far East and South America and also for brief exposure in tropical Africa. Personnel carried mefloquine/sulfadoxine/pyrimethamine (Fansimef) and, later, mefloquine (Lariam) as standby therapy for emergencies. After an almost total adoption of the treatment dose recommendation, there was no significant increase in the number of malaria cases, and standby medication was used by only 1% per year.[4]

Table 15–2. **Drug Regimens for Standby Emergency Treatment: Childrens' Dosages***

Mefloquine†			Sulfadoxine/ Pyrimethamine (500 mg/25 mg)		Chloroquine‡ (100 mg Base)				Artemether/Lumefantrine§‖ (20 mg/120 mg)				Atovaquone/Proguanil§ (250 mg/100 mg)			
Weight (kg)	Hr 1	Hr 6–24	Weight (kg)	Single Dose	Weight (kg)	Day 1	Day 2	Day 3	Weight (kg)	Day 1	Day 2	Day 3	Weight (kg)	Day 1	Day 2	Day 3
5–6	¼	¼	5–6	¼	5–6	½	½	½	—	—	—	—	—	—	—	—
7–8	½	¼	7–10	½	7–10	1	1	½	—	—	—	—	—	—	—	—
9–12	¾	½	11–14	¾	11–14	1½	1½	½	10–15	2×1	2×1	2×1	11–20	1	1	1
13–16	1	½	15–18	1	2	½	—	—	—	—	—	—	—	—	—	—
17–24	1½	1	19–29	1½	19–24	2½	2½	1	15–25	2×2	2×2	2×2	21–30	2	2	2
25–35	2	1½	30–39	2	25–35	3½	3½	2	25–34	2×3	2×3	2×3	—	—	—	—
36–50	3	2	40–49	2½	36–50	5	5	2½	—	—	—	—	31–40	3	3	3

Hr = hour(s).

* Given as tablet fractions.

† The total dosage (25 mg [base]/kg) is divided into two doses: 15 mg (base)/kg, followed by 10 mg (base)/kg 6 to 24 hours later.

‡ The total dosage is 25 mg (base)/kg divided over 3 days. (Tablets usually contain either 100 mg or 150 mg chloroquine base.)

§ There is a paucity of data on efficacy and tolerability of this drug combination in nonimmune travelers.

‖ On day 1, the tablets should be taken at 8-hour intervals; on days 2 and 3, at 12-hour intervals.

Travelers

The use of SBET by travelers has been reviewed[22] (Table 15–3). In earlier studies, some 4% of travelers to East Africa, where the attack rate is 0.2% to 1.5%, used their standby medication, which would suggest a 2.5- to 20-fold overuse of SBET. Conversely, when an SBET strategy (rather than prophylaxis) was recommended for travelers to areas of low transmission such as Thailand, only a small number (< 1%) of travelers used the standby medication.[23] This latter study examined the use of SBET in a cohort of 1,187 travelers who were prepared to self-treat malarial symptoms. Illness (with fever as the main indicator) was reported by 10.4% of the group; 6 people actually used the SBET carried, but only 1 of the 6 had proven malaria. A 1993 German study[24] followed up 3,434 travelers to areas of varying risk and showed a similar low use of SBET (1.4%), indicating that overuse of SBET by travelers is not a major problem.

NEGATIVE FEATURES

There are few data regarding the efficacy of SBET agents in the presence of resistant parasites, and carrying SBET should not lead the traveler to a false sense of security, as demonstrated by the reported failure of self-treatment with presumptive oral therapy (pyrimethamine/sulfadoxine) in U.S. travelers returning from Kenya.[25] Travelers must be aware that SBET is an interim solution only and that prompt medical advice is essential even after therapy has been successfully administered.

Travelers' knowledge and behavior remain major stumbling blocks, and many individuals, despite being made aware of the urgency of malarial treatment, choose to wait for their symptoms to resolve spontaneously rather than seek prompt medical attention, as demonstrated in a Zurich study[23] in which two-thirds of those who were ill failed to seek immediate medical attention. This problem was empha-

Table 15–3. **Travelers' Use of Malaria Standby Emergency Treatment**

Year	Agent	Travelers' Origin	Destination	Use (%)
1987/1988	SDX/PYR	Swiss	Africa	5.4
1989	MQ	Swiss	Africa	3.6
1991	MQ/SDX/PYR	French	Africa et al.	2.1
1992	MQ/SDX/PYR	Swiss	Asia, Americas	0.5
1992/1993	H, MQ, CL SDX/PYR	German	Asia Africa	0.3 1.0
1994	H, MQ, SDX/PYR	German	Asia Africa	1.0 5.0

CL = chloroquine; H = halofantrine; MQ = mefloquine; MQ/SDX/PYR = mefloquine/sulfadoxine/pyrimethamine (Fansimef); SDX/PYR = sulfadoxine/pyrimethamine (Fansidar).

sized in an earlier U.K. survey[26] in which over 23% of respondents would have acted inappropriately while experiencing malaria-like symptoms by taking extra prophylactic pills or by staying in bed until their symptoms resolved. However, the main problem inherent in the SBET strategy is the wide range of clinical presentations of malaria that complicate self-diagnosis and that can lead to over- or under-use of the medication and to a poor probability of correct use of SBET. Nothdurft and colleagues[24] found significant *Plasmodium falciparum* antibody levels in only 4 (10.4%) of 37 treatment users. Furthermore, data on the problems and frequency of treatment failures and nonmalarial fevers are lacking, and it is also unclear how nonimmune individuals will respond to therapy; most studies to date have been with semi-immune populations, and toxicity and efficacy profiles may differ.

NEW COMBINATIONS OF AGENTS

Two new combination treatments have been registered in Europe: atovaquone/proguanil (Malarone) and artemether/lumefantrine (Riamet). These therapies will undoubtedly play a major role in the treatment of malaria in endemic populations. The role of these agents as SBET in nonimmune travelers remains to be determined, and data are required for this indication.

Atovaquone/Proguanil

Fixed-combination atovaquone/proguanil (Malarone, formerly BW566C) has recently been approved in several European countries for the treatment of acute uncomplicated falciparum malaria in adults and in children weighing > 10 kg. Each tablet contains 250 mg of atovaquone and 100 mg of proguanil hydrochloride. The dosage for SBET is divided over 3 days (Table 15–1), and the medication should be administered with food to increase absorption and bioavailability. The components of the medication work synergistically, and although early clinical studies (in the United Kingdom, Thailand, and Zambia) with atovaquone monotherapy showed high rates of recrudescence, the combination with proguanil led to significantly improved cure rates[27] and was shown to be more effective than mefloquine in areas of multidrug resistance. A review of the safety data of the combination shows good tolerability compared to other antimalarials. AEs can be attributed to single entities or to the combination, and the most frequently reported events from clinical studies include headache (17% to 37%), nausea and vomiting (16% to 27%), and diarrhea (14% to 16%). In phase III studies with children, the most frequently reported events were coughing, headache, vomiting, abdominal pain, and anorexia. Serious AEs reported include anaphylactic shock, seizures in two patients with a prior history of epilepsy, and a severe hemolytic episode in a G6PD-deficient individual. A recent review of 10 open-label clinical trials concluded that atovaquone/proguanil is safe and effective for the treatment of malaria.[28] Further studies of the efficacy and tolerability of this combination in nonimmune travelers are required.

Artemether/Lumefantrine

The second new oral fixed combination, artemether/lumefantrine (Riamet, formerly CGP56697), or coartemether, was registered recently in Switzerland for treatment and SBET of acute uncomplicated *P. falciparum* infection or mixed malarial infections in adults and children. This new treatment is a fixed combination (1:6) of artemether (a derivative of artemisinin) and lumefantrine (formerly called benflumetol, a synthetic racemic fluorene derivative of the aminoalcohol class) as potentiation between these drugs was observed in combination experiments. (Riamet tablets consist of 20 mg of artemether and 120 mg of lumefantrine.) The recommended SBET dosage is an intensive 3-day administration (Table 15–1) and should be administered with food. Artemether is rapidly absorbed (C_{max}: 2 hours) and eliminated ($t_{1/2}$: 2 hours); its use results in rapid and considerable reduction of the parasite biomass and in the resolution of malaria symptoms whereas lumefantrine, with delayed absorption and slower clearance (C_{max}: 6 to 8 hours; $t_{1/2}$: 2 to 3 days), eliminates residual parasites in a "mopping up" process. The efficacy of the combination is therefore dependent on (a) the number of parasites remaining after artemether has been eliminated and (b) the duration for which lumefantrine plasma concentrations exceed the minimum inhibitory concentration. Dose-finding studies have indicated an efficacy of > 95% with a four-dose regimen in China and India but of only 76.5% in Thailand,[29] where a subsequently tested six-dose regimen produced cure rates of 98%,[30] similar to cure rates observed with the current mefloquine/artesunate standard regimen. The efficacy and tolerability of artemether/lumefantrine (AL) (4×4 regimen) compared to that of halofantrine was evaluated in travelers returning to the Netherlands and France. The recrudescence rate with the AL regimen was found to be unacceptably high (18%), and the investigators proposed a six-dose regimen over a 3-day period.[31] Clinical experience to date indicates rapid clearance of fever and parasites, high cure rates, and reduced gametocyte carriage rates. In a randomized controlled trial of AL versus pyrimethamine/sulfadoxine (P/S) for the treatment of uncomplicated malaria in 287 African children, AL cleared parasites more rapidly than P/S and resulted in fewer gametocycte carriers. The 15-day cure rate was, however, higher with P/S and is explained by the prophylactic effect of residual P/S levels.[32] A randomized open trial involving 260 Tanzanian children compared AL with the standard chloroquine regimen used in the area. Seven-day parasitologic cure rates were 94% in the AL group versus 35% in the chloroquine group. Gametocytes were also more effectively suppressed by AL than by chloroquine. No serious drug-related AEs occurred in either group, and there was no significant difference in symptom reporting. Drug-related AEs included rashes (3.8% with AL vs. 3.9% with chloroquine) and pruritus (0.8% with AL vs. 6.2% with chloroquine).[33] Other reports indicate that the most common AEs include headache, dizziness, insomnia, abdominal pain, and anorexia. One area for particular scrutiny is the cardiac effect of AL, particularly the prolongation of the Q-Tc interval, as lumefantrine has a chemical structure similar to that of halofantrine (both are classified as aminoalcohols). One randomized double-blind two-way crossover study assessed the cardiac effects of AL and halofantrine in 14 healthy male subjects after single oral doses of the respective antimalarial were administered with a high-fat meal. No prolongation of Q-Tc interval was observed with AL (480 mg : 80 mg) whereas halofantrine (500 mg) caused a significant increase in Q-Tc interval in all subjects.[34] This finding was confirmed in a prospective electro-cardiographic study, in which no evidence of cardiotoxicity was observed in 150 patients treated with AL.[35]

DIAGNOSTICS

The use of a malaria diagnostic test as an adjunct to the SBET strategy may be an attainable objective as previously proposed.[23] Such a development would enable the traveler to test a blood droplet for malarial infection. Two recent studies have examined the feasibility of the use of the rapid malaria tests ParaSight F and MalaQuick (ICT) by travelers,[36,37] with the objective of assessing whether travelers can perform such tests and interpret the results. Test performance was often poor. More importantly, both tests were associated with high levels of false-negative interpretations, especially at the low parasitemia levels commonly encountered in travelers, and the authors concluded that technical improvements in performance and interpretation are essential before such tests can be recommended for laypersons. These findings were reinforced by the poor results in both test performance and interpretation shown in a study on the Kenyan coast, where tourists presenting with malaria symptoms were asked to perform and evaluate the rapid malaria test.[38]

Despite these discouraging findings, rapid malaria tests will evolve and become easier to perform and interpret. This technology should be continuously evaluated with regard to its suitability for travelers.

CONCLUSION

Concise advice is necessary for travelers who consider SBET either alone or as a backup to continuous chemoprophylaxis. Those who advise travelers should stress the importance of medical consultation at the first sign of illness. Travelers' behavior and the difficulty of defining simple diagnostic guidelines are major delimiting factors in this strategy. In choosing a suitable SBET agent, the following must be considered: (1) level of malaria transmission at the destination, (2) type and intensity of resistance, (3) efficacy and toxicity of available options, (4) prophylactic agent used (if applicable), and (5) ease of administration of the standby therapy. Of the available WHO-approved agents, chloroquine is preferred in the limited geographic areas where this agent is still effective; otherwise, mefloquine appears to offer a good solution except for foci of multidrug resistance and for individuals with predisposing contraindications. The future points to the newer combination therapies of artemether/lumefantrine (AL) (Riamet) and atovaquone/proguanil (Malarone), which have recently been registered in several countries for this indication. The possible provision of a simple diagnostic test could mitigate the most negative aspect of the SBET strategy, namely, the self-diagnosis of malaria; however, currently available tests have proven unsuitable for travelers.

WEB SITES

http://www.safetravel.ch
http://www.who.int/ith
http://www.cdc.gov/travel

REFERENCES

1. Hien TT, White NJ. Qinghaosu. Lancet 1993;341:603–608.
2. World Health Organization. Health risks and their avoidance. In: International travel and health 1999. Geneva: World Health Organization, 2001.
3. Schlagenhauf P, Phillips-Howard PA. Malaria: emergency self-treatment by travelers. In: DuPont HL, Steffen R, editors. Textbook of travel medicine. Hamilton, London: B.C. Decker, 2001.
4. Steffen R, Holdener F, Wyss R, Nurminen L. Malaria prophylaxis and self-therapy in airline crews. Aviat Space Environ Med 1990;61:942–945.
5. Hatz C, Schlagenhauf P, Funk M, et al. Malariaprophylaxe für Kurzzeitaufenthalter. BAG Bulletin 2001;Suppl 1. [In press]
6. Bradley DJ, Warhurst DC. Guidelines for the prevention of malaria in travellers from the United Kingdom. Commun Dis Rep 1997;7:137–152.
7. Centers for Disease Control and Prevention. Health information for international travel. Atlanta: U.S. Department of Health and Human Services, 2001.
8. Weinke T, Trautmann M, Held T, et al. Neuropsychiatric side effects after the use of mefloquine. Am J Trop Med Hyg 1991;45:86–91.
9a. World Health Organization. Drug alert: halofantrine. Wkly Epidemiol Rec 1993;68:268–270.
9b. Irons D, Morrow J. Sudden death in a traveler following halofantrine administration-Togo 2000. Morb Mortal Wkly Rep 2001;50:169–179.
10. Rieckmann KH, Davis DR, Hutton DC. *Plasmodium vivax* resistant to chloroquine? Lancet 1989;2:1183–1184.
11. Murphy GS, Basri H, Purnomo P, et al. Vivax malaria resistant to treatment and prophylaxis with chloroquine. Lancet 1993;341:96–100.
12. Phillips-Howard PA, Behrens RH, Dunlop J. Stevens-Johnson syndrome due to pyrimethamine/sulphadoxine during presumptive self-therapy of malaria [letter]. Lancet 1989;9:803–804.

13. Fontanet AL, Johnson BD, Walker AM, et al. High prevalence of mefloquine resistant falciparum malaria in eastern Thailand. Bull World Health Organ 1993;71:377–383.

14. ter Kuile FO, Luxemburger C, Nosten F, et al. Serious neuropsychiatric adverse events following mefloquine treatment: evidence for a dose relationship? [Ph.D. thesis]. Amsterdam: University of Amsterdam, 1994.

15. Luxemburger C, ter Kuile FO, Nosten F, et al. Single day mefloquine-artesunate combination in the treatment of multidrug-resistant falciparum malaria. Trans R Soc Trop Med Hyg 1994;88:213–217.

16. Merkli B, Richle R, Peters W. The inhibitory effect of a drug combination on the development of mefloquine resistance in *Plasmodium berghei*. Ann Trop Med Parasitol 1980;74:1–9.

17. Weinke T, Loscher T, Fleischer K, et al. The efficacy of halofantrine in the treatment of acute malaria in non-immune travellers. Am J Trop Med Hyg 1992;47:1–5.

18. Bryson H, Goa K. Halofantrine: review of its antimalarial activity, pharmacokinetic properties and therapeutic potential. Drugs 1992;43:236–258.

19. Matson PA, Luby SP, Redd SC, et al. Cardiac effects of standard-dose halofantrine therapy. Am J Trop Med Hyg 1996;54:229–231.

20. Brewer TG, Grate SJ, Peggins JO, et al. Fatal neurotoxicity of arteether and artemether. Am J Trop Med Hyg 1994;51:251–259.

21. Grimmond TR, Cameron AS. Primaquine-chloroquine prophylaxis against malaria in Southeast Asian refugees entering S. Australia. Med J Aust 1984;140:322–325.

22. Schlagenhauf P, Steffen R. Stand-by treatment of malaria in travellers: a review. J Trop Med Hyg 1994;97:151–160.

23. Schlagenhauf P, Steffen R, Tschopp A, et al. Behavioural aspects of travellers in their use of malaria presumptive treatment. Bull World Health Organ 1995;73:2:215–221.

24. Nothdurft HD, Jelinek T, Pechel SM, et al. Stand-by treatment of suspected malaria in travelers. Trop Med Parasitol 1995;46:161–163.

25. Malaria in travelers returning from Kenya: failure of self-treatment with pyrimethamine/sulfadoxine. MMWR Morb Mortal Wkly Rep 1989;38:363–364.

26. Behrens RH, Phillips-Howard PA. What do travellers know about malaria [letter]? Lancet 1989;2:1395–1396.

27. Looareesuwan S, Viravan C, Webster HK, et al. Clinical studies of atovaquone alone or in combination with other antimalarial drugs for treatment of acute uncomplicated malaria in Thailand. Am J Trop Med Hyg 1996;54:62–66.

28. Kremsner PG, Looareesuwan S, Chulay JD. Atovaquone and proguanil hydrochloride for treatment of malaria. J Travel Med 1999; 6(S1):S18–S20.

29. Gathmann I, Xiu-Quing J, Wright S, et al. Co-artemether: integrated summary of efficacy [abstract P30]. Proceedings of the Conference Clone Cure and Control; 1998 Sep 14–18; Liverpool, U.K.

30. Van Vugt M, Looareesuwan S, Gathmann I, et al. A randomized trial of the six-dose regimen of artemether-benflumetol in comparasion with mefloquine-artesunate in the treatment of acute *Plasmodium falciparum* malaria [abstract P32]. Proceedings of the Conference Clone Cure and Control; 1998 Sep 14–18; Liverpool, U.K.

31. Van Agtmael M, Bouchaud O, Malvy D, et al. The comparative efficacy and tolerability of CGP 56697 (artemether + lumefantrine) versus halofantrine in the treatment of uncomplicated falciparum malaria in travellers returning from the tropics to the Netherlands and France. Int J Antimicrob Agents 1999;12:159–169.

32. von Seidlein L, Jaffar S, Pinder M, et al. Treatment of African children with uncomplicated falciparum malaria with a new antimalarial drug, CGP 56697. J Infect Dis 1997;176:1113–1116.

33. Hatz C, Abdulla S, Mull R, et al. Efficacy and safety of CGP 56697 (artemether and benflumetol) compared with chloroquine to treat falciparum malaria in Tanzanian children aged 1–5 years. Trop Med Int Health 1998;3:498–504.

34. Bindschedler M, Ezzet F, Degen P, Sioufi A. Comparison of the cardiac effects of the antimalarials co-artemether and halofantrine in healthy subjects after single oral doses given with a high fat meal [abstract P29]. Proceedings of the Conference Clone Cure and Control; 1998 Sep 14–18; Liverpool, U.K.

35. Van Vugt M, Ezzet F, Nosten F, et al. No evidence of cardiotoxicity during antimalarial treatment with artemether-lumefantrine. Am J Trop Med Hyg 1999;61:964–967.

36. Trachsler M, Schlagenhauf P, Steffen R. Feasibility of a rapid dipstick antigen-capture assay for self-testing of travellers' malaria. Trop Med Int Health 1999;4:442–447.

37. Funk M, Schlagenhauf P, Tschopp A, Steffen R. ParaSight F versus MalaQuick™ (ICT) for self-diagnosis of travellers' malaria. Trans R Soc Trop Med Hyg 1999;93:268–272.

38. Jelinek T, Amsler L, Grobusch M. Self-use of rapid tests for malaria diagnosis by tourists. Lancet 1999;354:1609.

Chapter 16

Odyssean and Non-Mosquito-Transmitted Forms of Malaria

Margaretha Isaäcson and John A. Frean

ABSTRACT

This chapter deals with the more unusual ways in which malaria may be transmitted and acquired. Odyssean malaria and its numerous manifestations (airport, baggage, container, port, taxi rank, and minibus malaria) are examples of malaria acquired by the bites of infected mosquitoes imported by mechanical modes of transport from malaria-endemic regions. Induced malaria is acquired by means other than a mosquito bite and includes transfusion malaria and needle malaria, the latter occurring either in a nosocomial setting or among intravenous drug users. Congenital malaria is acquired transplacentally by an unborn child from its malaria-infected mother. Further, all of these unusual forms have in common the fact that their diagnosis and specific treatment are often delayed due to the frequent absence of a history of exposure to potentially malaria-infected mosquito bites. Consequently, the incidence of severe, complicated, and fatal falciparum malaria is high.

Key words: airport; baggage; congenital; container; induced; malaria; needle; odyssean; port; runway; taxi; transfusion.

ODYSSEAN MALARIA

Historic Background and Nomenclature

The original term "paludisme aéroporté" was first coined by French workers during the 1970s to distinguish cases of malaria locally acquired through the bite of a tropical malaria-infected mosquito that has been imported by air into a non-endemic area from other cases of autochthonous malaria (i.e., malaria locally acquired from the bites of indigenous mosquitoes). This term arose from the recognition that all of the patients in 13 such cases in Europe had worked at or lived near international airports where infected mosquitoes were thought to have arrived aboard international flights.[1] The French term was correctly translated by Gentilini and Danis in their English summary as "airborne malaria." Two earlier French cases dating back to 1969 were found on review by Doby and Guiguen[2] in 1981 to have similar characteristics and were therefore believed to be the first cases of airport malaria to have been seen in France. However, Doby and Guiguen used the term "paludisme d'aérodrome," meaning "airport malaria," a name that has since been in general use for this subclass of autochthonous malaria in the international literature.

Guillet and colleagues[3] drew attention to the important observation that airport malaria occurs not only in airport employees and in residents in the vicinity of airports but also in persons living at some distance from an airport (after secondary transport of the vectors by road) and in persons bitten by vectors that have been transported in baggage or in freight containers.

In recent years, cases of malaria acquired in non-endemic areas by the bite of imported mosquitoes have come to be reported under a plethora of names based on the type of vehicle assumed to have transported an infected malaria vector or on the type of facility where such vehicles are parked, loaded, and unloaded. Thus, we now read of variants of airport malaria, such as container, baggage,[4,5] minibus, port,[6,7] and taxi rank[8] malaria, with undoubtedly more names to follow as the possibilities for mosquito transport have by no means been exhausted. The terms "luggage malaria"[3] and "suitcase malaria"[7] have been used as synonyms for baggage malaria. The great importance of the role of freight containers in harboring and transporting arthropod vectors has been highlighted by the results of epidemiologic and entomological studies.[3]

"Runway" malaria[9-12] is acquired when passengers en route from one non-endemic area to another are bitten by infected mosquitoes that have flown into aircraft during brief stopovers (usually 1 hour or less) at airports in malaria-endemic areas.[13] Runway malaria, being simply a variant of imported malaria (i.e., malaria acquired outside the area or country where it presents), fails to meet the definition of airport malaria,[3,14] nor is it (as has been suggested) a combination of imported malaria and airport malaria,[9] as the airport in "airport malaria" refers to the non-endemic airport at the destination of a tropical mosquito rather than the malaria-endemic airport of departure.

The volume of commercial road transport between malarious and nonmalarious areas suggests that this form of primary conveyance of infected mosquitoes may be of greater public health importance than air transport.[8] Motor vehicles may serve as a secondary means of transport, carrying infected mosquitoes from their primary port of arrival to destinations that may be far from international airports and harbors.[15] This may further complicate the early diagnosis of malaria in patients involved in such scenarios.

All the named variants of airport malaria have one factor in common, namely, the accidental relocation, by mechanical transport, of a malaria-infected mosquito that survives in a hostile environment to obtain the blood meal needed to ensure its progeny. However, due to adverse climatic conditions, the process of reproduction usually terminates prematurely. It should be noted that in the overwhelming majority of reported cases, the incrimination of an imported mosquito has been based purely on circumstantial albeit compelling evidence.

For the sake of simplicity, it has been suggested[16] that airport malaria and its variants should collectively be termed "odyssean malaria," after the mythic Greek hero Odysseus of Trojan War fame (who, on his journey to be reunited with his wife, Penelope, endured many dangerous hardships and unusual modes of transport).

The extent to which mosquitoes can make themselves at home in aircraft cabins is illustrated by the case of the "commuter mosquito."[17] A 35-year-old English woman flew, by Ethiopian Airways, from London's Heathrow Airport to Italy, where she developed a febrile illness 12 days later and was treated for what was thought to be enteritis. Seven days later, having developed a further febrile illness with respiratory and central nervous system (CNS) symptoms, she flew home and was admitted to hospital, where falciparum malaria with a high parasitemia was confirmed on the same day. It soon emerged that another passenger traveling from London to Rome on the same Ethiopian Airways flight had also developed falciparum malaria. This flight had arrived in London from Addis Ababa, and it was assumed that an infected mosquito had traveled on board all the way from Addis Ababa, via London, to Rome. In the process, the mosquito was probably disturbed while having a blood meal, and it continued its meal on a second passenger.[18]

Table 16–1 shows a classification of malaria on the basis of mode and locality of acquisition as well as locality of clinical presentation. Cases of malaria acquired by syringes or needles have also been referred to as accidental induced malaria.[19]

Table 16–1. **Classification of Malaria by Mode and Place of Transmission**

Mosquito-transmitted, locally acquired (autochthonous)

Indigenous: Natural to the area or country where it occurs. Can be endemic or epidemic.

Introduced: Acquired in a nonmalarious area, from local mosquitoes infected by having fed on individuals with imported malaria.

Odyssean: Acquired in a nonmalarious area, from the bite of an imported mosquito.
   Airport malaria
   Baggage (luggage, suitcase) malaria
   Container malaria
   Port malaria
   Taxi rank malaria
   Minibus malaria

Non-mosquito-transmitted

Induced: Transfusion malaria: acquired by transfusion of blood from a malaria-infected donor.
   Needle malaria: acquired by use of a malaria-contaminated needle or syringe.

Congenital: Transplacentally acquired by an unborn baby from its mother.

Incidence

Odyssean malaria is a rare phenomenon. During the 1970s and 1980s, airport malaria was virtually the only form of odyssean malaria to appear in the literature, and all cases were reported from European countries. Since then, cases have also been recognized further afield, for example, in Australia.[20] Gratz and colleagues[5] estimated a total incidence of 89 cases of airport and baggage malaria during the 30-year period of 1969 to 1999. This is probably a gross underestimate, as many cases (if not the majority of cases) are likely to be undiagnosed or unreported.

The rarity of odyssean malaria is illustrated by Italian data showing that of a total of 5,012 malaria cases presenting in Italy during the 11-year period of 1986 through 1996, only 17 cases occurred in people without a history of travel to malarious regions. Of these, 9 (0.18%) were cases of airport and container malaria, 7 (0.14%) were cases of transfusion malaria, and 1 was the case of an intravenous drug user apparently infected through the practice of needle sharing.[21]

Most cases of odyssean malaria seen in countries with a temperate climate occur during the warm and humid summer season, when conditions for the limited survival of tropical mosquitoes and the transmission of malaria parasites are favorable.

Clinical Features

The clinical details and management of malaria and its complications in nonimmune persons are dealt with elsewhere in this book (see Chapters 11, 12, 14).

Most cases of odyssean malaria have been reported from Europe and have been due to *Plasmodium falciparum*. Clinically, their initial presentation is similar to that seen with imported malaria in most nonimmune persons. There is usually a flulike picture, with fever, hot and cold shivers, nausea, vomiting, myalgia, and headache. Fever may occur in distinct bouts except in falciparum malaria, in which fever is often irregular and may show no signs of periodicity. The presence of a rash or lymphadenopathy should be regarded as an indication of an alternative or coexisting pathology.

Leukopenia is common except in the presence of a coexisting bacterial infection. Thrombocytopenia occurs in most patients with falciparum or vivax malaria. For example, in a series of 89 cases of imported falciparum malaria, thrombocytopenia and lymphopenia occurred in more than 60% of cases while anemia was found in only 15%.[22]

In untreated cases of falciparum malaria, the initial symptoms may be followed by features indicating the onset of complications such as cerebral malaria with coma and convulsions, hemolytic anemia, renal failure, metabolic acidosis, hypoglycemia, pulmonary edema, circulatory collapse, intravascular coagulation and hemorrhage, hyperpyrexia, hyperparasitemia, hemoglobinuria, and blackwater fever.[23] Hypoglycemia and pulmonary edema are common in pregnant patients.

Analysis of a 20-year series of 29 airport malaria cases in Europe showed that the duration of illness before hospitalization ranged from 2 to 30 days in 11 patients while the length of illness before diagnosis ranged from 4 days to more than 6 weeks.[14] Thrombocytopenia was present in 83.3% of cases. For 21 patients, it was established that 67% had severe or complicated malaria by the time malaria was diagnosed. Complications included cerebral malaria in 28.6%, jaundice in 38.1%, anemia in 23.8%, and renal failure in 19.0%. Of 24 patients for whom the outcome was known, 4 (16.7%) died, compared to an overall annual case-fatality rate not exceeding 4.97% among imported falciparum malaria cases in a large European study.[24] Of 14 airport malaria patients with severe or complicated falciparum malaria, 4 (28.6%) had a fatal outcome.[14] This high case-fatality rate (CFR) was similar to that ($\geq$ 20%) reported for severe cases of imported malaria in the United States.[25] The high CFRs among airport malaria cases is clearly related to the excessive delays in diagnosis and treatment.

Diagnostic Aspects

The importance of odyssean malaria cases is related to the frequent delayed or missed diagnosis of the cause of illness in affected patients, which often results in high rates of complications and mortality.[26] The absence of a history of travel to a malaria-endemic area is almost always responsible for this state of affairs. Although a high index of clinical suspicion may exist among some clinicians practicing in the vicinity of repeatedly affected international airports, the probability of a missed diagnosis is high for cases presenting far away from such airports.[3,27] In some cases, the diagnosis is only made at autopsy.

Malaria parasites should routinely be looked for in one or more successive blood films of any febrile patient in whom a diagnosis is not readily apparent. Until recently, the diagnostic problem was aggravated by the replacement of manual blood counts by an automated blood-counting apparatus that (unlike microscopy) was incapable of recognizing and reporting malaria parasites. However, more modern automated blood count analyzers using laser depolarization are capable of showing intracellular malaria pigment in blood. In a series of 224 blood samples received for malaria diagnosis, the overall sensitivity of this method was 72%, and overall specificity was 96%. However, for reasons that are as yet unclear, the sensitivity was 90% for blood from black patients and 43% for white patients whereas the specificity was identical (96%) for both groups.[28] These findings do not invalidate the usefulness of this source of serendipitous diagnosis in certain malaria patients, such as those with the odyssean or induced forms in whom malaria is entirely unsuspected, but they should not be relied on to the extent of replacing other, specific methods of malaria diagnosis. Clinicians should continue to specify malaria examinations and should not assume that these will automatically be done when a full blood count is requested.

Quantitative parasite counts should always be requested as these give an indication of the severity of illness and are useful in showing the response to treatment.

The presence of falciparum gametocytes on blood films is indicative of untreated or inadequately treated malaria of at least 10 days' duration (but frequently 3 weeks or longer).[14]

Management of Patients

The treatment of patients with odyssean malaria is similar to that of patients with imported malaria (see Chapter 14). However, a higher rate of severe and complicated illness should be anticipated in view of the frequently delayed diagnoses; facilities must therefore be readily available to deal with these more severe and complicated cases.

Preventive Measures: Aircraft Disinsectization

In the absence of known potential exposure to malaria vectors, there are no specific measures to prevent odyssean malaria. Persons working or living in the vicinity of international airports should be advised that they are at risk, albeit low, of exposure to imported infected mosquitoes during the summer season; in the event of an obscure febrile illness, such individuals should inform their medical practitioners of this possibility. The burden of prevention rests with the airline companies, which should strictly adhere to the international aircraft disinsectization recommendations.

The first reported presence of insects in an aircraft was in 1928, when no fewer than 10 species were discovered on plants carried on board the dirigible *Graf Zeppelin* on its arrival in the United States.[5] Prior to the advent of flight, insects were regularly carried aboard shipping. Indeed, in 1930, *Anopheles gambiae,* a major African malaria vector, was introduced into Brazil either by sea or by air and was subsequently responsible for some 300,000 cases of malaria that resulted in 16,000 deaths. This vector was eradicated at great expense by the Brazilian government. Repeated inspections of numerous aircraft have since yielded innumerable insects of many species.

Female mosquitoes in search of a blood meal, especially at night, are attracted into aircraft cabins prior to departure by the presence of light, warmth, humidity, and a raised level of carbon dioxide.[29] Despite vector control measures, 210 aircraft at a New Orleans airport yielded 81 mosquitoes on inspection of baggage compartments and cabins, 1,183 aircraft at Miami International Airport yielded 100 mosquitoes, and 89 aircraft in Honolulu yielded 32 mosquitoes.[5] Some 967 arthropods were collected from 592 aircraft arriving at Piarco International Airport, Trinidad and Tobago, West Indies.[30] As the usual rate of malaria infection is about 2% among African *Anopheles* mosquitoes,[5] the great majority of bites inflicted on people in flight or after landing at a non-endemic airport would be relatively harmless. Thus, during a 3-week period in 1994 when six cases of airport malaria occurred at Roissy-Charles de Gaulle Airport, it was estimated that 8 to 20 *Anopheles* mosquitoes were imported into France on each of 250 to 300 aircraft arriving from malaria-endemic areas in Africa. On arrival, only a small proportion of such mosquitoes find a host and favorable conditions for survival.

The chief objective of aircraft disinsectization is to minimize the importation of the vectors of yellow fever and malaria into non-endemic countries. Judging by comments and questions from travelers on this topic, there are numerous misinformed perceptions about the disinsectization of aircraft. Among the commonest are "they never sprayed the plane on my recent flight," "they only sprayed the plane when we were about to land at home," and "I am terribly allergic to the stuff they use for spraying, and so are most of my friends." Travel clinics and doctors advising their patients on travel-related concerns should therefore be informed about the facts of aircraft disinsectization methods. If disinsectization is carried out correctly, it does not present a risk to either human health or the environment.[31]

Three methods are currently in use:

1. Blocks-away method. Spraying is done with a knockdown single-use insecticide aerosol before takeoff, after the passengers have boarded and the doors have been closed. Passengers should be advised to close their eyes and cover their faces during spraying if they feel that it may cause them discomfort. The air-conditioning should be turned off during spraying, and toilets, galleys, and wardrobes should be included. Holds and wheelbays are sprayed before departure, and the flight deck is sprayed before boarding by the crew. The empty cans must be retained for inspection by the Port Health Authorities on arrival.
2. Preflight and top-of-descent spraying. Spraying is carried out with a residual insecticide aerosol before passengers board the aircraft and can therefore include the empty overhead baggage lockers. This procedure is followed by a further in-flight spraying with a knockdown insecticide, carried out just as the aircraft is about to start its descent to the airport of arrival.
3. Residual treatment. This involves the regular spraying of all internal surfaces of the aircraft (except for food preparation areas) with a residual insecticide at intervals determined by the insecticide used.

Adherence to these guidelines would significantly reduce the incidence of airport malaria.

NON-MOSQUITO-TRANSMITTED MALARIA ACQUISITION

Other unusual forms of malaria acquisition are known as induced malaria (which includes transfusion malaria and needle malaria) and congenital malaria. These forms have in common the fact that the infecting parasites are not sporozoites. As a result, a typical pre-patent period (the pre-erythrocytic phase) and true relapses are absent.[32]

Induced Malaria

The term "induced malaria" was first applied to the experimental transmission of malaria by parasite inoculation of animals and to the process of malariotherapy in humans. Malariotherapy involved the planned inoculation of malaria parasites into patients with neurosyphilis and was practiced from 1922 until the advent of penicillin revolutionized the treatment of that disease.[33] Accidental induced malaria may result from the use of malaria-contaminated needles or from the transfusion of blood or blood products, also known as transfusion malaria. Whole blood is the most common source of transfusion malaria, but concentrates of leukocytes and platelets and even fresh plasma have also been incriminated. Cryopreserved blood has been found to sustain viable plasmodia for at least 2 years. Common-source nosocomial malaria outbreaks have been traced to the use of multidose heparin vials,[34–36] and reports have also appeared of suspected malaria transmission by renal transplantation[34] and by contaminated catheters.[37] Reported cases of induced malaria are not common; for example, between 1957 and 1994, only 101 such cases were reported in the United States.[38]

As infecting parasites of *Plasmodium falciparum* origin may present in the peripheral blood in a well-synchronized manner, serial blood films must be prepared and examined during a period of 36 to 48 hours if the diagnosis of induced malaria is not to be missed.[33] Furthermore, the morphology of the plasmodia may be atypical, especially in transfusion malaria, in which plasmodial morphology may be affected by the underlying disease for which the patient is being transfused and by any other therapy that may be administered. In such cases, blood films should ideally be referred to a specialist. The same factors may also affect the clinical presentation. Thus, splenectomized patients may have unusually severe disease.[34]

The prevention of transfusion malaria by the exclusion of all potential blood donors with a history of travel to a malaria-affected area during the preceding 5 years is a practical measure to prevent falciparum and vivax malaria in nonmalarious countries. *Plasmodium ovale* infections may persist for up to 7 years, and *Plasmodium malariae* infection may be lifelong. Microscopic screening of blood is not recommended because the majority of healthy malaria carriers have very low parasitemias and would be missed by this method. Serologic screening for antibodies in potential donor blood to identify malaria-infected persons is feasible in countries with a relatively low malaria endemicity but becomes impractical in hyperendemic areas, where such screening would result in the exclusion of most would-be donors. In such situations, antimalarial drugs (the choice of preparation depending on the local drug resistance pattern) may be administered together with the blood to the transfusion recipient.

Needle malaria[33] (also called needle-induced malaria and needlestick malaria), the result of accidental needle transmission from a malaria patient to a health care worker collecting or preparing blood samples, is another form of accidental induced malaria. Such transmission has also occurred among laboratory workers while pro-cessing *Plasmodium falciparum* maintained in continuous culture in vitro. Needle malaria is frequently nosocomial but also occurs as a result of needle sharing by intravenous-drug users, in whom it causes a high rate of severe and fatal malaria.

Accidental induced malaria, like odyssean malaria, is also commonly associated with a delay in diagnosis and appropriate treatment. This is well illustrated by the report of a young English woman who, about 3 weeks after having visited southern Africa, was treated in an Italian hospital with intravenous fluids and antibiotics for fever and diarrhea.[39] Three days later, she returned to England; on the following day, falciparum malaria with a 30% parasitemia was diagnosed. Her doctor in Italy, who had suffered a needlestick injury while setting up her drip, became ill and died from falciparum malaria (diagnosed at necropsy) 1 month after the injury. He had no history of prior exposure to malaria.

Congenital Malaria

Congenital malaria is acquired directly by transplacental transfer of malaria-infected erythrocytes from the mother, either in utero or during delivery.[40] In malaria-endemic areas, congenital malaria should be diagnosed only when parasites are detected in the newborn within 7 days after birth. Findings of malaria parasites in the liver and spleen of stillborn infants indicate that infection may occur before rather than during birth. If parasites are found between 7 and 28 days after birth, the condition should be designated neonatal malaria, to indicate the possibility of transmission by mosquito bites.

Congenital malaria infection is rarely symptomatic, especially in infants born to malaria-infected semi-immune mothers, even though parasites have been found by microscopy in the cord blood of up to 47% of infants born to infected mothers.[41] Polymerase chain reaction (PCR) is likely to reveal even higher rates of cord blood parasitemia. Such a study in Kenya also revealed a high rate (five times greater than expected) of triple-species infection.[42]

The reasons for the rarity of symptomatic congenital malaria are incompletely understood. Since it is also a very uncommon condition in infants born to infect-ed nonimmune mothers, the placental transfer of passive immunity to the unborn infant is not likely to be a significant factor in the rarity of congenital malaria.

REFERENCES

1. Gentilini M, Danis M. Le paludisme autochthone. Med Mal Infec 1981;11:356–362.
2. Doby JM, Guiguen C. A propos de deux cas "Bretons" de paludisme autochtone, en realite, premiers cas Francais de "paludisme d'aerodrome." Bull Soc Pathol Exot Fil-iales 1981;74:398–405.
3. Guillet P, Germain MC, Giacomini T, et al. Origin and prevention of airport malaria in France. Trop Med Int Health 1998;3:700–705.

4. Castelli F, Caligaris S, Matteelli A, et al. "Baggage malaria" in Italy: cryptic malaria explained? Trans R Soc Trop Med Hyg 1993;87:394.

5. Gratz NG, Steffen R, Cocksedge W. Why aircraft disinsection? Bull World Health Organ 2000;78:995–1004.

6. Delmont J, Brouqui P, Poullin P, Bourgeade A. Harbour-acquired *Plasmodium falciparum* malaria. Lancet 1994;344:330–331.

7. Peleman R, Benoit D, Goossens L, et al. Indigenous malaria in a suburb of Ghent, Belgium. J Travel Med 2000;7:48–49.

8. Dürrheim DN. Taxi rank malaria. BMJ 1995;311:1507.

9. Conlon CP, Berendt AR, Dawson K, Peto TEA. Runway malaria. Lancet 1990;335:472–473.

10. Oswald G, Lawrence EP. Runway malaria. Lancet 1990;335:1537.

11. Bada JL, Cabezos J, Fernandez-Roure JL. Runway malaria. Lancet 1990;336:881.

12. Connor MP, Green AD. Runway malaria in a British serviceman. J R Soc Med 1995;88:415–416.

13. Csillag C. Mosquitos stow away on aircraft. Lancet 1996;348:880.

14. Isaäcson M. Airport malaria: a review. Bull World Health Organ 1989;67:737–743.

15. Whitfield D, Curtis CF, White GB, et al. Two cases of falciparum malaria acquired in Britain. BMJ 1984;289:1607–1609.

16. Isaäcson M, Frean JA. African malaria vectors in European aircraft. Lancet 2001;357:235.

17. Smeaton MJ, Slater PJ, Robson P. Malaria from a "commuter" mosquito. Lancet 1984;i:845–846.

18. Warhurst DC, Curtis CF, White GB. A commuter mosquito's second bite? Lancet 1984;i:1303.

19. Terminology of malaria and of malaria eradication. Report of a drafting committee. Geneva: World Health Organization, 1963. p. 1–124.

20. Jenkin GA, Ritchie SA, Hanna JN, Brown GV. Airport malaria in Cairns. Med J Aust 1997;166:307–308.

21. Baldari M, Tamburro A, Sabatinelli G, et al. Malaria in Maremma, Italy. Lancet 1998;351:1246.

22. Richards MW, Behrens RH, Doherty JF. Short report: hematologic changes in acute, imported *Plasmodium falciparum* malaria. Am J Trop Med Hyg 1998;59:859.

23. Warrell DA, Molyneux ME, Beales PF. Severe and complicated malaria. Trans R Soc Trop Med Hyg 1990;84 Suppl 2:1–65.

24. Muentener P, Schlagenhauf P, Steffen R. Imported malaria (1985–95): trends and perspectives. Bull World Health Organ 1999;77:560–566.

25. Kain KC, Harrington MA, Tennyson S, Keystone JS. Imported malaria: prospective analysis of problems in diagnosis and management. Clin Infect Dis 1998;27:142–149.

26. Giacomini T, Axler O, Mouchet J, et al. Pitfalls in the diagnosis of airport malaria. Seven cases observed in the Paris area in 1994. Scand J Infect Dis 1997;29:433–435.

27. Signorelli C, Messineo A. Airport malaria. Lancet 1990;i:164.

28. Mendelow BV, Lyons C, Nhlangothi P, et al. Automated malaria detection by depolarization of laser light. Br J Haematol 1999;104:499–503.

29. White GB. Airport malaria and jumbo vector control. Parasitol Today 1985;1:177–179.

30. Le Maitre A, Chadee DD. Arthropods collected from aircraft at Piarco International Airport, Trinidad, West Indies. Mosquito News 1983;43:21–23.

31. Recommendations on the disinsecting of aircraft. Wkly Epidemiol Rec 1998;15:109–111.
32. Garnham PCC. Malaria parasites of man: life-cycles and morphology (excluding ultra-structure). In: Wernsdorfer WH, McGregor I, editors. Malaria. Principles and practice of malariology. Edinburgh, London, Melbourne, New York: Churchill Livingstone, 1988. p. 61–96.
33. Wernsdorfer WH. Transfusion malaria and other forms of induced malaria. In: Wernsdorfer WH, McGregor I, editors. Malaria. Principles and practice of malariology. Edinburgh, London, Melbourne, New York: Churchill Livingstone, 1988. p. 903–912.
34. Lettau LA. Nosocomial transmission and infection control aspects of parasitic and ectoparasitic diseases. Part II. Blood and tissue parasites. Infect Control Hosp Epidemiol 1991;12:111–121.
35. Al Saigul AM, Fontaine RE, Haddad Q. Nosocomial malaria from contamination of a multidose heparin container with blood. Infect Control Hosp Epidemiol 2000;21:329–330.
36. Abhulrahi HA, Bohlega EA, Fontaine RE, et al. *Plasmodium falciparum* malaria transmitted in hospital through heparin locks. Lancet 1997;349:23–25.
37. Chen KT, Chen CJ, Chang PY, Morse DL. A nosocomial outbreak of malaria associated with contaminated catheters and contrast medium of a computed tomographic scanner. Infect Control Hosp Epidemiol 1999;20:22–25.
38. Zucker JR. Transfusion-associated malaria. Reply to F. Taylor. Emerg Infect Dis 1996;2:152.
39. Needlestick malaria with tragic consequences. Commun Dis Rep CDR Wkly 1997;7:247.
40. Chongsuphajaisiddhi T. Malaria in paediatric practice. In: Wernsdorfer WH, McGregor I, editors. Malaria. Principles and practice of malariology. Edinburgh, London, Melbourne, New York: Churchill Livingstone, 1988. p. 889–902.
41. Lehner PJ, Andrews CJ. Congenital malaria in Papua New Guinea. Trans R Soc Trop Med Hyg 1988;82:822–826.
42. Tobian AAR, Mehlotra RK, Mehlotra I, et al. Frequent umbilical cord-blood and maternal-blood infections with *Plasmodium falciparum*, *P. malariae*, and *P. ovale* in Kenya. J Infect Dis 2000;182:558–563.

Chapter 17

MALARIA VACCINES

Kimberly A. Moran and Kent E. Kester

ABSTRACT

The morbidity and mortality caused by malaria persist as a worldwide health concern despite concentrated efforts to control this devastating illness. Due to evolving parasite resistance to available chemoprophylaxis and therapeutics as well as vector resistance to insecticides, vaccine technology appears to be an ideal control measure, not only for those in malaria-endemic regions but also for travelers to these areas.

Malaria vaccine development has seen major advancements in the past decade. Current efforts focus on target antigens expressed during different stages of the parasite's life cycle. These vaccine strategies may include the use of recombinant proteins or synthetic peptides based on key target antigens, deoxyribonucleic acid (DNA) vaccines composed of a larger number of target antigens, or a combination of vaccine technologies to maximize the host immune response.

Although several attempts to develop an adequate malaria vaccine over the past number of years have resulted in suboptimal protection, the most recent studies of the various vaccine candidates have shown promise. Malariologists are optimistic that a vaccine ideal for immune and nonimmune populations is a realistic goal for the near future.

Key words: circumsporozoite protein; DNA vaccine; malaria; merozoite surface protein; NYVAC-Pf7; Pfs25; Pfs28; RTS,S; SPf66; vaccine.

INTRODUCTION

Malaria, caused by the multistage protozoan *Plasmodium*, has existed for centuries, continually evading multiple strategies devised for control. Although the majority of morbidity and mortality resulting from this parasitic infection exists in the developing regions of the world and is caused primarily by *Plasmodium falciparum*, there is a growing population of travelers who are also at risk. The number of visitors (including military personnel) from North America and Europe who travel to malaria-endemic countries continues to rise, resulting in an increased number of cases of nonimmune and imported malaria and creating a major health concern. To date, measures taken to protect travelers to malaria-endemic regions have been plagued with limitations. Chemoprophylaxis with medications such as chloroquine and mefloquine is increasingly ineffective and may result in toxic side effects, leading to noncompliance. Children and pregnant women, unable to take routine chemoprophylaxis, present a unique challenge for health care providers. Evolving parasite resistance to chemotherapy continues to threaten prophylaxis strategies as well as effective therapy following infection and has resulted in a reduced number of medications available for these purposes. While important adjuncts to parasite control, personal protection and vector control measures such as insecticides and insect repellents are not 100% effective in preventing infection. Compliance with these measures by travelers is typically not optimal, and vector resistance to insecticides has made these measures even less effective.

A vaccine for the prevention of malaria infection seems a logical solution to the persistent lack of control over this devastating disease. A concentrated effort to develop a malaria vaccine has taken place over the past four decades. While progress has been slow, there have been significant advances and discoveries made in the past decade, which allow for a renewed sense of optimism. Most of the current malaria vaccine research involves *Plasmodium falciparum* because this species is responsible for the majority of fatalities and the most severe clinical disease.

BACKGROUND

Vaccine development has made an enormous positive impact on morbidity and mortality, not only in developed countries but in developing countries as well. Unfortunately, vaccine development can be a prolonged and complicated process. Although the time required to produce a specific vaccine varies, it typically takes many years from the time an infectious agent is propagated to the development of an effective vaccine product. The amount of time required for vaccine development largely depends on the antigenic properties of the agent, on host interactions, and on the ability to grow the organism in culture. For example, *Streptococcus pneumoniae*, the organism responsible for the majority of community-acquired pneumonia infections, was discovered and cultured in 1881, but the vaccine for this infectious agent did not become available until 1977. *Bordatella pertussis*, the agent responsible for whooping cough, was first cultured in 1906, but it wasn't until the 1940s that a vaccine became available. In contrast, the hepatitis B virus was discovered in the 1940s and was cultured in 1973; the vaccine was released in 1981. Timelines reflecting years of research prior to vaccine availability are also seen in the development of vaccines for measles, mumps, rubella, and polio.[1] The ultimate success story, made possible through vaccine technology, is the global eradication of smallpox.

The length of this development process is largely dependent on multiple steps that integrate the results of basic scientific research with clinical application. In the past, once an infectious agent was identified, it was necessary to grow the agent in large amounts to advance to clinical trials with a live attenuated organism or crude antigen preparation. With the advent of recombinant DNA technology, this is no longer a requirement for vaccine production. This is of particular interest to malariologists due to the difficulty of mass production of malaria parasites in vitro.

The target of malaria vaccines varies, depending on the parasite's life cycle. The malaria parasite is notable for antigenic diversity, with many different antigens expressed during (and being specific for) different stages of the parasite's life cycle. Vaccine development has been dependent on the study of parasite surface antigens and on the discovery of potential target antigens recognized by the sera of immune adults.[2] There are currently three major areas of focus in *Plasmodium falciparum* malaria vaccine development, depending on stages of the life cycle (Figure 17–1).

After an infected female *Anopheles* mosquito takes a blood meal, sporozoites are introduced into the human circulation. They quickly (within minutes) enter hepatocytes, where maturation to schizont forms and production of merozoites occur. This process takes approximately 5 days for *Plasmodium falciparum* and is not associated with clinical disease in the host. *Pre-erythrocytic* vaccines consist of antigens or antigen subunits produced on the surface of sporozoites and/or the liver stage of the parasite. A fully effective pre-erythrocytic vaccine would prevent either

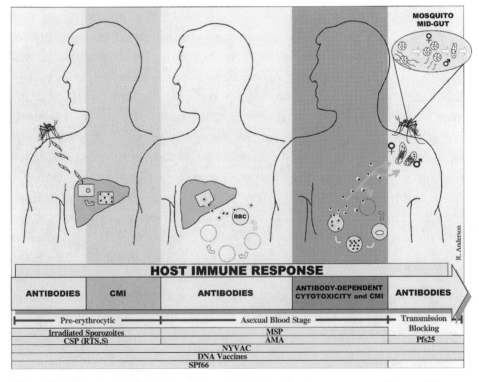

Figure 17–1. Malaria vaccine development in relation to host immune response and stages of the parasite's life cycle. (AMA = apical membrane antigen; CMI = cell-mediated immunity; CSP = circumsporozite protein; DNA = deoxyribonucleic acid; MSP = merozoite surface protein.) (See Color Plates)

the invasion of hepatocytes by sporozoites or the development of merozoites within the liver. The release of merozoites from infected hepatocytes results in the onset of clinical disease, with subsequent invasion of circulating erythrocytes. *Blood-stage* (asexual) *vaccines* are directed against the antigens produced (1) during the merozoite invasion and occupation of erythrocytes and (2) during the release of merozoites from erythrocytes. A proportion of the asexual blood-stage parasites (merozoites) develop into gametocytes and later enter the sexual stage of the parasite's life cycle, which is completed in the mosquito midgut after gametocytes are taken up in a blood meal. The antigens expressed on the surface of sexual-stage parasites are the focus of *transmission-blocking vaccines*.

Key obstacles hinder the development of an effective malaria vaccine. The inability to use the entire organism (due to culturing difficulties and practical considerations) results in the need for a subunit or synthetic peptide vaccine, developed through recombinant DNA technology. Suboptimal immunogenicity resulting from the production of synthetic antigenic peptides was an unexpected outcome in the early development of malaria vaccines using this technology and led to the use of newer more potent adjuvant systems to boost the vaccine-induced immune responses.[3]

The complexity of malaria parasite immune evasion and of the human immune response to infection is not yet fully understood. The immunity seen with natural infection or vaccination with whole irradiated parasites has been difficult to reproduce despite major technologic advances. For this reason, it is a common belief that a successful malaria vaccine will require multiple antigenic components from different stages of the parasite's life cycle, in contrast to a single stage-specific vaccine. In addition to the variable immunogenicity of antigens seen with various stages of the malaria parasite's life cycle, there are host-specific genetic factors (such as the human leukocyte antigen [HLA] haplotype) that affect the T-cell responses to specific parasite epitopes, resulting in varying degrees of immune control.[4] These genetic factors also appear to be age specific and may play a significant role in childhood infection.

There are three general approach strategies to malaria vaccine development. These approaches include (1) the use of recombinant proteins or synthetic peptides based on a few key target antigens, resulting in a primarily antibody and CD4-positive (CD4+) T-cell response, (2) the use of DNA vaccine technology to include a larger number of antigens, with a resultant antibody CD4+ and CD8+ T-cell response, and (3) a combination of vaccines to enhance as well as prolong the vaccinee immune response.

PRE-ERYTHROCYTIC VACCINE (SPOROZOITE LIVER STAGE)

The pre-erythrocytic vaccine is an ideal approach to immunizing travelers and military personnel against malaria. Inducing immunity at this stage of the parasite's life cycle would both prevent hepatocyte invasion by sporozoites and facilitate the destruction of those sporozoites that were able to enter the liver. A fully effective pre-erythrocytic vaccine would thus serve to eliminate the development of clinical malaria. There are two facets of the host immune response corresponding to this stage of the parasite's life cycle. Antibodies are produced in response to the introduction of sporozoites into the human circulation, and hepatic invasion is accompanied by a CD8$^+$ T cell–mediated immune response.

In the late 1960s, Nussenzweig and colleagues published the first reports of protective immunity from malaria challenge resulting from the injection of attenuated irradiated sporozoites, which could invade hepatocytes but were unable to mature within hepatocytes in both murine and primate models.[5–7] It was discovered that the immune response to sporozoites in the circulation was largely mediated by antibodies.[8] Simultaneously, results of studies in mice, as well as observations made in individuals from malaria-endemic regions with a history of natural malaria infection, indicated that high levels of sporozoite antibodies were necessary for the prevention of hepatic invasion by parasites. The circumsporozoite protein (CSP), so named due to its presence over the sporozoite surface, was described as the sporozoite antigen inducing the major antibody response following immunization with irradiated sporozoites or natural infection. This was originally detected using sera from immunized mice incubated with sporozoites, resulting in the observation of a morphological alteration of the sporozoites in vitro (known as the circumsporozoite precipitation reaction).[9] Due to the risks involved with injecting humans with sporozoites dissected from infected mosquitoes (i.e., mosquito tissue contamination or hypersensitivity), intact infected mosquitoes were irradiated and were permitted to feed on the hosts (originally mice), with the resultant development of antibodies to CSP and protective immunity.[10] Clyde and colleagues published the results of the first human trial of immunization with irradiated mosquitoes infected with *P. falciparum* in 1973.[11] In this study, three volunteers were each exposed to 379 infected irradiated mosquitoes over 84 days. Two weeks after completing the immunization phase of the study, the volunteers were bitten by 9 to 13 infected nonirradiated mosquitoes. One of the three volunteers developed CSP antibodies, as determined by immunofluorescent antibody assays (IFAs), and displayed protective immunity when challenged. The immunity was found to be species (*P. falciparum*) and stage specific, with no protection seen on challenge with blood-stage parasites. Despite the inability to calculate the immunizing dose of sporozoites and the difficulties with maintaining immunizations repetitively, this study established that complete immunity to malaria was feasible through vaccination. It was the cumbersome and impractical nature of this method that left malariologists searching for alternative means of immunization.

The genes encoding CSP for *P. falciparum* were cloned and sequenced by 1984.[12] CSP consists of 412 amino acids with a central region containing 37 repeats of the amino acid sequence asparagine-alanine-asparagine-proline (NANP) flanked by nonrepeat regions. This repeating unit was considered to be the immunodominant portion of the protein against which antibodies are produced. The first human clinical vaccine trials using either a synthetic peptide or a recombinant protein contained multiple copies of the *P. falciparum* CSP NANP B-cell epitope.[13,14] These initial studies revealed only partial immunity, with low antibody titers against sporozoites. Several human vaccine trials have targeted the pre-erythrocytic stage of the parasite's life cycle, incorporating synthetic CSP repeat sequences, and have resulted in somewhat discouraging antibody titers, cellular responses, and levels of protection from the sporozoite challenge. Due to the apparent necessity of high levels of antisporozoite antibodies to bestow protection on challenge, more-immunogenic vaccines were composed, using advanced adjuvants and carrier proteins. One of the more promising pre-erythrocytic-stage vaccines using recombinant DNA technology was inspired by the use of hepatitis B surface antigen (HBsAg) particles as a carrier matrix for the *P. falciparum* CSP B-cell epitopes found in the central repeat region.[15] Gordon and colleagues[16] were the first to conduct human trials with this promising vaccine named RTS,S. RTS is a single polypeptide chain containing amino acids 207 to 395 of *P. falciparum* CSP fused with a 226–amino acid polypeptide chain of HBsAg (S) (coexpressed in the yeast *Saccharomyces cerevisiae*), which assembles into antigenic particles. When formulated in the adjuvant known as AS02 (Glaxo SmithKline Biologicals, Rixensart, Belgium)—consisting of an oil-in-water emulsion, 3-deacyl-monophosphoryl lipid A and the saponin derivative and QS21—6 of 7 volunteers were protected from malaria sporozoite challenge.[17] A follow-up study to determine the duration of protection from sporozoite challenge revealed short-lived immunity (less than 6 months in the majority of volunteers) in the previously protected subjects, with no correlation between immune responses and protection.[18] The immune effector mechanisms of this vaccine remained unclear despite its ability to confer sterile immunity in human volunteers. For this reason, the immune responses of 10 volunteers immunized with RTS,S/AS02 were characterized.[19] RTS,S/AS02 was found to be a potent inducer of both cellular and humoral immunity. This vaccine was taken to Gambia for a phase I trial to assess safety and the immune response in 18 semi-immune adults.[20] Following three doses of vaccine (given at 0, 1, and 6 months), volunteers developed CSP-specific antibodies (the most significant rise being after the third dose) without evidence of significant toxicity or adverse events. The results of a number of human studies using the RTS,S vaccine, including safety and sporozoite challenge studies, support the potential efficacy of this vaccine in nonimmune and partially immune populations. There are ongoing clinical trials assessing the efficacy of RTS,S in these two populations, including a study in Gambia that is evaluating protection from natural infection following vaccination.[20,21]

In view of the limited time that sporozoites are present in the extrahepatic circulation prior to hepatocyte invasion, it is likely that antisporozoite antibodies, alone, are incapable of conferring complete immunity, as demonstrated in a number of field trials and natural-infection observations.[22,23] The hepatocyte has become a major target of vaccines developed for pre-erythrocytic-stage immunity. Major histocompatibility complex (MHC) class I and class II molecules present parasite-derived peptides on the infected hepatocyte surface to CD8+ and CD4+ T cells, respectively; however, it appears that the immune mechanism against the hepatic stage of the parasite is primarily CD8+ T cell–mediated. There is also recognized dependence on cytokines (such as interferon-γ [IFN-γ] and interleukin-12 [IL-12]) and other factors (including nitric oxide) for sterile immunity against challenge, as demonstrated by immunization with pre-erythrocytic antigens in various delivery systems in mice.[24] Earlier studies in mice demonstrated a loss of immunity after immune constitution via vaccination with irradiated sporozoites when treated with anti–IFN-γ or anti-CD8+ antibody, but this was not seen following treatment with anti-CD4+ antibody.[25,26]

In the late 1980s, Kumar and colleagues[27] established the presence of genetic restriction of the cytotoxic response and reported the mapping of T-cell epitopes to the variant region of the CSP. It was Hoffman and colleagues[28] who demonstrated in 1989 that the infected hepatocyte was the target for cytotoxic T-cell activity and that the epitope on the target cell surface was derived from the CSP. In 1994, Sinnis and colleagues[29] revealed that the highly conserved region (II+) of the CSP functions as a ligand for sporozoites to the liver cell receptor. It was the discovery of the T- and B-cell immunogenicity of nonrepeat regions of the CSP that resulted in the inclusion of these regions in more advanced vaccine development.[30]

On discovery of the required CD8+ T cell– and cytokine-mediated immunity for disruption of the infected hepatocyte, the focus of the pre-erythrocytic vaccine shifted to include parasitized hepatocyte surface antigens (a total of five have been identified to date: CSP, TRAP, LSA-1, Exp-1, and LSA-3), with a multiantigenic approach using alternative vaccine delivery systems (i.e., synthetic peptides vs. subunits vs. plasmid DNA injection). It is likely that a vaccine targeting this stage of the parasite's life cycle will contain CSP immunogens as well as other hepatocyte stage–specific antigens, perhaps using a combined approach of recombinant proteins or synthetic peptides with a DNA vaccine (see "Other Approaches," below). This collective method would achieve the recruitment of immunity mediated by antibodies, CD4+ and CD8+ T cells, and cytokines. A vaccine with these properties will be most beneficial to travelers and military personnel and will provide complete and sterile immunity with prevention of clinical disease.

BLOOD-STAGE VACCINE (ASEXUAL ERYTHROCYTIC STAGE)

The asexual erythrocytic stage of the malaria parasite's life cycle begins with the release of merozoites from infected hepatocytes. This is followed by rapid invasion of erythrocytes and further intraerythrocytic development, leading to the rupture of merozoites from the parasitized red blood cell (RBC), allowing the invasion of additional RBCs or later differentiation into the sexual stage of the parasite (gametocytes). Clinical disease caused by *Plasmodium* occurs during the erythrocytic or blood stage of the parasite's life cycle. Vaccines targeted against antigens or toxins produced at this phase would result in reduced morbidity and mortality by preventing disease without necessarily preventing infection. The immune mechanism against the erythrocytic stage is considered to be primarily antibody mediated with the added support of CD4$^+$ T-cell activity and cytokine production.[31-33]

In 1993, approximately 20 *P. falciparum* asexual blood-stage target antigens were under evaluation for potential vaccine development.[1] The majority of these antigens are polymorphic and express significant antigenic diversity, which could potentially limit the effectiveness of vaccines specific for this stage of development. Additionally, conformational characteristics of these antigens can be difficult to reproduce through synthetic production, leading to probable reduced immunogenicity.

Today, the leading candidates for *P. falciparum* asexual blood-stage vaccines include merozoite surface protein 1 (MSP-1) and apical membrane antigen 1 (AMA-1). MSP-1 was first identified through monoclonal antibodies to the merozoite surface proteins (MSPs) in 1988.[34] Studies in murine and primate models revealed protection following vaccination with purified MSP-1 from rodent and *P. falciparum* parasites, respectively.[35] Additionally, observation revealed the reaction of protective antibodies with an epidermal growth factor–like domain (19-kDa fragment) in the C terminus, MSP-1$_{19}$.[36] This fragment is a conserved region of the MSP molecule felt to play a crucial role in the invasion of erythrocytes.[37] The first clinical trial of an MSP-1–based vaccine using the MSP-1$_{19}$ fragment, assessing safety and immunogenicity, was conducted by Keitel and colleagues at Baylor University in the late 1990s. Adult volunteers received two or three doses of a vaccine containing the MSP-1$_{19}$ fragment fused to tetanus toxoid T-helper epitopes. Hypersensitivity responses were observed in three volunteers after the third dose, including a generalized reaction with hypotension. Serum antibody responses occurred in 31% (5 of 16) of those receiving 20 μg of MSP-1$_{19}$, 56% (9 of 16) of those receiving 200 μg, and 0% (0 of 8) of the control group.[38] Due to the suboptimal immunogenicity and hypersensitivity observed in experimental models, a larger polypeptide (MSP-1$_{42}$), which is cleaved within the parasite to produce MSP-1$_{19}$ and a 33-kDa fragment, is being studied by the group at the Walter Reed Army Institute of Research (WRAIR).[39] This larger fragment, formulated with the adjuvant AS02, was found to be safe and immunogenic when used to immunize Rhesus monkeys (unpublished data). There are ongoing clinical trials assessing the safety and immunogenicity of MSP-1$_{42}$ in healthy nonimmune volunteers.

A combination of three blood-stage surface antigens (MSP-1, MSP-2, and ring-infected erythrocyte surface antigen [RESA]) formulated in an oil-based adjuvant was administered in phase I and phase IIb double-blind randomized placebo-controlled trials in 120 children in a province of Papua New Guinea.[32,40] No severe adverse events were seen. In children who were not treated to clear infection prior to vaccination, parasite densities were reduced by 62% following immunization. The implication of this reduction in parasite density is not clear.

The immunogenicity of these blood-stage antigen vaccines, as well as their ability to reduce parasite densities in endemic populations, makes them attractive candidates in need of further development. Targeting the malaria parasite at the asexual blood stage of the life cycle would ultimately result in reduced morbidity and mortality and would be an important approach to disease control in malaria-endemic regions. An additional advantage to using this vaccine in endemic populations would be the immune boost resulting from repeat episodes of natural infection.

OTHER APPROACHES

Deoxyribonucleic Acid Vaccines

In 1990, Wolff and colleagues described the use of nonreplicating DNA plasmids containing reporter genes encoded for protein expression within muscle cells, following injection.[41] The concept of DNA vaccines began with the observation that gene transfer, using a variety of techniques, resulted in protein expression. Wolff and colleagues were the first researchers to describe direct intramuscular (IM) inoculation of plasmid DNA resulting in protein expression within muscle cells. There are several advantages to using this technique for vaccination and immunization purposes. Plasmid DNA purification is a relatively easy process, requires little time for production, and is very cost effective. No "cold chain" or series of refrigeration are required to maintain stability, eliminating major storage and distribution concerns. Instead of vaccination with protein subunits or specified epitopes, an entire gene encoding a protein can be mapped into a plasmid, optimizing the immune response and reducing the risk of genetic restriction. Last, the intracellular production and processing of antigen results in MHC class I–dependent cytotoxic T-lymphocyte (CTL) response, which cannot be achieved with synthetic peptide, subunit, or killed vaccines.[42,43]

DNA vaccines consist of the gene of interest cloned into a bacterial plasmid and resemble live or attenuated vaccines in their ability to induce both humoral and cellular immune responses; however, DNA vaccines do not prompt the safety concerns of the latter vaccines in terms of virulence. It is not entirely clear how the antigen encoded by the plasmid-inserted gene is processed and presented to the immune system after injection. Three likely mechanisms exist (Figure 17–2). First, somatic cells (such as myocytes or keratinocytes) may prime the immune response directly by antigen production and presentation to T cells. Second, the protein produced by the somatic cells may be taken up by "professional" antigen-presenting cells (APCs) or dendritic cells and presented to T cells. This mechanism has been supported by studies in mice.[44] Third, injection of plasmid DNA may lead to the

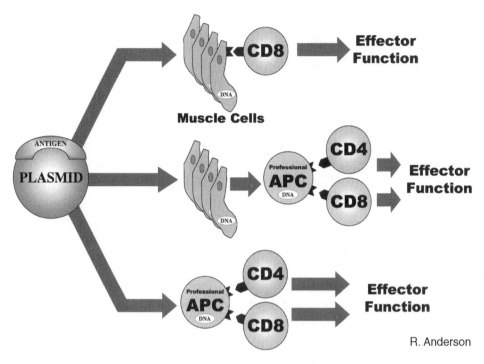

R. Anderson

Figure 17–2. (APC = antigen-presenting cells; DNA = deoxyribonucleic acid.) (See Color Plates)

direct transfection of APCs, which in turn present the antigen to T cells.[42–44] Transfected myoblasts, following IM injection with plasmid DNA encoding influenza nucleoprotein, were stably transplanted into naive mice. The transplanted mice produced high antibody titers and MHC class I CTL responses conferring protection from lethal-challenge influenza A. The induction of the CD8+ T cell–mediated CTL response is one of the major advantages of DNA vaccines.

Intracellular infections caused by microorganisms such as human immunodeficiency virus (HIV), herpes simplex virus (HSV), and parasites (i.e., malaria) likely require both humoral and cellular immunity for host protection. Cellular immunity, comprising primarily CD4+ and CD8+ T-cell responses, results from the recognition of foreign antigens processed and presented by APCs. Killed or inactivated pathogens, proteins derived from vaccines, or recombinant proteins are taken up by APCs through phagocytosis or endocytosis and are presented by MHC class II molecules to CD4+ cells, resulting in the generation of an antibody response. On the other hand, intracellularly produced antigens interact with MHC class I molecules for stimulation of CD8+ T cells and a resultant CD8+- specific CTL response seen only with DNA and live, less attenuated vaccines.[42,45]

The new revolutionary method of DNA vaccination attracted the attention of malariologists early in its developmental stages. It was not only the ease of production and storage that made this method appealing but also the ability of this technique to stimulate a CTL response, felt to be instrumental in malaria immunity.[46–48] DNA vaccines also offer the potential for entire gene expression and multi-antigenic formulations, which could enhance all properties of the immune response. In 1994, Sedegah and colleagues published data on the first malaria DNA vaccine in the *Plasmodium yoelii* rodent model.[47] Based on data from the irradiated sporozoite model and the identification of CSP as the target of immunity, a plasmid encoding *P. yoelii* CSP (PyCSP) was injected intramuscularly into mice. Induction of antibody production as well as CTL response directed against PyCSP were observed at higher levels than those produced following immunization with irradiated sporozoites. It was also illustrated that the protection conferred was CD8[+] T-cell dependent.

After the promising results with the *Plasmodium yoelii* rodent model, the focus shifted to the development of *Plasmodium falciparum* DNA vaccines against the pre-erythrocytic stage of the parasite. Given the genetic restriction of CD8[+] T-cell responses with host variable MHC class I components and known variation in CD8[+] T-cell epitopes among *P. falciparum* isolates worldwide, a multiantigenic vaccine with considerable redundancy was designed.[49–51] Studies in the rodent model have revealed specific target antigens produced in infected hepatocytes, resulting in protective CD8[+] T-cell responses. The *P. falciparum* homologues to these antigens have been identified as *P. falciparum* CSP (PfCSP), *P. falciparum* sporozoite surface protein 2 (PfSSP2, or thrombospondin-related adhesion protein [TRAP]), and *P. falciparum* exported protein 1 (Exp-1), respectively. A fourth antigen, *P. falciparum* liver-stage antigen 1 (LSA-1), and the above homologues have been recognized as CD8[+] T-cell targets after immunization with irradiated sporozoites and natural infection and were therefore chosen for initial nonhuman primate malaria DNA vaccine studies.[49–52] In 1998, Wang and colleagues conducted the first *P. falciparum* DNA vaccine studies with a mixture of four pre-erythrocytic-stage antigen-encoded plasmids in nonhuman primates.[51] The objective of their study was to determine if *P. falciparum* proteins (CSP, SSP2, Exp-1, and LSA-1) could induce CTL responses in Rhesus monkeys after individual IM vaccination with four different DNA plasmids encoding these proteins and immunization with a mixture of the four plasmids, assessing for potential alteration in immunity. The findings indicated immunogenicity to all four plasmids separately as well as in mixture, with subsequent production of CD8[+] T-cell responses to all components of the mixture. This was the first study to reveal the immunogenic properties of *P. falciparum* DNA plasmids in primates in addition to the effectiveness of a mixture of plasmids in inducing a CD8[+] T cell–directed CTL response.

On the basis of their success with rodents, Wang and colleagues proceeded with the vaccination of 20 malaria-naive human volunteers with plasmid DNA encoding PfCSP in a phase I safety trial.[53,54] Vaccinees received three deltoid injections of one of four doses (20, 100, 500, or 2,500 μg) of the PfCSP plasmid DNA at monthly intervals. All doses were well tolerated; the most common complaint was tenderness at the injection site, lasting less than 48 hours. No anti-CSP antibodies were detected in any of the several plasma samples collected throughout the study from all 20 of the volunteers.[55] On the other hand, antigen-specific genetically restricted, CD8[+] T cell–dependent CTL responses were induced in a significant number of the volunteers.[53] Immunization with 500 or 2,500 μg of plasmid DNA resulted in a significantly greater CTL response, compared to the lower doses of plasmid DNA.

The safety and CTL induction seen in this phase I malaria DNA vaccine trial are promising. These data provide the framework needed for future malaria vaccine studies using this innovative technology. This study has been described as the pilot study for a multiplasmid vaccine that ideally would provide protective immunity against various parasite antigens conferring resistance to challenge.[55] It appears that the ideal malaria DNA vaccine would be described as a multistage, multivalent, and multi–immune response vaccine.[46,47,55] Ongoing studies include human vaccine trials with a mixture of multiple DNA plasmids encoding various pre-erythrocytic-stage P. falciparum antigens. To date, however, no efficacy data related to DNA vaccines have been reported.

The rapid advances that have been made using DNA vaccine technology have left researchers optimistic (at minimum) about the potential of this technique. However, this technique being a new method of vaccine delivery, safety and long-term effects are not clearly defined. The most commonly mentioned safety concerns are integration of plasmid DNA into the host cell genome (insertional mutagenesis), which could potentially activate oncogenes or inactivate tumor suppressor genes, and immune alteration or autoantibody production.[56] There are few available data evaluating either of these possibilities; however, findings to date support the unlikelihood of these untoward events. In 1999, Martin and colleagues reported the results of a murine study determining "the structural nature of plasmid DNA sequences persisting in total muscle DNA at both 30 and 60 days" following IM injection with a DNA plasmid encoded for the PfCSP gene.[57] Polymerase chain reaction (PCR) assays were performed after linearization, using endonucleases of extracted DNA (to enable agarose gel size fractionation of all extrachromosomal plasmid DNA from mouse genomic DNA) to quantitate plasmid-specific DNA. The average amount of persistent plasmid DNA in muscle tissue was approximately 1,500 copies per 150,000 genomes. Agarose gel purification of mouse genomic DNA reduced plasmid DNA quantities to 3 to 30 copies per 150,000 mouse genomes. It was impossible to determine whether the remaining plasmid DNA was covalently linked to the genomic DNA. The authors argue that, assuming that the greatest number of plasmid DNA copies identified (30) were covalently linked to mouse genomic DNA and that each insert represented a mutation, the mutation rate would be 3,000 times less than the spontaneous mutation rate for mammalian genomes. Therefore, there does not appear to be a significant safety concern at this rate of integration. These findings followed a study in mice injected with DNA plasmid encoding for the influenza A nucleoprotein gene.[58] Using the purification techniques described above, the study revealed similar results (~1 to 7.5 plasmid DNA copies per 150,000 genomes).

Due to concerns that DNA vaccines may induce autoimmune disease (by production of anti-DNA or anti–muscle cell antibodies as well as clinical or serologic evidence of disease), studies have been conducted to rule out this possibility.[59] To date, there are no experimental data to support the development of autoimmune disease following DNA vaccination.

DNA vaccine technology has shown promise, with many advantages over other vaccine strategies against malaria, given its ability to induce CD8[+] guided CTL immunity and cytokine production. Additionally, this vaccine delivery system has the potential to include all immune targets (a total of 15 to date—5 hepatocytic, 10 eyrthrocytic). However, the limitations of this technique (i.e., the possible safety risks, which have not been extensively investigated) must be recognized.

Transmission-Blocking Vaccines

Transmission-blocking vaccines are sometimes referred to as "altruistic" vaccines due to their mission of reducing malaria infection within a community by preventing mosquito transmission without conferring specific benefit to individual vaccine recipients. The goal of transmission-blocking vaccines is to disrupt fertilization (and/or the production of sporozoites following fertilization) within the vector (i.e., mosquito), preventing later transmission to humans. This is achieved through the production or induction of antibodies against antigens present on the sexual stages of the parasite. An effective transmission-blocking vaccine will reduce morbidity and mortality and may eradicate the parasite altogether in some geographically isolated areas.

Laveran's discovery (in 1880) of the etiologic agent of malaria in the blood sample of an Algerian man coincided with the observation of exflagellation, in which intracellular male gametocytes form extracellular gametocytes in the infected blood specimen.[60] Despite this finding, it was not until the late 1950s that the concept of transmission-blocking vaccines (or antibody production against gametocyte surface antigens, preventing development within the mosquito midgut) was entertained. In 1958, Huff and colleagues reported the successful interruption of mosquito infection by vaccinating chickens (on which mosquitoes fed) with avian malarial whole asexual and sexual parasites.[61] This was followed (in 1976) by similar findings following vaccination with purified sexual-stage parasites alone.[62] In 1980, the first gametocyte target antigens were identified, using monoclonal antibodies, for the purpose of producing a transmission-blocking vaccine.[63] By 1985, the sequencing of genes encoding specific target antigens, allowing for expression by the use of recombinant DNA technology, began. Target antigens discovered to date fall into one of two categories: pre-fertilization antigens or postfertilization antigens. Pre-fertilization target antigens are synthesized predominantly on the gametocyte within the vertebrate host; examples include *P. falciparum* antigens Pfs230, Pfs48/45, and Pfg27.[64–66] Due to their production within the human host, the use of these antigens in transmission-blocking vaccines would likely boost transmission-blocking antibodies during natural malaria infection, perhaps resulting in long-term immunity. In contrast, postfertilization antigens are expressed only within the mosquito, late in the sexual development of the parasite and after fertilization; therefore, the immune response would not be boosted by natural infection. The major advantages of using postfertilization antigens are immunogenicity and the limited genetic diversity due to lack of selective pressure by the vertebrate immune system.[67] Examples of major postfertilization antigens present on the *P. falciparum* parasite include Pfs25 (the first malaria sexual-stage antigen gene to be cloned) and Pfs28.[68]

DNA vaccine technology has been used to test transmission-blocking vaccines in mice.[69] Gene sequences encoding Pfs25 postfertilization antigen and Pfg27 pre-fertilization antigen were inserted into plasmid vectors VR1012 or VR1020, both alone and in combination. The most potent antibody responses were seen with DNA vaccines encoding Pfs25 when administered intramuscularly, either alone or with Pfg27-encoded sequences. Up to a 97% decrease in oocyst production in the mosquito midgut and a 75% decrease in the rate of malaria infection were observed. A DNA vaccine encoding Pfg27 alone revealed less optimal effects in preventing oocyst production. This was the first study demonstrating an effective antibody response with the use of a transmission-blocking DNA vaccine. These results suggest that a combined approach, with a DNA vaccine encoding multiple antigens (including pre-erythrocytic, erythrocytic, and gametocyte [Pfs25]-stage antigens), may be an effective way to eradicate malaria.

Transmission-blocking vaccines will be most effective in geographically isolated regions endemic for malaria, where the human parasite and mosquito burdens are high; the usefulness of transmission-blocking vaccines for travelers is not clear. Currently, the most practical use for transmission-blocking vaccines appears to be in combination with personal protective and antivector measures (i.e., bednets) and with chemotherapy in areas endemic for malaria. Nevertheless, a multicomponent vaccine (or DNA vaccine) including gametocyte and postfertilization antigens is currently under investigation in animal models and will likely present a viable option for a multiantigen vaccine for use in both partially immune and non-immune (i.e., travelers and military personnel) populations.

Multiantigen Vaccines

As discussed previously, a multiantigenic approach to designing a malaria vaccine may be necessary to stimulate the complex immune response required for protection from this potentially fatal disease. Two such vaccines are NYVAC-Pf7 and SPf66.

NYVAC-Pf7 Vaccine

The NYVAC-Pf7 vaccine is a genetically engineered, multistage, multiantigenic, and highly attenuated vaccinia virus with the genes of seven *P. falciparum* proteins inserted into its genome.[70] The vaccinia virus is an attractive vaccine antigen delivery system due to its capability of incorporating and expressing exogenous DNA and due to the resultant stimulation of both humoral and cellular immunity. Antigens from all stages of the parasite's life cycle are represented in the NYVAC-Pf7 vaccine. These include two sporozoite surface antigens (CSP and PfSSP2, also known as TRAP); one antigen expressed only within the infected hepatocyte (LSA-1); three antigens expressed during blood and hepatic schizogony (MSP-1, serine repeat antigen [SERA], and AMA-1); and one sexual-stage antigen (Pfs25).[70] The NYVAC-Pf7 vaccine was found to be safe and well tolerated in Rhesus monkeys. Following inoculation, antibodies to the sporozoite, liver, blood, and sexual stages of the parasite were recognized. With the optimistic observation of antigen-specific immunity in primates after vaccination with NYVAC-Pf7, preparation for human trials began. In 1998, Ockenhouse and colleagues[71] published the findings from a phase I/IIa trial in 49 human volunteers. Each volunteer received at least two immunizations with the NYVAC-Pf7 vaccine. The vaccine was safe and well tolerated in all volunteers; however, the immune response observed was variable. Overall, the antibody responses were suboptimal while cellular immune responses were detected in greater than 90% of volunteers. After the completion of immunization, 35 subjects were challenged using the WRAIR sporozoite challenge model, which requires subjects to be bitten by five *P. falciparum*–infected *Anopheles* mosquitoes. Only one volunteer was protected from sporozoite challenge. The remainder of the volunteers displayed significant delay to parasite patency, compared to control volunteers. Although the NYVAC-Pf7 vaccine appeared to be safe and well tolerated in both primate and human trials, it appears that when this vaccine strategy is used, additional measures will be necessary to enhance the immune response in order to confer protection from infection.

SPf66 Vaccine

The SPf66 vaccine was the first multiantigen vaccine to undergo extensive field studies. This vaccine is a synthetic "hybrid construct" containing the amino acid sequences of three different fragments of the *P. falciparum* merozoite surface proteins and the NANP motif, derived from the CSP sequence.[72,73] The most recent condensed report, supplied by the Cochrane Collaboration, summarized the results of several randomized placebo-controlled field trials studying the immunogenicity and protection resulting from SPf66 immunization in various malaria-endemic regions.[74] The results of nine field trials were reviewed and subcategorized by geographic location. In the African trials (four trials conducted in children less than 5 years of age), there was no evidence that vaccination with SPf66 resulted in a reduced incidence of *P. falciparum* malaria. Five trials (conducted outside of Africa) that included both children and adults and that are notable for significant differences in scientific design demonstrated modest reductions in the incidence of documented malaria infection. There were no severe adverse effects resulting from vaccination with SPf66. Overall, given the reproducible lack of protective efficacy, there appears to be no role for further clinical evaluation of SPf66 in its standard formulation.

Prime-Boost Strategy

One of the most challenging obstacles in the development of an effective malaria vaccine is inducing an expanded immune response to include humoral and cellular components as well as cytokine production. The prime-boost strategy may be an alternative means of achieving an adequate immune response. A basic boosting immunization technique has been used for decades, as exemplified by repeated vaccination in series. Unfortunately, this technique is vaccine dependent and does not necessarily result in the CD8+ T-cell immunity felt to be necessary for protection from the intracellular malaria parasite. With the advent of more advanced vaccine technology such as DNA plasmid vaccines, there is greater potential for the prime-boost strategy by using vaccines in combination.[75] In the implementation of a prime-boost series, a vaccine recipient would undergo a primary immunization (prime) with a DNA vaccine, for example, followed by a boosting effect (boost) with an alternative vaccine such as a synthetic peptide, a vaccinia virus, or a specific T-cell epitope. Haddad and colleagues[76] reported the results of a study in which mice of varying genetic backgrounds received a plasmid DNA vaccine encoded for the blood-stage *P. falciparum* RESA, followed by boosting with either DNA vaccine or the corresponding recombinant protein in alum adjuvant. Higher titer and longer-lasting immunity were observed in mice that received the DNA vaccine and the protein boost than in controls receiving the first vaccine alone.

The prime-boost technique, including a combination of vaccine antigens or delivery systems, is still in developmental stages. There are ongoing safety and immunogenicity clinical trials of this strategy, including trials using multiantigen-encoded DNA vaccines followed by boosting with RTS,S vaccine in human volunteers. This strategy will likely play a role in enhancing the immune response, using the most effective vaccines identified to date.

CONCLUSION

Malaria, particularly falciparum malaria, is responsible for millions of deaths and cases of human disease annually. With increasing travel to malaria-endemic regions, North American and European individuals as well as military personnel are at risk for major health concerns. The mounting resistance of parasites to available medications and of vectors to insecticides has increased the threat to these populations. In 1993, 72 American soldiers returning from the Somalia humanitarian relief mission ("Operation Restore Hope") were diagnosed and treated for malaria, despite having received instruction in personal protective measures and prophylactic medication prior to deployment. According to the American Forces Press Service, malaria was the most common cause of troop casualties during this U.S. operation. One marine unit suffered a 10% malaria attack rate within a single month. Scenarios such as this create a major problem for military forces, reducing the number of available soldiers and ultimately disrupting combat readiness.

An effective malaria vaccine would be the ideal solution to both resistance issues and noncompliance with medication or personal protective measures. A malaria vaccine must induce multiple facets of the immune response, including humoral and cellular immunity, to be effective. A vaccine capable of inducing this range of immunity, conferring protection from parasite challenge, is unavailable at present. However, there are several ongoing clinical trials assessing the safety, the immunogenicity, and levels of protection of various potential vaccine candidates. With the advanced technology currently available, there is a new sense of optimism for the development of a successful vaccine in the near future.

REFERENCES

1. Khuran SK, Talib VH. Malaria vaccine. Indian J Pathol Microbiol 1996;39:433–442.
2. Alonso PL, Lindsay SW, Schellenberg JR, et al. A malaria control trial using insecticide-treated bed nets and targeted chemoprophylaxis in a rural area of the Gambia, West Africa—design and implementation of the trial. Trans R Soc Trop Med Hyg 1993;87:31–36.
3. Hoffman SL, Miller LH. Perspectives on malaria vaccine development. In: Malaria vaccine development: a multi-immune response approach. Washington (DC): American Society of Microbiology Press, 1996.
4. Garcia A, Cot M, Chippaux JP, et al. Genetic control of blood infection levels in human malaria: evidence for a complex genetic model. Am J Trop Med Hyg 1998;58:480–488.
5. Nussenzweig RS, Vanderberg J, Most H, et al. Protective immunity produced by the injection of X-irradiated sporozoites of *Plasmodium berghei*. Nature 1967;216:160–162.
6. Nussenzweig RS, Vanderberg JP, Sanabria Y, et al. Immunity in simian malaria induced by irradiated sporozoites. J Parasitol 1970;56:252.
7. Nussenzweig RS, Vanderberg J, Spitalny GL, et al. Sporozoite-induced immunity in mammalian malaria—a review. Am J Trop Med Hyg 1972;21:722–728.
8. Vanderberg JP, Nussenzweig RS, Sanabria Y, et al. Stage specificity of antisporozoite antibodies in rodent malaria and its relationship to protective immunity. Proc Helminthol Soc Wash 1972;39:514–525.
9. Vanderberg JP, Nussenzweig R, Most H. Protective immunity produced by the injection of X-irradiated sporozoites of *Plasmodium berghei*, V: In vitro effects of immune serum on sporozoites. Mil Med 1969;134:1183–1190.
10. Vanderberg JP, Nussenzweig RS, Most H. Protective immunity produced by the bite of X-irradiated mosquitoes infected with *Plasmodium berghei*. J Parasitol 1970;56:350–351.

11. Clyde DF, Most H, McCarthy VC, Vanderberg JP. Immunization of man against sporo-zoite-induced falciparum malaria. Am J Med Sci 1973;266:169–177.

12. Dame JB, Williams JL, McCutchan TF, et al. Structure of the gene encoding the immunodominant surface antigen on the sporozoite of the human malaria para-site *Plasmodium falciparum*. Science 1984;225:593–599.

13. Herrington DA, Clyde DF, Losonsky G, et al. Safety and immunogenicity in man of a synthetic peptide malaria vaccine against *Plasmodium falciparum* sporozoites. Nature 1987;328:257–259.

14. Ballou WR, Hoffman SL, Sherwood JA, et al. Safety and efficacy of a recombinant DNA *Plasmodium falciparum* vaccine. Lancet 1987;1:1277–1281.

15. Rutgers T, Gordon DM, Gathoye AM, et al. Hepatitis B surface antigen as a carrier matrix for the repetitive epitope of the circumsporozoite protein of *Plasmodium falciparum*. Biotechnology 1988;6:1065–1070.

16. Gordon DM, McGovern TW, Krzych U, et al. Safety, immunogenicity, and efficacy of a recombinantly produced *Plasmodium falciparum* circumsporozoite protein-hepatitis B surface antigen subunit vaccine. J Infect Dis 1995;171:1576–1585.

17. Stoute JA, Slaoui M, Heppner DG, et al. A preliminary evaluation of a recombinant cir-cumsporozoite protein vaccine against *Plasmodium falciparum* malaria. N Engl J Med 1997;336:86–91.

18. Stoute JA, Kester KE, Krzych U, et al. Long-term efficacy and immune responses follow-ing immunization with the RTS,S malaria vaccine. J Infect Dis 1998;178:1139–1144.

19. Lalvani A, Moris P, Voss G, et al. Potent induction of focused Th1-type cellular and humoral immune responses by RTS,S/SBAS2, a recombinant *Plasmodium falci-parum* malaria vaccine. J Infect Dis 1999;180:1656–1664.

20. Doherty JF, Pinder M, Tornieporth N, et al. A phase I safety and immunogenicity trial with the candidate malaria vaccine RTS,S/SBAS2 in semi-immune adults in the Gambia. Am J Trop Med Hyg 1999;61:865–868.

21. Kester KE, McKinney DA, Tornieporth N, et al. Efficacy of recombinant circumsporo-zoite protein vaccine regimens against experimental *Plasmodium falciparum* malaria. J Infect Dis 2001;183:640–647.

22. Saul A. Kinetic constraints upon the development of a malaria vaccine. Parasite Immunol 1987;9:1–9.

23. Hoffman SL, Oster CN, Plowe CV, et al. Naturally acquired antibodies to sporozoites do not prevent malaria: vaccine development implications. Science 1987;237:639–642.

24. Doolan DL, Hoffman SL. The complexity of protective immunity against liver-stage malaria. J Immunol 2000;165:1453–1462.

25. Schoefield L, Villaquiran J, Ferreira A, et al. Gamma interferon, CD8+ cells and anti-bodies required for immunity to malaria sporozoites. Nature 1987;330:664–666.

26. Weiss WR, Sedegah M, Beaudoin RL, et al. CD8+ T cells(cytotoxic/suppressors) are required for protection in mice immunized with malaria sporozoites. Proc Natl Acad Sci U S A 1988;85:573–576.

27. Kumar S, Miller LH, Quakyi IA, et al. The cytotoxic T-cell response to *Plasmodium falciparum* circumsporozoite protein is genetically restricted and maps to the vari-ant region of the protein. Vaccine 1989;89:305–310.

28. Hoffman SL, Isenbarger D, Long GW, et al. Sporozoite vaccine induces genetically restricted T cell elimination of malaria from hepatocytes. Science 1989;244:639–642.

29. Sinnis P, Clavijo P, Fenyo D, et al. Structural and functional properties of region II-plus of the malaria circumsporozoite protein. J Exp Med 1994;180:297–306.

30. White K, Krzych U, Gordon DM, et al. Induction of cytolytic and antibody responses using *Plasmodium falciparum* repeatless circumsporozoite protein encapsulated in liposomes. Vaccine 1993;11:1341–1346.

31. Miller LH, Hoffman SL. Research toward vaccines against malaria. Nat Med 1998;4:520–524.

32. Genton B, Al-Yaman F, Anders R, et al. Safety and immunogenicity of a three-component blood-stage malaria vaccine in adults living in an endemic area of Papua New Guinea. Vaccine 2000;18:2504–2511.

33. Berzins K, Perlmann P. Malaria vaccines: attacking infected erythrocytes. In: Malaria vaccine development: a multi-immune response approach. Washington (DC): American Society of Microbiology Press, 1996.

34. Smythe JA, Coppel RL, Brown GV, et al. Identification of two integral membrane proteins of *Plasmodium falciparum*. Proc Natl Acad Sci U S A 1988;85:5195–5199.

35. Holder AA, Freeman RR. Immunization against blood stage rodent malaria using purified parasite antigens. Nature 1982;294:361–366.

36. Chappel JA, Holder AA. Monoclonal antibodies that inhibit *Plasmodium falciparum* invasion in vitro recognize the first growth factor-like domain of merozoite surface protein-1. Mol Biochem Parasitol 1993;60:303–311.

37. Blackman MJ, Heidrich HG, Donachie S, et al. A single fragment of a malaria merozoite surface protein remains on the parasite during red cell invasion and is the target of invasion-inhibiting antibodies. J Exp Med 1990;172:379–382.

38. Keitel WA, Kester KE, Atmar RL, et al. Phase I trial of two recombinant vaccines containing the 19kD carboxy terminal fragment of *Plasmodium falciparum* merozoite surface protein 1 (MSP-1_{19}) and T helper epitopes of tetanus toxoid. Vaccine 1999;18:531–539.

39. Anders RF, Saul A. Malaria vaccines. Parasitol Today 2000;16:444–447.

40. Saul A. Human phase I vaccine trials of 3 recombinant asexual stage malaria antigens with montanide ISA720 adjuvant. Vaccine 1999;17:3145–3159.

41. Liu MA. Overview of DNA vaccines. Ann N Y Acad Sci 1995;772:15–20.

42. Gurunathan S, Klinman DM, Seder RA. DNA vaccines: immunology, application, and optimization. Annu Rev Immunol 2000;18:927–974.

43. Davis HL, Michel ML, Whalen RG. Use of plasmid DNA for direct gene transfer and immunization. Ann N Y Acad Sci 1995;772:21–29.

44. Ulmer JB, Deck RR, Dewitt CM, et al. Expression of a viral protein by muscle cells in vivo induces protective cell-mediated immunity. Vaccine 1997;15:839–841.

45. Benjamin E, Leskowitz S. The role of major histocompatibility complex in the immune response. In: Immunology, a short course. New York:Wiley-Liss, Inc., 1991.

46. Hedstrom RC, Sedegah M, Hoffman SL, et al. Prospects and strategies for development of DNA vaccines against malaria. Res Immunol 1994;145:476–483.

47. Sedegah M, Hedstrom R, Hobart P, et al. Protection against malaria by immunization with plasmid DNA encoding circumsporozoite protein. Proc Natl Acad Sci U S A 1994;91:9866–9870.

48. Hoffman SL, Doolan, DL, Sedagah M, et al. Nucleic acid malaria vaccines current status and potential. Ann N Y Acad Sci 1995;772:88–94.

49. Hedstrom RC, Doolan DL, Wang R, et al. The development of a multivalent DNA vaccine for malaria. Springer Semin Immunopathol 1997;19:147–159.

50. Hoffman SL, Doolan DL, Sedegah M, et al. Strategy for development of a pre-erythro-cytic *Plasmodium falciparum* DNA vaccine for human use. Vaccine 1997;15:842–845.

51. Wang R, Doolan DL, Charoenvit Y, et al. Simultaneous induction of multiple antigen-specific cytotoxic T lymphocytes in nonhuman primates by immunization with a mixture of four *Plasmodium falciparum* DNA plasmids. Infect Immun 1998;66: 4193–4202.

52. Hoffman SL, Doolan DL, Sedegah M, et al. Toward clinical trials of DNA vaccines against malaria. Immunol Cell Biol 1997;75:376–381.

53. Wang R, Doolan DL, Le TP, et al. Induction of antigen-specific cytotoxic T lymphocytes in humans by a malaria DNA vaccine. Science 1998;282:476–480.

54. Le TP, Coonan KM, Hedstrom RC, et al. Safety, tolerability and humoral immune responses after intramuscular administration of a malaria DNA vaccine to healthy adult volunteers. Vaccine 2000;18:1893–1901.

55. Doolan DL, Hoffman SL. Multi-gene vaccination against malaria: a multistage, multi-immune response approach. Parasitol Today 1997;13:171–177.

56. Hilleman MR. DNA vectors precedents and safety. Ann N Y Acad Sci 1995;772:1–13.

57. Martin T, Parker SE, Hedstrom R, et al. Plasmid DNA malaria vaccine: the potential for genomic integration after intramuscular injection. Hum Gene Ther 1999;10: 759–768.

58. Nichols WW, Ledwith BJ, Manam SV, Troilo PJ. Potential DNA vaccine integration into host cell genome. Ann N Y Acad Sci 1995;772:30–39.

59. Mor G, Singla M, Steinberg AD, et al. Do DNA vaccines induce autoimmune disease? Hum Gene Ther 1997;8:293–300.

60. Laveran A. Note sur un nouveau parasite trouvé dans le sang du plusiers malades atteints de fièvre palustre. Bull Acad Natl Med (Paris) 1880;9:1235.

61. Huff CG, Marchbank DF, Shiroishi T. Changes in infectiousness of malarial gameto-cytes. II. Analysis of the possible causative factors. Exp Parasitol 1958;7:399–417.

62. Carter R, Chen DH. Malaria transmission blocked by immunisation with gametes of the malaria parasite. Nature 1976;263:57–60.

63. Rener J, Carter R, Rosenberg Y, Miller LH. Anti-gamete monoclonal antibodies synergistically block transmission of malaria by preventing fertilization in the mosquito. Proc Natl Acad Sci U S A 1980;77:6797–6799.

64. Quakyi IA, Carter R, Rener J, et al. The 230-kD gamete surface protein of *Plasmodium falciparum* is also a target for transmission-blocking antibodies. J Immunol 1987;139:4213–4217.

65. Kocken CH, Jansen J, Daan AM, et al. Cloning and expression of the gene coding for the transmission-blocking target antigen Pfs48/45 of *Plasmodium falciparum*. Mol Biochem Parasitol 1993;61:59–68.

66. Wizel B, Kumar N. Identification of a continuous and cross-reacting epitope for *Plasmodium falciparum* transmission-blocking immunity. Proc Natl Acad Sci U S A 1991;88:9533–9537.

67. Kaslow DC. Transmission-blocking vaccines: uses and current status of development. Int J Parasitol 1997;27:183–189.

68. Kaslow DC, Quakyi C, Syin C, et al. A vaccine candidate from the sexual stage of human malaria that contains EF-like domains. Nature 1988;333:74–76.

69. Lobo CA, Dhar R, Kumar N. Immunization of mice with DNA-based Pfs25 elicits potent malaria transmission-blocking antibodies. Infect Immun 1999;67:1688–1693.

70. Tine JA, Lanar DE, Smith DM, et al. NYVAC-Pf7: a poxvirus-vectored, multiantigen, multistage vaccine candidate for *Plasmodium falciparum* malaria. Infect Immun 1996;64:3833–3844.

71. Ockenhouse CF, Sun PF, Lanar DE, et al. Phase I/IIa safety, immunogenicity, and efficacy trial of NYVAC-Pf7, a pox-vectored, multiantigen, multistage vaccine candidate for *Plasmodium falciparum* malaria. J Infect Dis 1998;177:1664–1673.

72. Amador R, Moreno A, Valero V, et al. The first field trials of the chemically synthesized malaria vaccine SPf66: safety, immunogenicity and protectivity. Vaccine 1992;10:179–184.

73. Amador R, Moreno A, Murillo LA, et al. Safety and immunogenicity of the synthetic malaria vaccine SPf66 in a large field trial. J Infect Dis 1992;166:139–144.

74. Graves P, Gelband H. Vaccines for preventing malaria. The Cochrane Database of Systematic Reviews Volume (Issue 3). The Cochrane Library, 2000.

75. Schneider J, Gilbert SC, Hannan CM. Induction of CD8+ T cells using heterologous prime-boost immunisation strategies. Immunol Rev 1999;170:29–38.

76. Haddad D, Liljeqvist S, Hansson M, et al. Characterization of antibody responses to a *Plasmodium falciparum* blood-stage antigen induced by a DNA prime/protein boost immunization protocol. Scand J Immunol 1999;49:506–514.

Chapter 18

IMPORTED MALARIA

Patricia Schlagenhauf and Patric Muentener

ABSTRACT

Malaria is frequently imported into non-endemic industrialized areas. This chapter examines malaria's mobility, with emphasis on trends and patterns of imported malaria cases in non-endemic areas. Data on reported malaria cases in industrialized countries for the period of 1985 to 1995 have been collated with main outcome measures such as incidence, case-fatality rates (CFRs), and attack rates in tourists to Kenya. The collated data showed gross under-reporting of imported cases in industrialized countries and marked heterogeneity in the type and availability of national data. In the United States, over 1,000 cases are reported annually. The total reported number of malarial infections in Europe increased from 6,840 in 1985 to 7,244 in 1995, with a peak incidence of 8,438 cases in 1989. Due to under-reporting, the real figures are probably at least three times the reported case numbers. The main importers in Europe are France, the United Kingdom, Germany, and Italy. In the former Union of Soviet Socialist Republics (U.S.S.R.), reported incidences dropped from 1,145 in 1989 to 356 in 1990 due to the cessation of activities in Afghanistan, but the situation in the Russian Federation is currently deteriorating. In industrialized countries, *Plasmodium falciparum* accounts for an increasing proportion of imported species, and CFRs range from 0% to 3.6%, with Germany showing consistently high rates. Attack rates in travelers to Kenya (1990 to 1995) are high, ranging from 18 to 207 per 100,000 travelers. Apart from tourist and business travelers, immigrant groups in industrialized countries are high-risk groups for malaria infection and are unlikely to seek medical advice prior to travel or to use chemoprophylaxis; they need to be especially targeted for preventive measures. Imported malaria in industrialized countries remains a public health problem associated with high CFRs.

Key words: case-fatality rates; immigrants; imported; malaria; travelers.

INTRODUCTION

The United States, Europe, Australia, and Canada are officially classified as non-endemic areas for malaria, but this was not always so. Malaria was formerly endemic throughout the continental United States; 600,000 cases were recorded in 1914. In industrialized countries, indigenous malaria receded in the middle of the 19th century,[1] and this "natural recession" has been attributed to the drainage of swampy areas, better animal husbandry, improved housing, greater availability of quinine, and general socioeconomic improvements. Indeed, the achievement of malaria eradication in Europe is viewed as a major success in the checkered history of global malaria eradication.[2,3] However, due to human migration and the tidal wave of tourist travel to malaria-endemic countries, malaria is often imported into industrialized areas that are classified as "malaria free."

A brief glance at travel statistics shows the spectacular growth in tourism worldwide.[4] Africa, the main global reservoir of malaria, had 17,875,000 international tourist arrivals in 1993 compared to 750,000 in 1960, for an average annual growth rate of 10.1%.[4] A high prevalence of antibodies against the circumsporozoite antigen of *Plasmodium falciparum* (6% to 49%, depending on the type of travel) has been observed in the sera of travelers returning from sub-Saharan Africa, which indicates a high rate of malarial infection.[5] However, only a small proportion of travelers to malaria-endemic areas will actually develop clinical infection. This situation poses two dangers. The first danger, primarily to the individual who has acquired the infection, is that this exotic disease will be undiagnosed or incorrectly diagnosed, with a resultant high risk of fatality. The second (albeit theoretic) danger is to the communities with which the traveler comes into contact at journey's end and is that competent malaria vectors and favorable environmental conditions could theoretically result in local malaria transmission. Several recent incidences of autochthonous malaria transmission have been reported in the "malaria-free" United States,[6-9] and transmission of malaria has occurred in Europe, resulting either from the introduction of infected mosquitoes by aircraft (airport malaria)[10] or from local European mosquitoes that have become contaminated by feeding on infected persons returning from endemic areas.[11-13] With global warming, malaria transmission could theoretically spread to wider-ranging areas and higher altitudes. However, this factor, while most important for current endemic areas and fringe areas of marginal endemicity, is considered unlikely to lead to widespread new transmission in areas where malaria has been eradicated because the principal factor in the eradication of malaria from previously endemic areas was not vector eradication (the *Anopheles* mosquitoes are still present) but rather better housing, protection against mosquito entry, and the amelioration of living standards.[14]

DATA FROM INDUSTRIALIZED COUNTRIES

Imported malaria refers to infection acquired in an endemic area by an individual (either tourist or indigenous native) and diagnosed in non-endemic industrialized areas after clinical disease has developed. Many national authorities consider their reported data to underestimate the true situation, and it is generally recognized that under-reporting is rampant. There is also wide variation in the type of data collected in industrialized countries (Table 18–1). In France, a mean of 1,230 cases were reported annually, but the true figure is estimated at approximately 3,900 cases per year.[15] There is marked heterogeneity in the quantity and quality of data available, in that certain key data variables (such as chemoprophylaxis used, traveler status and country of origin of infection, recovery, and deaths) are infrequently collected.

Table 18–1. **Data Collection in Industrialized Countries**[16]

Country	Mandatory Notification	Specific Notification Form	Reports from Laboratories	Confirmation of Parasite
Austria	yes*	yes	no	P, S
Belgium	yes[†]	yes	yes	P
Denmark	yes	no	no	P
Finland[‡]	yes	yes	yes	P
France[§]	no[‖]	yes	yes	P
Germany	yes	yes	yes	P
Greece	yes	yes	no[#]	P
Ireland**	yes	no	no	—
Italy	yes	yes	no	P
Luxembourg	yes[††]	yes	no	P
Malta	yes	yes	yes[‡‡]	P
Netherlands[§§]	yes	yes	yes	P
Norway	yes	yes	yes	P
Poland	yes	no	no[‖‖]	P
Portugal**	yes	yes	no	P, S
Spain	yes	yes	yes	P, C
Sweden	yes	no	yes	P
Switzerland	yes	yes	yes	P
U.K.	yes	yes	yes	P
Australia	yes	yes	yes	P
U.S.A.	yes	yes	yes	P
New Zealand	yes	yes	no	P

P = parasitology; S = serology; C = clinical.
* Since 1994 only.
[†] Only indigenous infection in Flemish part of country.
[‡] Estimates a level of under-reporting of 20%.
[§] Estimates a level of under-reporting of 55%.
[‖] Only indigenous infection.
[#] Hospitals also notify.
** No detection of duplicates and recurrent cases.
[††] Majority of cases reported by one national clinic.
[‡‡] Reporting is done by hospital and laboratory.
[§§] Estimates a level of under-reporting of 59%.
[‖‖] Rarely, laboratories send data.

Imported malaria in industrialized countries has been recently examined in detail, and many of the data presented here are based on this earlier publication.[16]

Table 18–2 shows a total of 77,683 reported malaria cases imported into Europe over the preceding 11 years. The overall trend in recent years is toward stable or increasing case numbers (see Table 18–2), with an overall increase of 5.9% in total reported malaria cases for 1995 versus 1985. The numbers vary from 0 cases in Malta to 2,332 cases in the United Kingdom in 1991 to an estimated 3,900 cases annually in France. Seventeen countries report 200 or fewer cases annually, six countries report 200 to 1,000 annual cases, and the United Kingdom and France usually report more than 1,000 cases annually. Outside Europe, only the United States reports slightly more than 1,000 malaria cases annually. In the former U.S.S.R., case numbers dropped from 1,145 in 1989 to 356 in 1990 due to the cessation of activities in Afghanistan.

TRENDS IN CASE NUMBERS

In the 11-year period surveyed in Table 18–2, only a 5.9% increase in reported imported cases was recorded, which was less than the increase in travel to malaria-endemic regions. Fluctuating malaria situations in endemic areas, changed compliance with and efficacy of chemoprophylaxis used, or reporting artefacts in the surveillance data also probably influenced the data on imported cases. The increased incidence observed excludes the former U.S.S.R. Between 1981 and 1989, a total of 7,683 cases of malaria were imported into the U.S.S.R. from Afghanistan, mainly by demobilized military personnel.[17] Notifications in many countries show an increase of cases in recent years, and the official notifications of many countries clearly understate the true position. In France, it is estimated that only about 32% of all cases are notified.[18] The problem of inconsistent malaria surveillance in European countries has been previously identified.[19] A recent publication by Legros and Danis addressed this question in detail for European countries.[15] Attack rates are also likely to be underestimates as they do not take into account cases that occur abroad or under-reporting in the home countries.

THE CHANGING PROFILE OF IMPORTED MALARIA

Species Profile

The reported proportions of *Plasmodium* species vary considerably among countries. *Plasmodium falciparum* is the predominant species, accounting annually for more than 50% of all cases (Table 18–3). France shows the highest proportion of cases due to *P. falciparum*, sometimes exceeding 80%. The lowest proportion of *P. falciparum* cases (approximately 40%) is recorded in the United States.

Table 18–2. **Reported Malaria Cases in Industrialized Countries, 1985 to 1995**

Country	1985	1986	1987	1988	1989	1990	1991	1992	1993	1994	1995	Annual Mean	Total Cases
						Europe							
Austria	82	92	52	83	98	112	111	58	89	75	80	85	932
Belgium	208	298	258	271	272	264	314	249	320	423	304	289	3,181
Czechoslovakia	9	11	20	26	28	7	8	7	8	n/a	n/a	14	124
Denmark	128	178	138	142	125	114	110	110	113	136	175	134	1,469
Finland	30	28	19	n/a	52	46	33	39	31	49	31	36	358
France	631	1,125	1,143	1,664	1,863	1,491	1,165	905	769	824	1,167	1,159*	12,747
Germany	591	1,137	794	1,030	1,143	976	900	773	732	830	941	895	9,847
Greece	34	39	47	52	48	28	45	29	35	27	24	37	408
Ireland	22	21	28	30	23	12	11	15	9	12	9	17	192
Italy	178	191	287	350	468	521	471	499	688	782	743	471	5,178
Luxembourg	7	3	5	n/a	8	7	5	1	4	6	6	5	52
Malta	4	5	2	2	10	3	5	0	4	2	6	4	43
Netherlands	137	167	153	259	244	248	272	179	223	236	312	221	2,430
Norway	53	68	47	53	52	60	71	36	76	73	80	61	669
Poland	15	14	16	21	22	21	16	17	27	18	20	19	207
Portugal	62	95	119	113	161	129	108	61	49	67	n/a	96	964
Romania	10	8	13	n/a	5	9	11	19	21	20	30	15	146
Spain	112	179	166	176	118	161	159	154	171	268	263	175	1,927
Sweden	140	147	155	172	180	205	149	124	143	160	161	158	1,736
Switzerland	200	196	192	322	340	295	322	261	285	310	289	274	3,012
U.K.	2,212	2,309	1,816	1,674	1,987	2,096	2,332	1,629	1,922	1,887	2,055	1,993	21,919
U.S.S.R. (former)	1,918	1,686	1,323	1,580	1,145	356	254	188	293	485	548	889	9,776
Yugoslavia	57	75	64	53	46	23	18	10	20	n/a	n/a	41	366
Total	6,840	8,072	6,857	8,073	8,438	7,184	6,890	5,363	6,032	6,690	7,244	—	77,683

* True mean figure is estimated at 3,900 cases per annum.
Continued on next page.

Table 18–2. **Reported Malaria Cases in Industrialized Countries, 1985 to 1995 (continued)**

Country	1985	1986	1987	1988	1989	1990	1991	1992	1993	1994	1995	Annual Mean	Total Cases
						Non-Europe							
Australia	421	696	574	601	770	874	939	743	670	710	610	692	7,608
Canada	314	436	515	307	284	417	674	407	483	n/a	637	447	4,474
Japan	53	50	40	48	49	49	52	49	51	64	n/a	51	505
New Zealand	n/a	n/a	n/a	n/a	27	32	39	29	58	34	41	37	260
U.S.A.	1,045	1,091	932	1,023	1,102	1,098	1,046	910	1,275	1,014	n/a	1,054	10,536
Total	1,833	2,273	2,061	1,979	2,232	2,470	2,750	2,138	2,537	1,822	1,288	—	23,383

n/a = not available.

Table 18–3. Malaria Cases Due to *Plasmodium falciparum* Infection, by Country

Country	Plasmodium falciparum *Cases* (% of all malaria cases)							
	1989	1990	1991	1992	1993	1994	1995	*Average*
Austria	64.3	47.3	43.2	34.5	56.2	56.0	57.5	51.3
Belgium	68.0	74.2	68.5	65.1	55.9	n/a	n/a	66.3
France	81.1	78.0	n/a	n/a	81.1	84.5	86.0	82.2
Germany	60.7	60.2	58.9	63.3	48.8	67.8	55.9	59.4
Greece	60.4	57.1	44.4	31.0	54.3	37.0	25.0	44.2
Italy	73.7	75.8	74.3	73.5	68.0	72.1	70.9	72.6
Netherlands	68.0	69.0	61.8	61.5	59.6	64.4	55.8	62.9
Portugal	82.6	79.1	79.6	55.7	36.7	n/a	n/a	66.8
Spain	59.3	54.0	64.2	55.8	51.5	71.6	60.5	59.6
Sweden	44.4	56.1	42.3	54.0	61.5	75.0	52.2	55.1
Switzerland	49.7	58.3	42.9	54.0	51.6	61.0	65.7	54.7
U.K.	56.2	52.3	56.3	57.4	54.5	62.4	54.1	56.2
U.S.A.	40.7	39.0	39.2	32.5	35.8	43.6	n/a	38.5
Annual mean	62.2	61.6	56.3	53.2	55.1	63.2	58.4	—

n/a = not available.

The actual profile of imported species varies considerably among countries, primarily reflecting the geographic source of the infection. In many countries, immigrant communities account for an increasing proportion of malaria cases (Table 18–4), and the geographic origin of the immigrants plays a major role in the determination of the predominant *Plasmodium* species. The United Kingdom traditionally has imported a large proportion of *Plasmodium vivax* infections because of the large number of immigrants from India and Pakistan.[20] In 1988, however, *Plasmodium falciparum* became the dominant imported species, reflecting the increased transmission of *P. falciparum* in Asia, the changing patterns of traveler origin, and drug resistance. In the United States, *P. falciparum* accounts for less than 50% of all imported infections as many Americans visit Central America and Asia as opposed to tropical Africa. Only 0.4 million American and Canadian travelers visit Africa, versus 17 million visiting Central America and 2.1 million visiting Asia,[21] both regions that are predominantly *Plasmodium vivax* transmission areas. In Italy, imported cases show a high prevalence of *Plasmodium falciparum* infections, mainly in African immigrants who revisit their country of origin and become ill with malaria after their return to Italy.[22,23] Data from the Italian Ministry of Health indicate that malaria from immigrant communities accounts for an increasing proportion of national malaria figures, its incidence rate having risen from 14% in 1986 to 40.4% in 1991.[23]

Table 18–4. **Studies of Immigrants as a Risk Group for Imported Malaria in Industrialized Countries**

Country	Cohort	Proportion of Non-Nationals
Spain*	Imported malaria at a referral center in Madrid	37.5%
Switzerland[†]	Hospital admissions for malaria in Basel (1970–1992)	27%
France[‡] (Moselle region)	Imported malaria cases treated in Moselle (1996–1999)	96% (64% from W. Africa)
Norway[§]	Imported malaria cases in Norway (1989–1998)	58% (26% from Pakistan, India, Sri Lanka)
Netherlands[‖]	Malaria cases treated at the Academic Medical Centre, Amsterdam (1991–1994)	40% (originally from endemic areas); 8% children born in the Netherlands to immigrant families

* Data from Lopez-Valez R, Perez Casas C, Martin-Arest J, et al. Clinicoepidemiological study of imported malaria in travelers and immigrants to Madrid. J Travel Med 1999;6:81–86.

[†] Data from Nuesch R, Scheller M, Gyr N. Hospital admissions for malaria in Basel, Switzerland: an epidemiological review of 150 cases. J Travel Med 2000;7:95–97.

[‡] Data from Talarmin E, Sicard JM, Mounem M, et al. Imported malaria in Moselle: 75 cases in three years. Rev Med Interne 2000;21:242–246.

[§] Data from Jensenius M, Ronning EJ, Blystad H, et al. Low frequency of complications in imported falciparum malaria: a review of 222 cases in south-eastern Norway. Scand J Infect Dis 1999;31:73–78.

[‖] Data from Wetsteyn JCFM, Kager PA, van Gool T. The changing pattern of imported malaria in the Academic Medical Centre, Amsterdam. J Travel Med 1997;4:171–175.

Despite a high risk of infection, returning immigrants are less likely to actually die from malaria infection and tend to have significantly lower parasitemia levels than those recorded in travelers despite the fact that immigrants rarely receive chemoprophylaxis. This suggests that in spite of a loss of immunity, some immunologic memory has a role in reducing the severity of the disease.[23] Retrospective analyses of the chemoprophylactic status of persons with malaria acquired abroad show that immigrants rarely use chemosuppressive drugs.[22] Immigrant groups in all industrialized countries are unlikely to seek medical advice prior to travel and need to be especially targeted for advice and protective measures.

Case-Fatality Rate Profile

Information on deaths due to malaria is inconsistently collected in the various European countries. In the industrialized countries, German travelers appear to have the highest CFR (mean from 1989 to 1995, 3.6%) (see Table 18–5). Incomplete data from Portugal indicated a very high CFR in 1993—11 deaths in 18 *P. falciparum* cases, a CFR of 61%—but this figure could not be confirmed. In contrast, the United Kingdom shows consistently low CFRs, averaging 0.7%.

Despite medical advances, it has proven difficult to reduce the CFR to below 1%. The difference in CFRs among countries is striking and can be only partially explained by surveillance inadequacies. Delayed identification of disease and/or inadequate treatment point to a deficit in medical awareness and expertise in the

Table 18-5. Case-Fatality Rates, 1989 to 1995 (*Plasmodium falciparum* Cases)[16]

Country	1989			1990			1991			1992		
	Cases	Deaths	CFR (%)	Cases	Deaths	CFR (%)	Cases	Deaths	CFR (%)	Cases	Deaths	CFR (%)
Austria	63	1	1.59	53	1	1.89	48	0	0.00	20	0	0.00
France*	1,511	18	1.19	1,163	15	1.29	n/a	20	—	n/a	11	—
Germany	694	22	3.17	588	19	3.23	530	10	1.89	489	21	4.29
Greece	29	0	0.00	16	0	0.00	20	0	0.00	9	0	0.00
Italy	345	7	2.03	395	7	1.77	350	6	1.71	367	7	1.91
Netherlands	166	2	1.20	171	1	0.58	168	2	1.19	110	2	1.82
Spain	70	0	0.00	87	0	0.00	102	2	1.96	86	4	4.65
Switzerland	169	2	1.18	172	3	1.74	138	3	2.17	141	2	1.42
U.K.	1,117	4	0.36	1,097	4	0.36	1,314	12	0.91	935	11	1.18
U.S.A.	448	4	0.89	428	2	0.47	410	0	0.00	296	7	2.36

Country	1993			1994			1995			1989–1995		
	Cases	Deaths	CFR (%)	Cases	Deaths	CFR (%)	Cases	Deaths	CFR (%)	Cases	Deaths	CFR (%)
Austria	50	2	4.00	42	0	0.00	46	1	2.17	322	5	1.55
France	624	10	1.60	696	12	1.72	1,004	13	1.29	4,998	99	1.98
Germany	357	17	4.76	563	28	4.97	526	18	3.42	3,747	135	3.60
Greece	19	0	0.00	10	0	0.00	6	0	0.00	109	0	0.00
Italy	468	4	0.85	564	4	0.71	527	5	0.95	3,016	40	1.33
Netherlands	133	0	0.00	152	2	1.32	174	2	1.15	1,074	11	1.02
Spain	88	1	1.14	192	3	1.56	159	5	3.14	784	15	1.91
Switzerland	147	3	2.04	189	2	1.06	190	2	1.05	1,146	17	1.48
U.K.	1,048	5	0.48	1,178	11	0.93	1,112	4	0.36	7,801	51	0.65
U.S.A.	457	8	1.75	442	4	0.90	n/a	n/a	—	2,481	25	1.01

CFR = case-fatality rate; n/a = not available.
* Incomplete data (U.S.A., 6 years; France, 5 years).

management of this infection. A Canadian report on imported malaria showed that about 59% of imported malaria cases are initially missed, which leads to high levels of morbidity and mortality.[24] For the period of 1977 to 1986,[19] the average CFR for Europe as a whole was 1.1%. The more recent survey detailed here[16] shows large intercountry variation, with Germany having a higher CFR; this could be partially explained by good mortality reporting in association with poor case reporting or detection and a lack of awareness in general practitioners. According to Zastrow and colleagues, fatalities occur almost exclusively in infections acquired in Africa and mainly occur in German short-term tourists to Kenya.[25,26] Tourists aged more than 60 years were shown to be especially at risk.

A Special Profile: Attack Rates in Tourists to Kenya

Studies have shown that short-term tourists to Kenya are particularly at risk of infection.[27,28] Tourists who visit Kenya without the protection of malaria chemo-prophylaxis develop malaria at a rate of 1.2% per month.[28,29] There was no international consensus with regard to recommendations for malaria chemoprophylaxis for travelers to Kenya during the period of study (1990 to 1995), and it is possible that the differences in attack rates can be attributed partly to the varying types of chemoprophylaxis used and/or to compliance with medication and antimosquito measures. Either mefloquine (United States and CH) or chloroquine/proguanil (United Kingdom and Sweden) was the regimen of choice for this destination.[30] Table 18–6 shows that rates were lower in countries where mefloquine was the first-choice regimen. Since 1993, when mefloquine was recommended for travelers to East Africa, the rate of imported cases from East Africa in the United Kingdom has fallen substantially.[31] At the same time, the number of malaria patients who report taking no chemoprophylaxis has remained steady. Taking malaria transmission levels into account, these observations were interpreted as evidence for the superior protective efficacy of mefloquine. Similarly, in U.S. civilians, the 38% decline in the number of *P. falciparum* infections acquired in Africa observed during 1991and 1992 was attributed partly to the increased use of the more effective mefloquine regimen.[32]

The highest attack rate for tourists to Kenya (160 per 100,000) was observed in Italian travelers in 1993. German travelers appear to be particularly at risk, with consistently high attack rates (mean, 128 per 100,000). Low attack rates (mean, 61 per 100,000) were observed in U.S. travelers.

COMPLIANCE WITH CHEMOPROPHYLAXIS AND SUBSEQUENT DEVELOPMENT OF SYMPTOMS

Information on compliance is only sporadically available, but several reports stress the importance of this factor.[30,33–35] Among U.S. civilians who had imported

Table 18–6. Attack Rates in Travelers to Kenya

Country	1990 Travelers	Cases	Cases per 10^5	1991 Travelers	Cases	Cases per 10^5	1992 Travelers	Cases	Cases per 10^5
Austria	15,100	20	132	15,350	8	52	14,041	6	43
Germany	123,100	188	153	126,740	140	110	109,973	167	152
Italy	41,400	63	152	40,130	33	82	35,105	22	63
Netherlands	n/a	20	—	15,720	23	146	12,628	12	95
Sweden	n/a	15	—	n/a	5	—	22,739	4	18
Switzerland	35,300	25	71	29,630	19	64	26,883	35	130
U.K.	105,100	128	122	141,420	176	124	117,458	129	110
U.S.A.	65,200	44	67	54,680	36	66	46,218	27	58

Country	1993 Travelers	Cases	Cases per 10^5	1994 Travelers	Cases	Cases per 10^5	1995 Travelers	Cases	Cases per 10^5	Average Rate per 10^5
Austria	16,607	9	54	9,650	12	124	13,880	9	65	78
Germany	130,000	105	81	132,300	197	149	108,707	136	125	128
Italy	42,000	67	160	55,000	80	145	34,701	72	207	135
Netherlands	14,936	7	47	n/a	7	—	12,482	4	32	80
Sweden	27,000	7	26	30,000*	27	90	24,476	16	65	50
Switzerland	32,000	31	97	30,200	46	152	26,574	36	135	108
U.K.	139,000	92	66	129,500	87	67	116,106	80	69	93
U.S.A.	55,000	34	62	59,700	32	54	45,687	n/a	—	61

n/a = not available.
* Approximately.

malaria, about 81% of infections occurred in persons who had not taken a chemo-prophylactic regimen recommended by the Centers for Disease Control and Prevention (CDC). In malaria cases imported to Germany (1987 to 1991), about 35% of infected individuals did not use any chemoprophylaxis.[26] Pryce and colleagues found poor compliance in travelers to Kenya, with only 16% of travelers using currently advised regimens.[27] Gyorkos and colleagues found that compliance with chemoprophylaxis was effective in reducing malaria risk.[34] Short-term travelers often use no protection, use inadequate regimens, or are noncompliant with their medication. Deaths occur more often in individuals who use no chemoprophylaxis, and prior chemoprophylaxis leads to a reduction in the severity of falciparum malaria.[35] Nuesch and colleagues showed that nonadherence to chemoprophylaxis was a major risk factor in hospitalized malaria patients.[36] This was reinforced by a Norwegian retrospective analysis that showed that noncompliance was significantly associated with the development of complicated disease.[37] Immigrants are even less likely to use chemoprophylaxis. In a recent analysis of malaria cases in Italian travelers,[38] only 36% of Italian and 4% of foreign malaria patients used regular chemoprophylaxis. Similarly, in Belgium, significantly fewer malaria patients of African origin used chemoprophylaxis during travel to high-risk areas, compared to Caucasians.[39] Appropriate effective chemoprophylaxis should therefore be recommended for risk areas, and the protective efficacy of respective prophylactic regimens needs constant monitoring. The increasing popularity of last-minute travel bargains will result in even more unprepared tourists abroad, and such spontaneous travel may well lead to an increased incidence of malaria.

CONCLUSION

The almost 10,000 imported malaria cases reported annually in industrialized countries (probably only one-third of the total cases) illustrate the need to target at-risk travelers and immigrant groups in regard to malaria awareness. Cooperation of the medical profession with the travel industry should lead to the development of preventive strategies to increase malaria awareness in travelers. The medical profession must be conditioned to consider malaria in the differential diagnosis of unexplained fever in travelers and immigrants and to act appropriately.

Inconsistent surveillance, lack of homogeneity of collected data, and lack of monitoring of drug response are major obstacles to the quantification of the actual problem of imported malaria in industrialized countries. Improved surveillance and reporting would serve to quantify absolute incidence rates, identify risk groups, and indicate the prophylactic efficacy of various regimens.

REFERENCES

1. Hackett LW. Malaria in Europe. London: Oxford University Press, 1955.
2. Bruce-Chwatt LJ, de Zulueta J. The rise and fall of malaria in Europe: a historical epidemiological study. Oxford: Oxford University Press, 1980.
3. Wernsdorfer W, McGregor I. History of malaria from prehistory to eradication. In: Malaria, principles and practice of malariology. New York: Churchill Livingstone, 1988.
4. Handszuh H, Waters SR. Travel and tourism patterns. In: DuPont HL, Steffen R, editors. Hamilton (ON): Textbook of travel medicine. B.C. Decker, Inc., 1997.
5. Jelinek T, Loscher T, Nothdurft H, et al. High prevalence of antibodies against circumsporozoite antigen of *Plasmodium falciparum* without development of symptomatic malaria in travellers returning from sub-Saharan Africa. J Infect Dis 1996;174:1376–1379.
6. Zucker JR. Changing patterns of autochthonous malaria transmission in the United States: a review of recent outbreaks. Emerg Infect Dis 1996;2:37–43.
7. Centers for Disease Control and Prevention. Mosquito-transmitted malaria—California and Florida, 1990. MMWR Morb Mortal Wkly Rep 1991;40:106–108.
8. Brook JH, Genese CA, Bloland PB, et al. Malaria probably locally acquired in New Jersey. N Engl J Med 1994;331:22–23.
9. Layton M, Parise ME, Campbell CC, et al. Mosquito-transmitted malaria in New York City, 1993. Lancet 1995;346:729–731.
10. Signorelli C, Messineo A. Airport malaria. Lancet 1990;335:164.
11. Marty P, Le Fichoux Y, Izri MA, et al. Autochthonous *Plasmodium falciparum* in southern France. Trans R Soc Trop Med Hyg 1992;86:478.
12. Gentilini M, Danis M. Le paludisme autochtone. Med Mal Infect 1981;11:356–362.
13. Simini B. First case of indigenous malaria reported in Italy for 40 years, news. Lancet 1997;350:717.
14. Reiter P. Global-Warming and vector-borne disease in temperate regions and at high altitude. Lancet 1998;351:839–840.
15. Legros F, Danis M. Surveillance of malaria in European Union countries. Eurosurveillance 1998;3:45–47.
16. Muentener P, Schlagenhauf P, Steffen R. Imported malaria (1985–95): trends and perspectives. Bull World Health Organ 1999;77:560–566.
17. Sergiev VP, et al. Importation of malaria into the USSR from Afghanistan: 1981–1989. Bull World Health Organ 1993;71:385–388.
18. Centre National de Référence pour les Maladies d'Importation. Bulletin No. 12, 1996.
19. Phillips-Howard PA, Bradley DJ. Epidemiology of malaria in European travelers. In: Steffen R, et al. Textbook of travel medicine. Proceedings of the First Conference on International Travel Medicine; 1988 Apr 5–8; Zürich, Switzerland. Berlin, Heidelberg, and New York: 1989.
20. Bradley DJ. Current trends in malaria in Britain. J R Soc Med 1989;82 Suppl 17:8–13.
21. World Health Organization. World Health Report 1996. Geneva: World Health Organization, 1996.
22. Raglio A, et al. Ten-year experience with imported malaria in Bergamo, Italy. J Travel Med 1994;1:152–155.
23. Di Perri G, et al. West African immigrants and new patterns of malaria imported to northeastern Italy. J Travel Med 1994;1:147–151.

24. Kain KC, Harrington MA, Tennyson S, Keystone JS. Imported malaria: prospective analysis of problems in diagnosis and management. Clin Infect Dis 1998;27:142–149.

25. Zastrow KD, et al. Reisekrankheit Malaria—Einschleppungen nach Deutschland 1988. Gesundheitswesen 1993;55:136–139.

26. Zastrow KD, et al. Malaria—Erkrankungen in Deutschland 1987–1991. Bundesgesundheitsblatt 1993;11:476–481.

27. Pryce DI, et al. The changing pattern of imported malaria in British visitors to Kenya. J R Soc Med 1993;86:152–153.

28. Lobel HO, et al. Recent trends in the importation of malaria caused by *Plasmodium falciparum* into the United States from Africa. J Infect Dis 1985;152:613–617.

29. Steffen R, et al. Mefloquine compared with other malaria chemoprophylactic regimens in tourists visiting East Africa. Lancet 1993;341:1299–1302.

30. Lobel HO, et al. Malaria incidence and prevention among European and North American travellers to Kenya. Bull World Health Organ 1990;68:209–215.

31. Behrens RH, et al. Impact of U.K. malaria prophylaxis policy on imported malaria. Lancet 1996;348:344–345.

32. Zucker JR, Barber AM, Paxton LA, et al. Malaria surveillance—United States 1992. MMWR Morb Mortal Wkly Rep 1995;44:1–17.

33. Cobelens FG, Leentvaar-Kuijpers A. Compliance with malaria chemoprophylaxis and preventative measures against moquito bites among Dutch travellers. Trop Med Int Health 1997;2:705–713.

34. Gyorkos TW, et al. Compliance with antimalarial chemoprophylaxis and the subsequent development of malaria: a matched case-control study. Am J Trop Med Hyg 1995;53:511–517.

35. Lewis SJ, et al. Severity of imported falciparum malaria: effect of taking antimalarial prophylaxis. BMJ 1992;305:741–743.

36. Nuesch R, Scheller M, Gyr N. Hospital admissions for malaria in Basel, Switzerland: an epidemiological review of 150 cases. J Travel Med 2000;7:95–97.

37. Jensenius M, Ronning EJ, Blystad H, et al. Low frequency of complications in imported falciparum malaria: a review of 222 cases in south-eastern Norway. Scand J Infect Dis 1999;31:73–78.

38. Romi R, Sabatinelli G, Majori G. Malaria epidemiological situation in Italy and evaluation of malaria incidence in Italian travelers. J Travel Med 2001;8:6–11.

39. Van den Ende J, Morales I, Van den Abbeele K, et al. Changing epidemiological and clinical aspects of imported malaria in Belgium. J Travel Med 2001;8:19–25.

Chapter 19

CLOSING THE CIRCLE

Jay Keystone and Phyllis Kozarsky

ABSTRACT

The trend in imported malaria in the 1990s was a reflection of an increase in the number of travelers to malarious areas, an increase in malaria transmission in various destination areas, and an increase in drug resistance. Most important for the present, however, are the lack of understanding among many travelers about the risk and serious nature of the illness and the resultant disinclination of travelers to seek pretravel health advice and to adhere to recommendations. These latter factors apply particularly to immigrants returning to their homelands to visit friends and relatives. In addition, health care providers often do not provide appropriate recommendations for malaria prevention. Since infection is often a result of nonadherence to prevention measures, one key to the solution is to use the Health Belief Model to help identify creative ways of communicating health advice to travelers so that they will begin to take greater responsibility for disease prevention. Also, there is a great need to improve culturally sensitive public education that encourages travelers to seek pretravel health advice and to improve continuing education for health professionals to insure that the advice they give is accurate and appropriate.

Key words: adherence; Health Belief Model.

HOW DID WE GET HERE?

Every case of malaria in travelers represents a failure: failure of the travel industry to promote awareness of the risk, failure of the health care provider to be knowledgeable about malaria prevention and thus to communicate risk effectively to the traveler, and/or failure of the traveler to adhere to malaria prevention measures. The trends of imported malaria are a reflection of these issues as well as several major influences, including an increase in the number of travelers to malarious areas, an increase in malaria transmission at travel destinations, an increase in drug resistance, and most importantly, the failure of travelers to adhere to appropriate recommendations for preventing the infection.[1–8]

The numbers are clear. As air travel becomes more accessible and less expensive, and as the traveler has the ability to reach any malarious region of the world within 48 hours, exposure to the disease has increased significantly. With the globalization of the economy, business travelers can remain virtually homeless, circling the globe indefinitely. Military intervention, as well as exotic, adventure, and "extreme" travel, brings individuals into greater contact with environmental challenges and with vectors of disease. Political upheavals and socioeconomic disasters have resulted in the mass migration of people from non-endemic to endemic areas as well as the return of migrants to their homelands after having lost their semi-immune status. Recent data from GeoSentinel, the global surveillance network of the International Society of Travel Medicine, indicate that the relative risk of acquiring malaria during travel varies widely according to the purpose of travel. Migrants going home to visit friends and relatives have an approximately eightfold increased risk when compared to usual tourists. More surprisingly, business travelers have a twofold increased risk, and those on research or academic missions have a threefold increased risk when compared to usual tourists. (Freedman DL, GeoSentinel Surveillance System. Personal communication to authors, Jan 10, 2001.)

Transmission of malaria in the 21st century approximates that seen in the earlier part of the 1900s. We have moved from "malaria eradication" in the 1950s and 1960s, to "malaria control" in the late 1960s and 1970s, to "Roll back malaria" in the year 2000.[9] This increase in malaria transmission has been due to the failure of public health programs, development schemes that have increased breeding sites for the vector mosquitoes, increased resistance of the mosquitoes to insecticides, and increased resistance of the malaria parasite to available antimalarial drugs. Compounding these problems has been the additional loss of prophylactic and self-treatment agents due to their lack of tolerability (e.g., severe cutaneous reactions from Fansidar, cardiotoxicity of halofantrine, agranulocytosis associated with amodiaquine, and neuropsychiatric problems due to mefloquine).

With few exceptions, the travel industry has not taken the responsibility of educating itself and its clients about the risk of malaria associated with travel. As a general rule, the travel industry is reluctant to use the words "health" and "travel" in the same message. What it fails to appreciate is that healthy travelers travel again and that unhealthy travelers do not travel again—nor do their friends, relatives, or colleagues.

Numerous studies of primary care physicians and even travel medicine specialists have demonstrated that their knowledge of malaria prevention measures is woefully inadequate.[10,11] Health care providers in many industrialized countries have little knowledge about the global disease burden of malaria, its epidemiology, and the changing patterns of drug resistance. Furthermore, these health care providers (who have had minimal training in the diagnosis and treatment of malaria) frequently fail to consider malaria in the differential diagnosis of illness in the returned traveler and do not appreciate the urgency with which the illness must be managed.[12]

Malaria chemoprophylaxis was straightforward when chloroquine was the single agent for the prevention and treatment of disease. However, with growing resistance and with an enlarging antimalarial armamentarium, the choice of a prophylactic drug for the traveler has become ever more complex. The difficulty faced by health care providers in making a decision concerning chemoprophylaxis has been magnified by the lack of consensus among various international and national authoritative bodies with regards to appropriate prophylaxis.[13–15] This problem is compounded by the Internet, through which travelers have access to a variety of travel health resources that contain both accurate and inaccurate information.

Irrespective of the issues outlined above, the key to the continued increase in travelers' malaria is the traveler. Although no antimalarial is 100% effective, the use of an appropriate antimalarial combined with personal protection measures virtually guarantees freedom from life-threatening malaria in travelers. In multiple reviews of travelers' malaria, an inappropriate regimen or the lack of adherence to the regimen was the major reason for infection.[16–22] There are a number of reasons why travelers may not comply with recommendations, such as ignorance of the risk and severity of malaria, confusion about which antimalarial to take, forgetfulness concerning the regular use of medication, cost and inconvenience, and concern about and experience with side effects.[23–27] Cultural perceptions of immunity to infection and exaggerated media reports about drug reactions have played major roles in influencing individuals in the decision whether or not to use antimalarials.[22,28–30]

In trying to better understand the crux of the problem of antimalarial use by travelers, it is useful to examine the Health Belief Model (Figure 19–1).[31] This paradigm is a theoretic framework for explaining the likelihood of an individual's undertaking a preventive health action. The theory argues that one's decision to take an antimalarial agent is dependent on one's perception of (1) the level of per-

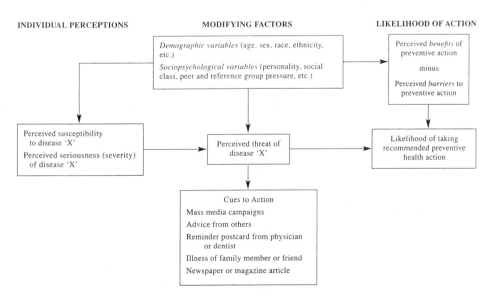

Figure 19–1. Original formulation of the Health Belief Model.

sonal susceptibility to malaria, (2) the severity of its consequences, (3) the potential benefits of chemoprophylaxis and personal protection measures, and (4) the other barriers or costs related to initiating these protective measures. The model also stipulates that a stimulus or a cue to action must occur to trigger the use of preventive measures by making the individual aware of his or her feelings about the threat of malaria.

Several studies have shown that travelers have inaccurate perceptions of the various health risks associated with travel. For example, 45% of 100 U.S. elderly travelers chose air travel as their greatest risk factor,[32] 70% of French travelers were concerned about snake or scorpion bites,[33] and 56% of Canadian travelers perceived their risk of illness to be less than 20% in a 1- to 4-week trip to Africa, Asia, or South America.[34] Focus groups and studies of the Nigerian and South Asian communities have shown that when returning to their countries of origin, these travelers, in particular, perceive their health risks as minimal.

WHERE SHOULD WE GO FROM HERE?

It is clear that the problem of travelers' malaria is not going to improve and will likely worsen over the next decade. Continued social strife and the lack of financial and human resources will impede malaria control programs. The annual budget for the World Health Organization malaria control program is less than the cost of one stealth bomber. The specter of global warming may increase the risk of disease in previously unaffected areas and lead to the deterioration of conditions in endemic zones.[35] Drug resistance shows no signs of slowing, and the pharmaceutical industry demonstrates little interest in developing new agents or insect repellents for the antimalarial armamentarium.

Is there any light at the end of the tunnel? The introduction of atovaquone/proguanil has brought renewed enthusiasm to the travel medicine community; however, this should be tempered by the cost of the drug and its unknown efficacy and safety in large groups of nonimmune travelers.[36] Most exciting is the possible introduction of tafenoquine, a drug that works in an analogous way to the military's "fire and forget." As with each introduction of a new antimalarial agent, however, how long will it be before the parasite takes the upper hand and develops resistance? Although a vaccine for preventing malaria holds great promise, it remains a fantasy. Until a vaccine is developed, travel medicine advisors must focus on the use of antimalarials and personal protection measures.

The availability of easy-to-use rapid diagnostic tests for malaria has fueled an interest in using these tools for the self-diagnosis of malaria in the field.[37] Unfortunately, studies have shown that these tests are not yet ready for use by the typical traveler but appear to be excellent for use in diagnostic laboratories.[38,39] This point cannot be emphasized enough as the diagnosis of malaria is fraught with undue

Table 19–1. **Clinical Utility Scores for Current Malaria Chemoprophylactic Regimens***

Drug	Efficacy[†]	Tolerance[‡]	Convenience[§]	Causal[‖]	Cost[#]	Total
Mefloquine	3	1	3	0	2	9
Doxycycline	3	2	2	0	3	10
Chloroquine/ proguanil	1	2	1	0	2	6
Azithromycin	2	2	2	0	1	7
Primaquine	2	2	1**	2	3	10
Atovaquone/ proguanil	3	3	2	2	1	11

* Scores and weighting are arbitrary and can be modified or individualized to specific travelers and itineraries.
[†] Efficacy: 1 = < 75%; 2 = 75% to 89%; 3 = ≥ 90% .
[‡] Tolerance: 1 = occasional disabling side effects; 2 = rare disabling side effects; 3 = rare minor side effects.
[§] Convenience: 1 = daily and weekly dosing required; 2 = daily dosing required; 3 = weekly dosing required.
[‖] Causal: 0 = no causal activity; 2 = causal prophylactic (may be discontinued within a few days of leaving risk area).
[#] Cost: 1 = > $100 per month; 2 = $50–$100 per month; 3 = < $50 per month.
**Requires a pretravel glucose-6-phosphate dehydrogenase (G6PD) level assessment, resulting in a lower convenience score.

delay and inaccuracies in most industrialized countries. Thus, rapid diagnostics could be useful even in health centers with little technologic sophistication. However, it will be the next generation rapid malaria diagnostic kits that should be more user-friendly and available at a reasonable price to the traveler for self-diagnosis of malaria.

Travelers' malaria is a failure, and the major cause of this failure is lack of adherence to prevention measures. As the source of the problem can be found by analyzing the Health Belief Model, so too can the solution. The key to the solution is identifying innovative and creative ways of communicating health advice to travelers so that they will be convinced of their vulnerability and will take responsibility for disease prevention. Education must be patient centered. This involves patients taking part in the decision-making process and may involve negotiating what is most reasonable, depending on variables such as cost, convenience, and adverse effect profile. In fact, the choices may not be optimal and may not even conform to the wishes of the health care provider. Moreover, culturally sensitive and culturally directed methods of communication (see Figure 19–1) will need to be developed to educate the traveler at greatest risk for malaria.

The predominant need is for studies to identify the most effective means of communicating malaria risk and preventative strategies to the travel industry and the health care provider, in addition to the traveler. This process can be assisted by the reduction of confusion and controversy through the development of uniform, evidence-based, globally accepted recommendations for malaria prevention. However, history has repeatedly shown that scientific evidence is not the sole determinant for official government recommendations of antimalarial drugs of choice. Geographic differences in culture, attitudes, experience, and risk perceptions play an important role in the decision-making process at the national level. On an individual level, the use of Clinical Utility Scores (Table 19–1)[40] seems at first glance to offer the most objective approach to choosing the optimal antimalarial drug. Once again, cultural and personal differences among travelers will have a significant influence on their acceptance of drug cost, convenience, efficacy, and side effects, thereby limiting the practical application of this scientifically based decision-making tool.

As health care providers entering the 21st century, we have an opportunity to use a different paradigm to look at the prevention of malaria. We know the epidemiology of malaria and the patterns of drug resistance. We have effective drugs, and we have effective measures to prevent mosquito bites. Effective strategies demand greater attention to the traveler, for it is only the traveler who can "close the circle."

REFERENCES

1. Handszuh H. Tourism patterns and trends. In: Dupont HL, Steffen R, editors. Textbook of travel medicine and health. 2nd ed. Hamilton (ON): B. C. Decker, Inc., 2001.
2. Muentener P, Schlagenhauf P, Steffen R. Imported malaria (1985–95): trends and perspectives. Bull World Health Organ 1999;77:560–565.
3. Hastings M, Alessandra U. Modeling a predictable disaster: the rise and spread of drug-resistant malaria. Parasitol Today 2000;16:340–347.
4. Steffen R, Heusser R, Machler R, et al. Malaria chemoprophylaxis among European tourists in tropical Africa: use, adverse reactions, and efficacy. Bull World Health Organ 1990;68:313–322.
5. Phillips-Howard PA, Blaze M, Hurn M, Bradley DJ. Malaria prophylaxis: survey of the response of British travelers to prophylactic advice. BMJ 1986;293:932–934.
6. Lobel HO, Campbell CC, Papaioanou M, Huong AY. Use of prophylaxis for malaria by American travelers to Africa and Haiti. JAMA 1987;257:2626–2627.
7. Cobelens FGJ, Leentvaar-Kuijpers A. Compliance with malaria chemoprophylaxis and preventative measures against mosquito bites among Dutch travellers. Trop Med Int Health 1997;2:705–713.
8. Behrens RH, Taylor RB, Pryce DI, et al. Chemoprophylaxis compliance in travelers with malaria. J Travel Med 1998;5:92–94.
9. WHO Expert Committee on malaria. World Health Organ Tech Rep Ser 2000;892:1–74.
10. Keystone JS, Dismukes R, Sawyer L, Kozarsky P. Inadequacies in health recommendations provided for international travelers by North American health advisors. J Travel Med 1994;1:72–78.
11. Hatz C, Krause E, Grundmann H. Travel advice—a study among Swiss and German general practitioners. Trop Med Int Health 1997;2:6–12.
12. Kain KC, Harrington MA, Tennyson S, Keystone JS. Imported malaria: prospective analysis of problems in diagnosis and management. Clin Infect Dis 1998;27:142–149.
13. Centers for Disease Control. Malaria. In: Health information for international travel. Atlanta: U.S. Dept. of Health and Human Services, 2000. p. 110–121.
14. World Health Organization. Malaria. In: International health and travel. Geneva: World Health Organization, 2000. p. 67–78.
15. Committee to Advise on Tropical Medicine and Travel. Canadian recommendations for the prevention and treatment of malaria among international travelers. Ottawa (Canada): Health Canada, 2000. p. 1–41.
16. Greenberg A, Lobel HO. Mortality from *Plasmodium falciparum* malaria in travellers from the United States. Ann Intern Med 1990;113:326–327.

17. Winters RA, Murray HW. Malaria—the mime revisited: fifteen more years of experience at a New York City teaching hospital. Am J Med 1992;93:243–245.

18. Froude JRL, Weiss LM, Tanowitz HB, Wittner M. Imported malaria in the Bronx: review of 51 cases recorded from 1986–91. Clin Infect Dis 1992;15:774–780.

19. Raglio A, Parea M, Lorenzi N et al. Ten-year experience with imported malaria in Bergamo, Italy. J Travel Med 1994;1:152–155.

20. Dorsey G, Ghandi M, Oyugi JH, Rosenthal PJ. Difficulties in the prevention, diagnosis and treatment of imported malaria. Arch Intern Med 2000;160:2505–2510.

21. Nuesch R, Scheller M, Gyr N. Hospital admissions for malaria, Basel, Switzerland: an epidemiological review of 150 cases. J Travel Med 2000;7:95–97.

22. Castelli F, Matteeli A, Caligaris S, et al. Malaria in migrants. Parassitologia 1999; 41:261–265.

23. Held TK, Weinke T, Mansmann U, et al. Malaria prophylaxis: identifying risk groups for non-compliance. QJM 1994;87:17–22.

24. Hoebe C, de Munter J, Thijs C. Adverse effects and compliance with mefloquine or proguanil antimalarial chemoprophylaxis. Eur J Clin Pharmacol 1997;52:269–275.

25. Huzly D, Schonfeld C, Beuerle W, Bienzle U. Malaria chemoprophylaxis in German tourists; a prospective study on compliance and adverse reactions. J Travel Med 1996;3:148–155.

26. Steffen R, Behrens RH. Travelers' malaria. Parasitol Today 1992;8:61–66.

27. Behrens RH, Curtis CF. Malaria in travelers: epidemiology and prevention. Br Med Bull 1993;49:363–383.

28. Dos Santos CC, Anvar A, Keystone JS, Kain KC. Survey of use of malaria prevention measures by Canadians visiting India. Can Med Assoc J 1999;160:195–200.

29. Epstein K. The Lariam files. The Washington Post 2000 Oct 10.

30. Winokur S. Some find malaria drug worse than disease. The San Francisco Examiner 1998 May 17.

31. Becker MI, Marman LA, Kirscht JP, et al. Patient perceptions and compliance: recent studies of the Health Belief Model. In: Haynes RB, Taylor DW, Sackett DL, editors. Compliance in health care. Baltimore: Johns Hopkins University Press, 1979. p. 79.

32. Olson PE, Mayers MT, Rumans L, et al. Misperceptions of travel risks by older travelers [abstract 58]. Proceedings of the Third International Conference on Travel Medicine; 1993 April 25–29; Paris, France.

33. Picot N, Receveur MC, Goujon C, et al. Real information needs of the traveler before his departure. Results of a survey by questionnaire. Bull Soc Pathol Exot 1993;86: 418–420.

34. McPherson DW, Stephenson BJ. Perception of risk in Canadian travelers [abstract 48]. Proceedings of the Third International Conference on Travel Medicine; 1993 April 25–29; Paris, France.

35. Lindsay SW, Birley MH. Climate change and malaria transmission. Ann Trop Med Parasitol 1996;90:573–588.

36. Shanks GD. New options for the prevention and treatment of malaria: focus on the role of atovaquone and proguanil hydrochloride. J Travel Med 1999;6 Suppl 2:S1–32.

37. World Health Organization. A rapid dipstick antigen capture assay for the diagnosis of falciparum malaria. Bull World Health Organ 1996;74:47–54.

38. Funk M, Schlagenhauf P, Tschopp A, Steffen R. Malaquick™ versus ParaSight® as a diagnostic aid in travellers' malaria. Trans R Soc Trop Med Hyg 1999;93:268–272.

39. Jelinek T, Amsler L, Grobusch MP, Nothdurft HD. Self-use of rapid tests for malaria by tourists. Lancet 1999;354:1609.

40. Kain KC, Shanks D, Keystone JS. Malaria chemoprophylaxis in an age of drug-resistance. Part 1: Currently recommended drug regimens. Clin Infect Dis 2001. [In press]

APPENDIX 1

Drug regimens for chemoprophylaxis (WHO guidelines)

Prophylactic schedules for children should be based on weight.

Chloroquine (common trade names: Aralen, Avloclor, Nivaquine, Resochin)

The recommended prophylactic regimen is **5mg base/kg weekly**. The following table is based on the administration of the commonly used tablets containing either 100 mg or 150 mg base.

Weight (kg)	Age (yr)	Number of Tablets/Week	
		100 mg Base*	150 mg Base
5–6	< 4 months	0.25	0.25
7–10	4–11 months	0.5	0.5
11–14	1–2	0.75	0.5
15–18	3–4	1	0.75
19–24	5–7	1.25	1
25–35	8–10	2	1
36–50	11–13	2.5	2
50+	14+	3	2

Note: Some authorities recommend a total weekly dose of 10 mg/kg divided into 6 daily doses (i.e., an adult dose of 100 mg base daily for 6 days per week).
*In the case of young children, more precise dosages can be obtained with tablets containing 100 mg base.

Proguanil (common trade name: Paludrine)

The recommended prophylactic regimen is **3 mg/kg daily** in combination with chloroquine. The following table applies to tablets containing 100 mg proguanil hydrochloride.

Weight (kg)	Age (yr)	Number of Tablets/Day
5–8	< 8 months	0.25
9–16	8 months – 3 years	0.5
17–24	4–7	0.75
25–35	8–10	1
36–50	11–13	1.5
50+	14+	2

Note: In several countries, a combination tablet containing 100 mg chloroquine base + 200 mg proguanil hydrochloride (common trade name: Savarine) is available, which may improve compliance in adults.

Mefloquine (common trade name: Eloquin, Lariam, Mephaquin)

The following regimens relate to the commonly used tablet containing 250 mg base to be taken for prophylaxis at a **single weekly dose of 5 mg/kg**. Patients prescribed the formulation available in the USA containing 228 mg base (i.e., 250 mg mefloquine hydrochloride) should take the same number of tablets but will receive a slightly lower weekly dose of the drug of the drug in terms of base.

Weight (kg)	Age (yr)	Number of Tablets/Week
< 5	< 3 months	Not recommended
5–6	3 months	0.25
7–8	4–7 months	0.25
9–12	8–23 months	0.25
13–16	2–3	0.33
17–24	4–7	0.5
25–35	8–10	0.75
36–50	11–13	1
50+	14+	1

Doxycycline (common trade name: Vibramycin)

The prophylactic dose is **1.5 mg salt/kg daily**, given as tablets or capsules containing 100 mg doxycycline salt as hyclate or hydrochloride. Doxycycline is mainly recommended for high-risk areas where resistance to mefloquine exists. It is also an alternative in high-risk areas with high levels of chloroquine resistance for persons unable to tolerate mefloquine.

Weight (kg)	Age (yr)	Number of Tablets/Day
< 25	< 8	Contraindicated
25–35	8–10	0.5
36–50	11–13	0.75
50+	14+	1

Atovaquone/proguanil (common trade name: Malarone)

In some countries, a combination tablet containing **250 mg atovaquone + 100 mg proguanil hydrochloride** (adult dose) is available for malaria chemoprophylaxis. It is also available in tablets containing 62.5 mg atovaquone + 25 mg proguanil hydrochloride for pediatric use. The regimen recommended by the manufacturer is 1 tablet daily (adult dose), starting 1 day before departure, and continuing for the duration of the traveler's stay in the endemic area and for 7 days after leaving the endemic area. Experience with this drug for chemoprophylaxis in nonimmune travelers is still limited. Atovaquone/proguanil is contraindicated in travelers with a hypersensitivity to the components of the drug, and in those with severe renal failure (creatinine clearance < 30 mL/min). Safety and efficacy of atovaquone/proguanil in pregnant and nursing women and in children weighing less than 11 kg have not been established.

Reproduced with permission from World Health Organization. International travel and health: vaccination requirements and health advice. Geneva: World Health Organ 2001:79–80.

APPENDIX 2

Drug regimens for standby emergency self-treatment (WHO guidelines)

Treatment schedules for children should be based on weight.

Chloroquine (common trade names: Aralen, Avloclor, Nivaquine, Resochin)

The total dose is **25 mg base/kg over 3 days**. The following table is based on the administration of the commonly used tablets containing either 100 mg or 150 mg base. If formulations of other strengths are used, the doses should be adjusted accordingly.

| | | Number of Tablets | | | | | |
| | | 100 mg Base | | | 150 mg Base | | |
Weight (kg)	Age(yr)	Day 1	Day 2	Day 3	Day 1	Day 2	Day 3
5–6	< 4 months	0.5	0.5	0.5	0.5	0.25	0.25
7–10	4–11 months	1	1	0.5	0.5	0.5	0.5
11–14	1–2	1.5	1.5	0.5	1	1	0.5
15–18	3–4	2	2	0.5	1	1	1
19–24	5–7	2.5	2.5	1	1.5	1.5	1
25–35	8–10	3.5	3.5	2	2.5	2.5	1
36–50	11–13	5	5	2.5	3	3	2
50+	14+	6	6	3	4	4	2

Sulfadoxine-pyrimethamine or sulfalene-pyrimethamine (common trade names: Fansidar for sulfadoxine-pyrimethamine, Metakelfin for sulfalene-pyrimethamine)

The following recommendations are for **single-dose treatment** with tablets containing 500 mg sulfadoxine or sulfalene plus 25 mg pyrimethamine.

Weight (kg)	Age (yr)	Number of Tablets
5–6	2–3 months	0.25
7–10	4–11 months	0.5
11–14	1–2	0.75
15–18	3–4	1
19–29	5–9	1.5
30–39	10–11	2
40–49	12–13	2.5
50+	14+	3

Mefloquine (common trade names: Eloquin, Lariam, Mephaquin)

Single-dose (15 mg base/kg) or split-dose (25 mg base/kg) treatment is recommended depending on the extent of mefloquine resistance in the area concerned. The following regimens are based on tablets containing 250 mg mefloquine base. The mefloquine formulation available in the USA, which contains 250 mg hydrochloride (equivalent to 228 mg mefloquine base), can be used according to the same regimens as regards the number of tablets, but the doses in terms of base will be slightly lower than recommended.

| | | Number of Tablets | | |
| | | | Split Dose* | |
Weight (kg)	Age (yr)	Single Dose[†]	Dose 1	Dose 2
< 5	< 3 months	Not recommended[‡]		
5–6	3 months	0.25	0.25	0.25
7–8	4–7 months	0.5	0.5	0.25
9–12	8–23 months	0.75	0.75	0.5
13–16	2–3	1	1	0.5
17–24	4–7	1.5	1.5	1
25–35	8–10	2	2	1.5
36–50	11–13	3	3	2
51–59	14–15	3.5	3.5	2
60+	15+	4	4	2

* Split dose (25 mg base/kg): areas with resistance to mefloquine, such as near the Thailand/Cambodia border. The split dose is given as 15 mg base/kg on Day 1 followed by a second dose of 10 mg base/kg 6–24 hours later.

[†] Single dose (15 mg base/kg): areas not affected by significant resistance to mefloquine.

[‡] Not recommended because data for this weight/age group are limited.

Quinine

Since many different tablet formulations of quinine salts are available, the following regimens are given in terms only of mg base/kg. The most common formulations are various strengths of quinine dihydrochloride, and quinine sulfate, containing 82%, 82% quinine base, and 82.6% quinine base respectively.

(a) Areas where parasites are sensitive to quinine:
quinine **8 mg base/kg orally 3 times daily for 7 days**

(b) Areas of high levels of resistance to quinine:

quinine **8 mg base/kg orally 3 times daily for 7 days,** accompanied by either doxycycline tablets or capsules 8 × 100 mg salt, over 7 days: 2 tablets on the first day, 12 hours apart, and 1 tablet daily for the next 6 days (not in children under 8 years of age and not in pregnancy)

or tetracycline 250 mg salt 4 times daily for 7 days (not in children under 8 years of age and not in pregnancy)

Reproduced with permission from World Health Organization. International travel and health: vaccination requirements and health advice. Geneva: World Health Organ 2001:83–4.

APPENDIX 3

Claudine Leuthold PH.D and Maia Funk-Baumann M.D.

Antimalarial Drugs: Synonyms And Trade Names

Due To Space Restrictions This List Is Incomplete.
Acridines And Sulfonamides (Except Combinations) Are Not Listed.

4- Aminoquinolines

Chloroquine
  Anoclor (ZA); Aralen (BR, CDN, P, PH); Aralen Hydrochloride (USA); Aralen Phosphate (USA);
  Arechin (PL); Avloclor (GB, ID, S); Avloquin (BD), Chlorochin (CH, D, GR, YU); Chlorocon (USA);
  Chloroquine (NL); Cidoquine (ET); Cloroc B (I), Clorochina (I); Clorochina Bayer (I); Cloroquina
  (BR, E); Chlorquin (AUS), Clorkin Vial (PH), Dagrinol (ET); Daramal (ZA); Delagil (CZ, H, SU);
  Diroquine (T), G-Chloroquine (BD), Genocin (T), Gromaquin (CH), Heliopar (SF); Jasochlor (BD),
  Klorokinfosfat (DK, N, S); Lagaquin (CH); Malarex (DK, ID, PH, S); Malarquine (Et); Mexaquin
  (ID), Nivaquine (B, CH, F, GB, ID, NL, RA, S, ZA); Nivaquine-P (BD), Novo-Chloroquine (CDN);
  Palux (BR); P Roquine (T), Resochin (A, CH, D, E, ID, NL, YU); Resochina (P); Riboquin (Id),
  Syncoquin (HK), Weimer (D)

Hydroxychloroquine
  Ercoquin (DK, N, S, SF); Evoquin (RA), Geniquin (TW), Hydroxychloroquine (USA); Metirel (RA),
  Oxiklorin (SF); Plaquenil (A, AUS, B, CDN, CH, CZ, DK, F, GB, GR, HK, I, MY, N, NL, PH, RA, RU,
  S, SF, SU, T, TW, USA); Plaquinol (P); Quensyl (D); Toremonil (J)

Amodiaquine
  Camoquin (CH, ET, P); Flavoquine (F)

Combinations
  Chloroquine + Proguanil: Savarine (F)

8-Aminoquinolines

Primaquine (Diphosphate)
  Primachin (SU), Primaquina (BR), Primaquine (CDN, GB, NL, S, USA), Eloquine

Tafenoquine
  Etaquine

Quninolinemethanols

Mefloquine
  Lariam (A, AUS, B, BD, CH, CZ, D, DK, F, GB, GR, H, HK, I, N, NL, PH, S, SU, SF, TW, USA); Mefliam
  (ZA); Mephaquin (CH, HK, P, S, T), Tropicur (Ra), Eloquine.

Combinations
  Mefloquine + Pyrimethamine + Sulfadoxine: Fansimef (CH)

Dihydrofolate Reductase Inhibitors (Antifolates)

Proguanil
  Paludrine (A, AUS, B, CDN, CH, D, DK, F, GB, I, MY, N, NL, S, SF)

Chlorproguanil Pyrimethamine
  Daramprim (TR); Daraprim (A, AUS, B, BR, CDN, CH, CZ, D, E, ET, GB, NL, RA, S, SU, T, USA, YU,
  ZA); Malocide (F); Pyrimen (PL); Pyrimethamin (D); Pyrison (BD), Tindurin (H)

Trimethoprim (List Not Complete)
  Abaprim (I); Alprimol (A); Alprim (AUS, MY, S); Idotrim (S); Infectotrimet (D); Ipral (GB);
  Monoprim (A); Monotrim (CH, DK, GB, NL, ZA); Motrim (A); Primosept (Ch); Proloprim (CDN,
  USA, ZA); Solotrim (A); Sulfadiazin+Tmp C25/5 (D); Syraprim (GB, P); Tediprima (E); Theraprim
  (ET); Tmp-Ratiopharm (CZ, D, SU); Trilaprim (YU); Trimesan (PL); Trimethoprim (A, CZ, D, NL);
  Trimetin (SF); Trimetoprim (N, S); Trimex Merckle (SF); Trimono (D); Trimopan (DK, GB, S, SF);
  Trimpex (USA); Triprim (ET, SU, ZA); Urotrim (YU); Utisept (T), Wellcoprim (A, B, F, NL, S)

Antifolate + Sulfonamide Combinations

Pyrimethamin + Sulfadoxin
   Fansidar (AUS, CH, F, ID, PH, USA); Madomine (MY, S); Malacide (S); Malex (BD); Methamar (PH); Saloprim (BD); Suldox (IN); Sulfamin (BD); Vivaxine (T)

Hydroxynaphtoquinone

Atovaquone
   Mepron (CDN, USA); Wellvone (A, B, CH, D, DK, F, GB, I, NL, P)

Atovaquone + Proguanil
   MALARONE (A, AUS, B, CH, DK, GB, S, T, USA)

Phenanthrenmethanol

Halofantrin
   HALFAN (A, B, CDN, CH, D, F, GB, NL, P)

Quinine (Salt) (Quinine Combinations Are Not Listed)

   Adco-Quinine (ZA); Aethylcarbonas Chinin (ID), Arsiquinoforme (F); Biquinate (Au), Chin Cl (I), Chin So (I), Chinina (I); Chinina Cloridrato (I); Chinina Solfato (I); Chininum Aethylcarbonicum (D); Chininum Dihydrochloricum (D); Chininum Hydrochloricum (D); Circonyl (CH); Endopalur (BR); G-Quinine (BD), Genin Tab (T), Jasoquin (Bd), Kanaquine (BD), Kinin (DK, S); Kinine (NL); Limptar (D); Myoquin (AUS), Paludil (BR); Quinaminoph (USA); Quinate (AUS), Quinbisul (AUS), Quinine (CDN, F, GR); Quinine-P (T), Quininga (LK), Quinoctal (AUS), Quinoforme (F); Quiphile (USA); Quinsul (AUS), Requin (BD), Sagittaproct (D); Strema (USA); Sulfato (BR); Sulfato De (BR)

Quinidine

   Apo-Quinidine (MY, CDN); Biquin (CDN); Cardioquin (CDN, NL, USA); Cardioquine (E, F); Chinid S Ifi (I), Chinidin (D, H); Chinidin-Duriles (A); Chinidina (I); Chinidini (SF); Chinidinorm (A); Chinidinsulfat (A); Chinidinum (H, PL); Chinteina (I); Cin-Quin (USA); Cordichin (D), Duraquin (USA); Galactoquin (A); Kiditard (GB, NL); Kinichron (CH); Kinidin (AUS, CH, CZ, DK, HK, N, PH, S, SF, SU, T, YU); Kinidin Duretter (DK); Kinidine (B, GR, NL); Kinidrin (GB); Kiniduron (SF); Kinilentin (CZ, DK, SF); Kinilong (SF); Longachin (I); Longacor (CH, E, F, P, TR); Longaquine (GR); Naticardina (I); Natisedina (E, I); Natisedine (BR, CDN, F, GR, P, TR); Neochinidin (I); Prosedyl (CDN); Quin Release (USA); Quinaglute (CDN, I, USA, ZA); Quinate (CDN); Quinicardina (E); Quinicardine (B, BR, GR, TR); Quinidex (CDN, USA); Quinidine (BR, CDN, ET); Quinidine Gluconate (CDN); Quinidurule (F); Quinobarb (CDN); Quinora (USA); Ritmocor (I); Systodin (N)

Sesquiterpen Lactone (Quinghuashu, Quinghoasu)

Artemether
   Artenam (B); Paluther (VR)

 Combination
   Artemether + Lumefantrine: Riamet (CH)

Artemisinine

Sulfones

Dapsone
   Avlosulfon (CDN, S, SF); Daps (RA), Dapson (D, DK, N, NL); Dapson-Fatol (D), Dapsone (AUS, ET, USA); Disulone (F), Dopsan (T), Servidapsone (T), Sulfona 100 (P), Sulfona Oral (E)

Sulfones Or Sulfonamides + Antifolate

Sulfadoxine + Pyrimethamine
   Fansidar (A, B, BR, CDN, CH, CZ, DK, F, GB, N, NL, PL, USA, ZA)

Tetracycline

Doxycycline (List Not Complete)
Abadox (I); Ak-Ramycin (USA); Ak-Ratabs (USA); Antodox (D); Apo-Doxy (CDN); Atridox (USA); Atridox 8,8% Zur (A); Atrisorb (USA); Azudoxat (D); Bactidox (D); Basecidina (E); Bassado (I); Bio-Tab (USA); Biocina (P); Biocyclin (A); Clinofug (D); Clisemina (E); Combaforte (GR); Curasol (CH); Cyclidox (ZA); Dagracycline (NL); Dagramycine (B); Deoxymykoin (CZ); Dinamisin (TR); Diocimex (CH); Doksiciklin (YU); Doksin (TR); Dophar (B); Doryx (CDN); Doryx Pellets (USA); Dosyklin (SF); Dotur (A); Doxakne (D); Doxiciclina (I); Doxiclat (E); Doxicrisol (E); Doximed (SF); Doximycin (SF); Doxina (I); Doxitab (ZA); Doxivis (I); Doxy (D, F); Doxy 100 (D); Doxy 200 (D); Doxy Basan (CH); Doxy Basf (D); Doxy Dagra (NL); Doxy Disp (NL); Doxy Eu (D); Doxy Komb. (D); Doxy M (D); Doxy S+K (D); Doxy-100 (B, D, F, USA); Doxy-200 (USA); Doxy-Acis (D); Doxy-Caps (USA); Doxy-Diolan (D); Doxy-Lemmon (USA); Doxy-Lichtenstein (D); Doxy-M-Ratiopharm (D); Doxy-N (D); Doxy-N-Forte (D); Doxy-Puren (D); Doxy-Tablinen (A); Doxy-Tabs (USA); Doxy-Wolff (D); Doxybene (A, DK, SU); Doxybiocin (D); Doxychel (USA); Doxycin (CDN); Doxyclin (CH, ZA); Doxycline (F); Doxycline Plantier (F); Doxycyclin (A, D, H); Doxycyclin-Ratiopharm (CZ); Doxycyclina (SU); Doxycycline (B, F, NL, PL, SU); Doxycyclinum (PL); Doxycyklin (DK); Doxycylin (A); Doxyderma (D); Doxydoc (D); Doxydyn (A); Doxyfim (B); Doxygram (F); Doxyhexal (D, H); Doxylag (CH); Doxylan (A); Doxylar (GB); Doxylets (B, F, ZA); Doxylin (N); Doxymerck (D); Doxymono (D); Doxymycin (ET, NL, ZA); Doxypharm (H); Doxyremed (D); Doxysol (CH); Doxytab (B); Doxytem (D); Doxytrex (P); Dumoxin (DK, N, NL, SF, ZA); Duradoxal (D); Esadoxi (I); Farmodoxi (I); Germiciclin (I); Gewacyclin (A); Ghimadox (I); Gram-Val (I); Granudoxy (F); Grodoxin (CH); Helvedoclyn (CH); Heska Perioceutic (A); Hiramicin (YU); Hydramycin (J); Iclados (I); Idocyklin (S); Impalamycin (GR); Ivamycin (GR); Jenacyclin (D); Lentomyk (GR); Liomycin (J); Logamicyl (B); Medomycin (SF); Mespafin (D); Microvibrate (GR); Minidox (I); Miraclin (I); Monocline (F); Monodoks (TR); Monodox (A, SF, USA); Monodoxin (I); Mundicyclin (A); Neo-Dagracycline (NL); Neo-Vibrin (CDN); Neodox (D); Nordox (GB); Novelciclina (E); Novimax (GR); Novo-Doxylin (CDN); Nymix (D); Otosal (GR); Pefaciclin (GR); Periostat (GB, USA); Pharmodox (NL); Pharmon (NL); Philcociclina (I); Pluridoxina (P); Radox (I); Reci-Dox (D); Relyomycin (GR); Retens (E); Rodomicina (E); Ronaxan 100 (D); Ronaxan 20 Ad Us.Vet. (D); Roxyne (B); Rudocyclin (CH); Samecin (I); Sigadoxin (A, CH, D, P); Sithruin (GR); Smilitene (GR); Solupen (E); Spanor (F); Stamicina (I); Supracyclin (A, CH, D); Tetradox (TR); Thedox (ZA); Tolexine (F); Unacil (I); Unidox (B, SU); Unidox Solutab (NL); Vibra (CDN, NL, SF, USA); Vibra-Tabs (CDN); Vibrabiotic (GR); Vibracina (E); Vibradox (DK); Vibramicina (BR, P); Vibramycin (A, CDN, CH, CZ, D, DK, ET, GB, GR, J, N, NL, S, SU, USA, YU, ZA); Vibramycine (B, F); Vibratab (B); Vibraveineuse (F); Vibravenosa (E); Vibravenös (A, CH, D); Visubiotic (GR); Zadorin (CH)

List Of Country Codes
A = Austria, AUS = Australia, B = Belgium, BD = Bangladesh, BG = Bulgaria, BR = Brazil, C = Cuba, CDN = Canada, CH = Switzerland, CS = Chechia (Old Code), CZ = Czech Republic, D = Germany, DK = Denmark, E = Spain, ET = Egypt, F = France, GB = Great Britain, GR = Greece, H = Hungary, HR = Croatia, HK = Hongkong, Bosnia-Herzegowina, I = Italy, ID = Indonesia, IL = Israel, IND = India, IRL = Ireland, J = Japan, L = Luxembourg, LK = Sri-Lanka, LV = Lithuania, MC = Monaco, MEX = Mexico, MY = Malaysia, N = Norway, NL = Netherlands, NZ = New Zealand, P = Portugal, PH = Philippines, PL = Poland, RA = Argentina, RC = P.R.China, RCH = Chile, RO = Rumania, RP = Philippines, S = Sweden, SF = Finland, SI = Slowenia, SK = Slowakia, SU = Russia, T = Thailand, TW = Taiwan, USA = USA, YU = Yugoslavia, ZA = South Africa

Claudine Leuthold PhD

ASTRAL

Rue Pedro-Meylan 7

CH-1211 GENEVA 17

INDEX

Page numbers followed by f indicate figure; those followed by t indicate table.